Public Health

Public Health

POLICY AND POLITICS

SECOND EDITION

Rob Baggott

palgrave
macmillan

First edition 2000
Reprinted 12 times
Second edition 2011

LEEDS TRI̶N̶ ̶A̶N̶D̶ ̶C̶O̶L̶L̶E̶GE

Published by
PALGRAVE MACMILLAN

Palgrave Macmillan in the UK is an imprint of Macmillan Publishers Limited,
registered in England, company number 785998, of Houndmills, Basingstoke,
Hampshire RG21 6XS.

Palgrave Macmillan in the US is a division of St Martin's Press LLC,
175 Fifth Avenue, New York, NY 10010.

Palgrave Macmillan is the global academic imprint of the above companies
and has companies and representatives throughout the world.

Palgrave® and Macmillan® are registered trademarks in the United States,
the United Kingdom, Europe and other countries.

ISBN 978–0–230–53793–4

Contents

List of Figures, Tables and Exhibits

Preface and Acknowledgements

Writing a second edition of any academic book is often considered a thankless task. Second editions are viewed as 'more of the same', lacking in originality. Yet, second and indeed subsequent editions provide an opportunity to develop ideas and issues further, to expand and update, and to engage in further reflection with the benefit of hindsight. Although the second edition of *Public Health: Policy and Politics* covers familiar territory, it is in many ways a different book, providing an updated and in-depth analysis of contemporary public health challenges.

Although the responsibility for this work is mine alone, I would like to acknowledge the help, support and advice of the following people: Lynda Thompson and Kate Llewellyn (Palgrave Macmillan); Kathryn Jones and Priti Meredith (Health Policy Research Unit, De Montfort University); Tim Brown (Centre for Comparative Housing Research, De Montfort University); Gill Perkins; Linda Norris and Bryony Allen; Merrill and Sheila Clarke, and Chris Nottingham (Glasgow Caledonian University). Many others, too many to name individually, also offered helpful advice along the way and provided references on specific topics. I would also like to thank the (anonymous) reviewers of the draft manuscript for their valuable comments. In addition, I am grateful to HMSO, the WHO European Region and the WHO Commission on Social Determinants of Health for permission to reproduce material in Exhibits 4.1, 5.2 and 17.2. As ever, the work has taken its toll on family life and I would like to express my thanks once again to Debbie, Mark, Danny and Melli for their support and forbearance.

The book draws on two decades of research into public health policy. It draws on material from several of my previous publications, including *Understanding Health Policy* (Policy Press, 2007) and a chapter in Alison Hann's edited volume, *Analysing Health Policy* (Ashgate Press). This new edition has taken over three years to produce. Ultimately, it is for the reader to judge whether this exercise has been worthwhile.

ROB BAGGOTT

Every effort has been made to trace all the copyright holders but if any have been inadvertently overlooked the publishers will be pleased to make the necessary arrangements at the first opportunity.

x

List of Abbreviations

ACMD	Advisory Council on the Misuse of Drugs	CAPIC	Collaboration for Accident Prevention and Injury Control
ACRE	Advisory Committee on Releases to the Environment	CASH	Consensus Action on Salt and Health
ADHD	Attention-deficit hyperactivity disorder	CCA	Climate Change Agreement
ADZ	Alcohol Disorder Zone	CCC	Committee on Climate Change
AHA	Area Health Authority	CCL	Climate Change Levy
AIDS	Acquired Immune Deficiency Syndrome	CCS	Carbon Capture and Storage
AICR	American Institute of Cancer Research	CDRP	Crime and Disorder Reduction Partnerships
APMS	Alternative Provider Medical Services	CFCs	Chloroflourocarbons
		CHC	Community Health Council
AQMA	Air Quality Management Area	CHD	Coronary Heart Disease
		CHI	Commission for Health Improvement
ASEAN	Association of South East Asian Nations	CHPP	Child Health Promotion Programme
ASH	Action on Smoking and Health	CHP	Community Health Partnership
BAT	Best Available Techniques	CIEH	Chartered Institute of Environmental Health
BATNEEC	Best Available Technology Not Entailing Excessive Cost	CJD	Creutzfeldt-Jakob Disease
BBC	British Broadcasting Corporation	CMO	Chief Medical Officer
		CND	Commission on Narcotic Drugs
BMA	British Medical Association		
BMI	Body Mass Index	CNO	Chief Nursing Officer
BPEO	Best Practicable Environmental Option	COMA	Committee on the Medical Aspects of Food
BSE	Bovine Spongiform Encephalopathy	COMARE	Committee on Medical Aspects of Radiation in the Environment
CAA	Comprehensive Area Assessment		
CAF	Common Assessment Framework	COMEAP	Committee on the Medical Effects of Air Pollutants
CAP	Committee of Advertising Practice	COSLA	Convention of Scottish Local Authorities
	Common Agricultural Policy	CPA	Comprehensive Performance Assessment

CPHVA	Community Practitioners and Health Visitors Association	DoE	Department of Environment
		DoH	Department of Health
		DPH	Director of Public Health
CPPIH	Commission for Patient and Public Involvement in Health	DTI	Department of Trade and Industry
		EAAP	European Alcohol Action Plan
CPP	Community Planning Partnership	EAC	Environmental Audit Committee
CPRS	Central Policy Review Staff		
CQC	Care Quality Commission	ECHR	European Court of Human Rights
CSA	Children's Service Authority		
CSR	Corporate Social Responsibility	ECM	Every Child Matters
		EEC	European Economic Community
CYPP	Children and Young People's Plan	EIA	Environmental Impact Assessment
DAAT	Drug and Alcohol Action Team	EFRAC	Environment, Food and Rural Affairs Committee
DAT	Drug Action Team	EFSA	European Food Safety Authority
DCIS	Ductal Carcinoma In Situ		
DCLG	Department for Communities and Local Government	EHO	Environmental Health Officer
DCMS	Department for Culture Media and Sport	EMCDDA	European Monitoring Centre for Drugs and Drug Addiction
DCRs	Drug Consumption Rooms		
DCSF	Department for Children, Schools and Families	ESA	Environmentally Sensitive Area
DEFRA	Department for the Environment, Food and Rural Affairs	ESRC	Economic and Social Research Council
DETR	Department of the Environment, Transport and the Regions	ETS	Emissions Trading Scheme External Tobacco Smoke
		EU	European Union
DFEE	Department for Education and Employment	FCTC	Framework Convention on Tobacco Control
DfES	Department for Education and Skills	FISS	Food Industry Sustainability Strategy
DfT	Department for Transport	FSA	Food Standards Agency
DHA	District Health Authority	FSS	Fat, Salt and Sugar
DHSS	Department of Health and Social Security	GATS	General Agreement on Trade in Services
DHSSNI	Department of Health and Social Security Northern Ireland	GATT	General Agreement on Tariffs and Trade
		GAVI	Global Alliance for Vaccination and Immunization
DHSSPS	Department of Health, Social Services and Public Safety	GDA	Guideline Daily Amounts
		GDP	Gross Domestic Product

GFATM	Global Fund for AIDS, TB and Malaria	IAG	Independent Advisory Group on Sexual Health and HIV
GM	Genetically Modified		
GMO	Genetically Modified Organisms	ICAS	Independent Complaints and Advisory Services
GMS	General Medical Services	IDeA	Improvement and Development Agency for Local Government
GOR	Government Office for the Region		
GP	General Practitioner	IHR	International Health Regulations
GUM	Genito Urinary Medicine		
HACCP	Hazard Analysis Critical Control Point	ILO	International Labour Organization
HAZ	Health Action Zone	IMF	International Monetary Fund
HCP	Healthy Child Programme		
HDA	Health Development Agency	INCB	International Narcotics Control Board
HDL	High-Density Lipoprotein	IOTF	International Obesity Task Force
HEA	Health Education Authority		
HEBS	Health Education Board for Scotland	IPC	Integrated Pollution Control
		IPPC	Integrated Pollution Prevention and Control
HEC	Health Education Council		
HFEA	Human Fertilization and Embryology Authority	IPPR	Institute for Public Policy Research
HFSS	High in Fat, Salt and Sugar	IRGC	International Risk Governance Council
HGAC	Human Genetics Advisory Committee		
HGC	Human Genetics Commission	JABS	Justice Awareness and Basic Support
HIA	Health Impact Assessment	JARs	Joint Area Reviews
HImPs	Health Improvement Programmes	JHIP	Joint Health Improvement Plan
HIMPs	Health Improvement and Modernization Plans	LA21	Local Agenda 21
		LAA	Local Area Agreement
HIV	Human Immunodeficiency Virus	LACORS	Local Authorities Coordinators of Regulatory Services
HMIP	Her Majesty's Inspectorate of Pollution	LDL	Low Density Lipoprotein
		LDP	Local Delivery Plan
		LEA	Local Education Authority
HOTN	Health of the Nation	LEAP	Learning, Evaluation and Planning
HPA	Health Protection Agency		
HPI	Happy Planet Index		Local Exercise Action Pilot
HPV	Human Papillomavirus	LEB	Life Expectancy at Birth
HRT	Hormone Replacement Therapy	LGA	Local Government Association
HSC	Health and Safety Commission	LGB	Local Government Board
		LGBT	Lesbian, Gay, Bisexual, and Transgender
HSE	Health and Safety Executive		

LHB	Local Health Board
LINk	Local Involvement Network
LPSA	Local Public Service Agreement
LSP	Local Strategic Partnership
LTP	Local Transport Plan
MAA	Multi-area Agreement
MAFF	Ministry of Agriculture Fisheries and Food
MAMOH	Metropolitan Association of Medical Officers of Health
MDGs	Millennium Development Goals
MMR	Measles, Mumps and Rubella
MOH	Medical Officer of Health
MoH	Ministry of Health
MRC	Medical Research Council
MRSA	Meticillin Resistant Staphylococcus Aureus
NACNE	National Advisory Committee on Nutritional Education
NAfW	National Assembly for Wales
NAO	National Audit Office
NEF	New Economics Foundation
NFER	National Foundation for Educational Research
NFU	National Farmers' Union
NGO	Non-Governmental Organization
NHI	National Health Insurance
NHS	National Health Service
NHSE	National Health Service Executive
NHSP	National Healthy Schools Programme
NHSS	National Healthy Schools Standards
NICE	National Institute for Health and Clinical Excellence
NOx	Nitrogen Oxides
NPCRDC	National Primary Care Research and Development Centre

NPH	New Public Health
NPHS	National Public Health Service for Wales
NRPB	National Radiological Protection Board
NSC	National Screening Committee
NSF	National Service Framework
NS-SEC	National Statistics Socio-economic Classification
NTA	National Treatment Agency for Substance Misuse
NTF	Nutrition Task Force
ODPM	Office of Deputy Prime Minister
OECD	Organisation for Economic Cooperation and Development
OFCOM	Office of Communications
Ofsted	Office for Standards in Education, Children's Services and Skills
ONS	Office for National Statistics
OSC	Overview and Scrutiny Committee
PAC	Public Accounts Committee
PAH	Polycyclic Aromatic Hydrocarbons
PALS	Patient Advice and Liaison Service
PATF	Physical Activity Task Force
PCBs	Polychlorinated Biphenyls
PCG	Primary Care Group
PCT	Primary Care Trust
PE	Physical Education
PHCTs	Primary Health Care Teams
PHIS	Public Health Information Service
PHLS	Public Health Laboratory Service
PHOs	Public Health Observatories
PHS	Public Health Service
PMS	Personal Medical Services
PMSU	Prime Minister's Strategy Unit

POPs	Persistent Organic Pollutants	SRB	Single Regeneration Budget
POST	Parliamentary Office of Science and Technology	SSA	Social Science Association
		STP	School Travel Plan
PPI	Patient and Public Involvement	TB	Tuberculosis
		UKCRC	UK Clinical Research Collaboration
PPIF	Patient and Public Involvement Forum	UKPHA	UK Public Health Association
PPF	Public Partnership Forum	UN	United Nations
PSA	Public Service Agreement	UNAIDS	The United Nations Joint Programme on HIV/AIDS
PSHE	Personal, Social and Health Education	UNDCP	United Nations Drugs Control Programme
PVC	Polyvinyl Chloride	UNDP	United Nations Development Programme
QoF	Quality and Outcomes Framework	UNEP	United Nations Environment Programme
RA	Regional Assembly		
RCEP	Royal Commission on Environmental Pollution	UNESCO	United Nations Educational, Scientific and Cultural Organization
RCP	Royal College of Physicians		
RDA	Regional Development Agency	UNICEF	United Nations International Children's Emergency Fund
RDPH	Regional Director of Public Health	UNODC	United Nations Office on Drugs and Crime
REACH	Registration, Evaluation, Authorization and Restriction of Chemicals	UV	Ultraviolet
		VAT	Value Added Tax
SARS	Severe Acute Respiratory Syndrome	VOC	Volatile Organic Compound
		WAG	Welsh Assembly Government
SBO	Specified Bovine Offal	WCH	Wales Centre for Health
SCS	Sustainable Community Strategy	WCISU	Welsh Cancer Intelligence and Surveillance Unit
SEA	Single European Act Strategic Environmental Assessment	WCRF	World Cancer Research Fund
SEU	Social Exclusion Unit	WHO	World Health Organization
SHA	Strategic Health Authority	WIC	Walk In Centre
SIRC	Social Issues Research Centre	WRAP	Waste Reduction Action Programme
SMAC	Standing Medical Advisory Committee	WTO	World Trade Organization
SOCA	Serious Organized Crime Agency		
SOLACE	Society of Local Authority Chief Executives		
SPS	Sanitary and Phytosanitary		

Public Health Concepts and Frameworks

What is Public Health?

There is no commonly agreed definition of public health. This is not surprising as the concept of health is itself multifaceted and contested (Blaxter, 2004). Health can be interpreted as the absence of illness or disease, as fitness or vitality, as an ability to perform certain functions. It can be perceived in terms of social relationships and psychosocial wellbeing. As Ewles and Simnett (2003, p. 5) observed, 'people's ideas of "health" and "being healthy" vary widely. They are shaped by their experiences, knowledge, values and expectations, as well as their view of what they are expected to do in their everyday lives, and the fitness they need to fulfil that role.'

Concepts of health are often divided into positive and negative approaches. The conventional biomedical perspective is negative in the sense that it conceives health as an absence of disease in individuals. In contrast, positive approaches highlight the social, environmental and psychological aspects of health (Aggleton, 1990). In modern times, negative concepts of health have predominated, largely because of the combined power of the medical profession and commercial health care interests (Hunter, 2003; Freeman, 2000; Moynihan, 1998). Even so, in recent decades the disease-based approach has been challenged by positive concepts. So much so that the medical profession more readily acknowledges the role of psychosocial factors in health, the importance of quality of life issues and value of holistic approaches to health. Meanwhile, commercial interests have sought to explore market opportunities in prevention and public health.

Perhaps the best-known positive definition of health is that formulated by the World Health Organization: 'a state of complete physical, mental and social well-being and not merely the absence of disease or infirmity' (WHO, 1946, p. 100). Although criticized for being utopian, this definition has been a rallying point for those seeking to shift the balance towards a more positive approach to health. These include Antonovsky (1979, 1996), who called for a refocusing of attention away from the causes of disease (the 'pathological paradigm') towards those factors that facilitate health (the 'salutogenic paradigm'). The salutogenic paradigm is based not on a dichotomy of health or disease, but on a continuum of states between 'health-ease and disease'. According to Antonovsky, a major factor influencing health, and determining one's location at the healthy end of the spectrum, is a 'sense of coherence.' This is derived from experiences through the life course that enable individuals to make sense of the world and cope with situations as they arise.

Wellbeing

Wellbeing is a key concept in positive approaches to health (see McAllister, 2005; Dolan et al., 2006; Felce and Perry, 1995; Searle, 2008; Kahneman et al., 2003; Huppert et al., 2005). It can be subjective; individuals assessing themselves in how satisfied or happy they are feeling. Alternatively, wellbeing may be objectively ascribed by others on the basis of specific criteria (such as economic resources, education, housing, access to public services). Wellbeing may be measured at the social and individual level. There are two main conceptual approaches to wellbeing. The first looks at the extent to which material, social and psychological needs are met. This is known as the hedonistic approach. Alternatively, the second, eudaemonism, focuses on the realization of potential and seeks to measure the extent to which people flourish as human beings. This may include criteria such as autonomy, personal growth, life purpose, mastery and positive relationships (see Ryff and Keys, 1995, cited in Dolan et al., 2006). Although there is disagreement over the relative weight that should be given to different types of wellbeing, there is much consensus on the domains that comprise overall wellbeing (McAllister, 2005): namely, physical, material, social, personal development and purposeful activity.

The current level of interest in wellbeing is based partly on observations that growing prosperity, as measured by conventional indicators (such as gross domestic product, GDP), has not yielded commensurate improvements in wellbeing (see Exhibit 1.1; Oswald, 1997; Easterlin, 1974; Layard, 2006; New Economics Foundation, 2004; James, 2007). It has also been stimulated by worries about climate change and sustainability (Dolan et al., 2006) and by evidence of the impact of social organization and structure on physical and mental health (Layard, 2006; Marmot, 2004). In addition, there has been specific concern about the wellbeing of children, arising from the increased regulation of childhood, child poverty, lack of protection from consumer capitalism, poor parenting skills and decline in the quality of family life (see James, 2007; UNICEF, 2007a; Bradshaw, 2002).

Exhibit 1.1

Measuring Wellbeing in the UK and Other Countries

There is evidence from the UK and other countries that levels of wellbeing, measured by surveys of life satisfaction, have not increased in line with increases in national income. In the UK, gross domestic product (GDP) doubled between 1973 and 2006 while the proportion of people who were satisfied remained stable. According to the Department for Environment, Food and Rural Affairs (DEFRA) (2007), 73 per cent of people in England rated their overall satisfaction with life at over 7 out of 10. Some aspects of life, however, received lower ratings. For example, although over 60 per cent of respondents said that they were satisfied with their community and their financial security, this was lower than the level of satisfaction with relationships, accommodation and standard of living, which achieved ratings of 80 per cent and over. Differences were found between different social groups (see also Blanchflower and Oswald, 2008). Middle-aged people, particularly men, are less satisfied with their lives than older and younger people. People in unskilled jobs or who are unemployed are also less satisfied with life.

Some have tried to add subjective measures of life satisfaction to other social indicators in an attempt to produce a broader quality of life measure. For example, the Happy Planet Index (HPI), used by the New Economics Foundation (2009), is based on three criteria – life satisfaction, life expectancy and environmental sustainability. Countries that achieve in these areas are given higher ratings and rankings than those that do not. On the basis of this index, the major industrialized countries are rated much lower than their economic wealth might suggest. In the 2009 rankings the UK came 74th out of 143 countries and the USA was ranked 114th. Some industrializing countries also fared badly, with India's and China's index falling over time. But this is not always the case: the HPI index for Brazil, which has undergone significant economic development in recent years, increased. There are also considerable differences between European countries, with Germany, Holland, Sweden, Switzerland and Austria ranked highest. Interestingly, among the top 10 countries ranked by HPI, all but one are in Latin America.

Definitions of public health reflect underlying debates about the meaning of health and wellbeing. In a narrow sense, public health refers to the longevity of a population and the extent to which it is free from disease. Public health is sometimes equated with 'public health medicine', that is the range of medical techniques, knowledge and interventions that are geared to preventing disease in individuals and in populations (see Chapter 6). Alternatively, reflecting positive perspectives on health, public health is perceived as primarily concerned with population health and wellbeing. According to Baum (2002, p. 14) 'the distinguishing feature of public health is its focus on populations rather than individuals'. Public health also incorporates a wider range of social interventions and collective action, reflecting Rosen's (1993, p. 1) observation that 'throughout human history, the major problems of health that men have faced have been concerned with community life'. This latter approach is captured by Winslow's classic definition:

> Public health is the science and art of preventing disease, prolonging life and promoting physical health and efficiency through organised community efforts for the sanitation of the environment, the control of community infections, the education of the individual in principles of personal hygiene, the organisation of medical and nursing services for the early diagnosis and preventive treatment of disease, and the development of social machinery which will ensure to every individual in the community a standard of living adequate for the maintenance of health. (C. E. A. Winslow, 1920, p. 23)

In the UK context, the Acheson report into public health (Cm 289, 1988) abridged this to 'the science and art of preventing disease, prolonging life and promoting health through the organised efforts of society.' Subsequently, the Wanless report on public health (HM Treasury, 2004) modified this definition in the context of consumerism, choice, pluralism and the personalization of public services to:

> the science and art of preventing disease, prolonging life and promoting health through the organised efforts and informed choices of society, organisations, public and private, communities and individuals. (Wanless, 2004, p. 27)

Public health is an extremely broad church. This is problematic because, as Griffiths and Hunter (1999, p. 1) observed, if public health encapsulates so much, it risks being a confusing and diffuse collection of ideas. Indeed, one reason why public health has lacked influence over policy and practice has been its lack of conceptual clarity leading to what some claim is an identity crisis (Hunter et al., 2010; Frenk, 1992). This is not a problem for the UK alone. Indeed, a study of terminology across a number of European countries did not find a common conceptual framework for public health (Kaiser and Mackenbach, 2008).

In an attempt to clarify the meaning of public health, Griffiths et al. (2005) outlined a conceptual model drawing on three distinct but interrelated domains of public health practice identified by the Faculty of Public Health (Griffiths et al., 2005): *health improvement* – such as information about healthy lifestyles or improvements to housing; *health service delivery and quality* – for example primary care services; and *health protection* – including immunization and screening. In another attempt to clarify the concept, Heller et al. (2003, p. 64) defined public health in terms of the types of knowledge required to meet the health needs of the public:

> [The] use of theory, information and evidence derived through the population sciences to improve the health of the population, in a way that best meets the implicit and explicit needs of the community [the public].

Efforts have been made to widen ownership of public health and share a common ethos across agencies and professional groups. Hunter and Marks (2005) promoted 'public health governance' which emphasizes the stewardship role of government and the participation of all relevant organizations in public health activities (see also Local Government Association et al., 2004). Similar recommendations have been made in other countries (Institute of Medicine, 1988, 2002; Canadian Institutes of Health Research, 2003). In this context, a distinction is often made between 'traditional' public health and 'new public health' (Baum, 2002; Ashton and Seymour, 1988; Ewles and Simnett, 2003). This dichotomy is examined more fully in subsequent chapters, but it is sufficient at this stage to note that the new public health (NPH) is perceived as a broader approach that acknowledges the importance of a wider range of environmental, social and personal factors. NPH is also viewed as being focused on promoting health and wellbeing in a positive sense rather than being concerned narrowly with the prevention of disease.

Health Promotion

Another key concept is health promotion (Naidoo and Wills, 2005). It too is a contested concept. It can mean, variously, a social movement, a means of addressing health needs, or a model of health (Bunton and Macdonald, 2002). According to the World Health Organization (WHO) (1986) 'health promotion is the process of enabling people to increase control over, and to improve their health.' This reflects the belief that health is a right and endorses a range of ways of improving the health of populations, communities and individuals (Lucas and Lloyd, 2005; Webster and French, 2002; Ewles and Simnett, 2003; MacDonald, 1998; Tones and Green, 2004). It can be contrasted with a narrow 'health education' approach, which focuses upon providing individuals with information about reducing the risk of disease, without addressing their wider social and environmental context.

Health promotion is a portmanteau term for a range of activities including health education, preventive health services, economic and regulatory activities, environmental health measures, organizational development, community-based work and healthy public policies (see Ewles and Simnett, 2003, p. 28). Some, however, believe that approach lacks coherence. They call for a more robust philosophy of health promotion to guide policy and practice. Antonovsky, previously mentioned, warned that health promotion risked becoming stagnant in the absence of a clear theoretical perspective. He developed the salutogenic paradigm as a means of highlighting factors promoting health rather than concentrating only on risk factors for disease. Similarly, Lucas and Lloyd (2005, p. 23) argue for a primary focus on 'improving the quality of people's day-to-day lives in areas which they have helped to identify', rather than solely aiming to prevent disease. In so doing, they and others identify the importance of empowerment: for example Tones and Green (2004, p. 3), for whom health promotion 'is a political endeavour and concerned with addressing issues of fundamental importance – particularly the pursuit of social justice and achievement of equity.'

The concept of 'health gain' is also relevant here. Health gain is defined as 'a measurable improvement in health status, in an individual or a population, attributable to earlier intervention' (Ewles and Simnett, 2003, p. 336). The relevance of 'health gain' lies in its focus on the outcomes of health promotion activities and as a basis for comparing different interventions (WHO, 1998b). Terms such as health improvement or health development are also used in the context of assessing the impact of health promotion activities (Ewles and Simnett, 2003).

Prevention

The focus of public health activities is aimed at preventing problems from emerging, or at least preventing their most serious consequences. The emphasis is on 'refocusing upstream', to tackle problems at or near their source (McKinlay, 2005). Prevention can be narrowly conceived as 'preventive medicine', incorporating techniques such as screening or immunization, or it may encapsulate a wider range of interventions such as regulation or taxation of potentially harmful products (Yarrow, 1986). It may be targeted at a small 'high risk' group or at the whole population (Rose, 1992). Three different types of prevention are usually distinguished: primary prevention – action to prevent ill health before it occurs; secondary prevention – identifying and treating people with early signs of illness; and tertiary prevention – halting or mitigating the effects of ill health already manifested (Cmnd 7615, 1979; Tones and Green, 2004, p. 21). Prevention is often justified with reference to improving welfare or saving budgetary costs (see, for example, Wanless, 2004), reflecting a belief that 'prevention is better than cure'. However, this is not necessarily the case. As we shall see, preventive interventions may involve significant additional economic costs as well as restrictions on choices and liberties.

So What is Public Health?

Debates about the meaning of public health are essentially political. Different interests favour particular interpretations of public health concepts. The interplay of these forces establishes meanings in policy and practice. Furthermore, these debates are linked to wider political debates, such as those surrounding the role of the state and the individual (Leichter, 1991). Meanwhile, public health policies are shaped by the interplay of political forces in government and in society (Mechanic, 2003; Rose, 1992).

A political analysis of public health is therefore potentially fruitful. This book adopts such an approach and is primarily concerned with political debates surrounding public health and their implications for the emergence, formation and implementation of public health policies. However, to avoid a purely descriptive account, a coherent analytical framework is required. Various frameworks exist (see Signal, 1998, for example). Three seem particularly appropriate: ideological perspectives on the role of the state and the individual; social and cultural theories of risk and expertise; and models of the policy process. Each will now be discussed in turn.

Ideological Perspectives

Public health reflects key ideological debates about the freedom of the individual, the authority of the state, and the balance between individual and collective responsibilities (see Mills and Saward, 1993; Leichter, 1991). The main perspectives are discussed below.

Paternalism and Utilitarianism

Much public health intervention occurred in the period before the era of the welfare state. This was often based on paternalist or utilitarian principles. Paternalism has been defined as 'the interference of a state or an individual with another person, against their will, and justified by a claim that a person interfered with will be better off or protected from harm' (Dworkin, 2005). Our main concern here is with state paternalism (also known as 'narrow paternalism'), but it can apply to employers, professionals, organizations, informal groups and between individuals as well (known as 'broad paternalism'). Paternalism is essentially a philosophy of intervention that is based on an inequality of power, authority and status coupled with an external assessment of individual needs by a higher authority (Dworkin, 1972).

Today, paternalism is a pejorative term, associated with the 'nanny state' and unnecessary interference with individual freedoms. This is perhaps unfair (Coote, 2004; Jochelson, 2005). There are strong reasons for intervening to protect children and other vulnerable groups, on the grounds that they are not in a position to make rational decisions for themselves (Gostin, 2007; Nuffield Council on Bioethics, 2007). There are circumstances where adults may not act rationally and a case can be made for preventing them from doing something they wish. Examples might include gambling, smoking, excessive alcohol consumption, and narcotic use. This justification might be taken further in the context of large-scale threats to health. It could be argued that as individual decisions are so embedded in society and shaped by their environment, the notion of free personal choice is illusory and can, in such circumstances, be justifiably overridden (Gostin, 2007). A further argument is that contemporary public health interventions could be justified on the grounds that with the benefit of hindsight those affected are likely to acknowledge that they have benefited (Cottam, 2005; Goodin, 1991).

Whether paternalism is justified or not depends on the degree and nature of coercion and the motives of those undertaking it (Wikler, 1978). In liberal democratic states, authoritarian paternalism is unacceptable except in the most extreme cases. Liberal forms of paternalism, which rely on 'softer' ways of influencing behaviour (such as taxation of harmful products, incentives to reduce risk, organizational rules, and the provision of information about risks, rather than legislative or punitive restrictions), and seek to steer people's choices in ways that will improve their welfare, are regarded as more appropriate to such political systems (Upshur, 2002; Nuffield Council on Bioethics, 2007; Weale, 1983; Sunstein and Thaler, 2003). Even so, there are occasions when an authoritarian approach is warranted, as in the case of an infectious disease outbreak carrying high potential for disability and death for example.

Public health measures have often been justified on utilitarian grounds. Indeed, Edwin Chadwick, who many regard as the father of the public health movement in Britain, was strongly influenced by utilitarian thinkers such as Jeremy Bentham (see Chapter 2). Utilitarianism is a diverse philosophy, but its fundamental principle is the maximization of happiness for the greatest number of people (Goodin, 1995; Scarre, 1996). It is a 'consequentialist' ethical theory that judges policy or action in terms of outcomes, principally costs and benefits. Utilitarianism can be used to justify policies/actions that are in the interests of the majority, even when this goes against the interests of the minority. It therefore provides a philosophical basis for interventions in public health and welfare that override individual choices and freedoms. Notably, utilitarianism went against the grain of the powerful laissez faire mentality of the Victorian era and provided the philosophical foundation for a range of social interventions in this period (see Chapter 2). Some of these interventions were undoubtedly in the public interest and benefited vulnerable groups in society (sanitary reform, protection of children, factory legislation) others (notoriously, the workhouses – Longmate, 2003) were certainly not. Utilitarianism also provided a broader rationale for reforms of government and public administration, including the rationalization of health and welfare services, which also had significant benefits for society.

Although utilitarianism has waned as an overt political ideology, it is still relevant today as a set of public policy principles (Goodin, 1995). The foundations of the modern state owe much to these principles. Moreover, many public policy decisions – including those affecting public health – are still made on the basis of calculations about overall costs and benefits. The influence of utilitarianism lives on.

The Liberal-Individualist Perspective

According to Leichter (1991, p. 10), 'health promotion policies often require a choice between good health and personal freedom'. The liberal-individualist perspective seeks to safeguard negative liberty. This can be defined as the freedom to pursue one's activities without interference from the state, providing that others are not harmed in the process (Mill, 1974; Berlin, 1969). Adherents of this perspective argue that an interventionist state is neither a benign nor a neutral force, but a hostile entity that coerces and disempowers citizens (Hayek, 1976, 1988; Nozick, 1974). They argue that individuals need greater protection from the state than from the vagaries of the market. Individual liberty can be saved only by strengthening the market sphere and increasing self-reliance among ordinary citizens. Neoliberalism – the revitalized version of this philosophy (King 1987; Green 1987) – provided a blueprint for political action to reverse the tide of paternalism and collectivism. This creed had a major influence over British governments during the 1980s and 90s (see Gamble, 1994). It is still influential today.

Specifically in relation to public health, liberal-individualists argue that it is unfair that the majority of individuals should sacrifice personal freedom for an illusory common good. They maintain that individuals must take responsibility for their own health, make their own choices and not be told what to do by the nanny state (see, for example, Bennett and Dilorenzo, 1999; Huntington, 2004; Booker and North, 2007). Should people wish to indulge in unhealthy behaviour, they must be 'free to be foolish' (Leichter, 1991). There are additional concerns about the cumulative impact of interventions upon personal freedom (House of Lords, 2006).

According to the liberal-individualist critique, the state bureaucracy has a vested interest in regulating and controlling people, and consequently has an incentive to exaggerate certain risks. It is argued that budgets, careers and status depend on expansion of bureaucratic and regulatory functions (see Booker and North, 1994, 2007; Berger 1991). But there is a high price to pay: regulatory overkill imposes high social costs, including restriction of liberties, discouragement of risk taking and enterprise, and a reduction in the efficiency and profitability of corporations (Neal and Davies, 1998; Power, 2004). From this perspective, the paternalist and collectivist approaches to public health are seen as pernicious, tantamount to 'an assault on pleasure'. Indeed, some argue that individual pleasures and social benefits of certain activities

(Future Foundation, 2005) – such as drinking alcohol for example – are totally discounted by government when it intervenes on public health grounds (Charlton, 2001).

There has been some disquiet about 'healthism' – where health is an end in itself, or becomes the ultimate goal (Ewles and Simnett, 2003; Crawford, 1980; MacDonald, 1998; Fitzpatrick, 2001; Skrabanek, 1994). Notably, this has not been confined to libertarians, but is shared by others who fear it could lead to victim-blaming and excessive state intervention. Such an approach may disempower individuals, undermining one of the key tenets of modern health promotion philosophy. A related concern is that while interference with personal freedom may be justified in terms of public health, it may mask moral judgements about people's lifestyles (see, for example, Leichter, 1991). The danger is that those seeking to influence lifestyles may be motivated more by an agenda of control and conformism rather than public health. It has been pointed out, somewhat ominously, that some of the worst totalitarian states in history have been enthusiastic supporters of 'healthism'. Skrabanek (1994) observes that in Nazi Germany, fascism was intimately connected with a set of beliefs about the state's role in public health and ideas about racial purity (see Procter, 1988; Davey Smith, 2004). However, such ideas have not been confined to fascists. At the beginning of the twentieth century similar beliefs had wide currency in liberal democratic states and were seen as providing solutions to problems of national efficiency (see Searle, 1976; Nottingham, 1999).

Collectivism and Socialism

Collectivists and socialists place great emphasis on the beneficial role of the state and other collective arrangements (such as mutual societies and cooperatives) and are highly critical of individualism (see Berki, 1975; Crick, 1987). They are particularly sceptical about the ability of isolated individuals to produce their own solutions to complex social problems. There is some foundation for this in the field of public health where, according to Rose (1985, p. 138), 'a preventive measure which brings much benefit to the populations offers little to each participating individual'. This 'prevention paradox' implies that left to their own devices, individuals have little incentive to contribute towards activities that improve public health (see also Rose, 1992).

'Public health', as Sears (1992, p. 65) has observed, 'was identified with the state from the outset.' Certainly the broader definition of public health discussed earlier justifies a key role for the state in protecting citizens' health while providing a rationale for specific health policy interventions. From a collectivist standpoint this includes ameliorating the health damaging consequences of individualism and tackling the socioeconomic causes of ill health generated by capitalism (Allsop, 1990; Doyal, 1979; Navarro, 1976; Havelock Ellis, 1892). Indeed as Beauchamp (1988) has argued, the protection of health depends in part on preventing the market from invading other spheres. Furthermore, the appeal to resist markets on health grounds is a powerful one. As Dicey (quoted in Weale, 1983, p. 806) observed, 'a collectivist never holds a stronger position than when he advocates the best ascertained laws of health'. From a socialist or collectivist perspective, equity in health is a key element of social justice. Intervention is justified not merely to protect individuals from specific threats to health, such as junk food or noxious emissions from factories, but to promote the health of everyone, irrespective of social class, income, gender, sexuality, age, or ethnic background.

Socialist and collectivist perspectives on liberty are used to justify certain types of public health intervention. In contrast to the conventional liberal approach, discussed above, greater weight is given to positive liberty (Green, 1911; Berlin, 1969). Positive liberty concerns the extent to which individuals are masters of their own fate and free from circumstances that limit opportunities. Hence state intervention and other forms of collective action can be justified on the grounds that such restrictions actually empower individuals to take control of their lives and make informed choices. This view is articulated by Beauchamp (1988), for example, who argues that advances in public health and prevention expand the liberties of citizens. Labonte (1998) pursues a similar line in relation to health promotion. He contends that arguments for social justice, reflecting notions of positive liberty, are more consistent with the historical practice of public health, with contemporary international health accords, and with current evidence on the impact of economic equality and environmental sustainability upon health. They therefore outweigh considerations about individual (that is, negative) liberties. However, Labonte stresses that libertarian theory offers an important caution against the undermining of individual autonomy by the state, and that a social justice approach must be complemented by 'deliberative democratic practice' in order to avoid interventions that marginalize and exclude socially disadvantaged groups. Similarly, Taylor and Hawley (2006, p. 20) argue that it is possible to see freedom in terms of empowerment, which 'affirms the importance of maintaining the sovereignty and integrity of the individual whilst recognizing that the state can facilitate individual and community development and support individuals in the choices they make.' Indeed, as Jochelson (2005) observed, it may be more appropriate to see the government's role in public health in terms of stewardship, setting new social standards, bringing about changes that individuals cannot make, protecting them from harm, and creating a framework that enables them to make decisions about their health. According to this view, the aim is to strengthen choice by encouraging independent judgement, not simply replace it by state direction (Rose, 1985, p. 117). A stewardship model was endorsed by the Nuffield Council on Bioethics as an ethical framework for public health intervention (see Exhibit 1.2).

Exhibit 1.2

The Nuffield Council on Bioethics: Public Health and Stewardship

In 2007, the Nuffield Council on Bioethics reported on ethical issues in public health. To guide its inquiries and to help it make recommendations, the Council devised an ethical framework. This was a revised liberal framework based on the notion of stewardship: that liberal states have responsibilities for the needs of people both individually and collectively. This implied that states must be more interventionist in public health matters than envisaged by a conventional liberal framework. However, unlike a conventional paternalistic approach, highly coercive measures would not be adopted unless there was a very strong threat indeed. The stewardship model was intended as a more sensitive framework, respecting individual preferences, being less intrusive and more proportionate to the risks involved.

According to this framework, public health programmes should aim to:

- reduce the risks of ill health that people might impose on each other
- ensure environmental conditions that sustain good health
- pay special attention to vulnerable groups, such as children
- provide information and advice but in addition provide support for people to overcome addictions and other unhealthy behaviours
- ensure that it is easy for people to lead a healthy life
- ensure that people have appropriate access to medical services
- reduce unfair health inequalities.

However, programmes should not coerce people into leading healthy lives; must minimize interventions introduced without individual consent or an adequate mandate; and seek to minimize interventions perceived as unduly intrusive and in conflict with personal values.

In addition, the Council identified 'third parties' having an important role in public health. These included publicly funded bodies and charities. The Council also considered the position of business organizations, arguing that in situations of market failure or where business fails to act responsibly, the state may intervene if the health of the population is at significant risk.

The Council also made recommendations on specific topics, such as alcohol, smoking and obesity, which are discussed in later chapters.

New Labour and the Third Way

The British Labour party leadership, out of office for almost two decades in the 1980s and 90s, abandoned its traditional socialist collectivism in effort to attract votes and gain office. Under the leadership of Tony Blair, it became 'New Labour'. The intellectual basis for this transformation was the Third Way, a combination of socialist notions of fairness, equity and community with neoliberal ideas about markets, competition, individual responsibility and choice (Giddens, 1998; Finlayson, 1999; Driver and Martell, 2002). Although there are different interpretations of the Third Way, its main principles are as follows.

The Third Way maintains that equality of opportunity rather than equality of outcome is crucial. It endorses an inclusive society, where citizens have both rights and responsibilities, and promotes values of self-reliance and voluntarism. The Third Way maintains that partnership with the voluntary and the private sectors is necessary in order to pursue the collective good. The state must be entrepreneurial in seeking new opportunities for wealth creation and solving social problems. Policy should be guided by what is effective rather than by ideological prescriptions as captured in the phrase: 'what counts is what works'. The Third Way also involves 'modernization' of government itself, with governing institutions seeking closer proximity to the people in order to be more responsive to their needs, preferences and choices. In addition, governing institutions must be prepared to work more efficiently and collaboratively to produce coherent policies and services ('joined up government').

The commitment to Third Way principles can be found in public health policy documents, including the white papers *Saving Lives* (Cm 4386, 1999) and *Choosing Health: Making Healthy Choices Easier* (Cm 6374, 2004). It is also evident in other documents, notably the Wanless report on public health (Wanless, 2004). The Third Way approach to public health acknowledges that the state has a legitimate role in shaping the environment within which people make healthy choices, through regulation, provision of services and information about health risks. But individuals themselves have a crucial role in taking responsibility for their own health and making healthy choices. Adherents to the Third Way perspective are strongly critical of the idea that social, economic and environmental factors determine health, and instead support the view that public health is about creating the conditions that will facilitate healthy individual choices (see Corrigan, 2007). Another key principle of the Third Way is partnership, between public sector organizations – such as the National Health Service (NHS) and local government – and between statutory, voluntary and private sectors. Again, this reflects the idea that government should not bear all the responsibility of improving health and that other bodies have an important part to play.

Green Ideology and Feminism

Those adopting a Green perspective oppose the destructiveness of industrial society, and its pursuit of economic growth at all costs. They are perhaps closer to the socialist and collectivist perspective regarding social justice and the belief in the countervailing power of collective action (see Ryle, 1988). Greens are suspicious of individualist-libertarian arguments, seeing them as an excuse for non-interventionism and corporate exploitation. At the same time they are wary of state power, believing that large state bureaucracies can be as oppressive towards individuals and as damaging to the environment as private corporations. Hence they place emphasis on the role of individuals and small, local groups in promoting a sustainable environment (see Porritt and Winner, 1989; Dobson, 1990). However, as Adams (1993, p. 318) has observed, 'while there is a good deal of consensus about what Greens are against, there is much less agreement about what Greens are for'. In practice there are many shades of Green, which differ considerably in their aims, ideas and prescriptions for change.

Green perspectives adopt an ecological model of health (Pietroni, 1991; Hancock, 1985; Draper, 1991). This highlights the complex and multiple sources of illness arising from the environment. In particular, mankind's interaction with the natural environment is seen as the crucial factor in the maintenance of health. Hence many of the major health problems of our time, such as foodborne illness and diseases linked to pollution, are viewed as a product of human exploitation of the environment. Greens believe that the social and economic structure of industrial society is corrosive, generating unhealthy lifestyles and working conditions, and producing socioeconomic inequalities that undermine health.

Greens endorse sustainable development policies, balancing economic, social and environmental considerations (Secrett and Bullock, 2002). They also support 'precautionary' principles – believing that early intervention on the basis of limited information is warranted to prevent serious damage to environment and health, rather than waiting for concrete evidence of irreversible and widespread harm (discussed further below). Despite criticism that their views are utopian, those adopting a Green perspective are prepared to endorse specific practical solutions, such as a ban on particular pollutants, which they believe will contribute to a healthier environment for all.

Feminism, like Green perspectives, is a movement that challenges dominant ideas, values, policies and practices. Although there is no single feminist perspective, there is a common belief that social systems, including the health care system, privilege men at the expense of women (Annandale, 1998; Doyal, 1995, 1998; Miles, 1991; Wilkinson and Kitzinger, 1994). In the health field one way in which this occurs is by the construction of the male body as 'normal' while the female is regarded as 'abnormal'. The female body is therefore pathologized, with particular attention focused on gynaecological and repro-ductive systems (Thomas, 1998). Feminists also argue that health care is male-dominated. Consequently, women are subject to male values and deci-sions, which can lead to control, exploitation and a failure to understand female needs.

Moreover, it is argued that medical practice continues to embody a mascu-line paradigm focused on disease, with little room for feminine and caring values (Davies, 1995). Medical research is also accused of downplaying the importance of women's perspectives on health (Doyal, 1998). With regard to public health, it is notable that many diseases affecting women have been addressed by prevention programmes (such as breast and cervical cancer). Nonetheless, the high profile of these interventions does not necessarily mean that women's public health needs are being met. Indeed, it may be argued that these technologies are a means of controlling women's bodies, have significant side effects (notably unnecessary treatment) and fail to address the fundamental causes of these diseases (discussed further in Chapter 8).

Risk

A second framework draws on social and cultural theories of risk. It is argued that we live in a 'risk society' where political conflict is defined in terms of risks linked to industrialization and globalization (Giddens, 1991; Beck, 1992; Lash et al., 1996; Bauman, 2007). A key feature of such societies is the identifi-cation and management of future threats. The precautionary principle – origi-nally designed to justify policy interventions in the environmental field (O'Riordan and Cameron, 1994) but now applied to other areas including public health (Calman and Smith, 2001; Pennington, 2003) is a fundamental concept. It presumes that intervention is justified in order to prevent harm, even when outcomes are uncertain. Meanwhile, the related principle of 'the polluter pays' means that those who cause potentially adverse consequences must take responsibility for reducing risks and bear the cost of doing so.

The precautionary principle and the assessment of risk that follows from its use have important implications for politics and policy. Because the future is uncertain and attitudes to risk vary, evidence is highly contested (Adams, 1995). In the health arena, for example, estimates of costs and benefits from interventions to prevent illness may turn out to be wrong. Much depends on how calculations are made and what factors are included in models predicting future trends. Indeed, it is often assumed that prevention is cost-effective, but this is not necessarily so (Cairns, 1995; Eurohealth, 2005; Rose, 1985). Closer analysis of specific prevention activities in areas such as obesity and smoking have shown that overall costs may rise due to people living longer (van Baal et al., 2008; House of Commons, 1977).

The media play a crucial role in the risk society, given their role in social definition and construction. They can exploit the uncertainty about future trends and exaggerate risks (Harrabin et al., 2003; Kitzinger and Reilly, 1997; Eldridge, 1999; Goldacre, 2008; Murdock et al., 2003; Booker and North, 2007). The media can be seen as part of a process of 'risk amplification' (Pidgeon et al., 2003; Kasperson et al., 2003), where relatively low risks can become a major public concern. They can also cover up important risks by not reporting on potential threats, particularly in situations where powerful commercial interests, including those of proprietors, might be adversely affected. The media can also affect public judgements about the credibility of government and experts as they seek to manage risks. This can promote public distrust in both, resulting in crises of confidence.

Experts are central to the process of risk identification and management. However, experts are not homogeneous. Some forms of expertise are more highly valued by government and by society than others. Some argue that there has been a shift whereby those whose expertise plays a key part in risk identification and management have become more powerful (Furedi, 1997; Power, 2004). In public health, for example, it is argued that epidemiologists have extended their influence over policy (Petersen and Lupton, 1996). Moreover, health researchers and health professionals have been accused of exaggerating health risks in order to consolidate their influence, even where evidence is thin (Furedi, 1997; Skrabanek, 1994; Bennett and Dilorenzo, 1999; Lee, 1994; Beaver, 1997; Feinstein, 1999; Le Fanu, 1994a, 1994b; Booker and North, 2007).

Governments see risk management as a means of governance and a way of managing demands from the public and pressure groups. In this context Hood and colleagues (2004) found that risk regulation was more strongly shaped by interest group politics than public opinion or by functional or market failure. Regulation of risks may be more about political perceptions than action. With specific reference to health, prevention policies have been seen as a means by which government can appear to be doing something about intractable health and social problems (Freeman, 1992, 1995; Fitzpatrick, 2001). This may reflect a broader process in modern societies, whereby increasingly powerless governments shift responsibilities for resolving problems onto individuals (Bauman, 2007).

The risk society has a number of consequences. The precautionary principle and risk management systems have been criticized for promoting an excessively cautious attitude to risk (House of Lords, 2006; Power, 2004). It is also claimed that the principles of risk management are applied inconsistently, unrelated to the actual levels of risk involved (Calman and Smith, 2001; House of Lords, 2006; Hood et al., 2004). For example, some have observed a particular tendency to place emphasis on the dangers of new technology while benefits are not fully weighted (Wildavsky, 1988, 1991; Douglas and Wildavsky, 1982). It is argued that an excessive approach to risk stifles innovation and creates an atmosphere of fear and distrust (Furedi, 1997). It may also be counterproductive, producing more serious adverse consequences in the longer term as people modify their behaviour in response to a 'safer' environment, a phenomenon known as risk compensation (Adams, 1995).

The risk society also involves greater surveillance of citizens. Skrabanek (1994) coined the term 'anticipatory medicine' to describe a new mode of surveillance involving the scrutiny of risk factors in the population as a whole as a basis for intervention. Similarly, Castel (1991) identified a shift in focus of policy from individuals manifesting signs and symptoms of impending illness, abnormality or social deviance, towards anticipating and preventing problems. As Petersen and Lupton (1996, p. 3) state 'the new public health can be seen as but the most recent of a series of regimes of power and knowledge that are oriented to the regulation and surveillance of individual bodies and the social body as a whole'. They contend that in modern societies public health is comprehensive in its scope, providing opportunities for the state to engage in moral regulation aimed at making subjects more self-regulating and productive in order to serve society's broader interests.

Related to this is the increased scope for controlling individuals and reducing their personal freedom. Risks and threats abound, and individuals are lured by promises of security to give up their freedom (Bauman, 2007). At the same time vast bureaucracies have developed to manage risk (Adams, 1995). Prevention policies have the potential to transfer power to government and professionals who control the technologies of health surveillance and flows of information and resources (Castel, 1991; Petersen and Lupton, 1996). Public health measures have always involved forms of control. According to Armstrong (1993), four different regimes of public health in history – quarantine, sanitary science, personal hygiene and new public health – are each linked to a mode of control. Quarantine represents a simple line of inclusion and exclusion; sanitary science regulates the movement between different spaces; and personal hygiene regulates a psychosocial space regarding attitudes and behaviours. According to Armstrong, the fourth regime – new public health – can be distinguished from previous regulatory approaches in the way it generalizes danger, increases the scope for surveillance and attempts to gear many aspects of behaviour to health objectives.

A further consequence of the risk society is the attribution of blame to certain social groups. Castel (1991), for example, argues that the preventive approach gives rise to greater social exclusion, arguing that such a regime provides the basis for differential modes of treatment for populations, which aim to 'maximise the returns on doing what is possible and to marginalise the unprofitable' (p. 294). But there is also a process of stigmatization at work as particular groups are blamed for their unhealthy behaviours. This has occurred in areas such as obesity, smoking and alcohol abuse.

The risk society itself has the potential for enormous adverse consequences, contributing to fear, distrust, loss of liberty, intrusive surveillance and the stigmatization of certain behaviours and people. On the other hand, it is acknowledged that governments and professionals have a duty to protect the health and welfare of the people. Moreover, the heightened awareness of risks need not necessarily frighten and disempower people. It may be possible to devise ways in which technologies, evidence and organization may be used in a positive way to enable people to improve their health, without being subject to excessive control from the state and experts.

Models of the Policy Process

A third framework explores the emergence of public health strategies within the policy process. It is helpful to analyse these processes by using models of policymaking (see, for example, Parsons, 1995; John, 1998; Hudson and Lowe, 2004). There are many different approaches to analysing public health policy and these are summarized below (see also Baggott, 2007).

Top-down and Bottom-up Models

Policymaking can be seen as a rational process, whereby central government makes policy, which is then implemented by lower tiers (see Simon, 1945). This idea underpins the 'stagist' approach to policy, which breaks the policy process down into discrete stages (such as agenda setting, policy formation, implementation and evaluation – see Hogwood and Gunn, 1984). This top-down approach has strongly influenced the understanding of policy implementation, which has been seen primarily as an 'add on' to the policy process (Pressman and Wildavsky, 1973; Dunsire, 1978). An important implication was that deviations between the intentions of policymakers and those charged with implementation were characterized as deficits or gaps. However, this approach – and rational models more generally – has been challenged by those who point out that policy is really more about compromise between different stakeholders (Lindblom, 1959). It is recognized that policy often involves mediation and negotiation between central decision makers and those who implement policies (Hill and Hupe, 2002; Barrett, 2004; Lipsky, 1979). Indeed, policies may be shaped as much from the 'bottom up' as by the intentions of policymakers at the top.

Parties and Elections

Policy can be seen in terms of competition and collaboration between political parties as they seek office. Parties can be regarded as 'battering rams of change' (Crossman, 1972), setting out new directions for policy. However, doubts have been expressed about the legitimacy of party programmes, particularly in the light of the broad and vague content of party manifestos, low turnout at elections and the unfairness of 'first past the post' electoral systems (used in the election of the UK Parliament, for example) – which give significant power to parties receiving only a minority of the vote.

Alternative views identify the constraints on parties and emphasize how parties in government retain elements of their predecessors' policies. Rose (1984) found that in practice policy develops in a more stable fashion as parties rotate in and out of office, characterized by what he called a 'moving consensus'. Meanwhile, others have pointed out how parties steal each other's ideas in search of electoral support (Webb, 2000; Bara and Budge, 2001). Parties also change their policies as a result of collaboration with each other. This is a feature of coalition politics, which occurs when parties cannot form a viable government on their own. Coalition governments are more common in systems of government based on proportional representation (including the devolved assemblies of Scotland, Wales and Northern Ireland). However, they can also happen elsewhere, as in the UK Parliament in 2010, when the Conservatives and Liberal Democrats formed a coalition government in an absence of an overall majority for one party. Related to this, the path dependency model (David, 1985; Berman, 1998) is based on a belief that institutions and previous decisions exert a strong influence over current policymaking, promoting incremental rather than radical change. Hence political parties and others wishing to change the direction of policy are heavily constrained by decisions and events from the past.

Policy as the Interplay of Interests

Another way of conceptualizing public health policy is to view it as a product of interaction between different interests articulated by pressure groups, organizations and social movements (Baggott, 1995; Grant, 2000; Coxall, 2001). A pressure group is an organization that seeks to represent interests or preferences in society, has a certain degree of independence from government and is not a recognized political party (see Baggott, 1995, pp. 2–3). There are several different approaches to the study of pressure-group politics, but most seek to explore how groups' resources, political contacts and status within the political process relate to their influence over policy. Studies of pressure groups also examine the environment within which groups interact with each other and with government, and how this affects their influence. Grant's distinction between insider and outsider groups is based on an acknowledgement that insider groups are given privileged access to decision makers in government and that this enhances their potential influence over policy. Others have since proposed modifications to this model, including Maloney,

Jordan and McLaughlin (1994), who argue that insider status (conferred by government) should not be confused with insider strategy (where a group decides for itself how it will pursue its campaign) and that insider status is further differentiated (into core, specialist and peripheral insider status, each of which carries different weight in the policy process).

Pressure group analysis is also concerned with how public support is mobilized (Jordan and Maloney, 1997; Ridley and Jordan, 1998), and how pressure groups relate to other 'pressure points' in the political system such as Parliament (Rush, 1990), supra-national decision makers and the media (Baggott, 1995). Pressure group analysts are interested in how groups, often with very different backgrounds and ethos, collaborate with each other, and form coalitions to press for a common policy. Social movements are also important drivers of policy change. They promote particular values among the population and often encourage direct action by constituent groups and individuals (Habermas, 1976; Byrne, 1997; Tarrow, 1998). Examples include the women's movement, the environmental movement and the mental health movement.

Policy Networks

The policy networks approach focuses on the processes of agenda setting, policy formation and policy implementation, and the ways in which these processes are influenced by relationships and procedures within and between governing institutions and other stakeholders (Marsh and Rhodes, 1992; Smith, 1993; Richardson and Jordan, 1979). These networks encompass pressure groups, government agencies and other participants having an interest in a specific policy area. The configuration of policy networks varies: some, known as policy communities, are exclusive, stable and highly integrated, and involve a high degree of interdependence between the participants. Others, known as issue networks, are less integrated, open and unstable, and participants are not interdependent. A key issue is whether or not the configuration of these networks can influence the development of policy (see Marsh and Smith, 2005; Richardson, 2000). Empirical work in this field has led to suggestions that policy networks vary and change over time and that this can have implications for policy development (Baumgartner and Jones, 1993; Heinz et al., 1993).

Policy Agendas and Policy Windows

In practice, the movement of an issue on to the political agenda is a complex process. Downs (1972) identified an issue-attention cycle, whereby issues attract public attention leading to pressure on government to intervene, only for the issue to subside once the costs of intervention become apparent. The emergence of an issue reflects the power of interests to shape the agenda (Bachrach and Baratz, 1962; Schattschneider, 1960; Lukes, 1974). The medical profession and commercial interests are particularly influential in this regard because of their influence over social values and the media (Navarro, 1978; Alford, 1975). Government also seeks to influence the media in order to distract attention away from 'difficult' issues (such as those that are intractable or involve taking on powerful interests). Hence much policy activity is symbolic (Edelman, 1977; Fairclough, 2000; Jones, 2002; Richardson and Moon, 1984). The media play a particularly important role in defining the agenda and can both advance and block policy developments (Baggott, 2007).

Also relevant here is Kingdon's (1984) notion of policy windows. Policy is shaped by an interaction between three streams: a problem stream comprises those issues that government is considering; a policy stream, where ideas about how to deal with problems circulate (within policy networks and among 'political entrepreneurs' who play a key role in selling policy ideas); and a political stream, which consists of public opinion, parties and pressure groups and government and various ways of building support and consensus. When these various streams come together, a 'launch window' is opened, enabling policy change to take place.

Policy Dynamics

Opportunities to promote policy change are limited. According to Baumgartner and Jones (1993), institutional arrangements can restrict access and inhibit the intrusion of new ideas. In effect a 'policy monopoly' is created which is resistant to certain interests and ideas. Such a monopoly can be challenged by redefining policy problems and setting new agendas in such a way that excluded interests have to be incorporated. Similarly, Majone (1989) has argued that discussion and argument are institutionalized and, as a result, choices of policy options are constrained. Furthermore, like Baumgartner and Jones, he acknowledges that institutional arrangements are not immutable. Actors can seek to change institutional arrangements 'that either give them new resources or increase the value of those they already have' (pp. 102–3).

Persuasion is also an important weapon within the policy process. But, as Majone observes, some policies are more highly resistant to change than others. Much seems to depend on how deeply rooted such policies are in the core beliefs of political actors. This view is endorsed by Sabatier (1987; see also Jenkins-Smith and Sabatier, 1994) who has attempted to explain policy change in terms of advocacy coalitions. Advocacy coalitions comprise actors within the policy process who share a set of beliefs about policy and who often act in concert. According to Sabatier, policy change can occur as a result of changes in the beliefs of advocacy coalitions, changes in the composition of a coalition, or a change in the relative strength of competing coalitions (which is in turn dependent upon resources such as money, expertise, number of supporters and legal authority). However, in the absence of external 'perturbations' (such as broader political or socioeconomic changes) fundamental policy beliefs are unlikely to change and this means that in practice the core policies of government are relatively consistent over time.

Experts and Policy

Empirical work on the role of expert policy advisors has confirmed that scientific findings are not automatically translated into policy, but filtered through a political process (Collingridge and Reeve, 1986; Barker and Peters, 1993a). Experts are valued by politicians not merely for their knowledge and advice, but because they give legitimacy to government decisions (Barker and Peters, 1993b). Indeed, as Fischer (1990) observed, as politics becomes a more technologically oriented task, the expertise of technocrats becomes a key resource in governance. For example, politicians may use their scientific findings to justify action or inaction, to gain public support for new policy initiatives or to reassure the public that all is well. Alternatively, the government may suppress findings, and in such situations doctors or other scientific experts may find themselves engaging in wider public debate in order to bring about policy change. As the earlier discussion on risk suggested, experts also have an important role to play in the formulation of policy responses to future threats, even where there is limited evidence.

Policy Transfer

Finally, any study of public policy, even if undertaken primarily within one country, must be aware of the comparative dimension, and in particular the tendency for policymakers in one country to borrow ideas from others (Leichter, 1991). This can occur by drawing lessons (such as drug decriminalization – see Chapter 14) from particular countries. Alternatively, supranational organizations, such as multinational companies, international pressure groups, or European or UN institutions, may actively promote particular policies at the global or regional level. By the same token, it is also possible for policies in one country to be rejected or discouraged as result of bad experiences elsewhere or because of opposition from international players. These transmission and inhibition mechanisms are important in the field of public health, given the role of the WHO and the existence of international health professional networks, not to mention powerful multinational corporations whose activities affect health.

Conclusion

The themes identified in this chapter will be explored in the context of a wide range of public health issues. In Chapters 2 and 3 the history of public health is outlined, focusing on the factors that have shaped public health intervention in the UK up to the 1990s. In Chapter 4, the development of health strategies in the 1990s is examined. Chapter 5 explores international developments. Chapter 6 looks at the public health functions of the NHS. This is followed by Chapter 7, exploring the role of other agencies in public health. Public health services are discussed in Chapter 8. Chapter 9 focuses specifically on public health aspects relating to children and young people, Chapters 10 and 11 examine environmental health issues and climate change. This is followed by a discussion of food policy in Chapters 12 and 13. The public health problems associated with alcohol, tobacco and other drugs are examined in Chapters 14 and 15, while Chapters 16 and 17 analyse the broader socioeconomic context of public health.

The Historical Context of Public Health

2

Rosen's (1993) historical account reveals that health promotion and disease prevention were undertaken by the earliest civilizations. Evidence from ancient sites in what is now part of India indicates that the importance of water and sewerage systems, paved streets and town planning was recognized as long ago as 2000 BC. Other civilizations, such as the Egyptians and the Incas, also recognized the importance of urban planning and sanitation. Some ancient civilizations sought to impose rules in an effort to promote health. The Babylonians had strict public health regulations governing personal behaviour, while the Egyptians promoted the value of good diet and hygiene (Inglis, 1965).

As Rosen explained, many ancient civilizations were concerned about cleanliness because of religious beliefs and practices. Disease was often associated in ancient cultures with divine retribution. It was not until the fifth century BC in Ancient Greece that a more rational, scientific approach began to emerge (Kitto, 1957). *Airs, Waters and Places*, attributed to Hippocrates, discussed the ecological balance between man and environment alongside the importance of climate, soil, water, and nutrition in the maintenance of good health. In so doing it provided not only an explanation for ill health but also practical recommendations for avoiding disease. The Romans too were aware of the health implications of the environment, and in particular sanitation. They built impressive aqueducts, public bathing facilities, and sewerage systems, and devised new techniques to purify water supplies. They also identified links between environment, occupation and illness.

As the Roman Empire declined, its system of public health decayed. The knowledge built up by classic civilizations was lost. In the Middle Ages epidemics struck regularly, often with terrifying severity – the Black Death of the fourteenth century being a prime example. The main response to such outbreaks was to isolate those infected. This was rarely undertaken with any clear plan in mind, although, as Rosen (1993) observed, quarantine methods began to improve from the middle of the fourteenth century, with large commercial ports such as Venice leading the way.

Limited public health measures were introduced in some cities from the twelfth and thirteenth centuries onwards (Simon, 1890). In London, a range of activities believed hazardous to health were regulated, including restrictions on pigsties and stray animals, regulation of 'offensive trades', street cleaning and the dumping of waste, and rules on animal slaughter. Some European cities, such as Paris and Prague, paved their streets, making them easier to cleanse. Some cities established municipal abattoirs to prevent offal littering the streets, while others established food inspection and market regulations to protect citizens against contaminated or dirty food. These rules were enforced quite vigorously, with severe penalties (Rosen, 1993).

Following the Black Death, European societies responded to the threat of disease in a piecemeal and reactive fashion. Even so, a more systematic approach to public health grew, albeit slowly, in line with greater understanding of the causes of illness. This was informed by studies of contagion and epidemics (Fracastoro, sixteenth century), diseases associated with particular occupations (Paracelsus, sixteenth century), and variations in death rates within the population (Graunt, seventeenth century).

Efforts to address underlying causes of disease increased during the Enlightenment period (the late-seventeenth and eighteenth centuries). For example, in order to combat the social ills attributed to cheap gin, depicted famously in Hogarth's *Gin Lane*, an Act of 1751 imposed a high tax and restricted availability. Also around this time, there was particular interest in improving the health of seamen and soldiers, although the authorities were slow to act on evidence (Inglis, 1965). James Lind demonstrated that scurvy – a seemingly unavoidable consequence of long voyages – was caused by a lack of vitamin C and could be prevented by issuing citrus fruit rations (although Lind's role has been subject to revision in recent years – see Bartholomew, 2002). Although Captain Cook successfully tested Lind's thesis, the Admiralty was not convinced until the early years of the following century. Meanwhile, Sir John Pringle identified a range of conditions – overcrowded accommodation, inadequate ventilation, poor sanitation – that were associated with common epidemics amongst military personnel, such as typhus for example. His recommendations on how to prevent outbreaks of disease were similarly ignored for many years. A further exponent of change in this period was the prison reform movement. The work of penal reformers such as John Howard is credited with giving an important impetus to the public health movement (Patterson, 1948). Prison campaigners examined the causes of diseases such as typhus and identified possible ways of preventing illness, such as improved hygiene, ventilation, sanitation, and the segregation of sick and healthy prisoners.

As the eighteenth century came to a close, however, public health was being taken more seriously by those in authority. Some municipal corporations sought to improve their civic environment and obtained legislative powers to this end (Rosen, 1993). They began to tackle specific problems, such as polluted water supplies and waste from trade. Nonetheless, towns and cities lacked a coherent system of public health administration. Efforts to introduce such a system (as in Manchester, which established a Board of Health in 1796) were rare and had limited success.

No historical account would be complete without mentioning the work of Edward Jenner (Fisher, 1991). In the last years of the eighteenth century, Jenner discovered that cowpox vaccination protected against smallpox. This represented an advance on the riskier practice of variolation, whereby pus taken from a smallpox sufferer was injected into a healthy person to prevent the disease. Controversially, Jenner proved the efficacy of cowpox vaccination by experiment: inoculating a child initially with cowpox and then subsequently with smallpox. Although the initial reaction of the scientific community was unfavourable, other doctors soon took an interest in vaccination. By Victorian times, vaccination against smallpox was commonplace, becoming compulsory in the 1850s.

The Victorians

The Victorians introduced many important public health reforms (see Simon, 1890; Flinn, 1968; Smith, 1979; Wohl, 1984). Two main phases of reform can be identified: the sanitary revolution and preventive medicine (Armstrong, 1993; Fee and Porter, 1992; Kickbusch, 1986).

The Sanitary Revolution

Some towns and cities took steps to improve their local environment long before the Victorians. However, the influx of people to the newly industrialized towns and cities (see Figure 2.1) created problems that even the most enlightened local administrations found difficult to manage.

Political elites were not completely oblivious to the social consequences of industrialization. Although limited attempts were made to confront the worst practices, there was no political will to undertake a comprehensive public health programme. A number of Acts concerning factories and workplaces were introduced before the dawn of the Victorian era. However, as Trevelyan (1973, p. 484) observed, they were 'not only very limited in scope, but remained dead letters for want of any machinery to enforce them'. Awareness of the public health problems associated with industrialization was plainly not enough: cause and effect had to be clearly established, feasible solutions identified, and the case for reform accepted by political elites. This was extremely difficult in an era dominated by liberal free market ideas and the powerful capitalist interests.

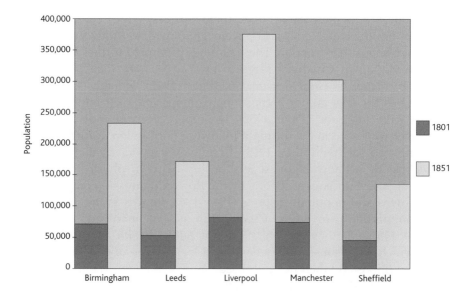

Figure 2.1 Population growth in the early nineteenth century

However, reformers had one thing in their favour: the obsession with rational solutions that characterized the Victorian period (Fraser, 1973). Research findings provided much impetus for sanitary reform. Local studies were conducted from the late eighteenth century onwards, for example such as in Chester and Carlisle. Those led the way for subsequent inquiries into the condition of the people in newly industrialized districts. For example, studies such as James Kay's (1832) research in the Manchester slums documented high levels of illness among the poor and pinpointed causes, notably a lack of sanitation.

These studies attracted the attention of the Poor Law Commission. This body was established in 1834, by the Poor Law Amendment Act, to oversee a new system of poor relief designed to reduce the burden on local taxpayers (Longmate, 2003). The key principle of this system was 'less eligibility': poor relief for the able-bodied would be given in conditions that deterred all but the destitute. Workhouses were built for this purpose, with 'outdoor relief' restricted to those who were aged, infirm or ill (although many of these ended up in workhouses). The regime was harsh and inhumane. Although some of its worst aspects were tackled in 1847, its key elements continued well into the next century.

Keen to explore avenues to further reduce the burden of the poor, the Poor Law Commission (prompted by Edwin Chadwick, its Secretary, who was to play a major role in sanitary reform) supported further studies into the link between illness and poverty. In 1838, three doctors, James Kay, Thomas Southwood Smith, and Neil Arnott, were appointed to study conditions affecting public health in London. These findings prompted further investigations, culminating in Chadwick's report on *The Sanitary Condition of the Labouring Population of Great Britain* (Chadwick, 1842). Notably, Chadwick was named as the sole author because the Commission itself refused to be associated with the report (Finer, 1952). The report received wide publicity: 20,000 copies were sold in the fortnight following publication. A further 3000 were distributed for free (Flinn, 1965). Chadwick's report set the terms of future debate by acknowledging a relationship between physical environment and disease. Subsequent reports by the Royal Commission on the State of Large Towns and populous districts (1844; 1845, known as the 'Health of Towns Commission'), in which Chadwick was also involved, provided detailed recommendations on sanitation and public health administration, many of which were subsequently enshrined in law. The documentation of physical conditions and their health consequences was augmented by reports from the Registrar-General's office, created in 1837. Its driving force was William Farr, a statistician with a medical background. Farr employed the vital statistics acquired through the registration process to illustrate the need for public health improvements. In particular, mortality rates of poorer areas were highlighted by comparison with healthier areas, giving further ammunition to public health reformers.

Evidence about links between the environment and ill health was given sharper focus by the death toll from infectious diseases. According to Hodgkinson (1967, p. 658), 'the chief importance of epidemics from the public health point of view was that they gave impetus to sanitary reform, for real panics made an ineffaceable impression'. Wohl (1984, p. 125) agreed, observing that such diseases drew attention to filthy conditions and to poverty, forcing the authorities to come to terms with public health. Of all the Victorian epidemics, cholera made the greatest impression (Longmate, 1966; Morris, 1976): according to Wohl (1984), out of proportion to its statistical importance. Certainly, other infectious diseases killed more people. Between 1837 and the end of the nineteenth century smallpox killed over 200,000 people (44,000 in the period 1871–3 alone), measles over half a million (including 16,765 in 1887 alone) and scarlet fever three quarters of a million (including 32,543 in 1870). Analysis of data from the period 1848–72 revealed that the average mortality rates for men and women from typhus, smallpox, measles, scarlet fever, whooping cough and tuberculosis (TB) were all higher than for cholera (Logan, 1950). Over the century, these diseases, along with typhoid, diphtheria, and influenza, represented a greater threat to health than cholera in terms of the numbers of people affected. But cholera epidemics induced a climate of fear. It was the classic 'dread disease', striking quickly, often killing people within hours. The belief that cholera was caused by filthy living conditions and poor physical environment added to the pressure for reform. The threat of further epidemics kept reform on the agenda when other political issues, such as the repeal of the Corn Laws and Chartist agitation might have removed it. The outbreak of cholera in 1848 undoubtedly 'scared society into the tardy beginnings of sanitary self-defence' (Trevelyan, 1973, p. 529).

Table 2.1 Cholera deaths in England and Wales: main epidemics in the nineteenth century

Year(s) of outbreak	Number of deaths
1831–32	21,866
1848–49	53,293
1853–54	20,097
1866	14,378

Source of data: C. Creighton (1965) *A History of Epidemics*, Vol. 2, London: Frank Cass

This response took the form of the 1848 Public Health Act, which permitted localities outside London to establish health boards responsible for regulating practices and conditions harmful to health (such as offensive trades and houses unfit for human occupation) and for managing sanitation, waste disposal and other services such as burial grounds, backed up with the power to levy rates. The Act also established a central authority – the General Board of Health – which could in certain circumstances compel localities to establish health boards. The main weapon against disease employed by this framework was sanitation, in particular the provision of clean water supplies and safe methods of sewage disposal. Over a hundred and fifty years later, sanitation is still regarded as one of the most important public health interventions. In 2007, in a poll carried out by the *British Medical Journal*, it was voted the greatest medical milestone of the last century and a half (www.bmj.com, 2007).

Cholera aside, other circumstances played a part in the emergence of the new legislation. The Reform Act of 1832 widened the franchise, in theory making governments more vulnerable to pressure from the electorate. However, this should not be exaggerated, as the vote remained restricted to a minority of men. More significant perhaps was the Chartist agitation of the 1830s and 40s, which forced an awareness of the grievances of the working classes on both government and Parliament. Wohl (1984) pointed out that the Chartists were not particularly interested in public health and actually opposed some sanitary measures. Nevertheless, as Woodward (1962, p. 147) correctly observed, 'this agitation of the poor compelled other classes to think about the condition of England', and strengthened the hand of those seeking to promote public health reform.

Battles were fought on other fronts, notably on working conditions. Here a similar story unfolded: the collection of evidence and organized pressure producing public outcry and then legislation to curb the worst evils. Legislation governing factories and mines provided further examples of how reform developed a momentum of its own. The 1833 Factory Act, which regulated hours of work, had limited impact. Adult hours of work were not covered by the Act, and only a small number of inspectors were appointed to enforce the law and they had limited powers. However, in 1840 a Commission was established to examine child labour in mines and factories. Its first report shocked the public with revelations of children and women working in barbaric conditions. This created a favourable political climate for the passage of the Mines Act (1842), vigorously contested by the mine owners, which prohibited the employment of all females and boys under 10 years of age underground, set age limits for those tending machinery, and created a mines inspectorate to regulate employment conditions. Another battlefront was the campaign against alcohol (Harrison, 1971; Dingle, 1980). Although not a central concern of the public health movement (Wohl, 1984), the health and social implications of alcohol consumption were widely acknowledged. A select committee found:

> That [the] following are only a few of the evils directly springing from this baneful source; destruction of health, disease in every form and shape, premature decrepitude in the old, stunted growth, and general debility and decay in the young, loss of life by paroxysms, apoplexies, drownings, burnings, and accidents of various kinds, delirium tremens ... paralysis, idoitcy [sic], madness and violent death. (Select Committee on Drunkenness, 1834, p. iv)

To place Victorian consumption levels in contemporary perspective, in Britain in 1870 the amount of alcohol consumed per person aged 15 and over was more than double that of the 1960s (for a discussion of Victorian attitudes to drink see Harrison, 1971). The temperance movement, initially a non-conformist-based movement concerned mainly with the immorality of drunkenness and its social consequences, focused on 'moral suasion' to persuade individuals to abstain from drinking (Dingle, 1980). Later, the movement expanded to include members of the established church, the Liberal party (then the main opposition to the Conservative party), and the medical profession. The temperance movement then began to campaign for 'legislative suppression' to restrict the alcohol trade including age limits for children, restricting hours of sale, higher taxes and imposing stricter conditions for licensing retail outlets. Some of these measures were enacted in the late Victorian period, and the rest during the first quarter of the twentieth century.

Ideas, Values and Ideologies

Public health reformers were at odds with two key principles of the Victorian age: laissez-faire in economic matters and local self-government (Fraser, 1973). Opponents of reform defended the status quo from these standpoints, arguing that government interference would damage the economy and undermine the rights of local communities. Such arguments barely covered the naked self-interest of industrialists and powerful local elites. However, they carried considerable weight, and required a careful response from reformers.

The fact that many reformers, including Chadwick, were inspired by Bentham's utilitarian principles, helped their cause. Bentham's principles were often used to justify the laissez-faire approach to economic and social matters. But, as Marquand (1988, p. 223) perceptively remarked, 'the reaction against full-blooded market liberalism took place under the same philosophical aegis as the movement towards it'. Edwin Chadwick's brand of utilitarianism was based on a desire to maximize public benefit. If it could be demonstrated that the market did not achieve this, then an enlightened bureaucracy would have to intervene. As Finer (1952) observed, 'Chadwick was instantly fired by any and every feature that caused unnecessary suffering, disease, and economic waste' (p. 3) and he realized that 'it was good economy to prevent the evils' (p. 152).

To see Victorian public health as a purely utilitarian response is far too crude, however. Indeed there are those who argue that Benthamite utilitarianism was less significant than 'administrative momentum' (see MacDonagh, 1977; Fraser, 1973). From this perspective, state bureaucracies, established in response to social problems, developed their own agendas and acquired greater powers of intervention. This occurred in an incremental and pragmatic manner rather than through an ideological 'master plan' of social reform. One should not overlook humanitarian motives, as reflected in the role of philanthropists such as Lord Ashley, the Earl of Shaftsbury. However, it has been argued that 'the argument for sanitary reform was not ... primarily humanitarian' (Tesh, 1988, p. 339). As Flinn (1965, p. 29) noted, apart from factory reform, the great Victorian philanthropists showed little interest in public health. Yet as the public health movement developed, it reached an accommodation with the broader notion of 'improvement', which was a major influence in the Victorian era (see Briggs, 1959; Walvin, 1987). As Wohl (1984) notes, the public health movement became a moral crusade to eliminate the visible signs of filth, with physical cleanliness and good health being viewed as a precondition for social and spiritual progress.

As these ideas and values became entrenched in the latter half of the Victorian period, the resistance to state intervention in the field of public health began to weaken. Meanwhile, a number of defenders of local self-government became transformed from enemies of public health to its staunchest supporters.

This transformation lay in the desire of local politicians to create a stronger civic identity by improving the physical environment of their towns and cities. The classic example was Birmingham, which, under its mayor, Joseph Chamberlain, developed a local strategy of social reform in the 1870s (see Judd, 1977). Chamberlain's motto – 'high rates and a healthy city' (Longmate, 1966) – was reflected in a range of programmes including the municipal provision of gas and water, housing improvements and welfare services.

Political Agents and Institutions

The public health improvements of the Victorian age did not occur simply because circumstances were favourable, or because certain ideas and values prevailed. Political agents had to employ ideas, promote values, and take advantage of circumstances. In today's political system, political parties play a key role in campaigning, selecting candidates and leaders, marshalling parliamentary majorities for and against legislation and shaping the political agenda. In the period before the second Reform Act of 1867, however, parties were much weaker. There was more internal dissent than today, where a rebellion by backbench MPs is still infrequent enough to be newsworthy. During the Victorian period, coalitions of support for legislation often cut across party lines, and public health issues were no exception. As MacDonagh (1977) observed, the political allegiance of those involved in the public health movement did not lie exclusively with any particular party.

In the early Victorian period, pressure groups rather than parties were the main vehicle for those seeking to influence government. For example, the Health of Towns Association was active in promoting public health reform among the middle classes, in Parliament, in the press, and within government (Patterson, 1948; Hollis, 1974). After achieving its main objective – the passage of the 1848 Public Health Act – the association was dissolved. However, local associations continued to press for further reform. Later, other organized groups became involved in public health debates, including the Social Science Association (SSA), the British Medical Association (BMA), the Metropolitan Association of Medical Officers of Health (MAMOH) and the Sanitary Institute. The SSA and the BMA were particularly influential in the establishment of the Royal Sanitary Commission in 1869. The Commission's recommendations (C 281, 1871) led to the reorganization of public health responsibilities (under the Local Government Board in 1871) and paved the way for the Public Health Acts of 1872 and 1875, which set the framework of modern public health administration. MAMOH (and its successor, the Society of Medical Officers of Health) was also involved, helping to draft the public health legislation and lobbying successfully for stricter requirements on the notification of diseases. Meanwhile, the Sanitary Institute, which acted as a professional body for sanitary inspectors, was regarded as an influential lobby group in the late Victorian period (Frazer, 1950, p. 233), deriving its authority from the expertise of its members.

However, other potential supporters did not play a major role. As Porter (1995, p. 59) argued, 'the medical colleges never gave an impetus to the public health movement'. He maintained that 'the organized medical profession played a surprisingly secondary and desultory role in the vast expansion of the Victorian state provision'. Indeed, medical professional bodies often took a negative view of public health measures, as exemplified by the criticism of the General Board of Health by the Royal College of Physicians. However, this should not obscure the fact that many doctors were very concerned about public health and participated in other lobby groups. Also, as mentioned, the BMA was active in the late Victorian period in pressing for reform.

Although pressure groups were important actors, the role of public servants, furthering the public health cause from the inside, was crucial. There were often close links between government insiders and pressure groups (Finer, 1952; Sheard and Donaldson, 2006). Flinn (1965) suggests that professional administrators within government played a key role in promoting public debate and government intervention. In the early Victorian period, the name of Edwin Chadwick looms large. He held a number of influential positions, secretary of the Poor Law Commission, secretary to the Health of Towns Commission, member of the General Board of Health. Southwood Smith was also an important figure in this period, and was involved in the inquiries into urban conditions of the 1830s. He was also a leading member of the Health of Towns Association, and sat alongside Chadwick on the General Board of Health. In the later phase of reform, the key figure was Sir John Simon (Lambert, 1963), a founding member of the Health of Towns Association, the first medical officer for London (1848) and the nation's first Medical Officer (1855). His achievement was to consolidate the earlier victories of the public health movement, while advancing state intervention into new areas. Simon's role is discussed in more detail later in this chapter.

Politicians played an important role in initiating legislation and steering it through Parliament, including Morpeth and Disraeli, both members of the Health of Towns Association. Morpeth, a member of the Whig cabinet during the 1840s, worked closely with Chadwick in framing public health legislation, including the 1848 Act. It has been argued that the contribution of some politicians to public health reform has been exaggerated. For example, the Public Health Act of 1875, introduced by Disraeli, was strongly influenced by the policies of the previous Liberal government. Moreover, it has been argued that Disraeli's government could have done more to promote public health, but was inhibited by an ideological commitment to local independence and private property rights (Smith, 1967).

Throughout the Victorian period, politicians and the vested interests they represented – such as the water companies – mounted a strong rearguard action against public health reform. They were successful in weakening the General Board of Health in 1854 and abolishing it in 1858. There are many other examples of business interests opposing public health reforms during the nineteenth century. One striking example occurred during the outbreak of cholera in Sunderland in 1831, where the local business community was so concerned about the impact of a possible quarantine on their trade that they forced the doctors to retract their diagnoses (Longmate, 1966, pp. 27–32). Later, a group of anti-quarantine businessmen secured control of the Sunderland Board of Health and were able temporarily to prevent the publication of new cases of the disease in a vain effort to avoid a quarantine being imposed. Local interests also resisted attempts by central government to introduce public health measures. For example, powerful London interests, and their representatives in Parliament, opposed central direction in public health matters and were successful in excluding the metropolis from the provisions of the 1848 Act. However, the City of London did appoint its own medical officer in 1848 partly in response to a fresh outbreak of cholera, and as the century wore on the powerful interests within the capital acknowledged the need for public health measures.

Other opposition came from civil liberties groups, particularly on the question of vaccination. Anti-vaccination groups flourished in the latter part of the nineteenth century following the imposition of compulsory vaccination against smallpox in 1853 (Blume, 2006; Wolfe and Sharp, 2002; Hobson-West, 2004). Strong local campaigns in over 50 cities and towns made it difficult to enforce the law and by 1896 around a fifth of districts failed to do so. In the 1890s the law was modified to allow conscientious objectors the right to decline vaccination. The Contagious Diseases Acts, passed between 1866 and 1869, also raised concerns about the intrusiveness of public health reform and its disregard for civil liberties. These Acts enabled the authorities to undertake compulsory medical examinations of alleged prostitutes in naval and military towns. Women found to be infected with venereal disease were subjected to compulsory detention and treatment. These diseases were a growing problem, particularly in towns where soldiers or sailors were stationed. Liverpool, for example, was described as 'a hot bed of syphilis' (Frazer, 1950, p. 200). Some, including members of the medical profession, wanted to see the Acts extended to other localities, and a pressure group was formed with this aim. There was, however, strong opposition from the National Association for the Repeal of the Contagious Diseases Acts, spearheaded by Josephine Butler, which successfully achieved a repeal of the legislation in 1886.

The press often saw itself as the guardian of individual liberty against the intrusion of the public health reformers, particularly in the 1840s and 50s. For example, the weakening of the General Board of Health in 1854 was greeted with glee in *The Times*:

> The British nation abhors absolute power. We prefer to take our chance with cholera and the rest than be bullied into health. (quoted by Longmate, 1966, p. 188)

However, from the 1860s onwards, the press became generally more supportive of intervention as opinion shifted strongly in favour of public health reform.

Although Parliament was a key battleground between public health reformers and their opponents in the Victorian era, local government was also an important arena. The 1848 Act was permissive in all but the most exceptional circumstances. This meant that decisions about public health were delegated to local communities, stimulating political divisions at this level. Efforts to impose a central framework for regulation were vigorously resisted. Indeed, according to some (Szreter, 1995, cited in Baum, 2002, p. 19) the 1840s were 'a false dawn' for the public heath movement, which failed to win over the governing classes. In the longer term, however, the impetus proved too powerful. The crucial change was the 1866 Sanitary Act, which imposed obligations on localities to cleanse their communities, although local communities continued to have considerable autonomy within this framework.

The Public Health Act of 1875 represented the culmination of the sanitary reformers' campaign. Although a consolidating measure, it set a clear framework for public health for the next fifty years. It also signalled the end of an era, for although legislation would still be used to improve the physical environment, attention was shifting towards other means of intervention aimed at improving social welfare generally and personal hygiene in particular.

Victorian Public Health: Preventive Medicine

In the latter part of the Victorian period, 'preventive medicine' replaced the 'sanitary idea' as the dominant philosophy of public health (see Armstrong, 1993; Kickbusch, 1986; Fee and Porter, 1992; Lewis, 1992). This was manifested in the 'medicalization' of public health; in a shift in the focus of attention from the general population towards specific subgroups and individuals, and in an increasing emphasis on access to health services. At the same time, the activities of the sanitary movement, while still contributing to public health debates, became more closely integrated with broader issues of social welfare.

It should be noted that Chadwick had a 'deep-seated distrust of curative medicine' (Finer, 1952, p. 157). Indeed, the early Victorian public health programme was 'fundamentally environmentalist' (Sheard and Donaldson, 2006, p. 1). Medicine played a secondary role to other professions, such as engineering for example. As already mentioned, medical professional bodies were less than enthusiastic about central government intervention. Nonetheless, individual members of the medical profession were an important driving force behind the sanitary revolution. Much of the early evidence about the extent of the problem was documented by individuals with a medical background, such as Farr, Southwood Smith and Simon.

As the century wore on, central government increasingly incorporated medical expertise. Doctors, alongside sanitary inspectors and surveyors, played an important role in the improvement of public health after the 1848 Act. The Act permitted the appointment of a local Medical Officer of Health (MOH), although this did not become compulsory until later (1855, in the case of metropolitan boroughs, 1872 for other local sanitary authorities, 1909 for county councils). As more and more localities employed MOHs, their influence grew. Initially, though, they had a precarious existence. In some places, opposition to sanitary reform led to their dismissal (see Wohl, 1984, p. 171). Posts were often part-time, salaries ungenerous and the duties often onerous. Even so, the local MOH began to exert leadership in health matters, partly due to the growing status of medicine, discussed in a moment. MOHs also began to exert greater influence at national level too. They formed their own separate association in 1856 and lobbied for improvements in legislation. As noted earlier, the MAMOH (and its successor, the Society of Medical Officers, formed in 1889) helped to draft public health legislation. Meanwhile, other professional organizations, the BMA in particular, became increasingly involved in campaigning on public health issues, both in relation to specific issues (such as vaccination) and with regard to reforming the system of public health administration (Bartrip, 1996).

The medical profession began to exert greater influence over public health matters within government. The appointment of a medical officer to the board of health in 1855 was a significant development. The first holder of this post, Sir John Simon, documented the main threats to health such as cholera, diphtheria, and TB, and their principal causes: bad housing, overcrowding, insanitary conditions, poor nutrition, difficult and dangerous working conditions. Simon's achievement was to place public health on a sounder scientific footing by establishing links between health and a range of social factors, which actually antagonized Chadwick and other sanitarians (see Sheard and Donaldson, 2006, pp. 148–9). This helped to establish a case for further government intervention in areas such as food quality, housing and sanitary reform. In a broader sense, Simon also helped to promote the influence of the medical profession, and its representative organizations, within government (Lambert, 1963).

The growing influence of the medical profession over debates about the future direction of public health provides only a partial explanation of the medicalization of public health. The other main reason was that medical knowledge was advancing, and this, along with the rising status of the profession (Parry and Parry, 1976), strengthened medical authority. The value of medical knowledge in relation to public health was demonstrated in two fields: epidemiology and bacteriology.

Epidemiology was exemplified by Snow's work on the cholera epidemic of 1854, which showed how the causes of ill health could be identified and measured (Baum, 2002, p. 138). Snow discovered that water supplies were associated with an outbreak of cholera in the Soho area of London, by marking reported cases on a map of the area. The resulting cluster highlighted a particular source of drinking water – the Broad Street pump. Further investigation revealed that the victims drank from this particular source. At the time, the medical establishment was reluctant to acknowledge Snow's findings – there was much controversy within the profession over whether diseases such as cholera were caused by noxious substances carried in the air or by contagion (Pelling, 1978). The discovery was subsequently hailed as a classic example of epidemiological detection.

Public health intervention has often anticipated scientific findings about the precise nature of disease causation. Snow's work provided circumstantial evidence about the causes of cholera and endorsed efforts to improve sanitation. But it preceded the identification of the disease agent (the cholera vibrio, discovered by Koch) by about thirty years. There are many other examples: the London County Council registered a nil return for typhus in their annual statistics three years before the transmission route of the disease – lice – was confirmed (Shryock, 1979, quoted in Inglis, 1965, p. 169). Furthermore, Lind's discovery of the link between diet and scurvy, discussed earlier, preceded identification of vitamin C deficiency as the cause by over a century.

Epidemiologists, such as Snow, and others such as William Budd (who developed a theory of causation regarding cholera similar to Snow's, and established that human excreta was associated with the spread of typhoid), legitimized improvements in sanitation that were already taking place and added further weight to the arguments of reformers. Yet it was only with the bacterial revolution of the 1880s that the scientific achievements of Snow, Budd and others came to be fully appreciated. The discovery of the bacteriological causes of infectious diseases placed preventive medicine on a sounder scientific basis. The endorsement of 'germ theory' had a number of other implications (see Fee and Porter, 1992; Lewis, 1992). First, it pinpointed the laboratory rather than society as the workshop for public health medicine. In future, public health would be increasingly the province of scientifically trained professionals. By implication, scientific knowledge would carry greater weight than other competing forms of knowledge. This in turn implied that public health intervention could no longer be justified solely on the basis of detective guesswork and circumstantial evidence but required hard, scientific evidence. This favoured quantitative laboratory studies over

qualitative studies. It also emphasized the importance of medical intervention, which could be more easily measured and quantified, over social intervention, which was more difficult to evaluate.

Another consequence of the growing dominance of germ theory was an
emphasis on the manifestation of disease in individuals and subgroups
within the population, rather than the health of the population as a whole.
As Starr (1982) observed in a US context, the concept of 'dirt' was in effect
narrowed by bacteriological discoveries. However, the emphasis on individuals and subgroups was not entirely new. For example, much of the
impetus for the sanitary movement arose from studies of the condition of a
subgroup: the poor. Moreover, personal health, particularly personal
hygiene, had long been an important focus for the movement. Local sanitary associations promulgated advice on the importance of cleanliness, and
from the 1860s employed 'visitors' (the forerunners of today's health visitors) to provide advice and education on health matters. Other groups, such
as the Ladies' Association for Diffusion of Sanitary Knowledge, disseminated advice to the lower classes. Meanwhile, the Association for Promoting
Cleanliness among the Poor lobbied successfully for legislation (the Baths
and Washhouses Act 1846) to improve the provision of washing and bathing
facilities in poorer communities.

The emphasis on personal health shifted attention away from environmental health concerns towards debates about the financing and organization
of health services. Indeed, the state's role in funding and providing preventive and treatment services became one of the central health issues as the turn
of the century approached. Yet concern about social and environmental
causes of ill health did not subside in the late Victorian period. It was rather
that the energies of public health campaigners became absorbed into a broader
movement to improve social welfare. This was reflected in part by the growing
demands for improved access to specific health services, particularly for
vulnerable people, such as mothers and children. It was also evident in
campaigns to improve housing and to tackle poverty and destitution.

According to Wohl (1984, p. 320), Victorian public health reformers failed
to challenge the fabric of society. He does not blame them, believing that to
have done so would have risked jeopardizing their position, thereby undermining the system of public health they had so carefully constructed. In the
earlier phase of reform, as Shryock (1979) remarks, sanitarians had sought to
break the cycle of poverty and disease. Only limited change to alleviate the
worst conditions was possible, given the prevailing values of early Victorian
society. In the later phase of reform, those seeking to advance public health –
such as Sir John Simon – readily acknowledged the role played by poverty in
disease. In his role as Medical Officer, he sought to draw attention to the
health consequences of poverty. However, within central government, as
Webster (1990) observed, the public health response was overshadowed by

the Poor Law. The creation of a Local Government Board (LGB) in 1871, which incorporated the Poor Law Board and the Medical Department of the Privy Council, rather than integrating health and local government administration, made it more difficult for those concerned about public health to initiate change (Sheard and Donaldson, 2006; Hodgkinson, 1967). As Honigsbaum observed (1970, p. 9), 'with few exceptions, the LGB's Poor Law functions smothered its concern for public health'. Eventually, in 1876, Simon resigned his post 'in frustration at the low status afforded to scientific authority in the Local Government Board' (Webster, 1990, p. 11).

The Poor Law system shaped public health at the local level in an adverse way. First, the philosophy that underpinned the Poor Law was often inconsistent with the sanitary idea. As Hodgkinson (1967, p. 637) notes, 'the Poor Law was a deterrent aimed at reducing costs and the public health movement by its obvious insistence on prevention, entailing large expenditure, was incompatible with Poor Law principles.' She goes on to observe that, apart from temporary cooperation brought on by the exigencies of epidemics, 'Poor law and public health continued side by side, each according to its own principles and ignoring the effect on the other' (p. 679).

The Poor Law deterred those needing treatment who were reluctant to submit to the workhouse test. Yet a system of relief that promoted earlier intervention would probably have had significant advantages for public health. During the late Victorian period, the conditions for medical relief were relaxed and it was increasingly given to those not technically destitute (Hodgkinson, 1967). Furthermore, in 1885 sick people were exempted from the strict Poor Law requirements by the Medical Relief Act. Despite these developments, the stigma of medical relief provided under the auspices of the Poor Law persisted.

The system of medical relief added to the complexity of health administration and seriously inhibited efforts to promote public health. Even when the poor law authorities subsequently developed public health functions (in relation to sanitation, vaccination, and the treatment of diseases, such as TB and venereal disease for example) these developed separately from public health authorities. The preventive work of Poor Law Officers and Medical Officers of Health was inhibited by the continuation of different administrative systems (even though in some areas Poor Law Medical Officers were also appointed as local Medical Officers of Health on a part-time basis).

Even where limited integration occurred, the Poor Law philosophy tended to dominate, to the detriment of public health. This domination continued well into the early years of the twentieth century (Honigsbaum, 1970). The development of schemes with a strong public health element – such as the inspection and treatment of schoolchildren – forced the LGB to take a greater interest in public health. But this shift in focus did not occur until the second decade of the twentieth century and was at any rate short-lived – the LGB's functions were taken over by a new Ministry of Health in 1919 (see Chapter 3).

To complete this chapter, it is important to mention two areas where reformers did begin to influence the social and economic conditions of the people in the latter half of the nineteenth century: housing and workplace legislation.

According to Wohl (1984, p. 327), 'Healthy housing was one of the cornerstones of the sanitary reformers' philosophy and programme.' Yet, apart from regulations on cellar dwellings and provisions for adequate drains for new houses, it was not until the late Victorian period that local authorities acquired significant powers to deal with problems of overcrowding and poor quality housing. Even then, much was left to voluntary activity, such as the housing schemes initiated by Octavia Hill (a grand-daughter of Southwood Smith). An Act of 1868 gave municipal authorities powers to force owners to repair or rebuild insanitary housing. This was followed by the Cross Act (Artisans' Dwellings Act, 1875), which enabled local authorities to undertake programmes of slum clearance, compensate owners and rehouse people. This legislation did not compel authorities to act. Few took up the challenge, as the costs were prohibitively high. Moreover, local authorities were not permitted to adopt the role of landlord until later legislation of 1885, 1890 and 1909. So although cities such as Liverpool and Birmingham set an example, municipal housing was by no means widespread by the end of the century.

Workplaces

Legislation to ameliorate some of the worst working conditions was the result of many years of hard campaigning. The Factory Act of 1833 and the Mines Act of 1842 have already been mentioned. A further Factory Act of 1844 limited the working hours of women and children in textile factories and set out regulations regarding the safety of machinery. The Ten Hours Act of 1847 placed a limit on the working hours of women and young people (and, by implication, placed a limit on the working hours of men too) working in the textile industry. A further Mines Act was passed in 1850, extending the powers of inspectors in construction and safety issues to enforce the law. Acts of 1864 and 1867 extended regulation to more industries and made provisions concerning the health and safety of the working environment. Although the legislation was consolidated in 1878, there remained exceptions, such as the notorious 'sweated trades', which were initially regulated in 1891, with more comprehensive legislation following in 1909. By the turn of the century, regulations had begun to address the problems of the working environment. There was growing interest in particular occupational diseases, but little was done to tackle these problems. As Wohl (1984) notes, physical conditions at work at the end of the Victorian era were still harmful to health in spite of these improvements.

Conclusion

This chapter has shown that the perceived importance of public health inter-vention has varied over time and between different societies. Although strong similarities in public health intervention can be found – the emphasis on sanitation by both the Romans and the Victorians being an example – there has been much variation in approaches adopted. In Britain, for example, from the Middle Ages up to the twentieth century, interventions fall into several phases, each of which emphasizes a particular model of public health: quar-antine; sanitary science: and personal hygiene. On closer inspection, however, as this chapter has shown, these phases are not so clear-cut, with different models co-existing in the same time period. It is therefore more appropriate to view each phase as being subjected to different influences, with one particular model having a stronger influence over public health policy and practice, but co-existing with others exerting less influence.

Public Health in the Twentieth Century

3

By the end of the Victorian era the public health movement had split into two main elements: the first committed to the promotion of general improvements in social conditions; the second more concerned with the provision of specific preventive and curative health services. This chapter examines how these elements influenced public health reform during the first half of the twentieth century and then discusses developments following the creation of the NHS in 1948, the impact of subsequent reorganizations, and the revival of interest in public health strategies from the 1970s onwards.

Public Health before the NHS

Poverty and the Poor Law

Social surveys, such as those undertaken by Booth (1902) in London and by Rowntree (1901) in York, stimulated awareness about poverty and health. Their findings reinforced arguments articulated by the national efficiency movement (see Searle, 1971), regarding Britain's inability to compete economically, technologically and militarily, because of the poor physical health, inadequate skills and limited educational ability of the British people. Such fears came to a head during the Boer War, when evidence came to light of the physical condition of recruits. Subsequently, the report of the Interdepartmental Committee on Physical Deterioration (Cd 2175, 1904), along with the Royal Commission on Physical Training in Scotland (Cd 1507, 1903) called for a range of measures, including systematic school medical inspections and facilities for feeding malnourished children. In 1906, local authorities were granted powers to provide meals to children in need and this was followed by a system of school medical inspections under the 1907 Education Act. This provided the basis for a compulsory school health service (Henderson, 1976; Leff and Leff, 1959; Gardner, 2008). The Children's Act of 1908 codified the law relating to children's health and welfare. Meanwhile, local authority health and welfare services for children began to expand.

The 'People's Budget' of 1909 introduced a more progressive tax system and enabled the state to finance its new social programmes. State pensions for the elderly were introduced. These measures were followed by the introduction of the National Insurance scheme, financed by the state, employers and workers. This provided financial benefits in times of unemployment for insured workers on a non-means-tested basis (and therefore lay outside the realm of the Poor Law system of relief), cash benefits for insured workers when they became ill, and a system of national health insurance (NHI), entitling them to free general medical services provided by general practitioners (GPs). Although a positive development, addressing an important link between poverty and illness, the NHI did not apply to non-working dependants (such as wives and children). Moreover, apart from TB treatment, specialist services lay outside its scope. Furthermore, because it dealt with people who were already ill, NHI had little impact on preventing illness.

The introduction of NHI outmanoeuvred two competing lobbies: those in favour of retaining the Poor Law in a modified form, and those clamouring for its abolition. In 1909, a Royal Commission had reported on this issue. Deep divisions between abolitionists and reformists on the Commission led to the production of two separate reports, each representing a different vision of social welfare and public health (Cd 4499, 1909; see also Bruce, 1968). The Commission's majority report was critical of aspects of the Poor Law but believed it could be refashioned. It argued that the stigma attached to the existing regime could be overcome by renaming the Poor Law as 'public assistance' and transferring its administration to local authorities. Another 20 years passed before this change was enacted. Some of the majority report's other recommendations, such as the creation of labour exchanges to help people find work and a system of unemployment insurance to cushion against hardship, were implemented more quickly.

The majority report wanted to see a more humane system of health care, recommending that sick people treated under the Poor Law should be accommodated in separate institutions from able-bodied persons, and acknowledging that the need for medical care should be assessed prior to assessment of financial means. Although it opposed giving people a right to free medical care, the majority report endorsed a scheme enabling poor people to have greater access to medical care in the community, funded by state subscriptions to existing insurance schemes. To administer health services for the poor, it envisaged the creation of a medical assistance committee under the auspices of each local public assistance authority.

In contrast, the Commission's minority report sought to address the causes of poverty and ill health by recommending that central government take responsibility for the labour market and unemployment. It recommended that Poor Law health services be combined with sanitary authorities to create a unified state health service. At local level, it proposed a health committee with wide responsibilities for illness prevention as well as service provision. The minority report called for health services to be free at point of delivery, assessment of means taking place only after treatment had been received, with the poor exempt from payment.

Although both reports were critical of the Poor Law, this system continued as the principal form of state assistance. It was not until the 1929 Local Government Act, according to Frazer (1950, p. 393) 'one of the important landmarks in the history of public health', that the Poor Law boards were replaced by local authority public assistance committees. The Act also gave local authorities discretion over the allocation of individual cases to specialist committees (such as education, health, and so on), transferred public health services provided by the Poor Law boards to local authorities, and allowed local health committees to take responsibility for Poor Law hospitals. Despite these important legislative and administrative changes, the remnants of the Poor Law system continued to influence health care and public health during the interwar period. On the eve of the Second World War, the majority of chronically ill people were still being cared for in institutions controlled by public assistance committees (Abel-Smith, 1964, p. 371).

Health and Welfare Services

One of the main reasons for the gradual decline of the Poor Law was the emergence of new health and welfare schemes. These included the NHI scheme, which challenged Poor Law principles by offering free services at point of delivery on the basis of contributions. The first two decades of the century saw the development of health and welfare services for babies and young children. These services, established by local authorities and voluntary organizations, included milk supplies and infant welfare centres. Local authorities began to organize community health services such as midwifery, district nursing and health visiting, working closely with voluntary associations and self-employed professionals. From 1912 onwards, the school medical service began to develop services such as school nursing, dental clinics, and the provision of spectacles. In 1918, following the Education Act of that year, a duty was placed on local authorities to provide treatment for certain diseases in schoolchildren, such as skin complaints and dental problems (Leff and Leff, 1959; Henderson, 1975). In the same year, the Maternity and Child Welfare Act clarified the law relating to local authority provision of services to expectant and nursing mothers and preschool children, facilitating the extension of schemes in this field (Frazer, 1950, p. 412).

During the 1920s and 30s, local authorities' responsibilities for health care continued to grow. As mentioned earlier, the 1929 Local Government Act allowed them to bring Poor Law hospitals under the control of their health committee. It also transferred other responsibilities of the Poor Law boards relating to maternity and child welfare, TB, immunization, blind people and mental deficiency to the local authorities, enabling them to develop a more comprehensive range of services in these fields. The expanding remit of local health committees and their medical officers of health (MOHs) in the interwar period explains why some saw it as a golden age of public health (Chave, 1974; Godber, 1986). Holland and Stewart (1998) argue that the 'period between the two World Wars was one of substantial progress for public health – a proud era' (p. 58). Indeed, there were positive developments in this period that should not be overlooked, such as the rationalization of maternal and child welfare services. The growing interest in health education was another important development. The Central Council for Health Education was established in 1927 and from 1936 local authorities acquired wider powers to provide public information about health and disease. Wider social reforms of the interwar period had positive implications for public health, such as housing improvement, discussed later in this chapter. Some, however, have questioned whether the acquisition of responsibilities actually improved public health in the interwar period. Lewis (1986, p. 16) observed that 'the public health departments added to their domain without questioning what was distinctive about public health'. She argues that this had important consequences. Public health doctors became preoccupied with their service delivery role at the expense of their traditional community watchdog role. There were also 'turf battles', notably between public health doctors and GPs.

Lewis's argument about the decline of the MOHs' community watchdog role is reflected in their failure to pursue immunization as readily as they might have done. She suggested that they and local health committees placed greater emphasis on the use of treatment facilities than prevention as a means of dealing with infectious diseases (Lewis, 1986, p. 30). Lewis also argues that the MOHs neglected their community watchdog role by failing to highlight the effects of long-term unemployment on nutritional standards and levels of morbidity and mortality. This is supported by Webster (1990, p. 15), who has stated that in the interwar period 'the public health mechanism failed to respond appropriately and showed itself incapable of resisting political pressures for falsification of the evidence relating to ill health and malnutrition.'

Webster refers to the dismal performance of the public health profession in this period (see also Webster, 1986). But is this a fair assessment? After all, local health authorities, to which MOHs were accountable, operated in a political environment that included powerful vested interests opposed to some public health measures. Although full-time MOHs could not be dismissed without the approval of the Minister of Health, they were often under great pressure not to upset their employing authorities and it is hardly surprising that some succumbed. But such pressures were not unprecedented in this field (Wohl, 1984). Moreover, although some MOHs were pusillanimous, others were not. The case of M'Gonigle, the MOH for Stockton on Tees in the 1930s, who painstakingly collected evidence on the health impact of malnutrition, shows the commitment of those seeking to highlight the socioeconomic causes of illness (Holland and Stewart, 1998, pp. 50–6). Similarly Welshman's (1997) study of MOHs in Leicester found that although some were complacent, others were innovative and imaginative, particularly in view of the constraints they faced.

Let us now examine the turf wars within the medical profession, which, as Lewis (1986) correctly observes, strongly influenced the direction of public health in the interwar period. The local authorities' involvement in primary care alarmed some doctors, particularly GPs, who foresaw the prospect of a state-run salaried general medical service. GPs were extremely vigilant about the 'encroachment' of local authority services (see Lewis, 1986, p. 10) on their role of delivering personal health services. A GP-centred model of primary care was central to the Dawson report, issued by the Central Council on Medical and Allied Services under the auspices of the Ministry of Health (Cmd 693, 1920). It envisaged the creation of a system of primary health centres focused on the maintenance of health rather than simply the treatment of illness. These centres would provide an accessible range of preventive and curative services, including community health services such as prenatal care, school medical services, and health promotional activities. They would bring together independent GPs, supported by nursing staff and technicians, who would have access to a range of diagnostic and treatment facilities. In addition, GPs would be assisted by visiting consultants and specialists, enabling a greater range of treatment to take place in this setting.

Although the Dawson report was never officially endorsed, it nevertheless had some impact. A number of local experiments reflected the report's emphasis on positive health and its desire to bring services under one roof. For example, the Peckham Centre, begun in 1926, went beyond a narrow medical approach and sought to establish health centres as an integral part of community life (Stallibrass, 1989). But more importantly, the Dawson report had an impact on debates within the medical profession, sending out an important signal to GPs to stake their claim to this territory.

Throughout the 1920s and 30s, tensions between the GPs and MOHs intensified, resulting in a fracturing of traditional medical solidarities (Porter, 1990). This intra-professional struggle revolved around status. In this period, both branches of the profession lacked prestige, although the status of GPs had risen following the introduction of NHI. By the outbreak of the Second World War, general practice rather than public health medicine had the edge.

GPs also had greater political clout, subsequently reflected in the organization of the NHS, which preserved their independent contractor status while at the same time removing key services from the MOH, as we shall see later.

The Ministry of Health

The public heath implications of the NHS will be considered later in this chapter. First, however, it is necessary to discuss an earlier development, the creation of a Ministry of Health in 1919. Calls to establish such a ministry can be traced to the early part of the previous century when Bentham proposed a health ministry responsible for sanitation, communicable diseases and the administration of medical care (Rosen and Burns, 1983). Although this suggestion was repeated on several occasions throughout the nineteenth century (its advocates included leading figures such as Sir John Simon), the closest Britain came was the short-lived General Board of Health (see Chapter 2).

During the second decade of the twentieth century, the case for a Ministry of Health intensified. It was argued that such a ministry would be able to clarify the aims of health policy and would overcome rivalries on health matters, for example between the insurance commissioners (who ran the national insurance system), the LGB and the Board of Education (Sheard and Donaldson, 2006). It was believed that a health ministry would effectively coordinate the network of public health services that had developed somewhat haphazardly: sanitation, the Poor Law, the municipal health services, the school health service and the NHI scheme. It was also seen as a means of liberating public health from the widely discredited Poor Law system.

The creation of a health ministry proved a difficult task, largely because of the political differences between the vested interests involved (see Honigsbaum, 1970; Gilbert, 1970). Four factors were crucial to its emergence. The First World War exposed once again the poor physical health of recruits, and produced renewed calls for improvements in health. Second, the alleged mishandling of an influenza epidemic in 1918/19 by the LGB added to pressures for change. A third factor was that government had to respond more sensitively to the demands of women's organizations following the enfranchisement of females over the age of 30 in 1918. These groups had campaigned for better services, particularly in the field of maternity and infant welfare, and had argued that a health ministry would help secure such improvements. Fourth, the government was willing to make concessions to powerful interests such as the local councils, Poor Law boards, friendly societies and insurance bodies and even other government departments. Hence an explicit commitment to abolish the Poor Law was shelved yet again, insurance companies received special rights of representation under the new arrangements, and the Board of Education retained its responsibilities for the school medical service. The casualty was the LGB, which was abolished, its functions absorbed into the Ministry of Health (Gilbert, 1970, p. 133).

The Ministry of Health was given a statutory duty 'to take all steps as may be desirable to secure the preparation, effective carrying out and co-ordination of measures conducive to the health of the people'. It had specific responsibilities for environmental health, child and maternal welfare, water supply and sanitation, housing, local government, the NHI scheme and the Poor Law. Although other health-related functions such as industrial hygiene (Home Office), health and safety at work (Board of Trade), and the school health services (Board of Education) were the responsibility of other departments, the health ministry was responsible for the overall coordination of health policies.

Despite an initial enthusiasm, the ministry's early initiatives came to little. This was partly because some of the key proponents behind its creation died, retired or moved to other posts, and partly because of restrictions imposed by the economic conditions of the 1920s. As Webster (1988, p. 19) commented, 'the ministry of health fell into a cautious and routine mode of operation consistent with the growing pessimism of the times'. Yet some important reforms were introduced, inspired by Neville Chamberlain's three spells as minister of health between 1923 and 1931 (Hyde, 1976). The most significant changes in this period concerned Poor Law reform, mentioned earlier, and housing. Legislation in 1923 and 1924 permitted subsidies to facilitate improvements in the housing stock. In 1930, the Greenwood Act required local authorities to draw up slum clearance plans and gave additional subsidies for this purpose, while the 1935 Housing Act set limits on overcrowding and made it an offence to breach them. As a result of these changes, the housing stock was expanded and improved, particularly in the latter part of the 1930s. Yet the problem of poor housing remained. As Gilbert (1970, p. 201) observed, the improved statistics for housing provision could not obscure the fact that 'the poor section of the population was probably little better housed at the end of the inter-war period than it had been at the beginning'.

Public Health and the NHS

The National Health Service

The creation of the NHS in 1948 can be regarded as a major public health achievement in its own right. The new service was comprehensive, inclusive and (until the introduction of charges) free at point of delivery. From a public health perspective, the NHS had a number of advantages over the previous system. As a national service, it emphasized the importance of public health as a national priority and responsibility. Also, by bringing together the whole range of health services within a national system, it raised the possibility of a more coherent and efficient health service. Furthermore, the NHS extended access to health services for those not covered by state insurance schemes: the dependants of workers, the poor and those requiring specialist services (Vetter, 1998). Some, however, were concerned that the NHS was constituted as a sickness rather than a health service and that it would concentrate on treatment rather than prevention of illness, which proved to be the case (see Lewis, 1992).

The Changing Role of the Medical Officer of Health

The creation of the NHS deprived local authorities of their municipal hospital services. MOHs instead focused on administering community health and social services, which remained in their remit (Frazer, 1950; Lewis, 1986). According to Ottewill and Wall (1990, pp. 85, 88), the performance of MOHs in expanding community health services was impressive. The amount of money spent on local health and social services rose by 170 per cent in real terms between 1949/50 and 1970/1, and by the end of this period accounted for a larger share of total NHS revenue expenditure. Much of this increase was associated with the provision of social welfare services. However, expansion created a momentum for further change as different professional groups sought independence from the MOH (Berridge, 2007). Social workers, for example, believed medical control inhibited their claims for professional status. The Seebohm committee, inquiring into the organization of personal social services in 1968, agreed, recommending new unified social service departments (Cmnd 3703, 1968). The implementation of this measure in 1970 removed a large part of the MOH's administrative empire, and undermined the future viability of the post (Webster, 1996, p. 296).

Public health doctors also faced increasing competition from GPs (see Lewis, 1986). During the postwar period, clinical work undertaken by public health doctors in the community was increasingly taken over by GPs. The position of GPs was further strengthened by policies that emphasized their pivotal role in the field of primary care. From the 1960s onwards, the encouragement of primary health care teams (PHCTs), where nurses and health visitors employed by the local health authorities were attached to general practices, further emphasized the leadership role of GPs at the expense of the MOH.

NHS Reorganization

Public health medicine was caught in a pincer movement between the GPs and the Seebohm reforms. Its future looked bleak. One possible solution was to redefine public health medicine as 'community medicine', and give practitioners specialist status, as envisaged by the Royal Commission on Medical Education (Cmnd 3569, 1968). In the event, changes were prompted by a reorganization of the NHS, which abolished the post of MOH, and transferred responsibility for community health services to new health authorities. The role of the public health doctor in this new structure was set out by the Hunter report (DHSS, 1972), which recommended that specialists in community medicine should promote effective integration of health and related services while acting as a link between administrators and the medical profession. It was envisaged that they would bring specialist skills, such as epidemiology and needs assessment, to enhance the planning and management function at all levels.

In 1974, community physicians were appointed to regional, area and district management teams in the NHS. In addition, specialists in community medicine were appointed to advise local authorities on a range of issues, such as child health and environmental health matters (Lewis, 1986). However, there was much confusion about the role of community physicians, not least among the post holders themselves. The granting of specialist status to community physicians did little to raise their status. Indeed, there is evidence that their skills and knowledge were inadequate for the tasks they were given (Strong and Robinson, 1990, p. 51). Moreover, the management role of the community physicians, particularly when associated with budget restrictions and service cutbacks, had a detrimental effect on their professional standing (Lewis, 1986). Their hospital colleagues regarded them with suspicion, and, rather than bridging the gap between medicine and management, community physicians became isolated from the rest of their profession. Managers also distrusted them, believing that they had greater loyalty to the profession than to the management team (Strong and Robinson, 1990, p. 52). All these factors contributed to growing demoralization among community physicians (Berridge et al., 2006).

The position of community medicine deteriorated with subsequent reorganizations of the NHS in the 1980s and they became an 'endangered species' (Berridge et al., 2006, p. 21). In 1982, area health authorities (AHAs) were abolished and the community physicians they employed were forced to seek posts elsewhere, usually in district health authorities, regarded by most as a downward career move (Lewis, 1986). This was followed by the Griffiths management reforms (DHSS, 1983), which led to the appointment of general managers and the reconstitution of management boards. Recommendations to give public health doctors a greater say on management boards were rejected by Griffiths (Berridge et al., 2006, p. 19). A consequence was that in many authorities community physicians were retained as advisors rather than in a managerial capacity and lost their places on management boards.

The Acheson Report

The parlous state of community medicine, underlined by a number of high-profile failures of the public health function at local level during the mid-1980s, discussed later in this chapter, led to the appointment of a committee of inquiry chaired by the then Chief Medical Officer, Donald Acheson. To address the confusion about the role of practitioners, the Acheson report called for community medicine to be renamed 'public health medicine' and set a target national rate for consultants in this specialty (of 15.8 per one million population). The report recommended that each health authority should appoint a director of public health (DPH) to lead the public health function. The DPH would act as a chief medical advisor and would advise on priorities, planning and evaluation; coordinate control of communicable disease; and develop policy on prevention and health promotion. The DPH would be expected to report annually on public health to the local health authority. Acheson also recommended that guidance should be issued to health authorities reminding them of their public health responsibilities. The report made recommendations to improve coordination between health and local authorities and establish clearer responsibilities for dealing with outbreaks of infectious disease. It also urged the government to revise current legislation on public health to provide robust statutory backing for the control of communicable disease and infection.

The implementation of Acheson's recommendations coincided with a period of great upheaval in the NHS. The introduction of the internal market in the early 1990s, divided purchasing (or as it became known, 'commissioning') of health services from their provision. It was envisaged that budget holders (namely, health authorities and fundholding GPs) would shift resources towards interventions that were cost-effective and demonstrated high levels of 'health gain' (Ham and Mitchell, 1990; Ovretveit, 1993). This proved hopelessly optimistic, largely because vested interests in treatment services had sufficient political influence to ensure that commissioners dare not cut their budgets. Their position was bolstered by government, which imposed restrictions on commissioners' freedom to switch resources away from existing service providers. Furthermore, budgetary restraints impeded investment in public health as commissioners had little flexibility to encourage the development of new preventive and health promotion services without threatening existing care and treatment services (Flynn et al., 1996; Levenson et al., 1997; Cornish et al., 1997).

Critics of the internal market argued that even if properly implemented, commissioning would have a detrimental effect on public health (Moran, 1989; Whitty and Jones, 1992). This was because commissioning invoked a narrow view of health gain, being based on an individualistic model of health care provision, rather than on a population-based approach to health promotion. Critics further pointed out that fragmentation caused by the division into commissioners and providers impeded a strategic approach to public health, both within the NHS and across local communities (Crown, 1999; Flynn et al., 1996; Nettleton and Burrows, 1997; see also Chapter 8). Another problem was that the contract culture of the internal market focused on measurable factors. There was some evidence that this drew professionals away from activities, including public health functions, where effects were often difficult or impossible to measure, especially in the short-term (McCallum, 1997).

The GP fundholding scheme, which enabled GPs to purchase health care services on behalf of their patients, attracted particular criticism. Although, in principle, fundholding could produce a shift in resources to health promotion and disease prevention in line with the needs of the population, this did not happen (Audit Commission, 1996). The negative consequences of fund-holding for public health were, however, more evident. GP fundholders could act in isolation without regard for local health priorities, although guidance was later introduced to address this problem. As the scheme was not universal, it was associated with inequities (see Kammerling and Kinnear, 1996; Dowling, 1997) although again efforts were made, by non-fundholders and health authorities, to counteract this. Fundholding was also criticized for strengthening GP domination of primary care, enabling greater control over the work of other primary care professionals, such as community nurses (Tinsley and Luck, 1998). Meanwhile, partly also due to other contractual changes, GPs began to employ more practice nurses, who developed a role in preventive care, such as immunization, health checks and disease prevention clinics (Broadbent, 1998). Although this was welcomed for increasing the capacity for health promotion activity in general practice, it may have stifled other nurse-led initiatives and population-based health promotion interventions (see Chapter 6).

The Need for a Strategy

One reason for the weakness of public health in the postwar period, both within national health policymaking and within the NHS, was that it lacked a strategic focus. Indeed, by 1951 the health ministry had ceded to other departments its responsibilities for financial assistance to the poor, pensions, town and country planning, environmental health, water supply, sewerage, land use, local government, housing and rent control. Some saw merit in this, for example Political and Economic Planning (PEP, 1937, quoted in Gilbert, 1970, p. 234) observed that the Ministry of Health 'too often allowed the non-health functions which it inherited from the Local Government Board to overshadow its public health duties'. However, the transfer of functions to other government departments had adverse effects (see Webster, 1996). First, it reduced the size and status of the Ministry of Health. Over the next twenty years it was not often represented directly in Cabinet. As a result, decisions were often made in the absence of health ministers. Second, the ministry's low status meant that (with one or two exceptions) it was difficult to attract ambitious ministers who might have given a stronger lead. Third, the removal of wider public health responsibilities (and the retention of community health services by local government) concentrated the ministry's focus upon hospital services (Sheard and Donaldson, 2006). As Macleod, a Conservative health minister of the 1950s commented, it was 'a ministry not for health, but for the NHS' (Webster, 1996, p. 39). This sentiment was echoed by others, notably Klein (1980) – who remarked that 'Britain has a health service but no policy for health'. The preoccupation with treatment services was accompanied by a lack of leadership on prevention and public health (Webster, 1988).

As Webster's (1996) official history suggests, the Ministry of Health was largely a non-interventionist department in the 1950s. This began to change in the following decade with the emergence of national plans for hospitals and for community health services. Efforts were also made to widen the focus of the department – a Department of Social Welfare was proposed at one stage (Webster, 1996, p. 40). Eventually, in 1968, the health department was merged with the Ministry of Pensions and National Insurance to form the Department of Health and Social Security (DHSS). However, this arrangement did not elevate public health. Ministerial attention was instead dominated by NHS reorganization and service plans for specific client groups such as elderly people, mentally ill people, and those with disabilities.

There were many examples during the 1950s and 60s where central government demonstrated a reluctance to intervene on public health issues. Perhaps the most obvious was the failure of the Conservative government of the 1950s and early 1960s to address the issue of smoking and health (see Chapter 15). Nonetheless, some important public health measures were introduced in this period (Yarrow, 1986; Webster, 1996), including an immunization programme against childhood diseases. There were important developments in health education (Berridge, 2007). A Clean Air Act was passed in 1956 in an attempt to reduce urban smog – a major cause of respiratory problems in industrial areas. Another significant measure, the Road Safety Act of 1967, introduced alcohol breath tests for motorists and led to a fall in alcohol-related motor accidents. Two years earlier, the government had responded to growing evidence of smoking-related illness by banning cigarette advertisements on television. However, such legislative interventions were few and far between and it was not until the 1970s and 80s that pressures for a more strategic approach to public health began to emerge.

Towards a Public Health Strategy

A key factor in the revival of public health in the 1970s was the 'the new public health' (Baum, 2002; Ashton and Seymour, 1988; Hunter, 2003). This was a revised philosophy of public health that moved away from the medical model, which concentrated on the prevention and treatment of disease in individuals, towards a social model that acknowledged the importance of environmental, social and personal factors in the promotion of health. The new public health also emphasized the importance of strategies, legislation and policy as means of intervention, the need for inter-sectoral and multidisciplinary action to tackle health problems, and the importance of community participation in health. It also promoted the notion of health as a fundamental human right and a social goal, and identified equity in health as an explicit aim.

This philosophy began to influence policy debates across the world, not just in the UK. In Canada, for example, an official report (Lalonde, 1974) called for a government health strategy based on awareness that health could be promoted through lifestyle and the environment, as well as health service provision and medical intervention. The report outlined the 'health field' concept, which identified four 'fields' that contributed to health: human biology, environment, lifestyle and health care. It maintained that while health care has received the majority of resources, the other fields had enormous potential to improve health.

Meanwhile, the World Health Organization began to formulate an international strategy on public health, reflected in the Alma Ata declaration on Primary Care (WHO and UNICEF, 1978) and the *Health for All by the Year 2000* strategy in 1981. These and subsequent statements (such as the Ottawa Charter of 1986 and the Healthy Cities initiative launched in the 1980s – see Exhibit 7.1) emphasized the importance of lifestyle and environmental factors in health and exhorted governments to devise strategies to promote good health (see Chapter 6).

The new public health challenged the orthodox medical model. It was inspired to a large extent by McKeown (1976) who contended that the contribution of medicine to the decline of disease had been exaggerated to the neglect of socioeconomic and environmental factors. He supported this by pointing out that the decline of major diseases such as measles, whooping cough and TB occurred before the advent of immunization and effective medical treatment. McKeown identified improvements in nutrition and rising standards of living as the key factors in the reduction of morbidity and mortality since the late nineteenth century. He also accepted that a healthier physical environment was partly responsible for the reduction in the death rate from the mid-nineteenth century onwards (see also Wohl, 1984). Furthermore, he pointed out that the major causes of ill health in industrial societies – cancer, heart disease and circulatory disease resulted largely from individual behaviour and environmental factors and could therefore be prevented. In contrast, orthodox medicine could only offer an inadequate and belated response, following conclusive evidence of specific disease processes.

Many of McKeown's conclusions attracted support (see Fuchs, 1974; McKinlay, 1979; Powles, 1973; Burkitt, 1973; Illich, 1977), although some challenged aspects of his thesis. Szreter (1988) disputed that rising nutritional and living standards were the main factors responsible for declining mortality rates. He argued that improvements in housing, education, working conditions, and health services played a major part. He also noted that members of the medical profession had an important role in preventing illness by participating in the Victorian public health movement and promoting the development of community health services at local level.

Sagan (1987), while sharing McKeown's scepticism about the impact of medical care, rejected the argument that public health measures or nutrition were primarily responsible for declining mortality. He argued that improvements in health resulted from higher levels of resistance to disease, determined by social factors. He identified a reduction in family size and modern parenting behaviour as the main reasons for the improvements in health. In his own words 'the smaller and more affectionate modern family has been a powerful factor contributing to improved health of individuals and to the historic fall in mortality rates' (p. 102). By the same token he suggested that changes in the postmodern family – marital instability, divorce, single parenting – have adverse implications for mental and physical health today.

McKeown's thesis has been attacked for failing to appreciate the contribution of modern medicine. Although scientific medicine in the Victorian period did little for patients, there were some important innovations – such as chloroform anaesthesia and the development of diphtheria anti-toxin – that laid the foundations for later discoveries and made possible the development of new and more effective forms of treatment (see Bynum, 1994). In addition, advances in medical technology improved the quality of life for many (Morris, 1980). Treatment does 'add years to life' as well. Bunker and colleagues (1994), examining the impact of medical care in the USA, found that the current effects of curative medicine added between 44 and 45 months to life expectancy, with an additional 18–19 months added by preventive medicine. Further analysis found that medicine contributed to improvements in health. Bunker (2001) estimated that half the 7.5 year increase in life expectancy since the 1950s could be attributed to medical care. On average, medical care contributed an additional five years of healthy life (measured by disability adjusted life years) for each individual. Subsequently, a review of the impact of health care on avoidable mortality across EU countries (Nolte and McKee, 2004) found that improvements in access to health care reduced deaths, particularly in infants and in middle-aged and elderly people (especially women). The reduction was greatest in countries with higher initial death rates.

Concern about the effectiveness of medicine provides only part of the explanation of why public health rose up the political agenda. The other reason is that governments themselves began to question the amount of resources used by the health services (Hunter, 2003). Even in the UK, where health care costs had been relatively low, health care funding became a preoccupation for politicians in the adverse economic circumstances of the 1970s. This continued in the neoliberal ideological climate of the following decade. The desire for economies in public sector budgets led governments to take a greater interest in public health in the hope of preventing treatment costs in the longer term (Lewis, 1992). Not surprisingly, the idea of prevention, particularly where it involved individuals taking greater responsibility for their own health, was endorsed by the Treasury in this period as a cost saving measure (Webster, 1996, p. 677) even though the evidence for this is mixed (see Chapter 1).

Towards a Health Strategy

By the mid-1970s the continued neglect of public health was not a realistic option (Webster, 1996). Public opinion was more favourable to intervention as people became aware of lifestyle and environmental health issues; pressure groups and experts were campaigning more effectively for a stronger lead from government on prevention (Yarrow, 1986; Webster, 1996). There was cross-party support for such a move (Webster, 1996), which was reflected in a parliamentary committee inquiry into preventive medicine (House of Commons, 1977) that made over 50 recommendations on policy, including stronger measures to tackle alcohol abuse, smoking, and diet as well as improvements in family planning, cancer screening, sport and exercise and health promotion. The committee served as a useful platform for experts and lobby groups seeking to influence policy (Webster, 1996, p. 676). In an effort to head off criticism, the then Labour government published a consultative document, *Prevention and Health: Everybody's Business* (DHSS, 1976a). This identified the following key areas for future intervention: inequalities in health status, heart disease, road accidents, smoking-related diseases, alcoholism, mental illness, drugs, diet and venereal disease. The document aimed to promote discussion rather than to outline a programme of action, and was described as 'hastily-compiled' and 'impressionistic' (Webster, 1996, p. 676). Although 'a new departure in health policy' and 'a thoughtful document', it had no real impact on the direction of policy (Hunter, 2003, p. 47). The Labour government did publish a white paper, *Prevention and Health* (Cmnd 7047, 1977), which disappointed those expecting a more strategic approach. Apart from a proposed increase in resources for health education, little was done to alter the balance of resources between prevention and treatment. Prevention did appear more prominently in policy documents from this time onwards, however. For example, the NHS planning and priority documents mentioned the importance of prevention (see DHSS, 1976b, 1977).

The Thatcher Government

The Conservative government led by Margaret Thatcher, elected in 1979, faced pressures to do more to improve public health. A Royal Commission, appointed by Labour in 1976 to examine the problems of the NHS, reported that prevention was not given sufficient priority or resources (Cmnd 7615, 1979). A year later the Black report identified the scale of health inequalities and acknowledged the range of lifestyle, socioeconomic and environmental factors that underpinned them (DHSS, 1980; Townsend et al., 1992).

Although the Thatcher government referred to the importance of prevention in its policy documents (DHSS, 1981a; Cm 249, 1987), it refused to address the socioeconomic and environmental factors that many experts believed harmful to public health. This government did not recognize health inequalities as a problem (see Chapters 16 and 17). Moreover, throughout the 1980s it was vehemently opposed to any form of central health strategy. Even so, the Thatcher government did approve of prevention policies that were consistent with its ideological predisposition – reducing public expenditure, promoting managerialism in public services, and encouraging individual responsibility (Berridge et al., 2006). More pragmatically, it endorsed policy initiatives that reassured voters that the NHS was safe in the hands of the Conservative party, such as cancer screening programmes, mass health education campaigns, and health promotion initiatives in general practice.

Some voices within the Thatcher government urged greater priority for public health and prevention. Usually this went with the grain of government policy. For example, health ministers including Norman Fowler and Edwina Currie promoted individually focused prevention policies (see Currie, 1989; Fowler, 1991) on issues such as healthy eating and exercise. There were also dissenting voices, such as Sir George Young, a junior health minister sacked by Thatcher for his tough approach to the alcohol and tobacco industries (Taylor, 1984; Baggott, 1990) and Donald Acheson, the Chief Medical Officer, who emphasized the importance of a broader public health perspective (Sheard and Donaldson, 2006, p. 171; Berridge et al., 2006). There were also the activities of the government's own agency, the Health Education Council, which infuriated ministers and was eventually disbanded for giving support to the Black report and criticizing government policies on public health and inequalities – see Chapter 17).

Faced with the government's refusal to formulate a national strategy, many local authorities and NHS bodies bypassed central government and established their own strategies (Berridge et al., 2006; Hunter et al., 2007a). Other parts of the UK also developed their own strategies (see Chapter 4). Wales, for example, developed a health strategy in 1989, while Scotland and Northern Ireland launched their own plans during the following years. Eventually, following Thatcher's departure, England followed suit with its *Health of the Nation* strategy in 1992, discussed in some detail in Chapter 4.

The English strategy resulted from additional pressures on government during the late 1980s. The Thatcher government was increasingly out of step with international developments, as other countries – encouraged by WHO – began to devise health strategies. There was 'bottom-up' pressure from the NHS and local government, which wanted clearer guidance and more resources in order to develop their public health strategies. Pressure was also created by the government's own economic and social policies which had led to increased inequalities and poverty. More specifically, the government's health policies created a rationale for public health policy. In 1987, a white paper on primary care had been introduced, which emphasized the importance of prevention in this field (Cm 249, 1987). Two years later, the internal market in the NHS was introduced (Cm 555, 1989). Both policies required a clearer public health framework. For example, primary care professionals needed to be aware of public health priorities in order to focus their prevention activities effectively. Health authorities, which under the internal market were now responsible for meeting the health needs of their populations, needed guidance on how best to achieve this.

There was also pressure from experts and academics who argued that a strategy was essential in order to improve health. A major study by the King's Fund (Smith and Jacobson, 1988) made a strong case for a health strategy. The government rejected its recommendations. A subsequent report from the Institute of Public Policy Research (Harrison et al., 1994, p. 3) criticized the 'unhealthy concentration on health services' and urged that health policy should give priority to health promotion.

Professional organizations used their insider contacts with the Department of Health and other government departments to raise concerns about the lack of a public health strategy and other specific issues. These included the Royal Colleges, the BMA and the Faculty of Public Health. Pressure groups also lobbied government on public health issues. These included groups such as the Public Health Alliance, formed in 1987, which brought together a range of individuals and organizations concerned about public health as well as 'single issue' groups such as Action on Smoking and Health.

Professional organizations and other pressure groups used links with the government and Parliament to advance their arguments. Evidence was given to select committees when they investigated aspects of public health policy (see for example, PAC (Public Accounts Committee), 1989, 1992; Agriculture Committee, 1989, 1990; Health Committee, 1990). Activities of pressure groups also shaped public perceptions by campaigning on health issues during the 1980s. Some of these received government funding (Berridge, 2007). The media also played a crucial role, by covering public health issues in depth and highlighting failures of policy, planning and regulation. Public health was rarely out of the news, given the high-profile coverage of issues such as HIV/AIDS, drug and alcohol abuse, smoking, food poisoning, and BSE.

The emergence of infectious disease outbreaks has been credited with creating ideal conditions for the revival of public health (Berridge et. al., 2006, p. 18; Hunter et al., 2007a). Fears of an HIV/AIDS epidemic brought public health to the top of the political agenda; it also forced government to devise an enlightened and comprehensive strategy in an area where it was, ideologically, reluctant to intervene (Day and Klein, 1989; Garfield, 1994a; Berridge, 1989). Also important were two major outbreaks of infectious disease during the mid-1980s, both of which received extensive media coverage. The food poisoning incident at the Stanley Royd Hospital in Wakefield, which resulted in 19 deaths (Cmnd 9716, 1986); and the outbreak of Legionnaire's disease at Stafford General Hospital, where 39 people died (Cmnd 9772, 1986). Both exposed failures of public health planning at a local level and a shortage of medical expertise in environmental health and led to the establishment of the Acheson inquiry, discussed earlier.

Although the media played an important role in publicizing perceived threats to public health, some sections – in particular the tabloid press – inhibited intervention by castigating public health campaigners as interfering busybodies. Politicians, increasingly fearful of the tabloids, were reluctant to take action that might lead to accusations of a nanny state. Although resonating with a significant 'fatalistic' strand of public opinion these newspapers actually operated against the tide of public opinion, which was becoming more concerned about lifestyle and environmental threats to public health. Evidence from successive British Social Attitudes surveys indicated a high level of public concern about such issues. For example, the 1987 survey reported that a large majority of people – 70 per cent of respondents – believed that they could alter their lifestyles to avoid heart disease, with younger people on average less fatalistic than their elders (Sheiham et al., 1987). The 1990 survey found a significant level of public concern about pollution and environmental health (Young, 1991; see also Young, 1985). More recent surveys into public views on health confirm that the majority of the population are keen to have greater regulation of factors influencing health. These include healthier school meals (90 per cent in favour), an advertising ban on junk food for children (73 per cent), action to reduce the price of fruit and vegetables (80 per cent) and laws to limit fat, salt and sugar in foods (72 per cent) (King's Fund, 2004).

Conclusion

This chapter has shown that for most of the twentieth century public health struggled to maintain its position on policy agendas compared with health service and treatment issues. Public health suffered from a lack of focus and identity. Its practitioners were politically weak and fragmented. Public health had a low profile within key institutions and structures of health policy-making and service provision. In the 1970s and 80s, however, there was greater awareness of the importance of public health issues and an acknow-ledgement of the need to strengthen policy and services in this field. Momentum built for a clearer strategic approach, even though in the UK the political context was largely unfavourable due to the advent of Thatcherism. Although the foundations for policy development were laid, the initial policy response was muted. As a result, public health strategy remained a low priority for the government and the NHS.

Health Strategies in the UK

4

During the early 1990s, the UK government began to adopt formal health strategies. This chapter examines the development of these strategies, first under the Conservative government of John Major and then subsequently under the New Labour governments of Tony Blair and Gordon Brown. It also discusses the similarities and differences between the strategies adopted in England and those in other countries of the UK.

The Health of the Nation Strategy

In 1991, the Major government published a green paper, *The Health of the Nation*, setting out proposals for a health strategy for England (Cm 1523, 1991). Its stated aim was to secure continuing improvement in the health of the population by 'adding years to life' – increasing life expectancy and reducing premature death – and by 'adding life to years' – improving the quality of life and reducing illness. This was to be achieved through the selection of key areas for improvement. Following consultation with a range of experts and pressure groups, a white paper was issued setting out the government's final strategy (Cm 1986, 1992). Five key areas – cancer, heart disease/stroke, mental illness, HIV/AIDS and sexual health, and accidents – were chosen. In each key area, two types of targets were identified: main targets, setting out planned reductions in the rates and levels of illness and mortality; and risk factor targets, aimed at the causes of these illnesses. These targets are detailed in Exhibit 4.1. The white paper set out how different agencies could help to achieve these priorities. Central government's main contribution was to coordinate the activities of the various departments of state. Guidance on policy appraisal was proposed as a means of assessing policies in terms of their consequences for health. A cabinet committee was established to oversee the implementation of the strategy for England and to coordinate health issues across the UK as a whole. This was supported by other committees, including an interdepartmental group of officials from all government departments with an interest in public health.

Health authorities were expected to collaborate with other local agencies to tackle the health priorities identified by national strategy. In an effort to promote collaboration, task forces were formed, incorporating individuals from government, business, the NHS, and academia. Their purpose was to formulate integrated plans of action, promote cooperation between the agencies involved, and ensure effective implementation. In addition, regional coordinators were appointed to assist with implementation by disseminating good practice.

Exhibit 4.1

The Health of the Nation: Main Targets and Risk Factor Targets

1   Main Targets

Coronary heart disease and stroke:

- To reduce death rates for both coronary heart disease (CHD) and stroke in people under 65 by at least 40 per cent by the year 2000 (1990 baseline)

- To reduce the death rate for CHD in people aged 65–74 by at least 30 per cent by the year 2000 (1990 baseline)

- To reduce the death rate for stroke in people aged 65–74 by at least 40 per cent by the year 2000 (1990 baseline)

Cancers:

- To reduce the death rate for breast cancer in the population invited for screening by at least 25 per cent by the year 2000 (1990 baseline)

- To reduce the incidence of invasive cervical cancer by at least 20 per cent by the year 2000 (1986 baseline)

- To reduce the death rate for lung cancer in the under-75s by at least 30 per cent in men and by at least 15 per cent in women by 2010 (1990 baseline)

- To halt the year-on-year increase in the incidence of skin cancer by 2005

Mental illness:

- To improve significantly the health and social functioning of mentally ill people

- To reduce the overall suicide rate by at least 15 per cent by the year 2000 (1990 baseline)

- To reduce the suicide rate of severely mentally ill people by at least 33 per cent by the year 2000 (1990 baseline)

HIV/AIDS and sexual health:

● To reduce the incidence of gonorrhoea by at least 20 per cent by 1995 (1990 baseline), as an indicator of HIV/AIDS trends

● To reduce by at least 50 per cent the rate of conceptions among the under-16s by the year 2000 (1989 baseline)

Accidents:

● To reduce the death rate for accidents among children aged under 15 by at least 33 per cent by 2005 (1990 baseline)

● To reduce the death rate for accidents among young people aged 15–24 by at least 25 per cent by 2005 (1990 baseline)

● To reduce the death rate for accidents among people aged 65 and over by at least 33 per cent by 2005 (1990 baseline)

2 Risk Factor Targets

Smoking:

● To reduce the prevalence of cigarette smoking to no more than 20 per cent by the year 2000 in both men and women (a reduction of a third) (1990 baseline)

● To reduce the consumption of cigarettes by 40 per cent by the year 2000 (1990 baseline)

● In addition to the overall reduction in prevalence, at least 33 per cent of women smokers to stop smoking at the start of their pregnancy by the year 2000

● To reduce smoking prevalence among 11–15 year olds by at least 33 per cent by 1994 (to less than 6 per cent) (1988 baseline)

Diet and nutrition:

● To reduce the average percentage of food energy derived by the population from saturated fatty acids by at least 35 per cent by 2005 (to no more than 11 per cent of food energy) (1990 baseline)

● To reduce the average percentage of food energy derived from total fat by the population by at least 12 per cent by 2005 (to no more than about 35 per cent of total food energy) (1990 baseline)

● To reduce the proportion of men and women aged 16–64 who are obese by at least 25 per cent and 33 per cent respectively by 2005 (to no more than 6 per cent of men and 8 per cent of women) (1986/87 baseline)

● To reduce the proportion of men drinking more than 21 units* of alcohol per week and women drinking more than 14 units per week by 30 per cent by 2005 (to 18 per cent of men and 7 per cent of women) (1990 baseline)

* One unit is approximately equal to a half pint of ordinary strength beer

Blood pressure:

- To reduce mean systolic blood pressure in the adult population by at least 5 mmHg by 2005 (baseline to be derived from new national survey)

HIV/AIDS:

- To reduce the percentage of injecting drug misusers who report sharing injecting equipment in the previous four weeks from 20 per cent in 1990 to no more than 10 per cent by 1997 and no more than 5 per cent by the year 2000

Source: Adapted from *The Health of the Nation*, Cm 1986, 1992, pp. 18–21, London: HMSO. Reproduced with permission.

The white paper also proposed 'healthy alliances' to stimulate joint working in public health. These would involve NHS organizations, local authorities, the Health Education Authority (HEA), the voluntary sector, the media and employers. Several settings were identified as possible arenas for health improvement: 'healthy cities', 'healthy schools', 'healthy hospitals', 'healthy homes', 'healthy workplaces', 'healthy prisons' and 'healthy environments'. Also, a series of measures was announced to improve the information base for public health decision-making, including surveys of health and illness, a public health information strategy, and a greater emphasis on public health research and development priorities.

The Impact of the Strategy

The *Health of the Nation* (*HOTN*) strategy appeared to have had a symbolic effect of placing health improvement and the prevention of illness on the political agenda (DoH, 1998; Hunter, 2003). However, it did not alter the outlook and behaviour of health authorities nor did it change the context within which they and other local agencies operated. Public health remained a low priority, for health authorities and their partners. However, the strategy's encouragement of alliances did in some circumstances have a small but positive effect on collaboration at local level.

Much criticism of *HOTN* focused on its use of disease-based targets. Some argued that targets downgraded health problems that were not easily quantified. The targets chosen reflected a narrow medical rather than a broader social perspective (Radical Statistics Health Group, 1991; Hunter, 2003). Although risk factor targets were included, they were secondary to disease targets and reflected individual rather than environmental or socioeconomic factors. By neglecting wider causes of ill health, the strategy alienated potential supporters and partners, in particular the local authorities (DoH, 1998; Hunter, 2003).

Some argued that the *HOTN* targets were too ambitious. Hockley and Bosanquet (1998) called for fewer core targets combined with a less directive and more inclusive approach bringing together a wider range of organizations, including the voluntary sector, while harnessing consumer power to raise health standards. Others, however, contended that the targets were too easy to achieve and that many would be met anyway if current trends continued (Mooney and Healey, 1991).

The impact of *HOTN* was disappointing. The National Audit Office (NAO, 1996a) discovered good progress in a minority of target areas. It found poor progress in three areas: women's alcohol consumption, smoking among children, and obesity in both men and women. The strategy had in fact stagnated (Hunter, 2003). The government was not prepared to address key public health problems, particularly where this upset powerful commercial interests such as food, alcohol and tobacco (see Chapters 13 and 15) or challenging socioeconomic inequalities (Chapter 17).

A further weakness was the lack of coordination within central government. Other government departments refused to prioritize public health and there was a failure to generate sufficient cross-departmental commitment and ownership (DoH, 1998). Although guidance on policy appraisal and health was issued, departments were not compelled to adopt it, and it fell far short of a comprehensive health impact assessment process (see Exhibit 11.2). The cabinet committee on public health was inactive and ineffective (DoH, 1998). Calls for a minister to coordinate public health across government were resisted (see Public Health Alliance, 1988).

Our Healthier Nation

Although the Labour party endorsed the idea of a national health strategy while in opposition during the 1990s, it was critical of the Major government's failure to acknowledge the impact of social, economic and environmental factors on health. It sought to incorporate these factors as part of an approach based on the Third Way (see Chapter 1), which emphasized both state intervention and greater individual responsibility in public health (Connelly, 1999).

Following Labour's victory at the 1997 general election, a minister for public health was appointed. Some were unhappy, however, that this was not a Cabinet-level position. The first appointee, Tessa Jowell, was given the position of minister of state. Disappointment increased in 1999, when Jowell was replaced by a minister of an even lower rank (parliamentary under secretary of state). The post was later upgraded to a minister of state appointment in 2006. At the time of writing, the post is once again being held by a parliamentary under secretary of state.

The Blair government introduced a raft of new initiatives, including an anti-smoking strategy (see Chapter 15) and an independent Food Standards Agency (see Chapter 12). There was greater acknowledgement of the importance of social, economic and environmental factors in ill health (see Chapter 17). The Independent Inquiry into Inequalities in Health (1998), chaired by Donald Acheson, was established. In addition, the government made a commitment to tackle social exclusion and abolish child poverty, and introduced regeneration programmes, tax breaks for working families with children, and Sure Start schemes (see Chapter 9).

An attempt was made to reorient the NHS towards public health objectives. National service frameworks (NSFs) were introduced, setting out standards for a range of diseases, conditions and client groups (for example heart disease, cancer, mental health, older people) covering prevention, care and treatment. The NHS planning system now gave greater emphasis to health improvement (see Chapter 6). A duty of cooperation on matters of health and welfare was placed on NHS bodies and local authorities. In addition, local authorities were required to formulate plans to improve their communities and received new powers to promote economic, social and environmental wellbeing (see Chapter 7). Meanwhile, health action zones (HAZs) were introduced in areas with high health needs to build collaboration between local agencies, improve health and reduce inequalities.

The Blair government's public health strategy was initially proposed in a green paper *Our Healthier Nation* (Cm 3852, 1998). Following a period of consultation, a white paper, *Saving Lives: Our Healthier Nation,* was published (Cm 4386, 1999). The two goals of the strategy were: 'to improve the health of the population as a whole by increasing the length of people's lives and the number of years people spend free from illness; and to improve the health of the worst off in society and to narrow the health gap' (Cm 4386, 1999, p. 5). Separate public health policy documents were introduced in Wales, Scotland, and Northern Ireland, discussed in more detail below (see Exhibit 4.2). There had for some time been a variation in public health policies between different parts of the UK, but with the advent of devolution, policy differences widened.

The main themes of the revised health strategy for England were, first, a 'new contract' between the state and the individual, involving government, local communities and individuals in partnership to improve health. This was portrayed as a 'third way' between a nanny state and victim-blaming approach, which the new government identified as features of previous public health policies. Second, the strategy maintained the focus on disease-based targets (Fulop and Hunter, 1999; LGA/UK Public Health Association, 2000). There were some changes, however. The headline national targets were now as follows:

- to reduce the death rate from heart disease, stroke and related illnesses among people under 75 years old by at least two-fifths

- to reduce the death rate from accidents by at least a fifth and to reduce the rate of serious injury by at least a tenth

- to reduce the death rate from cancer among people aged under 75 years by at least a fifth

- to reduce the death rate from suicide and undetermined injury by at least a fifth

Third, compared with the *Health of the Nation*, the revised public health strategy incorporated a greater acknowledgement of social, economic and environmental factors in ill health. The importance of health inequalities, a taboo subject under the previous Conservative government, was reflected in the second goal of the strategy, mentioned above. To the disappointment of some, however, the strategy did not set national targets for reducing health inequalities at this stage (see Chapter 17).

Fourth, ways of improving coordination on public health within central government and at local level were outlined. Public health was highlighted as a key element of central government policy. As already noted, a minister of public health was appointed to help coordinate policy. A dedicated cabinet committee of ministers drawn from 12 departments was also created to develop cross-departmental health policies. In addition, the government expressed an intention to gear other policies – in fields such as welfare, housing, crime, education, transport and the environment – to the achievement of public health objectives, promising health impact assessment for key policies. Meanwhile at local level, the government sought to advance public health by identifying a number of settings where health promotion initiatives could develop: schools, workplaces, and neighbourhoods. Changes to planning processes and new responsibilities to collaborate on health, mentioned earlier, were expected to strengthen such initiatives.

A Health Development Agency was created to maintain and disseminate the evidence base for health improvement, to advise on standards for public health and health promotion, and to commission and carry out health promotion campaigns. This new agency replaced the Health Education Authority, which disappointed some observers given its role in promoting government action on public health issues. The government also proposed that each region would have a public health observatory, linked with universities, to monitor health trends, highlight areas for action and evaluate progress by local agencies. In addition, proposals were set out to improve training in public health, to strengthen the public health roles of nurses, midwives and health visitors and to create a new post of Specialist in Public Health, open to professionals outside medicine.

The NHS Plan and its Aftermath

Although initially public health was high on the Blair government's agenda, attention quickly shifted to health care issues. Originally the new government intended bringing out its public health strategy prior to announcing plans for NHS reform. In the event, the white paper on the NHS: *The New NHS; Modern, Dependable* (Cm 3807, 1997) preceded the publication of the *Our Healthier Nation* policy documents. Furthermore, as the government came under increasing pressure on its handling of the NHS, public health remained a relatively low priority. This was in spite of the Health Secretary's declared aim of taking public health 'out of the ghetto' (Milburn, 2000). The continued marginalization of public health was further reflected in the government's NHS Plan of 2000, which was essentially a plan for health services. As Hunter (2003, p. 64) observed, 'a slim chapter buried deep in the plan was devoted to improving public health and reducing health inequalities'. Evans (2004, p. 68) summarized the views of many when he commented that 'from a public health perspective, the NHS Plan was disappointing'. Notably, the equivalent plans for the NHS in other parts of the UK gave a much higher priority to public health issues (see Exhibit 4.2 below).

Nonetheless, the NHS Plan for England did contain some important public health commitments (see Hunter, 2003). These originated from one of the subcommittees established by the government to provide new ideas for reform. In a reversal of previous policy, the government announced it would now introduce national inequalities targets (see Chapter 17). Other important proposals included: local strategic partnerships (LSPs) to coordinate action across different agencies and programmes (see Chapter 8), a new sexual health strategy, implementation of a teenage pregnancy strategy, an expansion of Sure Start and a new Children's Fund (see Chapter 9), schemes to increase the consumption of fruit and vegetables, action to combat obesity through physical exercise (Chapter 13), an expansion of smoking cessation services (Chapter 15), and Healthy Communities Collaborative projects to disseminate good practice. The NHS Plan also proposed the introduction of integrated public health groups across NHS and other regional authorities, the implications of which are discussed in Chapter 6.

A Loss of Momentum?

The Health Committee (2001) was concerned that the NHS Plan did not give sufficient attention to public health, commenting that 'for all the laudable Government rhetoric about dragging public health from the ghetto, in the race for resources it runs the risk of trailing well behind fix and mend medical services'. The committee called for a better balance between health and health care. It also wanted improvements in public health leadership at all levels, along with clearer responsibilities. The committee recommended that sufficient resources be available for organizations with public health responsibilities. It urged a more robust evidence base for public health interventions, stronger health partnerships between agencies, greater efforts to integrate, coordinate and implement policies, and more community involvement in public health projects. The Health Committee recommended the creation of stronger incentives for health improvement, better performance management systems, and warned of the dangers of structural reorganization, which it believed could impede efforts to improve public health.

On the same day as the Health Committee published its report, the government issued a much-delayed report on the public health function, commissioned from the former Chief Medical Officer, Kenneth Calman (DoH, 2001a). Publication was prompted by criticism of the delay from the Health Committee and others (Hunter, 2003). The CMO's report set out recommendations for improving coordination and collaboration in public health. The implications of the report are discussed more fully in Chapter 6.

Mindful of the mounting criticism of its public health strategy, the government published a progress report, *Vision to Reality* (DoH, 2001b). Essentially a restatement of policy, its primary purpose was to convince critics that the government remained committed to public health (Hunter, 2003). Meanwhile, the implementation of the NHS Plan, combined with a new initiative to 'shift the balance of power in the NHS to the front line' (DoH, 2001c) had serious implications for the public health function (Evans, 2004; Hunter, 2003). NHS regional offices and health authorities, both of which had important public health responsibilities, were abolished. After some deliberation, responsibilities were allocated to the new strategic health authorities and primary care trusts (PCTs). Even so, this reorganization caused significant disruption to the public health function (see Chapter 6).

Another relevant policy stream related to health inequalities (Evans, 2004). Building on the momentum of the 1998 Acheson report (see above), the work of the Social Exclusion Unit, and the government's commitment to end child poverty, a cross-government review of health inequalities was launched (DoH, 2003a). This set out a strategy that clarified commitments and responsibilities in areas such as housing, fuel poverty, physical exercise, child poverty, nutrition, smoking and drug abuse (see Chapter 17). This period also saw changes to the framework for public health protection (DoH, 2002a). A new Health Protection Agency was established bringing together bodies responsible for monitoring and managing communicable disease and environmental threats (such as biological hazards, radiation and poisons). These arrangements are discussed further in Chapter 8.

Meanwhile, health ministers reiterated the importance of public health. In 2002, the Secretary of State for Health made a further speech underlining the importance of action on public health and inequalities in which he called for a 'sea change in attitudes'. This was accompanied by increased public and media interest in lifestyle-related illness, including smoking, obesity, alcohol abuse and sexually transmitted diseases. The pressure to respond to these problems was increased by critical reports from the Health Committee and others (see Chapters 13 and 15). Another factor was a series of reports on health and social care undertaken by Sir Derek Wanless. In 2001, Wanless was invited by the Treasury to assess the level of resources required to secure high-quality health services in the future. He reported that the projected cost varied considerably according to the extent to which people became engaged with improving their own health and the level of responsiveness of health services to their needs (Wanless, 2002). He concluded that more responsive services and investment in health promotion would lead the way to a 'fully-engaged scenario', curbing increases in the future demand for health care and, correspondingly, minimizing the rise in expenditure on health care services. Subsequently, Wanless was asked to investigate this issue further. His report recommended a shift in the focus of the NHS 'from a national sickness service, which treats disease, to a national health service which focuses on preventing it' (Wanless, 2004, p. 183). He called for a clear national framework of objectives for all key health risk factors and the introduction of joint targets for the NHS and local authorities, reinforced through performance management and inspection systems. His report underlined the importance of collective action to prevent illness, highlighting the need for clear principles of action and a framework for assessing the role of policy instruments. Wanless also stressed the importance of individual choice and the need for high-quality personalized information to enable people to make informed choices about their health. Other key recommendations included: a stronger cross-government approach based on an assessment of the impact of policies on public health, an integrated approach to the assessment of the cost-effectiveness of interventions across disease and condition areas, an emphasis on health outcomes that would enable a comparison of the effectiveness of prevention and cure, a more effectively coordinated approach to public health research, clearer responsibilities within central government for health education, and a strategic plan for developing the public health workforce.

Choosing Health

Following the Wanless report on public health, the government embarked on the production of a further white paper, *Choosing Health: Making Healthy Choices Easier* (Cm 6374, 2004). This focused on specific risk factors: smoking, alcohol abuse, sexual lifestyles and obesity. It also emphasized the importance of reducing health inequalities. The policy was underpinned by a public service agreement (PSA) between the Treasury and the Department of Health (DoH), introduced in the summer of 2004, which included targets for life expectancy, health inequalities, obesity, teenage pregnancy, and smoking. The white paper sought to address these targets by setting out an overarching strategy and key policy initiatives. For example, smoking policies included proposals to further restrict tobacco promotion, smoking in public places and tobacco sales along with stronger health warnings, new anti-smoking campaigns and enhanced smoking cessation services (see Chapter 15). For obesity, the government proposed initiatives on food labelling, healthy eating, restrictions on marketing to children, and the promotion of sport and exercise (see Chapter 13). In the case of alcohol, building on an earlier cross-government initiative, the government pledged to tackle binge drinking through education campaigns and law enforcement and by extending alcohol misuse prevention services (Chapter 15). On sexual health, the white paper promised to improve education, prevention, early diagnosis and access to services.

The key aim of the white paper was to support individuals in making healthy choices (McKee and Raine, 2005). The focus was primarily on the individual: Secretary of State for Health, John Reid stated in evidence to the Health Committee (2005a) that 'the primary dynamo of social change is the individual'. Ministers saw the government's role as providing opportunities for individuals to improve their own health. The white paper proposed new support services such as health trainers (people accredited by the NHS to offer practical help on changing individual behaviour) for example. The other key role of government was to provide information. The white paper announced new campaigns on smoking, obesity, binge drinking and sexual lifestyles alongside more accessible forms of health information for the individual. It strongly endorsed the 'social marketing' approach to health promotion (see Chapter 8), tailoring health education and information to people's context and circumstances to maximize behavioural change.

Regulation, to alter the environment within which individuals make decisions, was only to be used when absolutely necessary. Indeed, rather than adopt an adversarial approach, the government sought to enlist the help of industries whose products and practices were associated with public health problems. The food, alcohol and advertising industries were therefore offered a role in improving public health. Direct regulation was not ruled out, particularly in the case of smoking, but even here the government had been sensitive to the needs of industry, as revealed by its earlier defence of certain forms of tobacco sponsorship and opposition to a total ban on smoking in public places (see Chapter 15).

Improved coordination between agencies was a key theme of the white paper. It identified networks of local health champions (consisting of people in the NHS, local government, and the voluntary and private sectors) as a means of sharing good practice. A new innovations fund was proposed to pump-prime new initiatives, along with a pilot scheme – Communities for

Health – to encourage integrated working on local health priorities. Local area agreements (LAAs), overseen by local strategic partnerships (see Chapter 7), were proposed as a way of providing a common framework of funding and performance management across health and local government bodies.

Another key theme of *Choosing Health* was the health of children and young people. Consistent with initiatives on child poverty and integrated services for children (see Chapter 9), the white paper emphasized joint working between agencies, including the NHS and local government. Health promotion was defined as a key responsibility of the new children's centres being established across England to bring together ante- and postnatal care, routine and preventive health services, family support, day care, and learning services. Schools were also identified as a key setting for health promotion. All schools were expected to achieve 'Healthy Schools' status by 2009. Other initiatives in this field included changes to the school inspection regime to assess their contribution to health, improved school meals standards, and restrictions on unhealthy food on school premises. Previous commitments to extend sport and physical exercise in schools, and to encourage cycling and walking to school, were reiterated.

Choosing Health sought to reorient the NHS towards health promotion. PCTs were expected to promote health as part of their public health responsibilities. Their progress would be closely monitored as part of the performance management regime. Furthermore, PCTs in the most deprived areas were later identified as spearhead areas, piloting new initiatives. In addition, the white paper announced new training programmes to enable health care professionals to identify and help people with unhealthy lifestyles. School nurses and health visitors were promised an expanded role in prevention. New job descriptions were identified, such as the new health trainers, already mentioned, and also community matrons, who would lead personalized care and give health advice for people with complex health problems. These developments were proposed in the context of a forthcoming national health improvement workforce plan (see Chapter 6).

The government also announced that health would be more integrated in central decision-making, by incorporating health aspects into regulatory impact assessment of new legislation. A new cabinet subcommittee, chaired by the Secretary of State for Health, was to coordinate the strategy. In addition, *Choosing Health* set out plans for strengthening the knowledge, information and evidence base for public health through increased research funding and an extension of the role of the National Institute for Clinical Excellence (NICE) to cover health improvement. NICE became the National Institute for Health and Clinical Excellence (while retaining its original acronym). More funds were promised for the regional public health observatories. A review of NSFs was promised in an effort to promote an integrated prevention framework across condition areas and client groups.

The government pledged over £1 billion over three years to fund these commitments. Additional amounts were pledged for initiatives on school sport and transport. Local authorities were promised reimbursement for additional costs arising out of the white paper. Even so, additional resources were relatively small compared with the scale of the task and by comparison with the investment in curative, care and treatment services. There were doubts that areas with high health needs would receive the level of funding necessary (Raine et al., 2003). There were also fears that public health budgets might be raided to meet other NHS priorities, which is exactly what happened (see Chapter 6).

Notwithstanding the provisions of the white paper, there was much scepticism about the ability of the NHS to transform itself into a genuine health service, focusing on prevention and early identification of illness. It was pointed out that the NHS had little incentive to prioritize public health (Hunter and Marks, 2005; King's Fund, 2005). Furthermore, the white paper's efforts to 'join up' public health were a continuation of previous practice rather than a radical new departure. Integrated planning and performance management systems for local agencies were seen as an improvement but no substitute for clearer public health responsibilities and powers (LGA et al., 2004; Chartered Institute of Environmental Health/Royal Society for the Promotion of Health, 2004). It was widely believed that local authorities should have a larger and more explicit role in public health (BMA, 2004a; LGA et al., 2004; Chartered Institute of Environmental Health/Royal Society for the Promotion of Health, 2004; Socialist Health Association, 2005; UKPHA, 2004). Arguments were also made that the government should adopt proposals to improve coordination at the national level by making public health a Cabinet-level responsibility (UKPHA, 2004; LGA et al., 2004; BMA, 2004a; Socialist Health Association, 2005; Association of Directors for Public Health, 2005; Royal College of Physicians, 2005a).

The white paper's emphasis on choice was criticized for not placing sufficient attention on the socioeconomic and environmental factors that shape people's behaviour (King's Fund, 2005; Socialist Health Association, 2005; McKee and Raine, 2005; Raine, et al., 2004; LGA et al., 2004; UKPHA, 2004; BMA, 2004a). The white paper made little mention of deprivation, transport, pollution, and poor housing (although the government claimed these were covered by other strategies). It also failed to address the fundamental social and economic inequalities that persisted, and in some respects deteriorated, under the Labour government (Chapter 17).

Despite the government's emphasis on an evidence-based approach to public health, it appeared to ignore its own prescriptions when it came to policy. For example, it ignored the extensive evidence on the role of socioeconomic and environmental factors, while backing mass education campaigns in an effort to change individual behaviour – in spite of the large body of evidence about their ineffectiveness (McKee and Raine, 2005). Others were critical of the new health trainers (UKPHA, 2004; Socialist Health Association, 2005) believing that there was insufficient evidence about their added value (see Visram and Drinkwater, 2005 for a discussion of the evidence).

Some were sceptical about partnership with commercial interests. While it was possible that collaboration might improve health by harnessing self-interested profit-seeking behaviour – such as launching high margin, low alcohol drinks or healthy food options – this could not be guaranteed (UKPHA, 2004; King's Fund, 2005). Indeed, these powerful industries could use their position and influence to shape the pace, direction and content of public health initiatives in a way that undermines the public interest. Critics argued that public health problems were so serious that a more forceful regulatory response was warranted. This would take a precautionary approach and place the onus of proof on industry (LGA et al., 2004). There was support in such quarters for radical policy options such as higher taxation of alcoholic drinks and products high in fat, salt and sugar, as well as bans, and tighter restrictions on the marketing of such products, including advertising bans (UKPHA, 2004; Chartered Institute of Environmental Health/Royal Society for the Promotion of Health, 2004; BMA, 2004a; Socialist Health Association, 2005). In the one area where the government proposed stronger regulation – smoking – it was criticized for not going far enough. It later relented under pressure, extending the proposed partial ban on smoking in public places (see Chapter 15). On the whole though, the government appeared very reluctant to strengthen regulation, fearing accusations of 'nanny statism' (Raine et al., 2004).

Developments since Choosing Health

Delivering Choosing Health (DoH, 2005a) set out further targets and actions. Specific action plans were produced for diet and physical activity (see Chapter 13). These implementation plans are discussed in more detail in later chapters in the context of specific health issues. However, it should be noted at this stage that shifts in emphasis became apparent. Mental health, which some believed had received insufficient attention in the white paper (UKPHA, 2004; Socialist Health Association, 2005; Rethink, 2005) was given greater prominence. The implementation plans also specified ways of improving older people's health, following criticism that the needs of this important group had been ignored in the white paper (Help the Aged, 2005).

Despite the momentum built by the *Choosing Health* programme, attention quickly shifted back towards health care provision. Financial problems in the NHS, new forms of service commissioning, reorganization and service reconfiguration drew ministers' attention away from public health. The status of public health issues correspondingly declined. For example in 2006, it was revealed that when the Department of Health was finalizing a new policy document for NHS commissioning, the CMO was asked to insert a reference to public health at only two hours' notice (Mooney, 2006a). There was increasing disquiet about the department's leadership in public health. The government's own reviews found weaknesses in the Department of Health's leadership, particularly in the way it worked across government on public health matters (Cabinet Office, 2007). The BMA (2007a) called for the department to develop a stronger focus on public health and for substantial improvements in the way in which the government as a whole worked together on these issues.

There were some positive developments, however. The minister of public health was promoted to a more senior rank, an indication perhaps that the government was seeking to raise the profile of public health. Greater prime ministerial interest in the public health agenda was also evident. The 'Small Change, Big difference' programme, launched by Blair himself, sought to encourage small lifestyle changes in individuals in an effort to produce aggregate improvements in population health. The focus on healthy lifestyles continued with the National Lottery allocating funding to projects tackling childhood obesity, healthy eating, physical activity and mental wellbeing.

In 2006, a new white paper, *Our Health, Our Care, Our Say* (Cm 6737, 2006) was published focusing on community health services. This reiterated the *Choosing Health* principles, highlighting prevention and early intervention, while emphasizing the promotion of health and wellbeing (rather than simply tackling 'health risks'). The new white paper developed proposals on how to prioritize health and wellbeing within the NHS and across other agencies. It focused on how best to integrate plans and service provision, such as more joint appointments and integrated staffing arrangements between PCTs and local authorities, and closer alignment of budgets, planning cycles and performance frameworks. It sought to encourage joint commissioning of services, leading to a new framework discussed in later chapters. The white paper proposed other measures focused on health promotion and public health including life checks to enable people to assess their lifestyle, greater emphasis on health and wellbeing in performance frameworks, clearer strategies for prevention at local level, greater emphasis on tackling inequalities, and a review of preventive health spending.

The *Choosing Health* strategy was relaunched in the autumn of 2006 with the publication of a further document *Health Challenge England: Next Steps for Choosing Health* (HM Government/DoH, 2006). This reviewed progress and set out future plans. In so doing, it repeated the same key principles and policies: individual choices, education and information, and voluntary action by industry. These dovetailed with the *Our Health, Our Care, Our Say* commitments on commissioning and collaborative planning. Further initiatives were mentioned, such as the creation of a central support team on public health for

PCTs and local authorities, based in the DoH. The document also referred to greater responsibilities for local government in relation to health. There was a renewed emphasis on the contribution of the voluntary sector to health objectives and the scope for greater community-based action, which had been raised initially in *Choosing Health*. Efforts to improve the socioeconomic structure and the environment had a low profile. Regeneration and efficient transport were mentioned as important aspects of policy, but little detail was given about how these might fit with the broader health strategy. The document also mentioned the relatively few areas where government had introduced stronger regulation such as school meals, the marketing of junk food to children, and smoking in public places, in all cases due to strong pressure from the public health lobby.

In 2007, the government introduced a fresh PSA agreement on the promotion of better health and wellbeing (HM Government, 2007a). This heralded a more locally led and incentive-driven system, emphasizing the role of local targets and agreements. Key national targets would, however, remain. The key to health improvement was identified as commissioning, both within the NHS (see Chapter 6) and increasingly jointly with local authorities and others (see Chapter 8). The regional tier was to be strengthened along with the local partnership arrangements that underpinned joint working on public health issues.

A further development was the Darzi review, which is discussed in more detail in Chapter 6. Amid concerns about reconfiguration of local health services, service quality and a lack of engagement with staff and patients, the government established a review of the NHS. Although focused on service issues, it considered a number of areas relevant to public health including patient safety, fair access to services, personalization of services and support for people to stay healthy. These elements were incorporated in regional and local plans and provided impetus for further service development in public health.

Did We Choose Health?

Reports have shed light on the impact of public health initiatives introduced by the Labour government. Derek Wanless (2007) examined the extent to which there had been progress towards a fully engaged scenario, where people took greater responsibility for their health and services were more responsive to their needs. He was particularly critical of the weaknesses of the public health function, noting that it had a relatively low priority. With regard to indicators of health, he observed that evidence was mixed, with some improvements in smoking prevention, diet and exercise but increasing levels of obesity. Wanless's overall conclusion was that progress fell short of the fully engaged scenario. The Healthcare Commission and the Audit Commission (2008) produced an evaluation of progress on improving health and reducing health inequalities. They pointed out that there had been some significant improvements, for example reductions in cancer and heart disease deaths, in smoking rates and teenage pregnancy. But progress was not uniform. Health inequalities persisted (see Chapter 17), there was uneven performance between different geographical areas in the attainment of targets, and in some policy areas, notably obesity and alcohol misuse, problems had deteriorated. The Healthcare Commission/Audit Commission report recommended:

- clear, consistent, ambitious and measurable public health targets
- relevant, reliable and up to date public health information
- a consistent focus on public health across the NHS and other areas of government
- putting evidence about what works into practice
- sufficient resources and incentives to support the delivery of health improvement programmes
- commissioning of services based on local need
- clear accountabilities for commissioning and delivery

These issues are discussed further in Chapters 6–8. It is interesting to note, however, that the elements of success identified by the Healthcare Commission and Audit Commission are hardly new, echoing previous reports. This raises the question as to why government has not acted on similar observations made previously.

A further report, on the topic of health inequalities, by the Health Committee (2009), made further observations on the government's overall health strategy. The committee was critical of the failure of government to evaluate interventions adequately and to learn lessons from the evidence. It also criticized poor coordination across government on public health issues. The detailed recommendations of the committee are mentioned in other chapters (see Chapters 11, 13, 15 and 17).

Following a change of government in 2010, further changes in policy can be expected. The Conservative–Liberal Democrat government, led by David Cameron, stated that it would introduce a new strategy on public health. It was envisaged that this would include a new public health service, ring-fenced public health budgets and significant new responsibilities for local government. These proposals are examined in later chapters.

Exhibit 4.2

Other National Health Strategies in the UK

As Greer (2007, 2009a) observed, devolution of powers to elected assemblies in Scotland, Wales and Northern Ireland brought divergence in public health policy-making. Even prior to this there were policy differences between the countries of the UK. Wales became the first to launch a public health strategy (Welsh Office NHS Directorate, 1989, 1992). The Welsh Office identified priority areas for achieving 'health gain': sustained improvements in health. These were: cancer, maternal and child health, mental handicap, mental distress and illness, injuries, emotional health, respiratory illness, cardiovascular diseases, healthy environments, and physical disability/discomfort. However, this ambitious plan did not achieve its desired outcomes (NAO, 1996b), due to several factors: a lack of leadership, too many targets, inadequate monitoring of performance, and difficulties in releasing resources for investment in areas where health improvement could be maximized.

In the late 1990s, Wales further developed its distinctive approach (Coyle, 2007; Drakeford, 2006; Greer, 2005). A new strategy – *Better Health, Better Wales* – was launched (Cm 3992, 1998; Welsh Office, 1998), which focused more sharply on the economic and social context of health than its English counterpart. The Welsh strategy endorsed a broad range of health gain targets, including back pain, arthritis, dental health, the consumption of fruit and vegetables, alcohol consumption, smoking, and breast, cervical and lung cancer. Following the NHS Plan for England, the Welsh Assembly revised its own plans to improve health and health services (NAfW, 2001). The Welsh plan, *Improving Health in Wales*, strongly featured public health objectives, health promotion and the reduction of health inequalities. These themes were taken forward in a further document, *Wellbeing in Wales* (Welsh Assembly Government, 2002a), and in the Welsh Assembly Government's (2003a) overarching strategy, *Wales – a Better Country*. Building on earlier efforts to create healthy alliances at local level, new joint 'health, social care and wellbeing strategies' were introduced (Welsh Assembly Government, 2003a), which sought to improve collaboration on public health across NHS bodies, local authorities and other relevant partner organizations, such as the voluntary sector. Local health promotion activities were undertaken within an evolving strategic framework, with the establishment of an All Wales Health and Wellbeing Council, an action plan to promote healthy lifestyles, a strategy for children and young people's wellbeing, and a food and wellbeing strategy (Welsh Assembly Government, 2003b, 2003c; Food Standards Agency/Welsh Assembly Government, 2003). Wales has placed particular emphasis on reducing health inequalities (see Chapter 17). It has also developed a distinctive institutional framework in this field, including a national public health service, providing expertise on public health issues (see Exhibit 6.1).

Debates about the performance of health and social care services, and about the increasing future demands upon them (Audit Commission, 2004a; Wanless, 2003), have led to greater pressures for health service reform in Wales. They also reinforced arguments that the public must be engaged in the process of health improvement and disease prevention. This was a key theme of Health Challenge Wales, a new campaign launched in 2004, which sought to raise awareness about the determinants of health and wellbeing, to enable people to make healthy choices by signposting information and activities, and to demonstrate how organizations can work together in this field. Improving health was also a key theme in the revised strategy for health and social care in Wales, *Designed for Life* (Welsh Assembly Government, 2005a). This reiterated the importance of prevention, partnership working and reducing inequalities and aimed to ensure full public health engagement at local and national levels. Specific commitments included extending breast cancer screening, eliminating smoking in public places and increasing the coverage of healthy schools schemes as well as a revised health inequalities strategy. The strategy also reiterated the importance of health gain targets in five areas: coronary heart disease, cancer, mental health, health of children and older people.

In Scotland, separate health targets were set for coronary heart disease and cancer during the early 1990s (Scottish Office, 1991, 1992). In addition, specific strategies, with targets, were introduced in a number of areas including smoking, alcohol, diet, breast-feeding, and oral health. Following a green paper on the subject (Cm 3854, 1998), a new Scottish health strategy was outlined in the white paper, *Towards a Healthier Scotland* (Cm 4269, 1999). This set out a number of action areas to improve health: life circumstances (such as poverty, poor housing, limited educational achievement), lifestyles (smoking, diet, drug and alcohol misuse), and tackling health inequalities. In addition, targets were set for cancer, heart disease, dental health, smoking, alcohol misuse, and teenage pregnancy and for diet, physical activity, and strokes. Other key areas for intervention were mental health, child health and accidents. In addition, four demonstration projects at a cost of £15 million were launched to promote sexual health, reduce coronary heart disease, prevent cancer, and promote the health of preschool children.

Devolution gave Scotland considerable scope for developing a distinctive approach to public health (Donnelly, 2007; Stewart, 2004; Greer, 2005, 2009a). Subsequent developments included a diet action plan, a sexual health strategy, a new approach to mental health promotion, a ban on smoking in public places (the first country in the UK to do this), new initiatives to strengthen the public health role of nurses, and the appointment of public health practitioners to local health bodies to improve leadership and coordination. Scotland also established a public health institute to coordinate efforts to improve health (see Exhibit 6.1). The Scottish NHS Plan (Scottish Executive, 2000a) placed a high priority on health promotion. A renewed public health strategy, *Improving Health in Scotland* (Scottish Executive, 2003a), was subsequently introduced alongside further proposals for health service reform set out in *Partnership for Care* and *Building a Health Service Fit for the Future* (Scottish Executive, 2003b, 2005a). Four specific themes of action were identified: early years, teenage transition, workplace and communities. In addition, a number of priority topics were specified: physical activity, healthy eating, smoking, alcohol, mental health and wellbeing, health and homelessness, and sexual health. The strategy aimed to establish health improvement at the top of the government's agenda and integrate it across all programmes. A new health improvement director was established in the Scottish Executive. Efforts were made to strengthen coordination between Scottish government departments and agencies. There was an attempt to improve coordination of health promotion campaigns. There was greater integration of health improvement in public sector planning, and learning networks to spread good practice were developed. New integrated programmes were launched in the priority topic areas. These were underpinned by joint health improvement plans, agreed between local stakeholders. Later, community health partnerships (CHPs) were established to strengthen coordination within the NHS and between other organizations in the field of primary and community services, such as local authorities and the voluntary sector (see Exhibit 6.1).

Following the election of a minority Scottish National Party government in 2007, further initiatives were introduced. The new government's health plans included a new initiative on health inequalities (see Chapter 17). It also announced measures to reduce smoking, alcohol problems, drug abuse and obesity. A further priority was to improve the health of children, measures including extending entitlement to free school meals, an increase in nursing and healthcare support in schools, and new targets for breast-feeding (Scottish Government, 2007a, 2007b).

In Northern Ireland, two key documents were published in the late 1990s: *Well in 2000* (DHSSNI, 1997) and *Health and Wellbeing: Towards the New Millennium* (DHSSNI, 1996). These set out a distinctive strategy placing greater emphasis on health inequalities and health impact assessment when compared with other UK strategies at the time. Public health targets in the Province related to a relatively wide range of issues (covering for example child health, the health of elderly people and people with learning disabilities). Between 1999 and 2002 Northern Ireland was granted devolutionary powers. Following a political crisis these were suspended but have since been restored. This has added to the complexity of policymaking and implementation. The 'on–off' nature of devolution in the Province has made it difficult to develop public health policies, partly because strategic responsibilities passed back and forth between the UK government and the devolved assembly and executive, and partly because policy development has played second fiddle to the need to establish workable governance arrangements and maintain peace and order (Wilde, 2007; Greer, 2005, 2009a). Other factors have also been important. A wide-ranging review of public administration in Northern Ireland prompted reorganization of the NHS and local government, currently being implemented. A review of public health was also commissioned (DHSSPS, 2004a), which led to the establishment of a Northern Ireland public health agency (see Exhibit 6.1) A further source of policy change is the increased collaboration between the North and the South on public health matters (indeed, an all-Ireland Public Health Institute was established in 1999 to promote cooperation and share expertise).

Northern Ireland has in some respects pursued a more vigorous public health policy compared with England (Wilde, 2007), perhaps understandable given its relatively higher levels of ill health and the role of socioeconomic factors such as poor housing, poverty, unemployment and social division. The promotion of health and wellbeing has been identified as a key priority by the Northern Ireland government (Northern Ireland Executive, 2008). Public health interventions have been explicitly linked to social welfare programmes such as *Targeting Social Need* and *Promoting Social Inclusion* (www.ccruni.gov.uk/equality/docs/newstsn.htm). The most recent Northern Ireland public health strategy, *Investing for Health* (DHSSPS, 2002a, 2004b), emphasized stronger partnership working and improved joint planning arrangements between NHS and local government bodies. It also set demanding targets for reducing health inequalities. *Investing for Health* was taken forward subsequently by a regional strategy document, *A Healthier Future* (DHSSPS, 2004c). At the time of writing the Northern Ireland Executive is reviewing the *Investing for Health* strategy.

Conclusion

Health strategies are undoubtedly a useful guide for action. Their very existence is an important development, indicating a shift in emphasis from the provision of health care services to promoting public health. Their impact should not, however, be exaggerated. Indeed, health strategies have been criticized on a number of grounds including design flaws, implementation failure, unwillingness to tackle vested interests, problems of coordination, and inability to fully address the social, economic and environmental causes of ill health, and for being inadequately resourced. Strategy is meaningless without the will to achieve objectives. Goals and targets can set direction, but cannot guarantee success. Much more depends on specific activities in a wide range of policy areas: the NHS, local government, partnership bodies, food policy, addictions, environmental policy and social inequalities. It is in these crucial battlegrounds where the commitment to the new public health perspective has been tested. Before moving on to these issues, however, it is important to first look at the broader international context in which national public health strategies, and for that matter local and regional strategies, are located.

Public Health in a Global Context

5

When considering public health policy, one cannot ignore the global context (Walt, 1994). Although, 'traditionally, public health has been a nationally focused endeavour' (Collin and Lee, 2007, p. 105), global trends now make it difficult to adopt a purely national response. It is true that external health risks are not entirely new, as exemplified by the spread of epidemics throughout history (Berlinguer, 1999). In the past, however, such risks were associated primarily with infectious disease. The main threats to health today are more complex, arising from a combination of factors associated with what some see as a process of 'globalization' (Labonte and Schrecker, 2004; Koivusalo, 2006; DoH, 2007b). These factors include climate change, population displacement, war and terrorism, increased international mobility, the communications revolution, ageing populations, rising levels of chronic disease, the concentration of capital and economic power, the spread of Western consumer culture across the world, trade liberalization, privatization and deregulation and increasing levels of inequality both within and between countries (Lee and Collin, 2005).

As Earle (2007a, p. 29) has observed, 'globalization is Janus-faced'. Although it poses threats to health, it may offer opportunities for improved prosperity and for the development of processes to combat health risks (Baum, 2002; DoH, 2007b). Indeed, it is widely acknowledged that global challenges to health cannot be tackled in isolation but 'can only be tackled when governments come together to confront shared problems' (McKee, 2007, p. 71). This goes beyond agreement on procedures for dealing with outbreaks of infectious diseases, to include action on wider public health threats, such as climate change, pollution, socioeconomic deprivation and inequity, and lifestyle-related illness.

This chapter explores the infrastructure for dealing with international health issues, beginning with an examination of the key institutions of public health governance at the global level and their policies. This is followed by an analysis of public health institutions and policies at the European level, which also have implications for domestic public health policies.

International Public Health

The World Health Organization

The World Health Organization (WHO) was founded in 1948 as a specialist agency of the United Nations (UN). Its main functions are to provide scientific advice on health matters, to set international standards, to prevent disease and to promote health. The institution had a strong public health ethos from the outset, reflected in its positive definition of health (see Chapter 1). Its early work focused on infectious disease and included the formulation of international health regulations (IHR) that required notification of specific diseases (plague, yellow fever and cholera). WHO played a major role in tackling major infectious diseases through education and vaccination programmes, notably with regard to smallpox (which it declared eradicated in 1977). WHO's work with regard to infectious disease continues today in the context of recent, new and emerging infections (HIV/AIDS, SARS, and new drug-resistant strains of influenza and TB). Notably, in 2005 the IHR was revised, extending WHO's role to any event that could constitute an international public health emergency (Nicoll et al., 2005).

WHO has sought to shift the emphasis of health policy towards disease prevention and health promotion. Its *Health for All by the Year 2000* principles were formulated during the 1970s and developed further at international conferences such as Alma Ata (WHO/UNICEF, 1978), Ottawa (WHO, 1986), Adelaide (WHO, 1988), Sundsvall (WHO, 1991), Jakarta (WHO, 1997a), Mexico City (WHO, 2000a), Bangkok (WHO, 2005a) and Nairobi (WHO, 2009d). These principles are as follows:

1　Health is a fundamental human right and a social goal. Health is defined in a positive sense, in line with the classic WHO definition, and comprises mental, physical and social wellbeing, not just the absence of illness or disease. Policies should be reoriented to focus on maintaining and improving health.

2　An equitable distribution of health resources, both within and between countries, should be a fundamental goal.

3　Health is shaped by many factors: social, economic, lifestyle, and environmental. Policymakers must construct 'holistic' and 'intersectoral' policies that take account of other sectors of decision-making which impinge upon health. Governments should adopt 'healthy public policies' which strongly reflect health priorities, coordinate the actions of government agencies, and which are based on assessments of their health impact (Milio, 1986).

4   Health policies must be pre-emptive and precautionary, the aim being to prevent the problems from arising at the earliest possible stage.

5   Health improvements require a community-wide response. This involves partnership between agencies drawn from all relevant sectors and at all levels. Health promotion must include and involve the community, responding to its concerns, while at the same time promoting healthy lifestyles and supportive environments.

6   Health services must be reoriented towards primary health care and geared to promoting health rather than simply treating illness.

7   Clear performance targets and review mechanisms must be adopted in order to guide health strategies and achieve their objectives.

These principles underpinned the *Health for All* strategy, which set global targets for the year 2000 (WHO, 1981). This represented an attempt by WHO to drive global health policy (Kickbusch, 2002, 2003). The WHO regional offices adopted their own strategies and targets, tailored to the specific health problems of their part of the world (the WHO European Region strategy is discussed further in Exhibit 5.2). WHO and its regional offices monitored the development of national policies and progress towards targets. Although WHO could not dictate to member states, the monitoring process created some gentle peer pressure. This was reflected in the number of countries that began to develop health strategies, examples of which are shown in Exhibit 5.1.

The *Health for All* strategy was subsequently revised for the twenty-first century (see WHO, 1998a; Pappas and Moss, 2001). Although its basic principles remain intact, the emphasis of the strategy has shifted. Sustainable development and environmental health issues have higher profiles (see Chapter 11), and there is greater emphasis on promoting equity in health and addressing socioeconomic determinants. There has also been renewed emphasis on public engagement in the development of health promotion initiatives. The need for a robust infrastructure of health promotion has been another key theme, underpinned by better coordination between levels of government as well as between different policy sectors. There has also been an emphasis on partnership working, with an acknowledgement that the private sector too has a role to play in improving public health. Finally, as will become clear in later chapters, WHO has become more proactive in recent years in promoting policies to combat specific threats to health from socioeconomic factors, including commercial interests; examples include the Framework Convention on Tobacco Control (FCTC – see Chapter 15), the establishment of a Commission on Social Determinants and Health (see Chapter 17), a global initiative on diet, physical activity and health (Chapter 15) and a global action plan for the prevention and control of non-communicable diseases (WHO, 2008a).

Exhibit 5.1

Health Strategies in the USA and Finland

Many countries now have a health strategy, setting out targets for reducing key illnesses and addressing the main risk factors. The USA was one of the first countries to do so. Following the Surgeon General's (1979) report on health promotion and disease prevention, a strategy was devised (US Department of Health and Human Services, 1980). This set over 200 targets in fifteen priority areas to be achieved by 1990. Subsequently a revised strategy, *Healthy People 2000,* was introduced (US Department of Health and Human Services, 1991) with further objectives and targets. Although the first two strategies had some success, notably reducing infant mortality and child death rates, the overall outcome was disappointing. An evaluation of *Healthy People 2000* found that only a fifth of targets were met (National Center for Health Statistics, 2001). In 2000 a further strategy, *Healthy People 2010*, was launched, its goals being to increase life expectancy, improve quality of life, and eliminate health disparities between different population groups (US Department of Health and Human Services, 2000). This strategy set out 28 focus areas (such as cancer, environmental health, nutrition) with associated targets (for example smoking reduction). It had over 900 objectives and 10 key indicators, reflecting key priorities: physical activity, overweight/obesity, tobacco, substance abuse, sexual behaviour, mental health, injury and violence, environmental quality, immunization, and access to health care. Progress reports showed that less than a fifth of objectives were met (these included cancer mortality, child vaccination and accidents at work), although in most some progress was made. In over a fifth of objectives the trends moved in the wrong direction (for example tooth decay in children, high blood pressure in adults and obesity levels) (Sondik et al., 2010). A revised framework, *Healthy People 2020*, is currently being formulated. Although the USA was among the first nations to adopt a health strategy, its public health policy has been criticized on the following grounds (see Institute of Medicine, 2002; Tilson and Berkowitz, 2006; Raphel and Bryant, 2006; Beaglehole and Bonita, 2004; David, 2000; Raphael, 2008): that it is too heavily focused on disease risks related to individual lifestyles rather than broader socioeconomic or environmental determinants; that there are too many action areas and targets; and that implementation of public health strategies is poor. There has also been criticism of a failure to clarify the responsibilities of federal government and other agencies, a lack of coordination between agencies, the variable quality of local public health agencies, a lack of capacity in the public health workforce, and an inadequately resourced public health system. The failure of public health priorities to influence other government policies has also been noted.

Finland also pioneered the use of health strategies. In 1986 it adopted the *Health for All* approach in its national plans (Tervonen-Gonçalves and Lehto, 2004). The Finnish national strategy is credited as having an inspirational effect on health policy, supporting the shift from treatment to prevention and encouraging health promotion activities. The most recent version of this strategy was introduced in 2001. This strategy, *Health 2015*, sets out a range of objectives to be achieved by 2015 (Ministry of Social Affairs and Health, 2001). There are eight key areas, some of which are population-wide (for example increasing healthy life expectancy by two years). Others are focused on specific subgroups (for example to reduce smoking rates for young people aged 16–18 to under 15 per cent). The strategy is closely monitored, with evaluations every four years.

Finland is recognized as a world leader in the field of public health. However, room for further improvement has been identified, including the need for stronger leadership by central government, improved coordination and cooperation between national agencies, stronger leadership at local level, systematic sharing of good practice, and increased capacity of the public health system (WHO Regional Office for Europe, 2002).

WHO has attracted criticism from various sources. Commercial interests, such as the food, alcohol and tobacco industries, have attacked its initiatives on lifestyle-related illness. It has been criticized by libertarians and adherents of free markets. It has also received criticism from governments, particularly those like the US and the UK, which are strongly influenced by neoliberal ideologies and commercial interests. On the other hand, others have been critical of WHO for being bureaucratic, lacking leadership and failing to stand up to hostile governments and corporations (Koivusalo and Ollila, 1997; McCarthy, 2002; Yamey, 2002a). Some believe that WHO has ceded its leadership of international health, with other bodies such as the IMF, World Bank and the World Trade Organization (see below) becoming much more powerful in this field (Earle, 2007a; Tudor Hart, 2006). WHO strategies have been criticized for lacking effectiveness, partly due to lobbying from vested interests (Beaglehole and Bonita, 2004; McCarthy, 2002). WHO's policy of promoting closer working partnerships with private corporations has been attacked (Ollila, 2005). More positively, it has been acknowledged that WHO has responded to criticism by reorganizing itself and refocusing its priorities, although the longer term impact of these changes is unclear (Beaglehole and Bonita, 2004; Kickbusch, 2003; Yamey, 2002b; McCarthy, 2002; Horton, 2006; Prah Ruger and Yach, 2005).

To be fair to WHO, it is operating in an environment that is politically much less conducive to its fundamental principles. The organization was born into the collectivist idealism of the immediate postwar period but now lives in a world dominated by pro-market neoliberalism. Moreover, WHO now inhabits a much more crowded policy environment than when it was formed (Prah Ruger and Yach, 2005). The international health policy community is increasingly fragmented and there is confusion surrounding leadership on global health matters (Kickbusch, 2002; Beaglehole and Bonita, 2004; Ollila, 2005). Indeed, it is possible that WHO could provide greater leadership and coherence in the future (Ollila et al., 2006; Horton, 2006).

Other International Bodies Concerned with Health

A wide range of other international bodies have an interest in health policy. In 2000, the UN General Assembly adopted the Millennium Development Goals (MDGs), which included several health objectives such as reduced child mortality, improvements in maternal health, the eradication of extreme poverty and hunger, tackling HIV/AIDs as well as malaria and other diseases, and ensuring environmental sustainability (UN General Assembly, 2000). Targets, to be achieved by 2015, included halving the proportion of people worldwide without access to safe drinking water and sanitation, halting and reversing the spread of HIV/AIDS and the incidence of malaria and other major diseases, reducing maternal mortality by three-quarters and mortality among children under five by two-thirds. The General Assembly has also considered specific health threats. For example, in 2001, it held a specific session on HIV/AIDs, the first time it had focused in depth on a specific disease (Beaglehole and Bonita, 2004, p. 90). It has subsequently deliberated other health issues including drugs, women's health, and road safety. The UN's growing involvement in environmental policy has also drawn it into the realm of public health. Concerns about ozone depletion, climate change and sustainable development have led to the creation of new international programmes and institutions (see Chapter 11).

Several UN agencies and bodies have an important stake in health policy. UNICEF, for example, has an interest arising out of its concern for child welfare. UNESCO has an interest in health education. There is a joint UN programme on HIV/AIDS (UNAIDS). Health also touches the agenda of other institutions and programmes such as the UN Development Programme, the Population Fund, the High Commissioner on Refugees, the High Commissioner on Human Rights, the Conference on Trade and Development, the Food and Agriculture Organization, the Drugs Control Programme and the International Labour Organization. Even the UN Security Council has considered health issues, in relation to war, terrorism, biosecurity and infectious disease (Lee and Collin, 2005).

Other bodies with an economic rather than a health, social, humanitarian or security brief seem to have acquired great influence in the health field. These include the World Bank, the International Monetary Fund (IMF), the OECD, and the World Trade Organization.

The World Bank and the IMF are autonomous institutions within the UN system, both established after the Second World War (Walt, 1994; Koivusalo and Ollila, 1997; Lee and Collin, 2005). Although their roles are principally economic and financial, they have influence over policies affecting social welfare and public health. Following postwar reconstruction, the World Bank turned its attention to financing long-term programmes in developing countries, although its policy prescriptions remain relevant to industrialized nations. The IMF lends funds to countries (not just developing nations) in return for certain conditions (for example on economic management, public finance and public service provision – including health and welfare budgets). It also gives financial guidance and issues reports about the state of their economies, which can affect investor confidence. Both the IMF and the World Bank sought to open up developing countries' economies to foreign investment and competition using neoliberal policies such as privatization, public spending cuts and deregulation. This often entailed cutting budgets for health and welfare. These policies were heavily criticized for impacting adversely on public health in these countries (Beaglehole and Bonita, 2004). This criticism seems to have had some effect. The World Bank now places greater emphasis on poverty reduction and social capital programmes, alongside its commitment to privatization and market forces. Significantly it has shifted its position on important health issues, such as tobacco (see Chapter 15). However, the IMF has been less open to change and it has been criticized for having continuing negative effects on health and welfare (Stuckler and Basu, 2009; Gilmore et al., 2009).

Another important organization is the Organisation for Economic Cooperation and Development (OECD). Its members constitute the main industrialized economies, accounting for two-thirds of world trade. The OECD was founded as a body to encourage postwar construction. Its current aims are to promote economic growth, improved standards of living and world trade through agreements between members, by undertaking research and by disseminating ideas about policy and reform. Like the IMF and World Bank, it tends to favour markets and neoliberal policies. Although it has fewer powers and resources than these bodies, OECD has a more subtle role, encouraging policy change through comparison, analysis and recommendation (Armingeon and Beyeler, 2004).

The World Trade Organization (WTO) was created in 1995 to negotiate, monitor and enforce trade agreements (Lee and Collin, 2005). It is not part of the UN, but has a close relationship with UN bodies. The establishment of the WTO was the latest phase in the attempt to liberalize trade, as part of the postwar General Agreement on Tariffs and Trade (GATT) and subsequently the General Agreement on Trade and Services (GATS). The WTO's rules and decisions are binding on members, who together account for 90 per cent of world trade. Although its membership extends beyond the wealthiest industrialized countries, these exert most power (Ostry, 2001).

WTO trade rules have enormous implications for health, in both developing and industrialized countries. This is acknowledged to some extent by the inclusion of health protection agreements within WTO rules. For example, under the WTO's sanitary and phytosanitary agreement (WTO, 1994), trade can be restricted to protect human, animal or plant life. However, the application of such restrictions can only occur when certain conditions are met: that

there is clear evidence of risk, that there is no discrimination against a particular country's products or services, and that the least possible restraint is
placed on trade. In practice, this may inhibit governments from regulating
where a threat to health exists but the evidence base is currently weak. It may
also prevent them from targeting producers in particular countries where
standards are low. The rules also contain a bias against strong forms of regulation (such as higher taxes or bans on products). From a public health
perspective, much criticism has centred on the implications of trade rules for
food safety. One of the key battles here has been the issue of opening up EU
markets to US and Canadian hormone-treated beef (see Chapter 12). A further
concern is that government measures that incidentally affect the supply of
services are now deemed restrictions on trade and require justification under
WTO rules. This opens up a wider range of government regulation in environmental health and safety to scrutiny for potential deregulation (Price,
2002). Another public health issue is raised by the impact of trade agreements
on the developing countries, notably with regard to regulations on intellectual property (Pollock and Price, 2003). Controversy surrounded the extension of these regulations to drugs, enabling pharmaceutical companies to
block cheaper generic products, with particularly serious implications for
poor countries. Although the WTO stated that intellectual property rules may
be overridden in order to meet public health needs, critics remained uncon-
vinced. Indeed richer countries have been able to negotiate bilateral trade
agreements with poorer countries that, in effect, reintroduce these rules (Lee
et al., 2009).

It has been pointed out that trade considerations dominate health and that
this is not good for global health, and could damage trade itself in the longer
term (Smith et al., 2009; Lee et al., 2009; Blouin et al., 2009). Critics have called
for a stronger health input into decisions about trade, including stronger
representation for WHO. It is also important that trade and health considerations are balanced more effectively at national level. Notably, the World
Health Assembly in 2006 called for national governments to demonstrate
greater coherence on trade and health policies. This prompted WHO, WTO,
the World Bank and others to develop a framework on trade and health to
enable policymakers to balance these interests. However, this does not address
the imbalance of health and trade considerations at the global level.

Global Initiatives on Health

The richest group of nations have taken a greater interest in global health
issues in recent years (Labonte and Schrecker, 2004). The G8 has played a
growing role in global health governance. It includes the richest countries,
accounting for around half of global GDP (France, the USA, the UK, Germany,

Italy, Japan, Canada and Russia). Successive G8 summits have set the direction for international public health policy with commitments to poverty reduction in the poorest countries and support for efforts to tackle specific diseases such as HIV/AIDS, TB and malaria. There is also an emerging role for the G20 group of nations – which includes those rapidly industrializing such as Brazil, China and India. This group has also begun to consider health matters, although it has yet to develop a clear role in this field of leadership (Batniji and Woods, 2009).

The wealthier nations have a particularly valuable part to play in stimulating partnership between different institutions and agencies. For example, the G8, along with the UN, World Bank, WHO and UNAIDS established a new Global Fund for AIDS, TB and malaria (GFATM). This is one of several new partnership arrangements in the field of public health, some of which involve non-government organizations and the private sector (Ollila, 2005; Lee and Collin, 2005). Another example is the Global Alliance for Vaccination and Immunization (GAVI), formed in 2000 with funds from the Gates Foundation, which makes vaccines more widely available in the poorest countries of the world.

Global initiatives reflect a heightened awareness among richer countries about the importance of health (see, for example, HM Government, 2008a). But motives are mixed. In the discourse surrounding global health there is an element of altruism, with enlightened politicians and charity lobby groups pressing for action on humanitarian grounds (Labonte, 2008). But there is also self-interest. The richer countries are acting partly in pursuit of economic gains. Improved health in developing countries creates the potential for new and expanding consumer markets. Moreover, the richer countries are concerned about their security, which could be adversely affected by diseases linked to climate change, conflict and poverty.

Progress made since 2000 has been considerable in some areas, such as vaccination against infectious disease. But commitments on poverty, maternal and child health and sanitation have been weaker (McCurry, 2008). There is additional concern in the light of the deep worldwide recession beginning in 2008 that the wealthier countries may renege on even these modest commitments.

Other International Players

Multinational corporations, such as pharmaceutical, food and alcohol companies, are increasingly involved in the international health policy arena as partners as well as lobbyists. The corporations argue that they wish to work with public health initiatives as part of their commitment to corporate social responsibility (CSR). Others are less convinced, seeing CSR as a front for enhanced policy influence (Bakan, 2005). Specific examples will be considered in the UK context in later chapters (see particularly 13 and 15). Other actors in this policy arena are non-government organizations (Earle, 2007a). These include charities and foundations, such as Oxfam and the Gates Foundation. In addition, there are single issue campaigning groups on specific concerns such as alcohol, smoking and diet, as well as environmental organizations, trade union bodies and anti-globalization groups which promote action across a wider range of issues related to public health.

Whose Interests are Served?

Global health policymaking is increasingly influenced by the industrial, trade and financial interests of the richest countries and the multinationals they host (Tudor Hart, 2006; Ollila, 2005; Fort et al., 2004; Lee et al., 2009). Above all, the USA is credited as being the single most powerful actor, able to reconfigure international institutions to suit its dominant market ideology and vested interests (McKee, 2007; Waitzkin et al., 2005). The growth of partnerships involving the private sector and the shift in power over health policy to economic and trade bodies is regarded as central to this process, which is seen as undermining national public health policies in both developing and industrialized countries (Ollila, 2005).

But perhaps the reality is more complex. The pluralistic nature of global health governance (Prah Ruger and Yach, 2005) does at least give countervailing groups opportunities to challenge the dominant interests. Charities, pressure groups and trade unions may not be on a level playing field, but they can gain access to a range of institutions in order to put their case. Some of these institutions are more sympathetic to their case than others. Furthermore, the fragmentation of the institution of public health governance makes it difficult for any single interest to dominate across the board. Hence it is possible for some international bodies to adopt policies and programmes that limit, ameliorate or even inhibit policies made by the economic, financial and trade bodies.

Exhibit 5.2

WHO European Region Targets for the Twenty-first Century

The WHO Regional Office for Europe takes forward health initiatives, often in collaboration with other European institutions with an interest in health policy, such as the European Commission's Directorate on Health and Consumers (see below). Over the years it has addressed a range of issues, including alcohol misuse, tobacco, and environmental health. The regional office has taken forward WHO's *Health for All* strategy and tailored it to the European context. In the 1980s, it launched the *Healthy Cities* project (Ashton, 1992, p. 4). This piloted the application of *Health for All* principles in selected cities across Europe in an effort to improve the health of disadvantaged people, reorient health systems towards primary care, and emphasize public involvement and partnerships. The *Healthy Cities* initiative has since spread across Europe and worldwide (see Exhibit 7.1 for further discussion of its impact within the UK).

The WHO region devised specific *Health for All* targets (WHO Regional Office for Europe, 1985); updated in 1991 (WHO Regional Office for Europe, 1993a) and later revised (WHO Regional Office for Europe, 1999). Further detailed targets accompany these main targets (some of which are discussed in later chapters in the context of specific health policy issues). The main targets are as follows:

1 By the year 2020, the present gap in health status between member states of the European Region should be reduced by at least one third.

2 By the year 2020, the health gap between socioeconomic groups within countries should be reduced by at least 25 per cent in all member states, by substantially improving the level of health of disadvantaged groups.

3 By the year 2020, all newborn babies, infants and preschool children in the Region should have better health, ensuring a healthy start in life.

4 By the year 2020, young people in the Region should be healthier and better able to fulfil their roles in society.

5 By the year 2020, people over 65 years should have the opportunity of enjoying their full health potential and playing an active social role.

6 By the year 2020, people's psychosocial wellbeing should be improved and better, comprehensive services should be available to and accessible by people with mental health problems.

7 By the year 2020, the adverse health effects of communicable diseases should be substantially diminished through systematically applied programmes to eradicate, eliminate, or control infectious diseases of public health importance.

8 By the year 2020, morbidity, disability and premature mortality due to major chronic diseases should be reduced to the lowest feasible levels throughout the Region.

9 By the year 2020, there should be a significant and sustainable decrease in injuries, disability and death, arising from accidents and violence in the Region.

10 By the year 2015, people in the Region should live in a safer physical environment, with exposure to contaminants hazardous to health at levels not exceeding internationally agreed standards.

11 By the year 2015, people across society should have adopted healthier patterns of living.

12 By the year 2015, the adverse health effects from the consumption of addictive substances such as tobacco, alcohol, and psychoactive drugs should have been significantly reduced in all member states

13 By the year 2015, people in the Region should have greater opportunities to live in healthy physical and social environments at home, at school, and in the local community.

14 By the year 2020, all sectors should have recognized and accepted their responsibility for health.

15 By the year 2010, people in the Region should have much better access to family- and community-oriented primary health care, supported by a flexible and responsive hospital system.

16 By the year 2010, member states should ensure that the management of the health sector, from population-based health programmes to individual patient care at the clinical level, is oriented towards health outcomes.

17 By the year 2010, member states should have sustainable financing and resource allocation mechanisms for health care systems based on the principles of equal access, cost-effectiveness, solidarity and optimum quality.

18 By the year 2010, all member states should have ensured that health professionals and professionals in other sectors have acquired appropriate knowledge, attitudes and skills to protect and promote health.

19 By the year 2005, all member states should have health research, information and communication systems that better support the acquisition, effective utilization, and dissemination of knowledge to support *Health for All*.

20 By the year 2005, implementation of policies for *Health for All* should engage individuals, groups and organizations throughout the public and private sectors, and civil society, in alliances and partnerships for health.

21 By the year 2010, all member states should have and be implementing policies for *Health for All* at country, regional and local levels, supported by appropriate institutional infrastructures, managerial processes and innovative leadership.

The WHO region plays an important role in building consensus among European states on public health strategies and actions. It also helps to promote a coordinated response to health problems in Europe. In some cases this has led to broad statements of intent, such as that which emerged from the ministerial conference in Talinn in 2008. This produced a charter, *Health Systems for Health and Wealth* (WHO Regional Office for Europe, 2008a), which acknowledged the importance of health systems in promoting social solidarity, wellbeing and wealth. It highlighted the contribution of disease prevention and health promotion to improvements in health. It also acknowledged that health systems should ensure attention is given to the needs of poor and vulnerable people. Member states committed to invest in health systems and in sectors that influence health. In addition, intergovernmental conferences under the auspices of WHO Europe have produced important policy statements and action plans on specific public health issues, such as children's health, obesity, alcohol, and food. These are examined in the context of later chapters.

Source: HEALTH21: the Health for All policy framework for the WHO European Region. Copenhagen, WHO Regional Office for Europe, 1999.179–201 (European Health for All Series No. 6), (http://www.euro.who.int/InformationSources/Publications/Catalogue/20010911_38)

European Institutions and Public Health

The European Union

Until the early 1990s, the involvement of European Union (EU) institutions in health matters was tightly restricted (Randall, 2001; Duncan, 2002; Montgomery, 2003). Under the terms of the 1957 Treaty of Rome, which established the European Economic Community (EEC), health was reserved as a matter for member states. However, there was some scope for health-related initiatives under the Treaty's social policy provisions. The EEC's efforts to harmonize employment and trade regulations across member states also provided opportunities to improve health and safety (Nugent, 2003). As a result, policy initiatives developed in areas such as occupational health and safety, cancer prevention, heart disease, HIV/AIDS, and drug abuse.

A major turning point was the Single European Act (SEA) of 1987, which sought to create a more competitive market for goods across the European Community. The SEA stated that harmonization of trade must be based on regulations offering a high level of health protection. This had implications for policy in a number of areas, including food labelling and food safety, tobacco regulation, and health and safety at work. The SEA also extended the European Community's powers in environmental policy. This led to the creation of a special European Environmental Agency in the 1990s and to plans and programmes on environmental health (covering issues such as chemical contamination, water pollution, air quality and noise levels (see Chapter 10).

Subsequently, the Maastricht Treaty of 1992, which created the European Union, established a new community responsibility for public health (Treaty on European Union, 1992; Booker and North, 2005; Nugent, 2003). Article 129 stated that 'the Community shall contribute towards ensuring a high level of human health protection by encouraging cooperation between member states and, if necessary, lending support to their action' and that 'health protection requirements shall form a constituent part of the community's other policies'. The legitimate areas for community action were specified as the prevention of disease through research, information and education. Paragraph 4 of the Article excluded harmonization of legislation, although incentive measures (grants, for example) were permitted. Another key clause in the treaty was that member states 'shall foster cooperation with third countries and the competent international organizations in the sphere of public health', which legitimized the EU's links with international bodies on public health matters.

The Maastricht Treaty also included a Social Chapter, which covered social policy and employment issues, and therefore had implications for public health in a wider sense. The Chapter was based on a Charter of Fundamental

Social Rights drawn up by the European Community in 1989. This included living and working conditions, health and safety, employment rights and other social protection issues. The UK refused to adapt the Charter and secured an opt-out from the Social Chapter of the Maastricht Treaty. However, in 1997 the Blair government signed up to the Charter and became party to the Social Chapter of the Amsterdam Treaty, discussed further below.

Following the ratification of the Maastricht Treaty, the EU developed a framework for action on public health. On the basis of this, a network for the control and surveillance of communicable diseases was established. In addition, in 1995 the Council of Health Ministers agreed plans to initiate programmes in cancer prevention, HIV/AIDS and drug addiction. Subsequently, approval was given for programmes in other areas: health monitoring, pollution-related disease, injury prevention and rare diseases (Randall, 2001). The emphasis remained on the provision of funds, research and information rather than on regulation. This was hardly surprising given the desire of member governments to retain control over health policy and the existence of powerful commercial lobbies intent on resisting EU-level public health policies that might adversely affect their interests. However, a tougher regulatory approach did emerge in some areas, notably on smoking (see Chapter 15) and food safety (see Chapter 12).

Pressure for a more coherent European approach increased following the BSE/CJD crisis, which revealed that the EU had neglected its public health responsibilities (see Chapter 12). This led to a reallocation of responsibilities within the European Commission (Randall, 2001). A new Directorate of Health and Consumer Protection was created, with a stronger focus on public health. Subsequently, the Amsterdam Treaty of 1997 increased the powers of the EU in this field. It stated that 'a high level of human health protection *shall be ensured* in the definition and implementation of all Community policies and activities' (European Union, 1997, emphasis added). Community action was extended to include measures 'directed towards improving public health, preventing human illness and diseases and obviating sources of danger to human health'. The Treaty also included powers to introduce new minimum standards for blood products and human organ donation. Measures relating to veterinary and phytosanitary practices directly related to public health were also permitted. In addition, greater cooperation was agreed in a number of areas including health monitoring and epidemiological surveillance of infectious disease. However, the EU was still not empowered to use 'the harmonization of laws and regulations of member states' as a means of improving public health (European Union, 1997, p. 40).

In the early years of the new millennium, public health continued to rise up the European agenda. This was due to several factors (McKee, 2005; Neroth, 2004; Koivusalo, 2005; Byrne, 2004; Nugent, 2003): an acknowledgment that migration and the accession of economically poorer countries into the EU would present significant health challenges for the EU; a recognition of the link between health, economic efficiency and competitiveness (as part of the Lisbon agenda linking social policies to economic competitiveness); and a growing awareness of global health threats to the EU emanating from beyond its borders (notably, infectious diseases such as avian flu and SARS). There was also a belief in some quarters that because health was a major issue for citizens across Europe, the EU's involvement could help it reconnect with the public, thereby bolstering support for its institutions.

In 2002, the EU introduced a public health strategy with a budget of E353 million. This set out a six-year programme of work (2003–8) aimed at improving health information and knowledge for the development of public health; enhancing the capacity to respond rapidly to threats to health; and addressing health determinants (Decision of the European Parliament and of the Council, 2001). Following a call by the Director General for Health and Consumer Protection (Byrne, 2004) to place health at the centre of EU decision-making, a further programme was agreed in 2006 (Decision of the European Parliament and of the Council, 2006). This had three objectives: to improve citizens' health security, to promote health for prosperity and solidarity, and to generate and disseminate health knowledge. Specific areas of action were identified: responses to communicable disease; action on patient safety; efforts to address health inequalities, greater cooperation on cross-border issues; action on lifestyles related to ill health, such as alcohol consumption, smoking and illicit drug use; and efforts to improve social and physical environments related to ill health. The EU also sought to improve health monitoring across member states, to develop tools and indicators, and provide better health information for citizens. This ambitious programme went too far for some member states. Following pressure, including from the UK government, the programme budget was substantially cut back.

Nonetheless, EU public health policy continued to develop. In 2004, the European Centre for Disease Prevention and Control was established as a specific agency to identify, assess and communicate about the threat of infectious disease. In the same year, the EU agreed a new treaty establishing a European constitution. This reiterated the commitment to ensure a high level of human health protection in all policies and set out new areas for action. However, this treaty was not ratified by all member states as required (Booker and North, 2005; Treaty Establishing a Constitution for Europe, 2004). In 2007, the Lisbon Treaty was introduced in an effort to salvage the constitutional provisions. This process was delayed by the Irish Republic's rejection of the Treaty in a referendum of 2008. Eventually, the Lisbon Treaty was accepted by all member states and entered into force in 2009.

The Lisbon Treaty amends the existing EU article on public health in similar ways to the Constitutional Treaty. The new provisions involve:

- an explicit reference to wellbeing as well as physical health

- a particular emphasis on encouraging cooperation between member states to improve the complementarity of health services in cross-border areas

- possible actions to include monitoring, early warning and combating serious cross-border health threats

- initiatives to promote coordination among member states, to include guidelines and indicators, organizing exchange of good practice and preparation of necessary elements for periodic monitoring and evaluation. The European Parliament must be kept fully informed of these activities

- EU legislation to include measures setting high standards and quality for blood products, organ transplants, medicinal products and devices where there are common safety concerns

- clarification of EU powers to adopt incentive measures to protect and improve human health. In particular these could be used to combat cross-border health scourges, measures to monitor, early warning of and combating cross-border threats to health, and measures to combat alcohol and tobacco-related problems. However, this must not involve any harmonization of laws or regulations of member states

In addition the Lisbon Treaty refers to a Charter of Fundamental Rights, based on rights and freedoms contained in the European Convention on Human Rights, the Council of Europe's Social Charter (see below) and other charters and conventions. Although not part of the Lisbon Treaty, the Charter may possibly provide the basis for legal challenges to domestic health policies, and decisions even in member states that have explicitly rejected it.

In the meantime, the European Commission introduced a further health strategy in the form of a white paper (Commission of the European Communities, 2007c). This set out the fundamental principles of EU action in health: shared health values; health as a prerequisite for economic activity; and the integration of health in all policies. Several strategic aims were identified: fostering good health in an ageing Europe; protecting citizens from health threats; and supporting dynamic health systems and new technologies. Proposed actions included: the adoption of a statement on fundamental health values; a system of European health indicators; further work on reducing health inequities; health literacy programmes; a programme of analytical studies exploring the relationship between health and economic growth; strengthening the integration of health concerns across all policies across the EU; and strengthening cooperation between the EU and other international actors in the health field. The commission also included plans

for: measures to promote the health of older people, the workforce and children and young people; actions on tobacco, nutrition, mental health, environmental and socioeconomic factors affecting health; new guidelines on cancer
screening; a review of the European Centre for Disease Prevention and
Control; and action on health aspects of climate change. The Commission also
proposed a new structured cooperation implementation system to provide
advice and promote coordination within the EU on health issues.

It is possible that public health will have a much higher profile within EU
decision-making in the future, perhaps with the development of a comprehensive health strategy at this level. Although the EU involvement in health
is likely to increase (Koivusalo, 2006; McKee, 2005; Greer, 2009b), member
states have jealously guarded their sovereignty on such issues and this is
unlikely to change. Furthermore, the expansion of EU membership is likely
to make agreement on health issues even more difficult given the increased
diversity of member states. Despite the developments of recent decades, the
EU's explicit powers in health policy remain restricted. It has only a small
health budget (less than one per cent of its entire budget), which limits its
influence. Moreover, it is strongly influenced by economic interests (agriculture, alcohol, food and tobacco), which continue to exert a powerful influence over decision-making and frustrate health campaigners. In addition,
the EU remains relatively disorganized on health policy. Although the creation of the Directorate of Health and Consumers, as it is now known, was
an important advance, this remains a relatively weak directorate (Greer,
2009b). As a result, calls persist for a specific European Commission body
on health, with its own commissioner (European Health Policy Forum,
2003; European Parliament, 1999). Other, more powerful directorates, such
as those responsible for agriculture, social affairs and the internal market,
also have interests in health, although these are poorly coordinated (Greer,
2009b). However, a gradual and lower profile extension of EU activity in
public health is likely. The EU's powers are likely to be extended through
the 'back door' in the form of regulations in areas such as health and safety,
food standards, trade and the environment, and through its social policy
programmes (Greer, 2009b).

The main EU institutions relevant to health policymaking (see Baggott,
2007; Greer, 2009b) include the Council of Ministers, the key legislative body
on policy matters. This comprises ministers from the member states having
relevant responsibilities for the issue being discussed. The European Commission, often regarded as the civil service of the EU, proposes and oversees the
implementation of legislation and policy. The European Parliament, which
consists of directly elected members from each state, has some legislative
powers and is charged with holding the Commission to account. The European Court of Justice makes judgments on cases brought under EU law and
given the supremacy of this body of law, has an impact on policy, including

health. There is also a European Council, which consists of the heads of state of member countries. This body sets the direction for overall policy, which can include health issues. There are also high-level advisory bodies – the Economic and Social Committee and the Committee of the Regions, but these do not appear to have had a significant role in health policy (Greer, 2009b).

The Lisbon Treaty has altered the EU decision-making process in a number of ways that should be mentioned. The Parliament now has new powers over legislation, the budget and international agreements. Also, the Council of Ministers will make more decisions by qualified majority voting, making it more difficult for individual states and smaller blocs to veto decisions. Even so, it should be noted that with regard to health, the overt powers of EU institutions remain quite restricted, and enforced harmonization of laws and regulations is explicitly ruled out. Public health organizations and campaigners seek to influence the EU policy process and now devote more resources to this. There are a variety of ways in which they can put their views across. The Commission, for example, has standard consultation processes where health groups can seek to influence policy. For instance, a European Health Forum was established to improve communication between the Commission and health groups, although some believe that this is more tokenistic than representative (Greer, 2009b, p. 33). The European Parliament is also open to lobbying by health groups. It should be noted that EU institutions are also subject to lobbying from interests that seek to limit EU public health policy, such as the alcohol, food and tobacco industries. The relative influence of the public health and industry lobbies over EU policy is considered in the context of specific issues in later chapters.

The Council of Europe

The Council of Europe, although not an EU body, is relevant to European public health policy. Founded in 1949, it has 46 member states. The Council of Europe aims to uphold democracy, human rights and the rule of law. To this end, it seeks to develop common responses on issues of concern relating to politics, culture, society and the law. One of its key functions is to promote charters protecting human rights. This began with the 1950 European Convention on Human Rights. Signatories, including the UK, are bound by its provisions. Individual citizens in such countries may pursue cases in the European Court of Human Rights (ECHR) or in their domestic courts if their country has incorporated the Convention into its laws. The UK incorporated the Convention when it implemented the Human Rights Act 1998. The importance for public health is that this brings within the scope of the courts decisions by authorities affecting life and liberty. For example, cases may be brought if they involve public health decisions that restrict liberty (such as a ban on activities involving health risks) or those that fail to protect life (Montgomery, 2003).

A further document issued by the Council of Europe (1996), and signed by countries including the UK, is the European Social Charter. This places several public health responsibilities on states, which could form the basis of legal challenges if not fulfilled (Montgomery, 2003). Its provisions include the removal wherever possible of the causes of ill health, the provision of advisory and educational facilities for health promotion and the prevention of infectious and other diseases, and of accidents. The Council of Europe issues guidelines and standards in a variety of fields relevant to public health, which includes the regulation of hazardous chemicals, transplants and blood products. The Council has also encouraged citizen engagement in health. It has promoted action in areas such as palliative care and nutrition and has encouraged policies to help vulnerable groups such as elderly and disabled people and people with HIV/AIDS. Although the Council of Europe has no direct influence on policy, it does have a role in building cooperation on health matters across Europe. It has a health department that works with the European Commission and WHO European Region on issues of common interest. Areas of cooperation in recent years have included school health promotion, the quality and safety of blood products and organs, and drug dependence.

Conclusion

As noted at the outset, the globalization of public health has both advantages and disadvantages. On the one hand it is associated with increased threats to health posed by our more complex, resource-hungry, fast-moving and interconnected world. It is also linked to the predations of narrow financial and commercial interests, the ideologies of governments, and global institutions dominated by these interests and governments. All of which can prevent or inhibit national and local efforts to improve public health. But there is also a positive side. The globalization of public health brings opportunities to reflect upon and respond to these various problems (Beaglehole and Bonita, 2004). Indeed, it is increasingly argued that health is a global public good that must be protected by collective action via international bodies, joint action and agreements (Smith et al., 2003). Furthermore, international public health governance processes yield opportunities for public health interests to advance their policies (Princen, 2007). The playing field may not be level, and the opponents are formidable, but there are sufficient opportunities for countervailing groups to mobilize and advocate change. If these challenges are successful, this will help build a stronger framework within which national, regional and local public health policy can develop.

Public Health and the NHS

6

Although the NHS has contributed to improvements in health standards – by making care more accessible and providing specific preventive services such as immunization, screening and health education – public health has not been a major influence on NHS policies and practice (Hunter et al., 2007a, 2007b, 2010; Holland and Stewart, 1998). This chapter explores why this is so and how recent governments have sought to address this problem. The first part explores the position of public health within NHS structures and processes. The second looks at problems linked to the public health capacity and workforce. The final part examines the relationship between public health and primary care services. Although the focus is primarily on England, important variations between the different parts of the UK are discussed (see Exhibits 6.1 and 6.2).

NHS Structures and Processes

As Chapter 3 demonstrated, public health perspectives have had little influence within the NHS since its creation. Changes introduced by the Blair government, however, created opportunities to strengthen public health considerations in health service decision-making. Public health priorities were included in new public service agreements (PSAs) agreed between the Treasury and the DoH. They also featured in planning guidance to the NHS, alongside clinical service priorities. In addition, health authorities were required to produce health improvement programmes (HImPs – later renamed as health improvement and modernizations plans – HIMPs), setting out how they intended to improve public health and reduce inequalities, again alongside other service priorities.

New primary care organizations were established to replace GP fund-holders and other commissioning arrangements introduced as part of the previous Conservative government's internal market reforms. Each country of the UK adopted a different structure (see Exhibit 6.1). In England, primary care groups (PCGs) were created to develop primary care and commission health services on behalf of all general practices in each area (Cm 3807, 1997). Although dominated by GPs, these bodies also included nurses, a lay member and representatives from the health authority and local social services department. Their broad objectives were to improve the health of their local population, address health inequalities, develop primary care and community health services and improve integration between them, and advise on the commissioning of health services. It was envisaged that PCGs, which initially operated under the wing of their health authority, would eventually become primary care trusts (PCTs), statutory bodies in their own right. The move to PCT status would be gradual, reflecting different organizational capacities and capabilities. However, following the NHS Plan and a subsequent initiative to devolve powers to 'the front-line', this process was speeded up and PCTs were established in all areas in 2002 (Evans, 2004). At the same time health authorities were abolished, and their functions reallocated to PCTs and to new strategic health authorities (SHAs).

The new PCTs were larger than PCGs in terms of population covered, geographical size and resources but smaller than the old health authorities. Most of the PCT budget was, in principle, allocated without strings from the centre. However, the imperatives of national priorities, targets and quality standards reduced their autonomy in practice (Baggott, 2007).

PCTs acquired important public health functions. Each was required to appoint a director of public health (DPH), who would be a member of the PCT board, supported by a public health team. For the first time, comprehensive and explicit responsibility for promoting public health and reducing health inequalities was given to organizations with a clear primary care focus (NHS Alliance, 2002; Peckham and Taylor, 2003; Iliffe and Lenihan, 2003; Woodhead et al., 2002). Moreover, following changes to the NHS resource allocation formula, PCTs with populations having poorer levels of health received above-average increases in funding. The additional funds provided greater scope for developing new initiatives to improve health and reduce inequalities.

The cumulative impact of the changes introduced by the Blair government seemed positive. Health improvement appeared to gain higher priority within PCGs and PCTs as they developed (Wilkin et al., 2002; Regen et al., 2001). PCG/Ts contributed to local health improvement plans, established subcommittees to develop this aspect of work, and designated lead roles for health improvement and inequalities. PCG/Ts allocated resources to public health initiatives, such as accident prevention schemes, exercise programmes and community development projects (Wilkin et al., 2002). But there was much variability. Some PCG/Ts showed enthusiastic commitment to health improvement, while others did not (Abbott et al., 2001). Moreover, significant shortcomings were identified. The involvement and impact of PCG/Ts within higher level planning processes (notably, the health authority's HImPs and HIMPs) was variable (Regen, et al., 2001). There was concern that PCG/Ts lacked information about local health needs and had limited capacity, resources and skills to address public health problems (Gillam et al., 2001; Health Committee, 2001). Meanwhile, it became clear that changes to the health planning process had failed to produce the shift in emphasis required (Hamer, 2000; Hunter, 2003).

The acquisition of key public health functions by PCTs in 2002 did not address these shortcomings. Although some effective initiatives were pursued (see NHS Confederation, 2004), a lack of systematic planning for health improvement remained evident and progress was limited (Audit Commission, 2004b; CHI, 2004; Healthcare Commission, 2006). In 2003, HIMPs were replaced by local delivery plans (LDPs), produced by SHAs and PCTs. These concentrated on service developments set out in the NHS Plan and did not place a high priority on public health (Evans, 2004).

Resourcing

Although more lipservice was being paid to public health, it was still perceived as under-resourced (Connelly et al., 2005; Healthcare Commission, 2006; Wanless, 2003; Hunter and Marks, 2005). There is considerable dispute as to the extent of under-resourcing, however. Much depends on how health promotion and prevention expenditure is measured. A narrow approach includes only specific preventive services (such as screening, health education, immunization), whereas a broader measure incorporates time spent by health professionals on health promotion and preventive work. Following the white paper, *Our Health, Our Care, Our Say* (Cm 6737, 2006), which identified a relatively low spend on prevention in the UK compared with other countries, an expert group was established to develop robust definitions and measures of preventive health spending. This was seen as an essential step towards setting prevention budgets and for shifting the balance between treatment and prevention budgets. This group published a report (Health England, 2009) that calculated prevention spending as 4 per cent of total health expenditure in 2006/7, which was above the average share of resources dedicated to disease prevention (2.8 per cent) across OECD countries.

Additional spending on public health was announced by the Blair government, including £1 billion to fund the new initiatives proposed in the *Choosing Health* white paper (Cm 6374, 2004). However, an ensuing financial crisis in the NHS led to public health budgets being raided in order to reduce deficits (Mooney, 2006b; BBC, 2006; Chief Medical Officer, 2006, 2007). This led to calls to ring-fence funds for public health expenditure (Crayford, 2007). Some have suggested that, in future, public health funds should be channelled through other agencies to prevent their being diverted to other services (Hunter et al., 2007b, p. 58).

Information and Capacity

Despite the greater emphasis on public health, a lack of information about local health needs continued to cause problems, inhibiting policy and planning (CHI, 2004; Peckham, 2003; Audit Commission, 2007; Healthcare Commission and Audit Commission, 2008). Capacity and skills shortages also remained major obstacles to progress (Audit Commission, 2004b; Fotaki, 2007; Abbott et al., 2005; Chapman et al., 2003; Connelly et al., 2005; Wanless, 2004). Indeed, this situation actually deteriorated because PCTs (being smaller than the health authorities whose public health functions they took on) found it difficult to sustain the full range of public health functions. As a result, public health expertise was both fragmented and, in some smaller PCTs, isolated (Chapman et al., 2005; Evans, 2004; Wirrmann and Carlson, 2005). An additional factor was the disruption caused by the 2002 reorganization itself, which led to considerable uncertainty and poor morale within the public health workforce (Chapman et al., 2005; Connelly et al., 2005). As a result, the changes were criticized for being 'not wholly thought through' (Evans, 2004, p. 69) and 'not ... designed with public health in mind' (Abbott et. al, 2005).

As a possible solution to problems of capacity, fragmentation and isolation, public health networks were proposed (Hunter et al., 2007a, 2007b; Evans, 2004). Their aim was to pool expertise and skills, but they were patchy and slow to develop (Chapman et al., 2005). There was a lack of consensus about their purpose and composition (Abbott and Killoran, 2005; Fahey et al., 2003; Chapman et al., 2005; Connelly et al., 2005). They were criticized for being ineffective (Connelly et al., 2005; Abbott et al., 2005; Audit Commission, 2004b) and of little benefit and, consequently, a low priority (Fotaki, 2007).

A further NHS reorganization in 2006 appeared to address the problems of capacity and fragmentation. PCTs merged, their numbers were halved, producing larger organizations covering a wider area. It also led to a higher degree of coterminosity with local government authorities (that is, common boundaries with councils – around two-thirds of PCTs are now coterminous with local authorities). However, the reorganization had potentially adverse consequences for PCT links with communities, as they were now larger and more remote bodies, similar in size to the former health authorities. The restructuring process, on balance, undermined public health functions. A critical parliamentary report (Health Committee, 2006a) was scathing about the lack of consultation in the reorganization plans and noted that the public health implications were largely ignored. Problems of capacity remained and public health functions were seriously disrupted (Hunter et al., 2007b). The reorganization was blamed for disrupting public health functions and disturbing interagency relationships (see Chapter 7). Morale was again adversely affected by job insecurity among public health professionals. It transpired that the reorganization plans had been announced without the involvement of senior public health professionals, including the CMO.

Despite the problems of the 2006 reorganization, it held potential opportunities for public health. Some advantages were perceived in the stronger focus of PCTs on strategic planning, needs assessment and commissioning (Wade et al., 2006). However, by separating key parts of the public health function (that is, the staff involved in commissioning and those involved in providing services), this could create additional problems of fragmentation and possible skill shortages. Further guidance from central government called on PCTs to commission not just for health care needs but for health and wellbeing, and to reduce inequalities (Cm 6737, 2006; DoH, 2006a, 2007a). This represented an important shift in policy towards health promotion and public health. The identification of spearhead PCTs, to pilot new public health initiatives (Cm 6374, 2004), was also seen as a positive move. These PCTs, located in the most deprived areas of the country, were given additional funding to improve health and reduce inequalities. Greater emphasis was placed on joint working with other agencies, such as local government and the voluntary sector, to achieve these objectives (see Chapter 7).

However, other changes to commissioning were less conducive to health improvement. The government's NHS reforms aimed to create a market in health care (Baggott, 2004), with more choice for patients and financial incentives for providers of care and treatment. As long as the emphasis on personalized choice and payment for specific care and treatment episodes prevailed, it would be difficult for commissioners to shift resources away from health care services towards public health objectives (Hunter and Marks, 2005; Hunter et al., 2007b). The creation of foundation trusts, whose existence depended on generating revenue from contracts for care and treatment, was also seen in some quarters as inhibiting a shift towards prevention and health promotion (Hunter et al., 2007b). Foundation trusts were promised greater autonomy, potentially undermining collaboration on public health issues. Another possible threat was practice-based commissioning. By giving practices delegated budgets to commission services for their patients, similar in some respects to the previous Conservative government's GP fundholding scheme (Aswani, 2007; Audit Commission, 2006), it held similar dangers that practices would fail to prioritize public health objectives and produce greater inequalities (Hunter and Marks, 2005; Hunter et al., 2007b).

In an effort to reinvigorate commissioning, an ambitious new initiative was introduced in 2007. This aimed to make commissioning the driving force behind service improvement. Named somewhat grandiosely as 'World Class Commissioning', the aim was to transform commissioning skills in a range of areas: leadership, engagement, knowledge management, strategy development, market development, contracting and procurement and finance. Interestingly, this was not simply aimed at improving health care services.

The vision for World Class Commissioning included improving health and reducing health inequalities. Its remit also included partnership working, public engagement and needs assessment, all of which are important in the delivery of public health objectives. Like the other areas covered by this initiative, commissioners were required to achieve levels of competence, while satisfying higher tier authorities and regulators that they were developing these competences. It is too early to assess the impact of this initiative. However, the inclusion of key public health aims and activities was a positive sign and had potential to strengthen the profile of these issues on local health agendas.

The Cameron coalition government, which came to office in 2010, proposed radical changes to the NHS structure and to commissioning (Cm 7881, 2010). Adopting a decentralist approach, the government stated that SHAs and PCTs would be abolished within two years, and their commissioning functions taken on by a national commissioning board and local consortia of general practices. Public health functions would be transferred to local authorities and to a new public health service (see below and Chapter 7). At the time of writing, the likely impact on public health is unclear. However, one thing is obvious, the devolution of commissioning to localized groups will make it difficult to coordinate commissioning across larger geographical areas and populations. In the absence of strong coordination, incentives and regulatory mechanisms, it is likely that commissioning for public health (rather than health care) will suffer.

Regional Developments

Important structural changes have taken place at the regional level. The regional public health function was originally located in Regional Health Authorities. When they were abolished in 1996, their functions were relocated into new Regional Offices, part of the Department of Health (DoH). A further change occurred in 2002, when Regional Offices were themselves abolished. Regional directors of public health and their teams were transferred to Government Offices for the Regions (GORs), encouraging a more joined-up approach to public health (see Chapter 7). In 2006, SHAs, established four years before as intermediary bodies between the DoH and PCTs (with responsibilities for strategic management, performance management and coordinating the public health function) were reduced in number, becoming in effect regional health authorities. Also, the posts of regional director of public health (RDPH) and SHA director of public health (DPH) were combined (DoH, 2006c). As noted earlier, the SHAs are to be abolished, which removes an important public health function from the regional level.

Renewed Priorities

The DoH attempted to restore the emphasis on public health by issuing further guidance requiring LDPs to cover the *Choosing Health* white paper priorities. At the same time there was an attempt to strengthen joint planning between the NHS, local authorities and the voluntary sector on public health issues, discussed further in Chapter 7. The NHS performance management regime introduced by the Blair government already included health improvement and tackling health inequalities as criteria. Even so, these did not carry the same weight as those relating to access and efficiency, which were regarded by managers as crucial (Hunter et al., 2007b; Wanless, 2004). Gradually, however, public health performance indicators achieved greater prominence. For example, a third of the targets for PCTs in the 2002–5 NHS performance framework related to public health (Evans, 2004).

Following mounting criticism of its target culture (see, for example, Hunter, et al., 2007b), central government modified its approach to performance management across public services. This was given further impetus following the replacement of Blair as Prime Minister by Gordon Brown. Although Brown was an architect of the 'top-down' performance regime in his previous role as Chancellor of the Exchequer, the time was now ripe for a system that identified fewer central targets, more flexibility for local authorities to determine their own priorities, and a greater emphasis on incentives and outcome indicators. This was evident from the new generation of PSA delivery agreements issued in the autumn of 2007, one of which covered the promotion of health and wellbeing (HM Government, 2007a). This set out five key indicators: overall mortality rate; differences in mortality between the average and the most deprived areas; smoking prevalence; proportion of people supported to live independently in the community; and access to psychological therapies. Previously set disease targets for cancer, heart disease and stroke, suicide and health inequalities (see Chapters 4 and 17) remained in place. Public health indicators and targets also appeared in other PSA delivery agreements (for example relating to childhood obesity, drug and alcohol misuse, and climate change).

Within the NHS, moves to change the performance management system chimed with the Darzi review, launched in 2007. This emphasized a devolutionary approach, giving local health care bodies greater ownership of service changes and more flexibility to respond to local circumstances and challenges. The final report of the review stated that the NHS should focus more on improving health and that PCTs specifically must commission comprehensive prevention and wellbeing services, in partnership with other bodies such as local authorities (Cm 7432, 2008). Although the main emphasis of the review was upon high-quality services, particularly relating to health care, it did not exclude public health services. Indeed, these are included in new systems of quality assurance currently being developed. The Darzi review also considered the development of primary care services, emphasizing the importance of access and quality in primary care (see below) and calling for a greater emphasis on prevention of illness and the maintenance of good health.

Following Darzi, a new operating framework was established (DoH, 2008a). This stated that there would be three tiers of priorities: national 'must dos', national priorities and local actions. The first two tiers were mandatory and related to specific indicators ('vital signs') and targets. The third tier was in effect a menu of indicators, from which local PCTs could choose. However, even the local action indicators were set by national government. Moreover, choice of indicator was not purely at the whim of the PCT but must be negotiated with local partner agencies and regional bodies. The operating framework included public health priorities and indicators, including the reduction of health care related infections, keeping adults and children well and improving health while reducing inequalities as national priorities. These were reiterated in subsequent guidance (DoH, 2009a; Cm 7775, 2009), alongside specific 'vital signs' for national requirements (for example MRSA and C. *difficile* infection rates), national priorities for local delivery (for example overall mortality rates, obesity in primary schoolchildren, smoking prevalence) and local action (for example hospital admission rates for alcohol-related harm, healthy life expectancy at age 65, breastfeeding rates at 6–8 weeks). Almost half (29 out of 63) vital sign indicators in the 2010/11 NHS operating framework related to public health, health improvement or health inequalities. These topics accounted for six out of thirteen national (tier one) requirements and thirteen out of seventeen national priorities for local delivery (tier two).

The Cameron government pledged to reduce unnecessary NHS targets (Cm 7881, 2010). However, it stated that it would retain targets that had clinical value and which were geared to improving outcomes for patients and the population as a whole. It seems likely that the Conservative–Liberal Democrat coalition will retain some health targets. A public health white paper, expected later in 2010, will outline the details of the government's public health strategy.

Standards

In 2005, the Healthcare Commission, then responsible for NHS standards, included public health as one of its seven key areas (Williams, 2007; Healthcare Commission, 2006). Each area (or 'domain' in the Commission's terminology) contained specific core standards, used as a basis for determining overall performance ratings for NHS organizations. In public health, for example, health care organizations had to 'promote, protect and demonstrably improve the health of the community served and narrow health inequalities' through partnership and cooperation and by 'ensuring that the local director of public health's annual report informs their policies and practices' while 'making an appropriate and effective contribution to local partnership arrangements'. Other core public health standards related to disease prevention, health promotion programmes and arrangements for health protection, meeting requirements of national service frameworks and national plans, with particular regard to obesity, smoking, substance misuse and sexually transmitted infections. A third core standard related to protecting the public by preparing for possible incidents and emergencies. In addition, a developmental standard was set as a basis for service improvement. In order to meet this, health care organizations had to demonstrate that they were identifying and acting upon significant public health problems and inequality issues, implement effective programmes to improve health and reduce health inequalities while conforming with best practice, and to protect populations from identified new and current hazards to health. They would also be expected to take into account both current and emerging policies and knowledge in the development of public health programmes, health promotion and prevention services and commissioning and provision services.

The Healthcare Commission explored standards across the NHS by undertaking reviews of specific public health interventions (on issues such as obesity, sexual health and smoking cessation). These highlighted shortcomings and good practice, and provided impetus for improvement. The Healthcare Commission's functions have since been transferred to a new body, the Care Quality Commission (CQC), which is responsible for regulating standards across health and (adult) social care. It inherited the Healthcare Commission's core standards as an interim arrangement, but is introducing a new statutory system of registration and standards that will eventually apply across all NHS bodies (including independent contractors such as GPs and dentists). The status of health improvement standards in this new regime is at present unclear. There are fears that the new system will focus on the regulation of health care commissioning and provision. If so, this will be a retrograde step from a public health perspective, as the emphasis on population-wide health promotion and disease prevention may be reduced.

Standards are also informed by the work of the National Institute for Health and Clinical Excellence (NICE), which is responsible for reviewing the evidence base for public health interventions (a role it inherited from the Health Development Agency following the latter's abolition in 2005). NICE reports on specific areas of intervention, such as obesity, alcohol misuse and smoking cessation. NICE also has a role in relation to quality standards in general practice, discussed further below. Standards are also derived from national service frameworks (NSFs), which set out guidelines for prevention, care and treatment in a particular condition area (for example heart disease) or for a specific client group (for example older people). In 2004, the government proposed a review of NSFs, both to strengthen the role of prevention within each individual NSF and to integrate prevention guidelines across them. It was expected that a new prevention framework would be forthcoming, but this did not materialize.

Regional public health observatories (PHOs), established following the *Saving Lives* white paper (Cm 4386, 1999), have an important role in establishing the evidence base for public health interventions. They support interventions by monitoring health and disease trends, identifying gaps in health information, developing measures and indicators, advising on methods for health and inequality assessments, highlighting particular health issues, evaluating progress in improving health and reducing inequalities, giving early warning about future health problems and developing capacity for measuring and interpreting health statistics (Wilkinson, 2007; Wanless, 2004, p. 43). PHOs produce local health profiles, which have been published since 2006 for every local authority area. These profiles contain vital information about health trends, which enable local authorities and NHS bodies to set priorities. PHOs also have an important role in supporting skills development in areas such as equity audit and health impact assessment, for example.

A lack of research about the effectiveness of public health interventions has been identified as a key problem (Health Committee, 2009; Wanless, 2004; Millward et al., 2003; UKCRC, 2008). Doubts have been expressed about the quality of research in this field (Macintyre evidence in Health Committee, 2001), and a failure to disseminate existing evidence into practice (DoH, 2001a). Serious problems of capacity, under-resourcing and a lack of strategy in public health sciences have been found, despite their importance to public protection, service provision and health improvement (Public Health Sciences Working Group, 2004). *Choosing Health* attempted to address the gap in the evidence base by establishing a new public health research initiative. This included a consortium of policymakers and researchers to focus efforts on strengthening the evidence base for interventions. A national prevention research initiative was also established in collaboration with research funders in the fields of cancer, heart disease, and diabetes. Five new public health centres of excellence were created in 2008, focusing on issues such as diet, nutrition, smoking, alcohol, drugs and tobacco. A new NHS public health research programme was also launched. Additional funding was made to NICE to enable it to expand its work on public health interventions, and to the regional observatories to support their enhanced role in strengthening the evidence base.

The Impact of Change

It is difficult to assess the impact of NHS changes on public health. It appears that despite early progress momentum was lost both after 2002 and 2006, partly as a result of NHS reorganizations and funding problems. This is surprising given that no fewer than three white papers made major policy commitments on public health from 1999 onwards. More optimistically, it appears that some progress was made from 2007/8. The Healthcare Commission and Audit Commission (2008) found some improvement in overall performance among NHS bodies on public health standards. There was, however, some variation with a small minority of health care organizations not compliant with core standards. However, the narrow concept of public health (based on measurable improvements) adopted by this report did not give a clear enough picture of NHS performance to make an accurate assessment.

Exhibit 6.1

Public Health Systems in Other Parts of the UK

As noted in Chapter 4, Wales endorsed the new public health agenda earlier than other parts of the UK. As a result, efforts to reorient the NHS began much earlier. Devolution gave the Welsh government further scope to develop a distinctive approach. The organization of the NHS in Wales has been shaped by public health considerations. Local health boards (LHBs) have a wide membership and include significant representation from local authorities and the voluntary and community sectors. They along with local authorities have a statutory duty to produce health, social care and wellbeing plans, in conjunction with partnership organizations, such as the voluntary sector (see Exhibit 7.4). LHBs employ directors of public health. At national level, Wales established a National Public Health Service (NPHS) to provide public protection, disease surveillance and public health expertise. Another organization, the Wales Centre for Health (WCH) was established to provide advice on public health to the Welsh Assembly Government and to support the public health function through information about health protection and health promotion, research, public engagement and support for health promotion networks. The WCH's brief also included the development of the public health workforce, through the provision of training and the dissemination of national occupational standards. Other organizations involved in public health included the Welsh Cancer Intelligence and Surveillance Unit (WCISU) and Screening Services Wales.

Wales has recently reformed its NHS and public health structures. This occurred in the light of a report on health and social care in Wales, which recommended that more could be done to prioritize prevention and early intervention (Wanless, 2003). Also, a review of the public health function in Wales found a lack of clarity in current arrangements and significant overlaps between the responsibilities of the various national bodies (Wright et al., 2006). There is now a unified national public health body for Wales (which includes WCH, Screening Services Wales, WCISU and NPHS). This body, now known as Public Health Wales, was established as an NHS trust. In addition, the current NHS structure of local health boards and trusts has been replaced by a smaller number of integrated health boards responsible for all services in their areas.

Scotland sought to strengthen its public health function following devolution (Donnelly, 2007; Stewart, 2004; Greer, 2005, 2009a). A Public Health Institute for Scotland (PHIS) was established in 2001, following a review of the public health function in the late 1990s (Scottish Executive, 1999a). This was not established as an executive body, but to provide support and coordinate efforts to improve public health. In 2003, the PHIS, along with another body, the Health Education Board for Scotland (HEBS), was subsumed within a new special health board – NHS Health Scotland – in an effort to create a more strategic approach to health improvement. Another organization, Health Protection Scotland, established in 2004, is responsible for dealing with infectious disease and environmental health hazards.

In Scotland, health boards have overall responsibility for the NHS at local level – there are no NHS trusts. Each has a director of public health who heads a public health department. Health improvement is one of several criteria against which health board performance is measured and plans for health improvement are included in the local health plan. Under the aegis of each board are community health partnerships (CHPs), which coordinate planning, development and provision of NHS services within a specific local area. They play an important part in developing joint health improvement plans and are expected to work closely with local authorities and the voluntary sector (see Exhibit 7.4). The Scottish government has allocated additional resources towards public health interventions. These include national demonstration projects (in areas such as children's health and wellbeing, sexual health and heart disease) and programmes in areas such as exercise promotion, food and health, community development, smoking cessation and alcohol misuse prevention. Scottish health boards are required to develop an integrated workforce development plan that includes health improvement, in consultation with other stakeholders such as local authorities and the voluntary sector. A national public health workforce partnership group has been established to map the workforce, encourage professional development, map levels of training provision and apply competence frameworks. The NHS in Scotland has also set out competences for health promotion at local level (NHS Health Scotland, 2005).

The public health function in Northern Ireland is currently in a state of flux for reasons discussed in Exhibit 4.2. There have, however, been some important institutional developments, including a Northern Ireland-wide public health agency established in 2009. As noted, there is also increasing cross-border cooperation between the North and South of the island of Ireland. An all-Ireland Public Health Institute was created to share intelligence and build collaboration on common issues.

The Public Health Workforce

Public Health Medicine

Public health has been dominated by medicine (Holland and Stewart, 1998; Evans, 2003; Hunter, 2003) with senior public health posts restricted to doctors until fairly recently. However, despite its pre-eminent position, public health medicine has been in crisis for many years. There have been tensions between the various roles performed by public health doctors (Goraya and Scambler, 1998). They are: *health strategists* (providing advice on priority-setting, service planning and evaluation of outcomes); *health promoters* (developing and evaluating disease prevention and health promotion services); *health experts* (monitoring and managing outbreaks of infectious disease); *health advisors* (to decision makers and the wider population regarding risks and threats to public health); and *health bureaucrats* (managing public health services). Concern was expressed that senior public health doctors were too closely involved in the management of clinical services rather than providing leadership on health promotion and disease prevention (Holland and Stewart, 1998; Beaglehole and Bonita, 2004; Health Committee, 2001). Attempts have been made since to clarify the nature of public health medicine. Organizational changes described earlier led to clarification of the strategic role of senior public health doctors (such as regional and local directors of public health). Clearer job descriptions, based on specific competences (see below) are now the norm.

A further problem is a decline in the independence of public health medicine. Although historically Medical Officers of Health (MOHs) were never completely free from political pressures and administrative constraints (see Chapters 2 and 3), they did have considerable independence. Their modern equivalents, DPHs, are currently directly responsible to the chief executive of their employing PCT and, in the case of joint appointments, there is accountability to the local council. They also have corporate responsibility for decisions taken by management bodies on which they sit. This places additional emphasis on their managerial and commissioning roles, weakening their role as health promoters and advocates (McCallum, 1997; Goraya and Scambler, 1998; Davies, 1997; Holland and Stewart, 1998). However, some efforts have been made to clarify their independence (see Exhibit 7.3). Meanwhile, RDPHs (who currently double as SHA directors of public health) are located in Government Offices for the Regions. Arguably, their independence is even more circumscribed (Chadda, 1996; Ashton, 2000). One idea to protect the independence of public health doctors and other practitioners is to bring them under the aegis of a national public health body (Public Health Alliance, 1988; Sram and Ashton, 1998). This would operate with a high degree of independence from government. Its main functions would be to set national strategies, supply specialist public health services, and accredit relevant training programmes. It would be multidisciplinary, integrating public health expertise. Wales (see Exhibit 6.1) has already gone down this route, with the creation of a unified public health service, drawn from different organizations. The Conservative–Liberal coalition government has decided to introduce a new public health service in England, integrating existing national public health bodies. The exact constitution of this body, however, has yet to be revealed.

Another problem has been the low status and morale of public health medicine. Although again not new, it is surprising that this situation has persisted in a period where public health has risen up the political agenda (Holland and Stewart, 1998; Wanless, 2004). Attempts have been made to raise status and morale. The Acheson report (see Chapter 3) tried to do this by renaming the speciality, clarifying its functions and relationships, reasserting its leadership role, and by recommending a target level of specialist manpower. This was unsuccessful. Since then, the multidisciplinary nature of public health has been more fully acknowledged. Some see this as the saviour of public health medicine, enabling it to survive with its leadership role intact while others see it as the ultimate threat to their hegemony within the field.

Multidisciplinary Working

During the 1990s, the creation of multidisciplinary public health departments at district level was actively encouraged by the government. The publication of the report on the Chief Medical Officer's (CMO) project to strengthen the public health function (DoH, 2001a) provided further impetus. It identified three broad categories of the public health workforce:

1   Public health consultants and specialists working at a senior level of management or with a high level of expertise.

2   Professionals spending a major part of their time in public health practice, such as health visitors, environmental health officers and community development workers.

3   Professionals who have a contribution to make to public health, but may not recognize this. Examples include teachers, social workers, housing officers and some health care professionals.

The CMO's report urged that the contribution of the wider public health workforce must be recognized. It maintained that public health leaders and specialists would in future be drawn from a wider range of professional backgrounds (including nursing, social science and environmental health). Among its many recommendations were: to form a national public health forum involving the broad public health community, strengthening public health networks and using them more systematically; to maintain progress with multidisciplinary approaches to public health; and to ensure that the public health workforce is properly skilled, staffed and resourced. It also recommended core competences for public health specialists and standards of accreditation, discussed further below. The CMO's report also called for national workforce targets and development plans to be put in place, which were not published, allegedly because of their financial implications (Evans, 2004).

It is possible to create effective multidisciplinary arrangements (see Levenson et al., 1997; Hunter et al., 2007b; Chapman et al., 2003). There is now wide support for a power-sharing model, where many professionals join together to tackle the social, economic and environmental factors affecting health. However, confusion remains over what multidisciplinary public health actually means and what exactly constitutes a public health specialist (Hunter et al., 2007b; Chapman et al., 2003), although this is now being addressed (see below). There is also concern that many professional groups and workers who could contribute to the public agenda are still not engaged (Evans, 2003; Mallinson et al., 2006; Hunter et al., 2007b). The public health workforce is fragmented and sections of it remain isolated (Chapman et al., 2003; Evans, 2004; Naidoo et al., 2003). There are also continuing problems of under-resourcing, skill shortages, undercapacity and poor morale (Chapman et al., 2005; Wanless, 2004, 2007; Hunter et al., 2007b; Hunter and Marks, 2005; Faculty of Public Health, 2008).

Added to this is continued resistance from some doctors who fear that other forms of expertise are encroaching on their territory (see Chapman et al., 2003; Scally, 1996; Kisely and Jones, 1987; McPherson et al., 2001; Wright, 2007). Previously, this produced an isolationist response, reflected in a decision in 1996 not to extend membership of the Faculty of Public Health Medicine to those outside the profession (Crown, 1999, pp. 219–20). However, things have since moved on. In 1998, the Faculty approved a new category of membership for non-medical professional groups. Full membership was opened to them in 2001 (Evans, 2003, 2004). To reflect an increasingly multidisciplinary focus, it was renamed the Faculty of Public Health in 2003. A voluntary register for specialists in public health, open to those from both medical and non-medical backgrounds, has since been introduced. *Saving Lives* had earlier proposed the creation of public health specialist posts of equivalent status to medically qualified consultants in public health medicine. In 2002, non-medical public health specialists were allowed to become Directors of Public Health. Even so, elements of medical hegemony remain (Hunter et al., 2007b). Although half of public health specialists are non-medical, they are still a minority among DPHs. In 2002, less than a fifth of PCT DPH's came from disciplines other than medicine (Evans, 2004). Furthermore, non-medical public health directors are appointed on a lower pay scale (Naidoo et al., 2003, p. 81) and doctors retain a strong influence over accreditation, training and standard setting in public health (Evans, 2003).

Competences and Skills

A number of important developments have taken place since the CMO's report. The key domains of public health practice have been clarified: health improvement; health protection; and health service delivery and quality (see

Griffiths et al., 2005). UK national standards for specialist practice in public health were developed to provide a basis for standards, accreditation and practice (Healthwork UK, 2001; Wright, 2007). This covered ten key areas: surveillance and assessment of population health and wellbeing; promoting and protecting population health and wellbeing; developing quality and risk management within an evaluative culture; collaborative working; developing health programmes and services, and reducing inequalities; policy and strategy development and implementation; working with and for communities; strategic leadership; research and development; ethically managing self, people and resources.

These were later developed into a framework of national occupational standards for public health (Skills for Health, 2004, 2007), covering a wider range of public health practitioners. This set out competences in various areas of public health work including: collecting data and information about health and wellbeing; leading others in improving health and wellbeing; planning, implementing, monitoring and evaluating strategies for improving health and wellbeing of the population. Furthermore, a skills and career framework in public health was devised (Skills for Health/Public Health Resource Unit, 2008). This is intended as a multidisciplinary 'route map' for public health covering specialists, practitioners and the wider workforce. It identifies public health competences, both core (those needed by anyone working in public health) and defined (those applying to specific areas or disciplines), and the knowledge base for each level from entry to senior professional. The core competences are: surveillance and assessment; assessing the evidence; policy and strategy; leadership and collaborative working. The defined competences are health protection; health improvement; public health intelligence; academic public health; and health and social care quality. The intention is that the framework will help to identify career paths, specify posts, underpin accreditation, and inform education and training of the public health workforce across organizations. It will also provide a basis for further moves to register and regulate those working in public health.

Workforce Planning

Public health workforce planning has been neglected (Wanless, 2004; Dawson et al., 2007). *Choosing Health* (Cm 6374, 2004; DoH, 2005a) proposed that public health workforce planning be included in future workforce strategies, not only in the NHS but in partner organizations too (such as local government and the voluntary sector). In order to instil public health across the wider workforce, the government stated it would seek to align public health workforce plans with mainstream NHS workforce initiatives such as *Modernising Medical Careers*, *Agenda for Change* and the *Knowledge and Skills Framework* (see Wright, 2007).

SHAs and PCTs were expected to identify and address deficits in public health capacity at regional and local level as part of their workforce plans.

Action to expand specialist capacity in public health was planned, including an expansion in training posts, strengthening public health elements in undergraduate curricula, offering new career pathways, improving retention of specialists, developing workforce capacity; assessing possible new areas of specialist practice; and recruiting managers to support the delivery of health improvement. The government also stated an intention to develop academic public health, which had experienced a serious decline (Gray, 2007).

Subsequently, 'teaching public health networks' were established in 2006 in each NHS region to improve and integrate public heath education and training. These aimed to bring together public health teaching and practice, build collaboration between different agencies who require training for their staff, and strengthen public health competences and accreditation. National Leadership programmes in public health have also been introduced. Public health roles of existing professional groups are being extended and new public health workers created. School nurses and health visitors were promised an expanded role in public health and the public health role of other community-based nurses has also been emphasized (see Exhibit 6.2). The government issued a strategy on pharmaceutical public health (DoH, 2005b) and modified pharmacist contracts to encourage involvement in public health. The public health role of dentists was also acknowledged, the government claiming that new contractual arrangements would encourage prevention. Meanwhile, other practitioners (including GPs, nurses, midwives and allied health professions) were offered opportunities to develop special interests in health improvement.

In addition, a new occupational group, health trainers, was proposed (see also Visram and Drinkwater, 2005). It was envisaged that these workers would be drawn from local communities and would be accredited to give people advice and support on healthy lifestyles. A national core curriculum and training modules were promised to train these new workers. Initially they would be appointed in areas of highest need, before being extended elsewhere.

Although *Choosing Health* placed great emphasis on health promotion functions, including new social marketing programmes and an expansion of community-based health improvement services, health promotion specialists as a workforce group were neglected. Subsequently, however, the DoH and the Welsh Assembly funded a project to develop the specialized health promotion workforce. It recommended greater recognition and advocacy of this group of staff, improved capacity and funding, clearer career progression, development of skills and competency and better supervision, accreditation and regulation (Griffiths and Dark, 2006).

These policies and initiatives have had a limited impact (see Gray and Sandberg, 2006; Faculty of Public Health, 2008; Wanless, 2007). Indeed, it appears that the capacity of the public health workforce was actually reduced in the years immediately following *Choosing Health*. Public health training was particularly badly affected by cuts in training budgets (Health Committee, 2006b; Gray and Sandberg, 2006). The total specialist public health capacity (excluding academics) fell (from 14.1 per million to 10.9 between 2003 and 2007 (Faculty of Public Health, 2008). In 2007 less than half (49 per cent) of respondents to a survey by the Faculty of Public Health (2008) reported that their team had adequate capacity. There is also concern that plans to establish training and skill development across agencies have been slow to develop (Healthcare Commission/Audit Commission, 2008).

The wider problems of NHS workforce planning did not augur well for public health either. A Health Committee (2006b) report criticized the 'boom and bust' in NHS recruitment and the adverse impact on capacity and training budgets. It identified 'a disastrous failure of workforce planning'. The committee found that insufficient thought had been given to workforce planning and that it lacked priority within the NHS. There was little attempt to plan long term and a failure to integrate plans across different professional groups. The fundamental problems identified by the committee, if not addressed, represented a major threat to specific plans for the public health workforce, which depend heavily on a long-term shift in capacity across several professional groups. More optimistically, however, the specific contribution of the public health workforce has been recently reiterated. The Darzi review issued specific guidance on workforce development, acknowledging the increasing demands on the public health workforce as a result of government priorities such as reducing obesity, heart disease and alcohol misuse, and emphasizing their importance to the key objective of helping people stay healthy. The review stated that 'we will address this by seeking to strengthen the numbers and skills of the public health workforce' (DoH, 2008b, p. 16). This was followed by a report from the NHS workforce review team (2009), a national body which works on behalf of the NHS to identify priorities in workforce development. The report identified the public health workforce as a key area for growth and development in the future, largely because of the increasing demands on these staff (from the 'staying healthy' and child health initiatives in particular, see Chapter 9). It is also possible that the new public health service in England, coupled with ring-fenced budgets for public health as promised by the Cameron government, may strengthen the public health workforce by improving its status, training and resources.

Primary Health Care

Although all aspects of the health care system have implications for public health, primary care perhaps has the greatest potential impact. There is much compatibility in principle between primary health care and public health (Green et al., 2007; Peckham and Exworthy, 2003). The vision of primary health care set out in the declaration of Alma Ata (WHO/UNICEF, 1978) was heavily influenced by public health principles. It emphasized a positive perspective on health, the reduction of inequalities, the promotion and protection of the health of the people, community participation and inter-sectoral working. According to this vision, primary health care should include a range of services to address health problems in the community, including preventive, promotional, curative and rehabilitation services. It should include health education, adequate food supply and nutrition, water and sanitation; maternal and child health care; immunization, disease prevention and control, treatment of common diseases and injuries and the provision of essential drugs. According to the Alma Ata philosophy, primary health care must contribute to the development of a comprehensive health care system, giving priority to those most in need. Health workers are expected to work in teams to meet health needs. Recently WHO (2008b) called for a renewal of these primary health care principles, with a particular focus on universal access and coverage in health systems, reorganizing services around primary care and social health protection, the pursuit of healthy public policies and improved governance, participation and accountability.

Primary health care has not lived up to this vision. In the UK, and in many other industrialized countries, primary health care is really a collection of professional health services rather than a system contributing to health improvement and equity (Green et al., 2007). The focus of primary health care reform is mainly on improving personal health services rather than adopting community-oriented primary care interventions (Iliffe and Lenihan, 2003). Primary care and public health tend to occupy separate worlds (Taylor et al., 1998; Meads et al., 1999; Ashton, 1990; Peckham and Exworthy, 2003). This has arisen for several reasons. There is a lack of agreement on key concepts between those working in primary health care and those in public health. There is often poor communication between these groups. Another factor is the dominance of primary health care by GPs, who tend to concentrate on disease manifested in individuals rather than on population health. Indeed, public health-oriented GPs have been in a minority (Tudor Hart, 1971; Widgery, 1988) and there has been substantial opposition if not hostility to public health initiatives within general practice (Fitzpatrick, 2001). As a result, primary care has neglected wider socioeconomic and environmental factors related to ill health. A further problem is a lack of public health capacity and skills among primary care professions and in primary care organizations.

Primary Care Reforms

Successive governments have tried to widen the focus of primary care to include health promotion. In the 1980s and 90s, a series of reforms were introduced that culminated in changes to GP contracts (Cmnd 9771, 1986: Cm 249, 1987). GPs received payments for: meeting targets on immunization and cervical screening; carrying out health checks on patients; and providing specific health promotion activities, such as special clinics for people with high risk of disease. In 1993, health promotion payments were replaced by a system targeted at the prevention of smoking, heart disease and stroke. Further changes, in 1996, led to GPs being paid according to locally agreed activities (see Le Touze and Calnan, 1996; Adams et al., 2001). The revised scheme did little to motivate practices beyond the minimum needed to trigger payments (Baeza and Calnan, 1998; Adams et al., 2001; Taylor et al., 1998; Health Committee, 2001). A minority of practices, however, did adopt a more positive approach to health promotion (see Cornish et al., 1997), for example undertaking assessments of the health needs of their practice population and building closer links with local public health departments.

Exhibit 6.2

Public Health Nursing

Nurses have great potential to contribute to health improvement (Butt, 2007; Standing Nursing and Midwifery Council, 1995; DHSSPS, 2003, 2005; DoH/CPHVA, 2003; Scottish Executive, 2001a; DoH, 1999a, 2004b; NAfW, 1999a). They are the largest professional group and have extensive contact with the public, offering many opportunities to promote health. Nurses interact with a range of other professionals, within and outside the NHS, enabling them to fulfil important networking and partnership roles in public health. They also have expertise, knowledge and information about health needs, which can be used to develop public health strategies and practices.

While all nurses can contribute to public health objectives, specialist nurses are particularly important:

- *Health visitors* are qualified nurses or midwives who, following a period of further training, specialize in providing advice and support for preschool children, disadvantaged children and families. Some also work with other vulnerable groups, such as homeless people, asylum seekers and elderly people. Although most of their workload involves specific individual or family cases, they are aware of structural factors affecting health and health inequalities and can promote community-wide interventions (UKPHA, 2009; Lowe, 2007; Cowley et al., 2007).

- *School nurses* are concerned with the health of school-age children and are the lynchpin of school-based health programmes. Their precise tasks include health surveillance, screening, immunization, counselling and health promotion. They also provide support for schoolchildren with complex health needs and have a role in child protection (Ball and Pike, 2005).

- *Midwives* have an important function in monitoring and promoting the health of women and their babies both during pregnancy and in the period following childbirth.

- *Practice nurses* working in GP practices now undertake a range of important health promotion tasks, such as health promotion and disease prevention clinics, immunization, and screening (see Eve et al., 2000; Broadbent, 1998; Audit Commission, 2004b).

- *Occupational health nurses* specialize in workplace health, in particular the minimizing of risks of physical injury, rehabilitation of sick or injured employees, and promoting positive health and wellbeing in the workforce.

- *District nurses* work with people with long-term, chronic illness in the community. This gives them an important role in maintaining and promoting the health and wellbeing of these people (Arnold et al., 2004).

- *Communicable disease control nurses* and *community infection control nurses* are vital to preventing the outbreak and spread of infectious diseases, and minimizing the threat of other environmental hazards.

- *Community psychiatric nurses* support people with mental illness in the community and help to improve their health and wellbeing.

- *Other specialist nurses* (such as clinical nurse specialists, nurse practitioners and nurse consultants) may specialize in health promotion and disease prevention (for example sexual health, drug misuse).

However, the potential of nurses to contribute to public health has not been fully realized (DHSS, 1986; Billingham and Perkins, 1997; Winters et al., 2007; Hart, 2004; Lowe, 2007). There has been a lack of a 'public health philosophy' within nursing. Like medicine, nursing is dominated by care and treatment rather than prevention and health promotion. Although a substantial number of nurses undertake public health roles, they are in a minority. Furthermore, even these nurses are fragmented into different professional groups, leading to poor inter-professional relationships, rivalry, overlap and duplication, adding further to the lack of clarity about what public health nursing actually means.

Nursing remains dominated by medicine, which in turn is dominated by biomedicine. Most nurses are employed in roles subservient to doctors. Hence practice nurses have developed a health promotion role only insofar as GPs have allowed them to do so (Eve et al., 2000). Others – nurse practitioners, health visitors and school nurses – have enjoyed greater autonomy. But they have struggled to attain leadership positions in public health and have had little impact on public health policy. Moreover, there is a gap between policy rhetoric about the crucial role of nurses in public health and their daily professional experiences. In practice, their role is more narrowly defined (Mackenzie, 2008; Popay et al., 2004). They have limited opportunities for challenging existing ways of working and applying a broader public health perspective in their work.

Key public health professionals, notably health visitors, school nurses and district nurses, have faced an increasing workload not matched by additional resources. The number of health visitors, for example, fell between 1990 and 2008 despite increasing workloads (Derrett and Burke, 2006; Audit Commission, 2010a). At current levels of staffing, this workforce does not have the capacity to provide a universal service offering proactive health promotion and identifying additional needs (Cowley et al., 2007). There are also concerns about lack of training, both in terms of new training places and continuing professional development of qualified health visitors (Family and Parenting Institute, 2009). School nurses have also declined in number while facing high and increasing demands (Ball and Pike, 2005; and see Chapter 9). Meanwhile, district nurses have reported that increasing caseloads are a barrier to developing a greater public health role (Arnold et al., 2004). The failure to match increased workload with resources has meant that public health nurses concentrate on crisis management rather than on developing strategic responses to underlying causes of health problems. A further problem has been the reorganization of the NHS and local government, which has disrupted relationships between public health nurses and other agencies. Reorganizations have also failed to address fundamental problems of inadequate administrative support and the location of staff.

Policymakers and regulators have proposed ways of strengthening public health nursing. In England, the nursing contribution to public health has been explicitly endorsed in government policy documents (Cm 4386, 1999; Cm 6374, 2004; Cm 6737, 2006; DoH, 1999a, 2004b; *Every Child Matters*, Cm 5860, 2003). Public health nurses are seen as having key roles in assessing community needs, contributing to health strategies, leading multidisciplinary teams and coordinating inter-agency partnership working. In addition, standards of care for health promotion practice were produced (DoH, 2006b). Standards of proficiency for specialist community public health nurses have also been set out (Nursing and Midwifery Council, 2004). A commitment was made to modernize school nursing and develop a national programme for best practice. Additional resources were promised in order to allow PCTs to employ one full-time, all year round school nurse working with a cluster of primary schools and its related secondary school (see Chapter 9). New community matron posts were established to improve the health of people with complex health problems. Health visitors were promised a role in overseeing new child health promotion programmes. A review of health visiting was also commissioned (Lowe, 2007). Efforts to produce closer teamworking have been evident, particularly in relation to children's health and welfare. For example, government has encouraged the co-location of health visitors and other professionals, such as community midwives, in children's centres (see Chapter 9). Although these new policy commitments appear impressive, public health nursing continues to face considerable problems of lack of clear focus, fragmentation and under-resourcing (UKPHA, 2009; Derrett and Burke, 2006; Popay et al., 2004).

Other parts of the UK have also examined the scope for changes in public health nursing. In Wales, a review of primary care and community nursing (Irvine and Kenkre, 2004) confirmed the importance of a public health role for community-based nurses. However, it found a lack of clarity around roles and functions and the need to provide a stronger focus on prevention. It called for a clear strategy, backed by resources. The report recommended a school nurse for every school; increased recruitment and investment in school nursing; the development of multi-skilled teams in the school nursing service; the development of a specialist public health role; and nurse-led, first contact primary care to be coordinated and led by highly skilled nurse practitioners/ practice nurses; and improvements in education and training. At the time of writing, the Welsh Assembly Government is consulting on proposals to reform community nursing (Welsh Assembly Government, 2009b).

With regard to public health nursing in Northern Ireland, an all-Ireland approach was taken. This led to the development of a joint statement on public health nursing, a clearer definition of public health for nurses, an action plan, and an implementation phase that concentrated on specific areas of achievement: networking and leadership; education; practice development; and developing an electronic database to support these activities (DHSSPS, 2003, 2005). This provided a boost to public health nursing. However, it was acknowledged that more must be done to engage the nursing workforce in public health issues and integrate occupational standards for public health into education and training programmes.

In Scotland, a review of nursing recommended a strengthening of public health nursing in the community (Scottish Executive, 2001a). As a result, school nurses and health visitors were given the title of 'public health nurse'. Additional investment in recruitment and training for public health nursing was promised. A new strategy was introduced for school nursing, focusing on health improvement. New public health practitioner posts were appointed at local level to lead and coordinate on public health issues, most filled by nurses or health visitors. Early evidence showed that the public health practitioner scheme worked well, particularly in promoting collaborative working and community development, but that more could be done to strengthen their influence over strategy (MacGregor, 2006). Despite efforts to develop a broader public health role in Scotland, considerable barriers remain including the higher status of clinical duties, low priority of public health work, and a lack of adequate support and infrastructure (Cameron and Christie, 2007). The Scottish Executive subsequently backed moves to create a new community nursing service that aims to promote health, reduce inequalities, support people to live more healthily in their homes and promote self-care. This will be based on a generic community nurse role to supersede district nursing, health visiting and school nursing.

Further reform of professional contracts in primary care offered opportunities to strengthen the focus on public health. In the late 1990s, drawing on Conservative government legislation, the Blair government piloted new forms of locally negotiated primary care contracts for personal medical services (PMS). This was done to encourage new forms of service provision, such as nurse-led practices and salaried GPs. PMS contracts were seen as a way of facilitating the development of primary care services in deprived and underserved areas of the country. This had implications for public health, given that people with the highest needs are located in such areas. They were also thought to give greater scope for flexibility and innovation than the standard contract. Although some innovative PMS schemes emerged, evaluations found that the overall picture was less positive (Sheaff and Lloyd-Kendall, 2000; PMS National Evaluation Team, 2002). The level of experimentation was less than expected, contracts failed to link incentives to objectives, and performance monitoring was weak. Subsequent research found that although PMS contracts facilitated improvement in the quality of care, the mechanisms of change (effective management, clear objectives and changing professional relationships within the practice) were not unique to PMS practices (Campbell et al., 2005). Dissatisfaction with the pace and scale of change brought by PMS led to the introduction of alternative provider medical services (APMS), which enabled PCTs to contract with independent sector organizations to deliver primary care services. This provided further scope for developing new services in disadvantaged areas. However, the scheme was heavily criticized for giving a foothold to private corporations whose interests lay more in providing services for profit rather than promoting public health (Pollock et al., 2007).

Meanwhile, renegotiation of the standard general medical services (GMS) contract led to measures linking payments to GPs to the quantity and range of services provided (Aswani, 2007; Peckham and Hann, 2008). A new contract, introduced in 2004, specified three types of service that practices could provide: essential services (which must be provided – for example seeing patients in surgery for a consultation); additional services (which practices may opt out of – immunization, cervical cancer screening) and enhanced services (a range of additional specialized services that the practice wants to provide). Payments are now linked to a quality and outcomes framework (QoF). Initially, this outlined indicators in 10 clinical areas (coronary heart disease, asthma, chronic obstructive pulmonary disease, hypertension, stroke, mental health, hypothyroidism, epilepsy, diabetes and cancer). Other clinical areas were later added in 2006/7 (palliative care, obesity, chronic kidney disease, learning disabilities, smoking, atrial fibrillation, dementia, depression and heart failure) and existing indicators have been amended. In addition, practices are assessed on the basis of organizational performance (for example information and records, practice management), patient experience (for example patient satisfaction, length of consultations), holistic care (to measure the breadth of care across clinical areas) and (for those practices that provide them) additional services.

The emphasis on clinical performance indicators in primary care may seem a useful step towards improving public health, but there are several problems with the approach currently adopted (Peckham and Hann, 2008). First, it may disincentivize activities that are not included in the framework or which attract a lower financial reward. It has been argued that some important health problems (for example alcohol misuse) have been neglected as a result (Alcohol Concern, undated). Second, some indicators may not be appropriate. For example, in relation to depression, health consumers' and patients' organizations have argued that indicators fail to reflect the prevalence of depression across the population as a whole and must cover the longer term management of depression in general practice (Depression Alliance/SANE, 2007). It has also been shown that practices can earn additional payments for measuring cardiovascular risk factors but this does not necessarily reduce the risk of cardiovascular disease (Guthrie et al., 2007). In general, the indicators adopted by QoF reflect service provision and clinical processes rather than health outcomes. Third, there are concerns that QoF may contribute to increased health inequalities (Peckham and Hann, 2008). This could arise from the difficulties of identifying and measuring illness in deprived and ethnic populations, leading to their neglect. However, some studies have found that health inequalities narrowed following the introduction of the framework (Ashworth et al., 2008; Doran et al., 2008).

Pressures to reform QoF have grown. There have been calls for stronger incentives to reduce health inequalities and to improve health outcomes (Health Committee, 2009; Healthcare Commission/Audit Commission, 2008; Wanless, 2007). The Darzi review (Cm 7432, 2008) saw reform of QoF as a way of giving incentives to maintain good health. Subsequently, NICE was given the role of developing clinical and health improvement indicators. Its task is to produce reviews that assess the cost-effectiveness of new and existing indicators, which can then be considered for inclusion in future QoFs.

The current GP contract does not embody a clear strategy for developing, supporting or rewarding public health activity in general practice (Peckham and Hann, 2008). Indeed, some public health interventions may be discouraged by the contract. Cervical screening and immunization are included, but as additional rather than essential services, although it is expected that most practices will continue to provide them. Some interventions (for example alcohol interventions) are part of the enhanced service element. Although enhanced services could lead to some GPs developing special interests in areas of public health practice, which is likely to be of positive benefit, there remains a danger that by defining services as 'enhanced' many practices may decide not to participate in important areas of public health services provision.

As earlier, the Conservative–Liberal Democrat coalition government has placed great faith in GPs as commissioners of health care. However, it is unclear how and to what extent the new GP consortia will prioritize public health issues. The lesson from the past is that this tends to take second place to the diagnosis, care and treatment of individual patients.

Other Primary Care Initiatives

A range of other initiatives have been introduced with potential to improve public health. NHS Direct is a nurse-provided health care information and advisory service for the public. It was introduced in England and Wales in 1998, initially as a telephone service later extended to the internet (NHS Direct Online) and digital television. Scotland has its own version of the service (NHS 24). NHS Direct has a high level of contact with the public (over six million people a year contact it). This gives considerable scope to educate and inform the public about symptoms and health risks, with positive implications for public health. The service is adjudged as being of good quality overall (NAO, 2002; CHI, 2003), although problems with consistency of advice have been identified (Williams, 2000). Also, the service is least used by those people with the greatest health needs, such as elderly people and ethnic minorities, carrying implications for health inequalities.

Walk In Centres (WICs) were introduced in England in the late 1990s as a means of improving access to primary care. They are mainly nurse-led and provide information and minor treatment without appointment. WICs are placed in easily accessible locations, such as rail and bus stations. Their potential contribution to public health lies in their ability to provide easy access and early intervention in order to identify a health problem and prevent it from deteriorating (Grant et al., 2002). Recent evidence indicates that they do not necessarily provide quicker access to primary care (Maheswaran et al., 2007). Furthermore, they cannot guarantee continuity of care and may not have sufficient information to assess, refer and treat appropriately (Edwards, 2001; Chapple et al., 2000).

Another development was the introduction of NHS life checks (Cm 6737, 2006). As part of a drive to 'personalize' health services the 'Life Check' aimed to promote self-assessment of risks to health, particularly at critical stages in life, such as early years, childhood, early adulthood, working life and later years. It was envisaged that the Life Check would be in two parts: an initial self-assessment by individuals (and parents/carers where appropriate); advice and support for individuals to improve their own health (and referral to specialist services where necessary). It was proposed that self-assessments would increasingly be undertaken online (as part of NHS Direct Online) and form part of patients' electronic care records. The Labour government emphasized the importance of health checks to prevent illness (Brown, 2008). In 2009, it launched a mass programme of vascular disease checks (to prevent heart disease, stroke, kidney disease and diabetes) for those aged from 40 to 74, including height and weight measurements, blood pressure and cholesterol checks and lifestyle advice (DoH, 2009a; Cm 7775, 2009).

The Darzi Review and Primary Care

Following the Darzi review (Cm 7432, 2008), the government set out plans to improve primary health services. This entailed GP and dental practices being regulated in future by the new Care Quality Commission; a new strategy for the QoF (already mentioned above); investment in prevention by PCTs and their partners; and joint strategic assessment of needs (discussed in Chapter 7). A key proposal was the establishment of new GP-led primary care centres in each PCT area. These would offer longer opening times and bring together a range of services (including minor surgery and diagnostic tests). These would cater for registered patients and would offer a 'drop in' service for those not registered. Earlier, there had been controversy about the government's intention to create 'polyclinics', bringing together local primary care services. Many believed this could lead to the closure of existing practices and privatization of primary care. Although the idea of 'polyclinics' was replaced by 'GP-led health centres', anxiety about the impact of new arrangements on existing services remained.

The Labour government also sought to extend patient choice in general practice, making it easier for patients to switch GPs. It also aimed to reinvigorate practice-based commissioning. Both the choice agenda and practice-based commissioning, as noted earlier in this chapter, are difficult to reconcile with a broader public health focus.

Exhibit 6.3

The Wider Contribution of the NHS to Public Health

Much of the debate about the contribution of the NHS to public health has focused on how services might be reoriented to promote health rather than just treat illness. However, the NHS can help deliver public health improvements in other ways. As the largest single organization in the country and the largest employer, it has enormous potential to shape health, promote sustainable development and strengthen the socio-economic fabric of communities (Coote, 2002). The NHS can contribute across a range of areas including employment, provision of childcare, health and safety, the provision of food, procurement of goods and services; management of waste, transport, energy, capital investment and building works. However, this potential is not fully realized, notably with regard to sustainable development (see also Dooris, 2006) and the health of NHS staff (DoH, 2009b).

Hospitals have been particularly unresponsive to the public health agenda. Their primary focus on care and treatment tends to override considerations about community, environmental and public health. There have been attempts to address this, however. The Health Promoting Hospitals project, a WHO European Regional Office initiative, aims to strengthen the ability of hospitals to promote health and prevent illness (Gray and Hicks, 2007). Over 80 UK hospitals are part of this project, which particularly seeks to extend hospitals' role in disease prevention, health promotion and rehabilitation.

The Department of Health has proposed that the NHS should become an exemplary employer in terms of promoting good health, promising a national workforce strategy reflecting this aim. Although undoubtedly a step in the right direction, much depends on the extent to which strategies are implemented. A review of policies in this field found that much improvement was needed (DoH, 2009b). It recommended improved organizational performance in preventing ill health among staff, including the development and implementation of strategies by NHS trusts supported by senior management, training and performance assessment. The review also urged proper assessment of risk factors and, as well as core services to meet nationally specified standards, trusts should provide additional health and wellbeing services to meet their staff needs. In order to realize the full potential of the NHS to improve public health, the service must take into account the wider health implications of its own decisions and actions. For public health considerations to shape the NHS would be unprecedented, providing a major challenge to current practice.

Conclusion

There is now much more emphasis within the NHS on public health, health improvement and reducing health inequalities than was previously the case. There is a stronger policy framework in terms of commitment to public health objectives. In addition, efforts have been made to strengthen implementation through NHS planning processes, allocation of responsibilities for public health and performance management systems. Attempts have been made to clarify public health roles and competences, improve accreditation and training and plan for the future public health workforce. Problems of capacity, skill shortages and resourcing remain, however. These efforts will come to little if insufficient resources are provided to expand and develop public health capacity and skills.

The NHS remains an institution dominated by the biomedical approach to health. This is as true in primary care as in hospital and specialist services. Biomedical dominance remains a major barrier to developing the public health approach of the NHS. It is being challenged by some polices – incentivizing GPs to focus on health promotion, commissioning for health and wellbeing, including public health criteria in performance management systems, extending public health training to non-specialists and strengthening public health nursing. Other policies, however, are operating in the other direction, such as patient choice, markets and payment by results, and other reforms that fragment the NHS into competing organizations. The move to decentralize commissioning could also be a step in the wrong direction from a public health perspective. Until and unless these other, more powerful policy streams are geared to health improvement and the reduction of health inequalities, the achievement of public health objectives will be limited.

Public Health Beyond the NHS

7

Although the NHS can make an important contribution to public health, it cannot undertake this task alone. Many of the levers, skills and resources that affect health and illness are possessed by other public agencies, notably local government organizations. The voluntary and private sectors also have a potential role to play in improving health. Moreover, little can be achieved without the active involvement of communities themselves. This chapter explores the contribution of other agencies and the wider community to public health and examines efforts to create stronger partnerships in this field.

Partnerships

Essentially, a partnership is a joint arrangement between two independent bodies seeking to cooperate in achieving a common goal (Audit Commission, 1998). However, there is much confusion surrounding the term (Ling, 2000; Powell and Glendinning, 2002; Sullivan and Skelcher, 2002). Partnerships vary according to the formality of their arrangements, their degree of autonomy, inclusiveness, styles of interaction, and mode of governance. Furthermore, the features of a partnership can change as it develops (Lowndes and Skelcher, 1998). The diversity and dynamism of partnerships make it difficult to compare and evaluate them. Nonetheless, principles of successful partnership have been identified (Hudson and Hardy, 2002). They include: acknowledgement of the need for partnership, clarity and realism of purpose, commitment and ownership, development and maintenance of trust, clear and robust partnership arrangements, monitoring and review processes and organizational learning.

Partnerships between different agencies have been promoted both as a means of providing more coherent responses to social problems and improving service delivery (see Balloch and Taylor, 2001; Newman, 2001; Perri 6 et al., 2002; Sullivan and Skelcher, 2002; Glasby and Dickinson, 2008). Potentially they have benefits, including the ability to transcend narrow organizational perspectives; develop innovative approaches; enable pooling of resources, expertise and knowledge; improve coordination of activities and reduce costs of overlap and duplication. Partnerships were boosted by the Blair government's drive to promote 'joined up government' and area-based welfare initiatives that involved multiple agencies, including the private and voluntary sectors (Clarke and Glendinning, 2002; Craig, 2003; Perri 6 et al., 2002). Partnership was closely related to the Third Way philosophy adopted by the Labour administration, which emphasized holistic government, community-based action, voluntarism and a more pragmatic approach to social interventions, including a role for the private sector and markets (see Chapter 1).

The rationale for partnerships in public health has long been acknowledged. Partnership is seen as 'an essential ingredient of public health' (Peckham, 2003, p. 70), which can be adopted at international, national, regional and local levels (Davies and Foley, 2007). It is viewed as a means of tackling the key determinants of health, sharing responsibility for public health, avoiding overlap and duplication, and engaging with communities. At the international level, WHO has championed a positive and holistic approach to health, while emphasizing multi-agency action across a range of policy arenas, as well as the need to work with communities (see Chapter 5). This is reflected in international declarations and strategies, such as *Health for All*, and specific programmes and initiatives aimed at strengthening partnership working. An example is the *Healthy Cities* programme (see Exhibit 7.1). Another is the Verona initiative, launched in the late 1990s, which supports capacity building for multi-sectoral action to promote health. Partnership working on health matters has been driven by other international agendas, notably the environmental sustainability agenda (see below and Chapter 11). It is also increasingly important within EU decision-making in the light of commitments to include health considerations in all policies (see Chapter 5).

Successive UK governments have emphasized the importance of multi-sectoral working in health. Central government has sought to improve coordination between national departments and agencies with little success (see Chapter 4). It has also tried to build alliances, collaboration and partnerships in public health at regional and local level, discussed further below.

Exhibit 7.1

Healthy Cities

The *Healthy Cities* programme emerged from debates about the role of cities as a focal point for health promotion (Davies and Kelly, 1992; Ashton, 1992; Duhl, 1986). It was launched by the WHO European Regional Office, with three main elements: the improvement of the health of poor and disadvantaged people; the reorientation of health services towards primary care; and an emphasis on public involvement and partnerships between the private, voluntary and public sectors. By 1991, thirty cities had joined the programme, four from the UK (Belfast, Glasgow, Liverpool and the London Borough of Camden). This has since risen to over 600 municipalities world-wide (Lawrence and Fudge, 2007). Cities participating in *Healthy Cities* were expected to adopt specific interventions based on *Health for All* principles (see Chapter 5), to monitor and evaluate interventions and share their experiences. All agreed to focus upon interventions aimed at reducing health inequalities and to establish coordinating mechanisms involving agencies that could contribute to health promotion.

Studies of Healthy Cities (see Costongs and Springett, 1997; Green, 1992; Lawrence and Fudge, 2007; de Leeuw and Skovgaard, 2005; Berkley and Springett, 2006), identified several benefits, including: focusing attention on the needs of deprived populations, greater awareness of social and environmental factors in ill health, and some reported improvements in inter-agency relationships. They also revealed implementation problems, difficulties in coordinating action between agencies, professional barriers, limited resources and a lack of sustainability. Assessment of impact was impeded by a lack of good quality research evidence (Tsouros, 1990; Curtice, 1992; Hancock, 1992; Kelly et al., 1992; Costongs and Springett, 1997; de Leeuw and Skovgaard, 2005). Evaluation was impeded by the difficulty of demonstrating short-term benefits, the presence of confounding factors affecting health (such as growing social inequalities, increased migration and the decline of traditional industries) and the co-existence of area-based initiatives (such as Local Agenda 21, regeneration programmes and health action zones).

Regional Government and Partnerships

In the 1990s, Government Offices for the Regions (GORs) were created by amalgamating regional branches of several government departments (Departments of Trade and Industry, Education, Employment, Environment and Transport). The GORs were seen as centralizing bodies, coordinating and monitoring the implementation of national policies at regional and local level (Pearce et al., 2008). This perception of their role remained, despite efforts by central government to give them a strategic role in a less centralized system of performance management, discussed further below.

The GORs gradually incorporated some regional functions of other departments, including the Department of Health. In 2002, regional public health directors (RDPHs) and their teams were relocated to the GORs. This brought public health expertise closer to decision-making about key issues affecting health, such as economic development, housing and transport (Ross and Tomaney, 2001; Health Committee, 2001; Evans, 2003). In 2006, SHAs were reduced in number, so that most had boundaries coterminous with a GOR. In addition, the posts of SHA director of public health and RDPHs were combined. It was expected that this would further strengthen joint working across different departments and sectors. In 2006, the DoH issued guidance to

GORs and SHAs requesting them to agree specific aims and arrangements for improved health and wellbeing in their regions. However, the Cameron government plans to abolish the SHAs by 2013. At the time of writing, the future of GORs is also in doubt. It will be interesting to see how this impacts on health planning at the regional level.

GORs have also worked with other regional bodies. Regional Development Agencies (RDAs) were established to promote sustainable economic development and regeneration. Regional Assemblies (RAs), which scrutinised the work of RDAs, had additional powers and responsibilities including strategic planning on issues such as sustainable development, transport and waste (ESRC, 2005). At the time of writing, both RAs and RDAs are also to be abolished.

In London, the situation is different from the rest of England. A Greater London Authority is headed by an elected mayor, scrutinized by an elected assembly. The mayor has strategic powers in housing, adult education, waste management, environment and sustainable development, transport, economic development and policing. Public health also falls within the remit of the mayor, who has a specific duty to improve the health of Londoners (Ross and Tomaney, 2001). The mayor acquired the responsibility to produce a health inequality strategy. However, the mayor has no statutory powers and few resources in relation to health (although powers in other areas such as transport and economic regeneration have important public health implications). The mayor has influenced the agendas and actions of other bodies through partnership working (Ross and Tomaney, 2001; Hunter et al., 2005) and by setting out specific strategies on issues such as food and air quality. This activity has been driven to some extent by the Health Commission for London (which includes among others representatives of the NHS, local government and the King's Fund) and by the appointment of the London RDPH to the mayor's cabinet.

Outside London, there was also more emphasis than previously on reducing health inequalities and greater awareness of the social, economic and environmental factors associated with illness. Regions developed strategies for public health (see for example: East Midlands Regional Assembly, 2003; East Midlands, Public Health et al., 2009). Although varying in detail, they covered similar topics (for example smoking, obesity, health inequalities), reflecting national priorities, but also addressed specific regional concerns. Some regions were more advanced in developing plans and building partnerships than others. However, the proposed abolition of regional bodies will make it more difficult to develop a more coherent response to public health problems.

Local Authorities and Partnerships

As previous chapters have shown, local government contributed much to health improvement prior to the creation of the NHS. However, during the postwar period local authorities lost important responsibilities and their public health role declined. The case for re-establishing this role is strong (see Campbell, 2000; SOLACE, 2001; Cm 6939, 2006; LGA/UKPHA, NHS Confederation, 2004; LGA, 2008). Local authorities can lead their communities and shape the places where people live (Clarke and Stewart, 1994; Sullivan, 2007). They plan, regulate or provide a range of services that affect health and wellbeing. They are democratically elected, to some extent accountable and responsive to the local community. Local authorities gather information about health needs and preferences, useful in strategic and service planning. Their work brings them into contact with a wide range of local organizations in the public, voluntary and private sectors, giving them a key role as a coordinator of agencies. In addition, as significant employers (both directly and through subcontractors), local authorities can influence the health of a large proportion of the local population.

During the 1980s, a minority of local authorities sought to re-establish a leadership role in public health (Harrow, 1991). They did not have a national framework to guide and support them (except in Wales, where a collaborative model of health promotion was developed – see Exhibit 4.2). Some local authorities were directly inspired by international initiatives, including *Health for All* and *Healthy Cities*. Another driver was Local Agenda 21 (LA21), part of the Rio Summit's Agenda 21, which encouraged the development of holistic plans for sustainable development encompassing both environmental and public health matters (see Chapter 11).

The *Health of the Nation* strategy of 1992 emphasized collaborative working between the NHS and other agencies, including local authorities, through 'healthy alliances' to combat diseases such as cancer and heart disease. It generally had a positive effect on collaboration, especially where good local relationships between the NHS and local government already existed, or where national initiatives, including funding, were already in place – such as HIV/AIDS awareness programmes, smoking cessation and accident prevention (DoH, 1993; Scriven 1998; Trevett, 1997; Cornish et al., 1997; Levenson et al., 1997). Even so, the strategy was inhibited by a failure to engage fully with local authorities, which were seen as marginal rather than central to the new public health agenda (Hunter, 2003). Likewise, local authorities lacked ownership of the strategy and did not regard it as having much impact on their work (DoH, 1998). It turned out that local authorities were not sent copies of the *Health of the Nation* document on publication (DoH, 1998, p. 29). The marginalization of local authorities was exacerbated by the strategy's emphasis on disease and its neglect of environmental and socioeconomic factors in health (such as housing, pollution and poverty).

The relationship between the NHS and local government has been problematic, particularly with regard to the interface between the NHS and local authority social services (Glasby and Littlechild, 2004; Hudson and Henwood, 2002; Health Committee, 1999). Collaboration on public health, while receiving much less attention, has been similarly weak (Snape, 2004; Health Committee, 2001; Hunter, 2003; Hunter et al., 2007a, 2007b). The *Health of the Nation* strategy failed to address this. It could, for example, have set out new responsibilities to work in partnership, additional powers and extra resources, which might have stimulated greater collaboration. As a result, notwithstanding good examples of joint working, healthy alliances encountered fundamental problems, including fragmentation of responsibilities, poor collaboration between agencies, insufficient resources, and isolation from key planning and commissioning decisions (DoH, 1998; Ewles, 1993; Nocon, 1993; Cornish et al., 1997).

The Blair Government's Partnership Agenda

The Blair government tried to strengthen partnership working between the NHS and local government on a range of issues. The Department of Health produced joint guidance for the NHS and local government, including joint responsibilities in areas such as health inequalities. National service frameworks (NSFs), which set out key principles and service standards, included guidance on partnership working. At the local level, PCGs and PCTs were given responsibilities for improving health and reducing health inequalities (see Chapter 6) and expected to engage with local authorities and other stakeholders. To underpin this, a new statutory duty of partnership for the NHS and local authorities was introduced in 1999. This required their cooperation in improving health and welfare. Primary care organizations included representatives from local authorities and the community on their governing bodies. Pooled budgets were introduced, primarily for improving joint working in social care but applicable also to public health. Joint investment plans relating to health and local government services were established for specific groups, such as elderly people and people with mental illness. On top of this, performance management processes in the NHS and local government increasingly emphasized collaborative working as a means of achieving common targets (such as reducing childhood obesity, teenage pregnancy and health inequalities).

Joint working was encouraged by initiatives to promote health in deprived areas. Health action zones (see Exhibit 7.2) were introduced in the late 1990s to improve inter-agency collaboration in the identification of health needs, health improvement, the provision of services, the reduction of health inequalities, and the involvement of local people. Another programme, Sure Start (see Chapter 9), which aimed to improve the health and wellbeing of preschool children in deprived areas through additional, improved and integrated services, also entailed a multi-agency approach. Health was also identified as an element in multi-agency regeneration programmes, such as the Neighbourhood Renewal strategy (see Chapter 17). In addition, plans to promote closer working between agencies on issues such as children's welfare (see Chapter 9), crime prevention, youth justice and drug abuse gave further impetus to establish effective partnership arrangements (in these cases also involving other agencies, such as the police and probation services).

Exhibit 7.2

Health Action Zones

Health action zones (HAZs) were established in England in 1998 to improve inter-agency collaboration in areas of high health need (Powell and Moon, 2001; Barnes et al., 2005; Matka et al., 2002; Judge and Bauld, 2006). They existed as a separate programme until 2003, when they were absorbed by PCTs. Their aims were to: identify and address the public health needs of an area; ensure that services were efficient, effective and responsive; and develop partnerships for health improvement and service provision. The HAZs also had a brief to integrate services, reduce health inequalities, and engage with local communities. In all, 26 HAZs were created, covering 13 million people. Some schemes focused on integrating health and social care services for particular groups, such as elderly people or those with mental illness; some focused on improving access to primary and community services, while others were geared to health improvement, such as smoking cessation or accident prevention.

The diversity of HAZs, coupled with a failure to measure their impact on health outcomes, made them difficult to evaluate (HDA, 2004; Health Committee, 2009; Perkins et al., 2009; O'Dwyer et al., 2007). There was indirect evidence that HAZ areas had a positive impact on some mortality rates, but this was not conclusive (Bauld and McKenzie, 2007). Even if a significant reduction in mortality rates across the board had occurred, it would have been difficult to attribute to HAZs alone, because they often co-existed with other health promotion and regeneration initiatives (Berkeley and Springett, 2006). HAZs also aimed to encourage public involvement, although their achievements here were limited (Health Committee, 2001; Crawshaw et al., 2003). The main positive impact of HAZs appears to have been on partnership working. They were credited with strengthening the broader public health perspective, getting health-related issues onto local agendas, improving working relationships between the NHS and local government, and facilitating shared learning among local agencies and professionals (Bauld and McKenzie, 2007). They promoted experimentation and stimu-lated debates about changes to service provision. Their main contribution lay in promoting organizational and cultural change as a basis for long-term improvements in partnership working. Indeed, these 'intangible' benefits were significant and may have laid the foundation for long-term improvements (Boydell and Rugkåsa, 2007).

HAZs, like other community-based public health interventions, faced difficulties in proving their worth in the short term (see Coote, 2004). Their achievements were diluted by setting ambitious goals, in the context of limited capacity and modest resources (Judge and Bauld, 2007; Davies and Foley, 2007). They were also under-mined and outflanked by other reforms, notably the uncertainties created by NHS reorganization, the development of a performance culture based upon crude targets, and the emergence of other initiatives designed to strengthen partnerships in public health (notably, local strategic partnerships – LSPs).

Local authorities were promised a greater role in the health arena (Cm 4386, 1999; Cm 4014, 1998). In England and Wales, they acquired new powers to promote or improve the economic, social and environmental wellbeing of their communities alongside a new duty to formulate a community wellbeing strategy. Community strategies have since been renamed as sustainable community strategies, and are expected to relate to broader issues concerning sustainable development (see Chapter 11). A national evaluation of community strategies has since found that partnerships between local agencies both broadened and deepened following their introduction, but that significant barriers to joint working remained, including difficulties involving stakeholders, a lack of compatibility between organizational structures of partner agencies, differences in agendas and priorities and a lack of joined-up working in central government (Darlow et al., 2007; ODPM, 2005a). Over 90 per cent of community strategies referred to health and social care issues (ODPM, 2005a). Case studies revealed some good practice in partnership working on health improvement planning although this was by no means widespread (Hamer and Easton, 2002; Perkins et al., 2009). The primary focus of partnership working between the NHS and local government remained strongly on social care (Snape, 2004; Darlow et al., 2007). Meanwhile, local authority wellbeing powers were, initially at least, underutilized. However, this may have been partly due to their using existing powers, in areas such as housing or environmental health, to secure improvements in public health (Snape, 2004; ODPM, 2005a).

Planning and Performance Frameworks

The planning and performance framework for local authorities has been ambivalent, with some elements conducive to partnership, community leadership and innovation, and others discouraging this (Snape, 2004). The Labour government's 'Best Value' regime for local government, introduced in 1997, appeared to offer opportunities for councils to innovate and collaborate in areas such as public health by compelling them to review functions in terms of their efficiency, economy and effectiveness. Overall, however, the regime did not radically challenge existing practices. It concentrated on improving current services rather than developing new roles and partnerships. Local authority involvement in partnership working and community leadership was, however, stimulated by performance indicators, both under the Best Value regime and the comprehensive performance assessment (CPA) system introduced in 2002 (Healthcare Commission/Audit Commission, 2008). Even so, performance indicators highlighted service performance at the expense of health promotion activities. This has had two main consequences. First, it reinforced the interface between the NHS and local authority social care services as the most important partnership in health policy, at the expense of public health (Snape, 2004). Second, it deterred services such as housing, environmental health and transport from taking a bigger role in public health. Indeed, an analysis of environmental health services found their detachment from the public health agenda was partly due to an emphasis on performance management of service provision – although other factors such as increased workload, additional statutory duties and limited resources were also to blame (Burke et al., 2002). Others also found that environmental health services were isolated from the public health agenda, and had a poor relationship with the NHS (Shaw et al., 2006). Another element of the local government performance agenda, generally though seen as conducive to improvements in partnership working, is the beacon council scheme, introduced in 1999. This rewards and disseminates innovative and best practice by local authorities in a range of areas including public health. Its weakness, however, lies in its voluntary nature and that it lacked the clout of 'top-down' performance management systems (Snape, 2004). The beacon council scheme is to be replaced by a local innovations award scheme in 2010.

Further changes to performance management were implemented to increase local flexibility and encourage stronger partnership working. Local public service agreements (LPSAs), introduced in England in 2000, were based on negotiations between local authorities and central government. Service improvement targets based on local and national priorities were agreed, with local authorities rewarded for achievement. LPSAs were credited with improving local partnerships, although their ability to promote lasting service improvement was less clear (Sullivan and Gillanders, 2005). LPSAs were followed by the piloting of local area agreements (LAAs), which identified joint targets across local public authorities including the NHS and local government. LAAs are discussed further in a moment. There are also multi-area agreements (MAAs) which exist between public sector bodies. These are not confined to the administrative boundary of a particular council. MAAs focus primarily on economic improvement, but include issues such as housing and regeneration which also have implications for public health.

Overview and Scrutiny

Local government's health role was further extended by the introduction of statutory health overview and scrutiny committees (OSCs) in England and Wales in 2003 (Campbell, 2002; Martin, 2006; Coleman and Glendinning, 2004; Centre for Public Scrutiny, 2005; Edwards, 2006; NPCRDC, 2006). The NHS must consult OSCs when substantial changes in service are proposed and must supply information to them in the course of their inquiries. Although health service changes form an important part of the work of OSCs, they do have a broader remit to scrutinize services, which may include concerns about access and quality of care. OSCs have also explored the public health agenda, including issues such as health inequalities, mental health, obesity and teenage pregnancy. OSCs have been credited with improving communication between the NHS and local government, raising issues that are traditionally marginal to the NHS (for example transport and health), and raising the profile of health and wellbeing issues on council agendas. In some cases this has led to stronger public health leadership and partnership working at local level (see Health Care Commission/Audit Commission, 2008).

Rationalizing Partnerships

The 'plethora of partnerships' (Health Committee, 2001) in health and other related areas of policy, created problems of its own. There was little coordination between the various partnership bodies, which led to overlap, duplication and confusion. To bring greater coherence, local strategic partnerships (LSPs) were introduced in England as overarching bodies (similar bodies exist in other parts of the UK, see Exhibit 7.4). Initially, LSPs were required only in certain areas (those designated as Neighbourhood Renewal Fund areas – see Chapter 17). However, the government decided that they should be the umbrella body for partnerships in all local areas. LSPs seek to incorporate the range of partnership bodies and agreements and include representatives of local stakeholders such as NHS bodies and local authorities, as well as other public bodies such as the police, training and educational providers, the voluntary sector and businesses. Their actual membership varies considerably, as do their governing arrangements. The main task of LSPs is to produce the local sustainable community plan and ensure that all stakeholders sign up to and implement it. However, they cannot compel involvement in or compliance with plans and agreements. Some regard them as simply another layer of bureaucracy (Coaffee, 2005). They have limited resources and their accountability has been called into question. A wide variation in the overall quality of partnership working between different LSPs has also been noted (ODPM, 2003a, 2006; Geddes et al., 2007; Audit Commission, 2009).

The *Choosing Health* white paper (Cm 6374, 2004) attempted to further strengthen local partnerships in public health by reiterating the importance of LSPs and proposing that the plans of the NHS and local government, and other relevant local bodies, be brought together. To this end, LSPs were given a key role in developing and delivering outcomes of new local area agreements (LAAs), which were expected to become the key instrument for setting and achieving local targets. LAAs are based on agreements between local partners and the relevant GOR. They specify expected outcomes and resources alongside partnership working arrangements. Although it is too early to arrive at a full judgement about their effectiveness, early problems were encountered. There was initial confusion about their purpose among stake-holders, and it appears that the scale of the task faced in achieving joint outcomes may have been underestimated (see ODPM, 2005a, 2006). On a more positive note, LSPs and LAAs came to be seen as important mechanisms for strengthening partnership working (Healthcare Commission/Audit Commission, 2008; Hunter et al., 2007b).

Choosing Health aimed to promote partnerships in other ways. It exhorted local agencies to pool resources on issues such as diet and nutrition, alcohol misuse, smoking and sexual health. It endorsed the practice of joint appoint-ments of DPHs by PCTs and local authorities (see Exhibit 7.3) as a means of promoting integration. It was envisaged that partnership initiatives would be pioneered in the 'spearhead areas', those which faced the greatest public health challenges. A further commitment was to extend public health work-force planning and training to include local authorities and the voluntary sector in order to extend the capacity of the public health function (see Chapter 6), although this was slow to develop.

These themes were reiterated and developed in the *Our Health, Our Care, Our Say* white paper in 2006 (Cm 6737). This proposed closer alignment between the planning, budgeting and performance management systems of PCTs and local councils. It called for more joint appointments and the estab-lishment of multi-agency teams. LAAs were again identified as the main vehicle for aligning the plans of local agencies or stakeholders. It was envis-aged that PCTs and local authorities would in future be subject to joint performance assessment (see below). They were also expected to engage more fully in joint needs assessment and joint commissioning for health and wellbeing. The Department of Health (2007a) subsequently produced a framework for commissioning to guide the activities of PCTs and local authorities. The importance of joint needs assessment and commissioning was reiterated by the Darzi review (Cm 7432, 2008). Darzi's report called for joint working between local authorities and PCTs to promote and maintain health, greater investment in health promotion and comprehensive health and wellbeing services. Progress on joint strategic needs assessment and commissioning has been slow, but there are positive signs, notably with regard to closer working relationships between the NHS and local govern-ment and the identification of common interests in improving commissioning (Hughes, 2009).

The reorganization of the NHS in 2006 reduced the number of PCTs and led to greater coterminosity between local authorities and NHS bodies (see

Chapter 6). This was seen as a positive development in the main. However, some argued that the creation of larger PCTs could disrupt existing relationships with smaller district councils (which undertake important public health activities such as environmental health, housing and refuse collection) (see Health Committee, 2006a). A further development was the publication of a white paper on local government (Cm 6939, 2006), which sought to strengthen local authorities' 'place shaping' role and improve partnership working at local level. It proposed improvements to local authority scrutiny of the NHS and endorsed joint approaches to planning, budgeting and performance assessment. Legislative changes were introduced in 2007, placing additional statutory duties to cooperate on local partner agencies including NHS bodies, and requiring PCTs and local authorities to undertake joint needs assessment. Furthermore, comprehensive area assessment (CAA), a new system of performance assessment, which looked at services across local agencies, was heralded as a means of promoting a more coherent approach to cross-cutting issues and encouraging partnership working at local level, including public health (Healthcare Commission/Audit Commission, 2008). It involved bringing together judgements from six different inspectorates (the Audit Commission, the Care Quality Commission, Ofsted and the inspectorates for the police, prisons and probation services). CAA focused on areas as well as organizations, explored outcomes not just processes, and looked forward, focusing on improvements rather than simply past performance.

A further initiative to join-up public services in relation to health, and other issues, is Total Place. This was introduced in 2009 in a number of pilot areas. The initiative involves local authorities, NHS bodies, the police and other agencies collaborating on efforts to improve efficiency and outcomes in relation to specific priorities. Initially, 13 areas were selected. In Leicestershire, for example (one of the pilot sites), the focus was upon alcohol and drug misuse. The project involved measuring the funds coming into the areas and how to maximize their impact. Another theme was reducing the impact of alcohol and drug misuse through joint working. One of the key outcomes was a set of new strategic proposals to combat these problems in a more efficient and effective way, focusing on prevention, reducing alcohol availability, improving the late night economy, a multi-agency A&E pilot, treatment systems and pathways, and a treatment pathway in offender management. Another part of the project involved working with partners to improve how people can access information and request services from public bodies. As part of the project, a public services board was established incorporating all the main public service authorities in the area. It is intended that this body will further develop partnership working on local priorities.

Exhibit 7.3

Joint Appointments

Joint appointments between the NHS and local government are seen as a way of improving partnership working (Health Committee, 2001; Hampton, 2001). After 2000, Directors of Public Health were increasingly jointly appointed by PCTs and local authorities (Redgrave, 2007). However, there was much variation in the precise arrangements adopted. There was often a failure to clarify the responsibilities of jointly appointed DPHs. Uncertainties surrounding the accountability of DPHs were also apparent. Further problems arose from the challenging workload associated with 'serving two masters' (Hunter et al., 2007b). Guidelines were issued to clarify the role and responsibilities of jointly appointed DPHs.

Joint appointments were boosted by *Choosing Health* and *Our Health, Our Care, Our Say*, which proposed a more integrated approach to health planning and performance assessment across the NHS and local government. Both endorsed joint working arrangements, although the latter went further by proposing a redefinition of the DPH role, more joint appointments and multi-agency teams across organizational boundaries, and greater use of pooled budgets. The emphasis on joint posts continued in the context of joint needs assessment and commissioning across NHS and local government boundaries (Cm 7432, 2008).

In 2010, the Conservative–Liberal coalition government stated that it would establish a new public health service (PHS) and transfer important public health responsibilities to local authorities. It envisaged that in future DPHs would be appointed jointly by the PHS and by local authorities, with the latter as the employing organization.

Other specific initiatives have been introduced to promote NHS and local authority collaboration on public health. Healthy Living Centres were introduced in 1998 to improve health and wellbeing at local level. These centres, which vary according to local need and circumstances, were established with funding from the National Lottery. They aim to bring together a range of health and social services (such as crèches, counselling, employment advice, youth services, health promotion services). The centres are based on partnership working between the NHS, local government and the voluntary sector. Another scheme, the Healthy Communities Collaborative, launched in 2000, focused initially on preventing falls in elderly people, adopting a community-based, multi-agency approach. A similar approach was later applied to other issues, including improving the diet of socially deprived populations.

The Communities for Health programme, which began in 2004, consisted of local authority-led partnership initiatives, funded by DoH. Aimed particularly at disadvantaged areas, the programme supported pilot projects covering issues such as smoking, alcohol, sexual health, obesity, cancer, stress and diabetes. Some schemes were aimed at the whole population, others at specific subgroups such as children, elderly people, teenagers, homeless people or other vulnerable groups. Methods included community workshops, training schemes, surveys, information and communication (DoH, 2007c). A further round of projects was launched in 2007.

A later initiative was the Healthy Communities programme introduced in 2006. It aimed to build the capacity of local authorities to tackle health inequalities, provide leadership to promote wellbeing and promote a joined-up approach to health improvement across local partnerships. The programme was funded by DoH and managed by the Improvement and Development Agency for Local Government (IDeA). The intended outcomes of this project included the creation of a model enabling councils to assess the achievement of programme aims, the development of training for local government leaders on health improvement, and the development of a network of expert advisors for local authorities seeking to mainstream public health in their activities. The project also explored issues of performance management, sought ways of disseminating best practice and improving networking on public health, and provided support for local authorities seeking to integrate health improvement activities into their services. ODPM and DoH (2005) provided a practical guide to promote action on health improvement by local partnerships. The DoH also created national support teams to assist the development of joint PCT/local authority initiatives. In 2008, a further initiative, aimed specifically at improving healthy lifestyles, was announced. 'Healthy Towns' were allocated funding from central government to reduce obesity, improve diet and encourage physical exercise. Local agencies were expected to collaborate in order to advance these objectives (see Chapter 13).

Finally, there have been efforts to improve joint working between councils and the NHS in relation to specific client groups such as children, people with mental illness and elderly people. Although these initiatives are focused on social care, they have increasingly adopted a preventive approach.

Assessing the Impact of Partnership Initiatives

One of the problems with assessing the impact of local partnership initiatives is that they are not strongly evidence-based (Glasby and Dickinson, 2008; Coote, 2004; Health Committee, 2009; Perkins et al., 2009; O'Dwyer et al., 2007; and see Exhibit 7.2). Such initiatives are by their very nature long term and are not amenable to experimental research methods (Houston, 2008). They are also difficult to separate from other initiatives, involve multiple interventions, and their outcomes are often subjective and difficult to measure. The main outcomes of such initiatives are not confined to improved health outcomes (although it is important that this can in some way be demonstrated, even if only in the longer term). Also important are improvements in process such as learning from experience, interaction between agencies and responsiveness to community-defined needs (Dobbs and Moore, 2002; Bauld and Judge, 2002; Boydell and Rugkåsa, 2007).

There is some evidence to hand. There appears to have been an improvement in the local government–NHS relationship from the late 1990s onwards, illustrated by examples of good practice (for example Campbell, 2000; HDA, 2004; SOLACE, 2001). Other, more systematic evidence supports this. PCGs, and subsequently PCTs, increasingly engaged with local authorities on health improvement matters (NPCRDC, 2006; Hamer, 2000; Wilkin et al., 2002; Regen et al., 2001; Glendinning and Coleman, 2003; Peckham, 2003), meanwhile councils began to take a greater interest in the public health agenda (Snape, 2004; Hunter, 2007b; Health Care Commission/Audit Commission, 2008) and expressed greater satisfaction with joint working arrangements (LGA, 2000). Notably, partnership working began to develop in areas outside the dominant health and social care arena, and extended into regeneration, housing, education and, to a lesser extent, transport and planning (Glendinning and Coleman, 2003; LGA, 2000). There was greater commitment to the notion of partnership working on public health in both the NHS and in local government, although more could be done by both to prioritize this (Shaw et al., 2006; Commission for Health Improvement, 2004; Healthcare Commission, 2006; Audit Commission, 2007; Healthcare Commission/Audit Commission, 2008). Partnership working has been helped by the availability of better data on local health profiles and more evidence about the effectiveness of interventions (Burton et al., 2004).

Although this is a more positive picture than hitherto, key concerns remain (see Health Committee, 2001, 2009; HDA, 2004; Wanless, 2004, 2007; Snape, 2004; Banks, 2002; Hunter, 2007b; Shaw et al., 2006; Healthcare Commission/Audit Commission, 2008; Audit Commission, 2009). Despite the rising profile of public health partnerships, progress has been inhibited by the continued pre-eminence of the NHS/social services interface. Furthermore, performance management regimes in both the NHS and local government continue to prioritize health care and social care. Although the full impact of these regimes remains to be seen, there has been little progress in integrating performance management on public health across NHS and local government (Wanless, 2007). In addition, reorganization of both the NHS and local government has disrupted local partnership working on public health. A further problem is that the enthusiasm within local government circles for a greater role in health is not uniform and therefore the engagement of local councils with the public health agenda has varied considerably (Audit Commission, 2007; Healthcare Commission/Audit Commission, 2008).

The latest evidence supports the view that there is much room for improvement. A report on the first year of CAA found considerable variations in the performance of local areas (Oneplace, 2010). A 'green flag' was awarded to services which performed exceptionally well or which demonstrated innovations: these flags were given to 63 local areas – 10 green flags related to health, but others were awarded to health-related services such as housing (4), older people (8), environment (22), children and young people (20). Red flags were awarded to areas where there were concerns about outcomes and future prospects for improvement: these were received by 48 local areas – 21 red flags related to health, 23 to children and young people, 17 to housing, 6 to older people and 4 to environment. The report highlighted some good examples of improved outcomes in health and related areas. It also pointed out that many areas had given priority to improving health outcomes and some had adopted innovative approaches. However, it also found that inequalities in health persisted and that only a few areas were addressing the multiple challenges of economic regeneration, environmental sustainability and persistent inequality.

A number of possible improvements have been suggested. These include clearer strategies and action plans, clearer accountability arrangements, greater use of flexible budgetary powers to pool resources for public health interventions, better evaluation, improvements in data and information systems and better arrangements for sharing intelligence on public health problems (Audit Commission, 2005, 2007, 2009; Healthcare Commission, 2006; Healthcare Commission/Audit Commission, 2008). Extending and increasing joint appointments has also been suggested as a way forward (see Exhibit 7.3).

A more radical approach is to reconfigure functions and responsibilities across partnerships (Perkins et al., 2009). Some have suggested transferring public health responsibilities from the NHS to local government (for example LGA, 2008). The Cameron government decided to adopt such a policy. In 2010, it announced that local government would be given new responsibilities for health improvement. In future, local authorities will employ DPHs, responsible for a ring-fenced public health budget. Local authorities will be given duties and responsibilities for joining-up health improvement. They will also be expected to work with the new PHS, which will bring together existing health improvement and protection bodies.

Partnership working will also be affected by the Cameron government's broader programme of local government reform. At the time of writing, the details of its policies in this field are being developed. However, it has already begun to dismantle regional government and has ended CAA as part of its plan to return powers and responsibilities to local government. The government has also indicated that it will return planning and housing powers to local government and introduce a general power of competence that will enable local authorities to act in the best interests of their communities.

Exhibit 7.4

Partnerships and Engagement in Scotland, Wales and Northern Ireland

Since devolution, policymakers in Scotland have highlighted the importance of partnership working (Scottish Executive, 2000a, 2003b). A special group (the Joint Future Group) was established to improve joint working between the NHS and local authorities, initially to improve services for elderly people (Scottish Executive, 2002a). The Scottish Executive subsequently established health and social care partnerships between the NHS and local government, encouraging closer alignment of budgets, a joint performance management framework and local partnership agreements. At national level, the partnership agenda was driven by the Scottish Executive, the Scottish NHS and the Convention of Scottish Local Authorities (COSLA). A further development was the creation of community health partnerships (CHPs) in 2005. These are statutory bodies operating under each health board. Their aims are: to integrate primary care and acute services, bring together community-based health care and social care, integrate children's services, promote closer working between the NHS and local authorities, improve health and reduce health inequalities. There are several different models of CHPs. Some focus on health services, while others seek greater integration between health and social care services (some have a single management structure for these services and are known as Community Health and Social Care Partnerships or Community Health and Care Partnerships).

Scottish health partnerships form part of a broader framework of community planning partnerships (CPPs) at local level. In 2003, local authorities became responsible for initiating, maintaining and facilitating CPPs. Other public bodies, such as the NHS, have a duty to participate in CPPs, alongside the voluntary and private sectors. CPPs draw up a community plan, bringing together the plans of various local partnerships, on health, regeneration, and so on. Each CPP must also produce a joint health improvement plan (JHIP).

CPPs seek to promote community development (Exhibit 7.5), recognized as a vital component in tackling local health and social problems. There is a Scottish Community Development Centre, which provides expertise, support and advice. This body has established national standards for community development, which local bodies and partnerships must achieve. Also relevant is the Scottish system of patient and public involvement (PPI), which differs from England. Each CHP has a public partnership forum (PPF), which replaced the former local health councils. PPFs are a mechanism through which local people can be engaged in planning, decision-making and service development. A national body, the Scottish Health Council, monitors PPI and seeks to ensure that the views of patients, carers and the public are taken into account by the NHS. It has local offices based in each health board area, which monitor local services and offer support on PPI issues, as well as local advisory councils, which can raise issues with the national body. In addition, the Scottish government decided in 2008 to pilot direct elections to NHS boards. Two NHS boards were chosen to trial these new arrangements.

These Scottish systems of partnership and engagement are relatively new and it is too early to judge their effectiveness. Although some initial studies have found weaknesses in community planning, joint health improvement planning and community engagement in health, this should not detract from the efforts north of the border to address these difficult issues (Audit Scotland, 2006; Scottish Health Council, 2007; Bauld and Judge, 2005).

Efforts to strengthen partnership working have also taken place in Wales (see Entwhistle, 2006; NAfW, 2001; Welsh Assembly Government, 2005a). A statutory duty was imposed on local health boards (LHBs) and local authorities to work in partnership with each other, and with other stakeholders, on public health, health care and social care issues. They are jointly responsible for formulating and implementing strategies on health, social care and wellbeing. Additional funding was provided to promote partnership working. The NHS and local government have scope for pooling and delegating budgets on public health and other areas of partnership working. There are also local health alliances, which bring local agencies and voluntary groups together to determine priorities and actions on health improvement. Formerly LHBs had coterminous boundaries with individual local authorities. This facilitated (but did not guarantee) improved partnership working. However, LHBs have since been reorganized and as a result their boundaries no longer coincide with individual local authorities.

Wales established local community strategy partnerships, to provide an overarching partnership at local level. These were responsible for producing local strategies across service boundaries. The Welsh Assembly also sought to build stronger partnerships at national level between the NHS, local government and other stakeholders such as the voluntary sector. It adopted an explicit policy of non-government sector inclusion in partnerships. With regard to public and community involvement, Wales has pursued community development as a means of improving public health and wellbeing. It has its own national body, Community Development Cymru, which led the creation of a new national strategic framework for community development for Wales in 2007. A community and voluntary sector grant scheme exists to develop capacity and capability in public health improvement. In the specific field of PPI, Wales retained community health councils (CHCs) and strengthened their role. NHS bodies in Wales are required to consult and involve the public and must undertake assessment of public and patient involvement activities. The Welsh Assembly has produced good practice guidance for PPI. The activities of local NHS bodies are monitored through the NHS Wales performance framework.

Although Wales made great strides to improve partnership working, both between agencies and when engaging with the community, problems remained (Wanless, 2003; Beecham Review, 2006; Entwhistle, 2006) – in particular, differences on key issues between agencies. Partnerships have struggled to address issues that cut across different policy and institutional agendas. Further reforms have been implemented, including local service boards and local service agreements to integrate planning, performance management and delivery across public service organizations in each area (Welsh Assembly Government, 2006a).

Partnership working has been a key policy aim in Northern Ireland for many years. Indeed, the Province was a pioneer of joined-up working, with the establishment of integrated health and social service boards in the 1970s (Heenan and Birroll, 2006).

The emphasis has been mainly upon partnerships in health and social care, although public health strategies have also promoted stronger partnerships between the NHS, local government and other stakeholders (DHSSPS, 2002a, 2004b). Specific initiatives include the establishment of 'Investing for Health' partnerships in each local area (which bring together statutory and voluntary sector bodies in order to address social, economic and environmental determinants of health), the production of local health improvement plans, health action zones and healthy living centres. Community development is a key priority, not only for promoting health and wellbeing, but to secure broader objectives such as promoting community cohesion and equality. There is a Community Development and Health Network, which supports and informs those working in this field and promotes community development in health and social policy. Northern Ireland also has its own PPI system, which is undergoing changes. The local Health and Social Services Councils (similar to CHCs) will be replaced by a new Patient and Client Council.

Currently, Northern Ireland is undergoing wide-ranging reform of public administration, which provides further scope for improving inter-agency working and community engagement. These reforms seek to address some of the problems encountered in partnership working, notably a large number of councils and other public bodies and a surfeit of partnership bodies (Policy Innovation Unit, 2005). A more coherent system of partnership working may also arise from proposals to give new local authorities more powers to lead community planning and to promote community wellbeing.

Partnership with Communities

Although local government, NHS bodies and other public bodies have a key role in interpreting local needs and coordinating action to improve public health, they cannot achieve their goals without the cooperation and involvement of the wider community. It is increasingly recognized that policymakers and practitioners must work more closely with communities and their organizations. However, these efforts encounter a range of conceptual, political and practical difficulties.

Community Participation

Community participation is, superficially, a simple concept. In the context of public health, it means involving people in the decisions and actions affecting their health and wellbeing. On closer inspection, it is far more complex, largely because the terms 'community' and 'participation' are themselves open to wide interpretation. The term 'community' is highly contested. It is used rhetorically to conjure up the notion of a closely-knit and supportive framework that satisfies individual and social needs (Baum, 2002). In reality, the community is difficult to discern amid the fragmentation of society into groups, networks and interests (Higgins, 1989; Gilchrist, 2006). Furthermore, in the context of public health, the community is often expressed using a variety of other terms, each having a different meaning: 'the public', 'citizens', 'patients', 'consumers', and 'service users' (or, in the field of mental health, 'survivors'). Although some terms are used interchangeably, they have different connotations and are often contested (see Hogg, 1999; Coulter, 2007; Wait and Nolte, 2006). For example, the use of the term 'consumer' in a health context is controversial, some arguing that it reduces the scope of participation in health to market relationships (Morley and Campbell, 2003; Needham, 2003; Rogers and Pilgrim, 2001; Williamson, 1992). However, even the term 'patient' has been criticized for prolonging an outdated, passive role for service users, especially in the field of mental health and maternity services where paternalistic practices have been strongly challenged (Baggott et al., 2005).

There is also disagreement over the meaning of 'participation'. Other terms, such as involvement and engagement are also used interchangeably, although they have different nuances (Wait and Nolte, 2006). Another term, consultation, is also subject to various interpretations, although most agree that it implies a passive form of participation (Cook, 2002). In an effort to provide some clarity, models have been devised that specify different levels of participation. The best-known perhaps is 'Arnstein's ladder' (Arnstein, 1969), which identifies a hierarchy of participation ranging down from those that give a degree of power (citizen control, power and partnership); those that are tokenistic (placation, consultation, and information) and those that are primarily a means of elite control (therapy and manipulation). Another model (Baum, 2002, p. 351) identifies a continuum of participation in public health ranging from *structural participation* (where community control predominates), *substantive participation* (where people are actively involved in determining priorities and implementation, but initiatives are externally controlled), *participation as means* (used to achieve a defined end), and *consultation* (where people's opinions and reactions to policy plans are simply gauged).

These approaches, which identify levels or continuums, have been criticized for being rather one-dimensional. In contrast, Charles and De Maio (1993) have conceptualized participation in health care as a three-dimensional activity. They identified three degrees of citizen involvement (consultation, partnership and citizen control) and argued that involvement could take place in three domains (macro-level policy, service design and resources, and individual treatment). They also identified a further dimension, reflecting different community perspectives (a narrow patient perspective or the wider public interest). Charles and De Maio's model is more useful as it allows for the complexities of community participation in health and the possibility of different approaches predominating in different domains (Baggott, 2005).

The Rationale for Greater Community Participation in Health

There are two main arguments for extending community participation in health (Wait and Nolte, 2006; Coulter, 2003; DoH, 2004c; Farrell, 2004; Anderson et al., 2002). The first is a broader democratic argument that health (and health care) decisions should have greater legitimacy and be more accountable to the community and responsive to its views and needs. Second, it is argued that greater community participation has a positive impact on health outcomes.

The assumption that the health of the community will improve as a result of increased participation is implicit in several policy documents, notably the Wanless (2002) report, which identified people's engagement with their own health as a key factor in shaping the future demand for health care. There are a number of possible ways in which health may be improved by an increase in community participation (see Naidoo and Wills, 2005; LGA et al., 2004; Anderson et al., 2002; HDA, 2000; Florin and Dixon, 2004; Tritter and McCallum, 2006). By participating in health, the community can take ownership and responsibility for dealing with health issues. It can bring lay knowledge to bear. Other resources may be mobilized, such as the skills of volunteers, for example. Furthermore, community participation may strengthen norms and values and build consensus for action on health issues. It may also facilitate the creation and strengthening of networks and social capital. Community participation can further our understanding of health needs and perspectives, particularly among disadvantaged and so called 'hard-to-reach groups' in society, enabling policies and services to be tailored accordingly. Moreover, the very act of participation could itself improve self-esteem and wellbeing in communities.

Although these are reasonable arguments, the evidence base linking participation to improved health is weak (Florin and Dixon, 2004). There is evidence linking health service improvement to participation, but impact on public health outcomes is less clear (Farrell, 2004; Daykin et al., 2007). This is largely because of an absence of systematic studies and the difficulties of carrying out research in this area. Nonetheless, there is plenty of evidence in the form of case studies to support the idea that participation improves health and that it plays an important part in building the capacity of communities to improve health (see below).

Social and political trends over the past few decades have encouraged participation (Williams and Calnan, 1996; Williamson, 1992; Kendall, 2001; Laverack, 2005). These include greater levels of health literacy, the greater availability of information about health, especially through the electronic media, the increase in media coverage of health issues, the rise of consumerism, the growing acknowledgement of the lay voice and experiential knowledge. There has also been a greater willingness to form voluntary associations and indulge in participatory politics. This has been combined with a decline in deference and trust in government and other institutions, including the professions, although trust in health professions remains relatively high (Ridley and Jordan, 1998; Sampson, 2004).

Other trends include the rise of new social movements, such as those dissatisfied with conventional models of health care (such as the mental health and childbirth movements) and those, such as the environmental movement, concerned with broader issues that have implications for health (Brown and Zavestoski, 2004; Byrne, 1997). Such movements have called for greater participation by the public along with a more holistic and preventive approach to public health problems. Another trend has been the activities of international organizations such as WHO. For example, the *Health for All* strategy and *Healthy Cities* both emphasized community participation. There has also been a specific concern about a democratic deficit in state health systems, including the NHS (Cooper et al., 1995). Other drivers include sustainable development strategies, such as Agenda 21, also based on principles of community participation.

Another key trend, perhaps surprisingly, has been the managerialist agenda, promulgated by neoliberal governments since the 1980s (Clarke and Newman, 1997). Indeed, policies aimed at extending participation emerged out of the new public management approach, which sought greater legitimacy by developing systems incorporating the perspectives of service users and the wider public (Clarke and Newman, 1997). These efforts were aimed more at securing legitimacy than extending democratic control over services but actually provided a basis for institutionalizing public and patient involvement (Baggott et al., 2005).

The recent history of public and patient participation in the UK is complex and is examined in detail elsewhere (Hogg, 1999, 2008; Baggott et al., 2005; Baggott, 2005). The first wave of reform involved the establishment of community health councils (CHCs) in England and Wales in 1974 (Pickard, 1997; Moon and Lupton, 1995; Gerrard, 2006). Until their abolition in 2003 (in England – CHCs still exist in Wales), these bodies tried to hold the local NHS to account by monitoring services and strategies (Gerrard, 2006). On a more practical level, they supported patients and the public by giving information and helping with complaints. But CHC powers were limited and they had few resources. They lacked democratic legitimacy and had difficulty maintaining their independence from NHS bodies. They were focused more on health care than public health, although some did get involved in public health and health promotion campaigns.

During the 1980 and 90s, CHCs were supplemented by other forms of participation. Many reflected managerialist and consumerist agendas, such as public satisfaction surveys and focus groups. Other activities included community development work (which has a longer history, see Exhibit 7.5), citizens juries to explore specific issues, and the creation of local advisory forums for patients and citizens. These indicated a more serious attempt to involve the community. However, even these arrangements were mainly used to consult on existing plans rather than engage with the community. There was much scope for manipulation, selectivity and bias in selecting community representatives and responding to their views. Indeed, such bodies were often seen as attempts to legitimize management decisions rather than respond to the view of the community (Jewkes and Murcott, 1998; Milewa et al., 1998; Barnes et al., 1999).

Despite the variety of initiatives to engage with the community, these arrangements were confused, fragmented, and unstable (NHSE et al., 1998). There was a high degree of tokenism, with professional and management views tending to predominate. Patient and public participation was under-resourced, focused mainly on health care services rather than public health and failed to involve the wider public. Indeed, the task of participation tended to fall on small groups of lay people, often characterized as 'the usual suspects', who, though invariably highly committed, were unrepresentative of the community at large (Anderson et al., 2002).

Following from commitments by the previous Conservative government (NHSE, 1996), New Labour reformed patient and public involvement (DoH, 1999c; Cm 4818, 2000). Although widely welcomed in principle, there was controversy, notably over the abolition of CHCs. Eventually CHCs were replaced by several different bodies: PALS (patient advice and liaison services), based in trusts and PCTs, giving advice and information to patients; ICAS (independent complaints advocacy services) supporting patients in the complaints process; PPIFs (patient and public involvement forums) advising PCTs and trusts on the views of patients and the public and monitoring the quality of services and OSCs (see above) based in local councils. A new national body – the Commission for Patient and Public Involvement in Health (CPPIH) – was established to provide a framework for local forums and represent patients and the public at national level. In addition, a statutory duty was imposed on NHS bodies to consult and involve the public. Meanwhile, other policies, such as HAZs, included requirements to involve the community and service users. Public involvement was identified as a function of PCG/Ts at the outset, and was included as a criterion in the framework for assessing the quality of NHS services.

Despite some good local examples of patient involvement and community development (see Exhibit 7.5), PPI had low priority within the NHS (Health Committee, 2003a). Most effort was focused on service provision rather on planning or public health. Indeed, participation in public health raised a number of key tensions, including how to balance 'uninformed' public views with 'expert' evidence about the effectiveness of interventions (Hunter et al., 2007b). There was a lack of understanding about how to involve the public;

even community-based initiatives failed to sufficiently involve local people (Health Committee, 2001). The new system of PPI, like its predecessor, was under-resourced, confusing, highly fragmented and dominated by professional and managerial concerns (Baggott, 2005; Hogg, 2008; Health Committee, 2003a, 2006c). Concerns about the independence and representativeness of those speaking on behalf of the community remained (Hogg and Williamson, 2001). The government responded in 2006 by proposing yet another round of reform, including the abolition of CPPIH and the PPIFs and the creation of a new system of local involvement networks (LINks) commissioned by local government. This new system was introduced in 2008.

As a footnote to this, the Conservative–Liberal Democrat coalition government stated that it would reform PPI. It proposed a new national body, Healthwatch England, to act as a consumer champion. It was proposed that this body would be part of the health service regulator, the Care Quality Commission. Local LINks would be renamed as 'Local Healthwatch'.

Community Participation beyond the NHS

From the 1990s onwards, other public authorities faced similar pressures to engage with citizens and service users, including local authorities (Bochel, 2006; Lowndes et al., 2001a, 2001b; Sullivan et al., 2004; Select Committee on Public Administration, 2001). Community participation was included as a specific requirement of regeneration and welfare programmes, such as Sure Start and the Neighbourhood Renewal strategy (see Chapters 9 and 17).

Local authorities and other public bodies increased their activities: undertaking surveys and focus groups, establishing advisory forums, consulting more regularly with citizens (sometimes using innovative methods, such as interactive websites), establishing citizens' juries and other participative forums. They also engaged in community development work and sought to build social capital in their communities (see Exhibit 7.5).

Despite this extensive activity, community participation in local government attracted similar criticisms as the NHS. Community engagement has been described as variable, with some authorities showing stronger commitment than others (Audit Commission, 2007; NAO, 2004a). Among the problems identified are limited capacity and overload, with consultation fatigue remaining a common complaint (Select Committee on Public Administration, 2001; Cook, 2002; Bochel, 2006; Taylor, 2006; Skidmore et al., 2006). There have been concerns about poor feedback to communities and a fear that much participation activity is tokenistic, with councils ignoring public views (Select Committee on Public Administration, 2001; Cook, 2002). The difficulties in overcoming public apathy and gathering the views of 'hard to reach' populations are also acknowledged (Select Committee on Public Administration, 2001; Cook, 2002; Gilchrist, 2006; Taylor, 2006). There have also been similar concerns about the representativeness of participants and dependence on the 'usual suspects' (Cook, 2002; Gilchrist, 2006). These problems also affect community participation in partnership and area-based initiatives (Burton et al., 2004).

Several possible solutions have been proposed to improve community participation in health (Glasby et al., 2006; Morley and Campbell, 2003). These include radical structural reforms, bringing responsibilities for public health under the aegis of local government, as discussed earlier in this chapter. Alternatively, health authorities could be democratized, perhaps even directly elected (currently being trialled in Scotland). A further suggestion is to improve partnership working on community participation, including greater efforts to coordinate consultation and engagement processes (see Campbell, 2000; Hamer and Easton, 2002). Notably, LSPs have a brief to improve coordination across agencies on issues such as community participation, although they have had limited success in this field (Taylor, 2006).

Other recommendations have focused on extending involvement beyond the 'usual suspects' to include people drawn from the wider community or at least to make sure that the minority who do get involved are able to contribute effectively and represent their communities (Skidmore et al., 2006; NICE, 2008a). This, however, requires a better understanding of the community, and involves working with existing community organizations, and investment in capacity through community development (see Exhibit 7.5).

Exhibit 7.5

Community Development

According to the Standing Conference for Community Development (2001, p. 5), 'community development is about building active and sustainable communities based on social justice and mutual respect. It is about changing power structures to remove the barriers that prevent people from participating in the issues that affect their lives.' Community development involves professionals, lay individuals, organizations and informal groups working on the basis of values that include social justice, participation, equality, learning and cooperation. Community development is relevant to a range of policy areas including anti-discrimination, environment, regeneration and poverty and social exclusion. With regard to health it has been defined as 'active engagement with a defined group of people over an extended period of time in order to identify and tackle some of the social, economic, environmental and political issues that determine their health and quality of life' (Naidoo and Wills, 2005, p. 123).

Community development has been described as a form of health promotion (Gilchrist, 2003). It places emphasis on empowerment, partnership, informal networks, respect for lay perspectives, and capacity building and is based on a holistic social model of health (Amos, 2002). Professionals and statutory organizations play a major role in community development, including health professionals, community development workers, local authorities and other public bodies. Much community development activity is undertaken by formal organizations, such as voluntary organizations, business organizations and partnership bodies. Community development in health has its recent origins in the new social movements of the 1960s and 70s, the community health movement of the 1970s, and the *Health for All* and sustainable development initiatives (Dalziel, 2008; Taylor, 2003; Amos, 2002; Laverack, 2005). It has deeper historical roots as well, in Victorian paternalism, the self-help movement and municipal enterprise in the field of community health.

A wide variety of activities can be classified as community development. Typically, they involve local health professionals, social and community workers working closely with community organizations to identify needs and address some of the key determinants of health (see examples from Salford, Falmouth and Sandwell in Handsley, 2007a; Morgan and Popay, 2007). Community development approaches have been used in several areas of health and wellbeing, including smoking cessation (Ritchie et al., 2004) for example. A number of models have been devised to provide a more systematic framework for community development (Naidoo and Wills, 2005): *Achieving Better Community Development* (ABCD) is based on four key principles: that planning and evaluation must be context-specific and built into projects; that evaluation must include ways of defining and measuring participation; that organizations need to be able to learn and adapt; and that the community is a key partner in evaluation. Another model, *Learning Evaluation and Planning* (LEAP), emphasizes that evaluation must be an integral part of promoting community health and wellbeing, that both providers and users should take part in planning and implementation, and that future work must be informed by lessons learned.

Government has acknowledged the contribution of local communities, groups and organizations to public health (Cm, 6374, 2004; Cm 6737, 2006). This has been reflected in national policies such as HAZs, Sure Start, sustainable development and regeneration initiatives, as well as in specific local projects. It is also evident in government endorsement of the role of the voluntary sector in public health. Even so, several criticisms of community development policy remain (see, for example, Mackereth, 2006; Naidoo and Wills, 2005; Baum, 2002). The overall approach chosen remains 'top down' with an emphasis on state and professional intervention. A distinction has been made between community development, where power is shared between professionals and lay people, and community-based outreach work, where professionals remain firmly in control (Dalziel, 2008; Gilchrist, 2003). Professionals lack skills in community development. It is difficult to secure the active involvement of apathetic and sceptical communities. Projects are often piecemeal and not sustained in the longer term, partly due to resource constraints. Partnership working between statutory and voluntary sectors remains problematic. There is also still a failure to evaluate community development initiatives, and to learn from good and poor practice, although there is now more guidance available on good practice (see Burton et al. 2004; Standing Conference for Community Development, 2001; NICE, 2008a). 'Reinventing the wheel' remains a common complaint. Finally, and more fundamentally, community development is criticized for not challenging the structures of inequality and disadvantage that lie behind health problems faced by many communities (Crawshaw et al., 2003).

The Voluntary and Private Sectors

In practice, working with the community usually means partnership with organizations that claim to represent the community. These include voluntary and community organizations and, in some cases, business organizations (Handsley, 2007a).

The voluntary sector can influence public health through health promotion, research, the provision of services and support, campaigning on health issues and by articulating the concerns of communities and disadvantaged groups (Wanless, 2004; LGA et al., 2004). Voluntary organizations can make a major contribution to community development, by acting as a bridge between public authorities and the people. A vibrant voluntary sector is regarded as a key indicator of social capital (Putnam, 2000).

Since the 1970s, governments have encouraged the voluntary sector in health and welfare, through provision of resources and by giving them a clearer role in planning and service delivery (Kendall, 2003; Wyatt, 2002). Although this offered greater opportunities for voluntary groups to play a fuller role, several problems were evident (Taylor, 1999; Craig and Taylor, 2002; Sullivan and Skelcher, 2002; LGA et al., 2004). These included: fears that the sector was being used to reduce the costs of service provision or as a form of privatization, undermining public services; tensions between voluntary organizations' service provider and campaigning roles; difficulties in maintaining their financial and political independence from the state; failure to include them as full partners in planning, especially at the strategic level; and under-resourcing of their activities.

In the late 1990s, national compacts were introduced in each part of the UK, setting out key principles and undertakings regarding the relationship between central government bodies and the voluntary sector (Morison, 2000). Subsequently, compacts were introduced at local level. LSPs were required to include community representatives and expected to work more closely with the voluntary sector (Taylor, 2006). Funding was provided to establish and develop the voluntary sector infrastructure, in the form of local community empowerment networks (NAO, 2004a). A task force was also established to identify barriers to the involvement of voluntary and community organizations in the provision of public services.

With regard to public health, initiatives such HAZs, Sure Start and regeneration initiatives emphasized the importance of partnership with the voluntary sector. The voluntary sector was mentioned as a partner in several health policy documents during this period (Cm 4386, 1999; Cm 6079, 2003; Cm 6374, 2004; Cm 6737, 2006). The DoH (2004c) drew up a specific strategic framework for the NHS and the voluntary sector and introduced guidance on patient and public involvement that acknowledged its role in service provision, health promotion and community representation. A unit was established in the DoH to coordinate policy on the voluntary sector and social enterprise (see below) along with a fund to encourage new initiatives.

What is the impact of these developments? The compacts, while important in building consensus and trust, had a symbolic value (Osborne and McLaughlin, 2002; Craig and Taylor, 2002), but were not crucial in shaping relationships between the voluntary sector and public authorities (Alcock and Scott, 2002; Baggott et al., 2005). More significant was the investment in infrastructure, reflected in greater voluntary sector activity within LSPs, and which in some areas has been translated into influence on decision-making (Taylor, 2006; NAO, 2004b). Even so, overall, the role of voluntary organiza- tions in planning processes remains peripheral and limited (Turning Point, 2004; ODPM, 2006; Shaw et al., 2006; NAO, 2004b). Moreover, where volun- tary organizations have become more involved in partnership activities, such as planning and public involvement, this has imposed a significant burden on them (Craig et al., 2004; Craig and Taylor, 2002; ODPM, 2006; Taylor, 2006). Notably, the voluntary sector contribution to public health is regarded as under-resourced (LGA et al., 2004).

Concerns about the independence of the sector have increased, as it has taken on a greater service provider role (Craig and Taylor, 2002). It is possible that voluntary organizations could be more open to manipulation by govern- ment and public bodies, stifling their advocacy and campaigning roles. Ulti- mately they may become more an arm of government rather than a representative of the community. However, there are broader concerns about their representative role (Craig and Taylor, 2002; Alcock and Scott, 2002; Baggott et al., 2005; Craig et al., 2004). There are major inequities within the voluntary sector, in terms of resources, public support and political networks. Consequently, some people have a stronger voice than others, while others lack organization and have no one to speak for them. A greater reliance on the voluntary sector may therefore reinforce existing inequities in the absence of measures to strengthen the voice of marginalized groups. Although recent initiatives have addressed this problem to some extent, with some programmes reaching new and previously unfunded groups, this remains a key issue (Taylor, 2006).

Private Sector

Increasingly, the private sector is seen as a legitimate partner in tackling public health problems. Historically, commercial enterprises have been seen as the enemy of public health. In modern times, the food and drink industries, alcohol and tobacco, and the great polluting industries such as oil, chemicals and motor manufacturing, are the 'bêtes noires' of health campaigners.

Furthermore, corporations are seen as inimical to public health because of their role in promoting economic and social inequalities and poor social conditions, and their opposition to government activities that might ameliorate them, such as regulation, taxation and welfare programmes.

Nonetheless, recent government policy in the UK has emphasized the contribution of business to health. It is argued that as people become more health conscious, demand for healthy products and services will increase, creating new markets that can be exploited by businesses. For example, trends towards healthy eating are already creating significant market opportunities (see Chapter 13). In addition to this approach, it is argued that businesses generally, and in particular those associated with products harmful to health, are preoccupied with public image. They are increasingly pursuing corporate responsibility policies, implying that they will not pursue profit to the exclusion of all other things, but are willing to undertake steps to limit adverse impacts they might have on the environment, health or society. In addition, some businesses may have knowledge, experience or resources that can promote or protect health. For example, they may have marketing skills that can be used to influence public attitudes or they may be able to convey health promoting messages to consumers (for example in stores, or on packaging).

In *Choosing Health* (Cm 6374, 2004), the government took the view that key industries such as alcoholic drinks and the food industry should be regarded as partners in health promotion. It envisaged that they would engage in self-regulation and share expertise, information and resources to support health promotion campaigns. This was highly controversial. While businesses may have an incentive to promote health, within a framework of regulation, the assumption that they will always act as good citizens was incredibly naive (Bakan, 2005). There was also broader concern about the influence of these industries over policymaking and their ability to block interventions that might be effective in improving health (see Chapters 10 to 15). There is certainly a role for the private sector as a partner and contributor to public health – examples include slimming clubs, private gyms and organic farmers – although even here there are concerns about 'profiteering' (Hunter et al., 2007b). Other businesses may also have a legitimate role in health promotion in view of their role as employers (see Chapter 10). But commercial interests can be very powerful and their involvement in health needs to be carefully managed and governed by clear principles.

Another aspect of business involvement relates to social enterprises. These businesses are driven by social or environmental objectives, which reinvest their profits to meet these objectives or to benefit the wider community rather than to enrich shareholders or private investors. There are over 60,000 social enterprises in the UK, some of which are making a contribution to health improvement. Examples include social enterprises providing care and support for vulnerable groups, which can help prevent health problems.

Some social enterprises focus on health promotion in specific population groups, for example people with mental health problems, young people, older people or ethnic minorities. Other social enterprises contribute to public health by focusing on issues such as recycling, promoting sport, transport, sustainable food, improving neighbourhoods and reducing crime (see www. networks.nhs.uk).

As a footnote to this, the Darzi review, as already mentioned, emphasized the importance of maintaining a healthy population. It proposed the creation of a coalition for better health. This would involve the public sector, businesses and the voluntary sector in efforts to improve health outcomes. It was envisaged that this would be achieved through a new set of voluntary agreements between these bodies, focused on key health improvement issues, beginning with obesity. Furthermore, the Cameron government is keen to work with businesses to promote health. It seeks to establish a 'responsibility deal' with business to share responsibility for health (Lansley, 2010b). Ominously, this implies a softer approach to the regulation of businesses that may undermine public health.

Conclusion

Recent analyses of public health in the UK have rightly pointed out the need to strengthen partnerships in this field. The benefits of better partnership working include a clearer strategic approach, greater coherence, less duplication, more resources and more effective interaction with the community. Although there appear to have been some improvements in both inter-agency partnership working and community participation, considerable problems and barriers remain. Participation remains highly tokenistic and is under-resourced, largely because of government fears of genuine community empowerment and local decision-making. Public agencies remain largely focused on their own mainstream concerns. This is partly the result of a failure to 'join-up' in central government, particularly with regard to different performance management regimes. A reassignment of public health responsibilities between the NHS and local government has, however, been proposed. It will be interesting to see how this pans out in practice. However, continued failure to mobilize public agencies and the community to achieve public health objectives may make it difficult to ignore more radical approaches to multi-sectoral working and community participation.

Public Health Services

8

This chapter explores the provision of public health services that aim to prevent disease and illness. It examines services in three areas: protection from infectious disease, screening, and health promotion. The chapter also contains two case studies of public health services: breast cancer screening and mental health promotion.

Protection from Infectious Disease

The Threat of Infectious Disease

During the middle of the nineteenth century infectious diseases were responsible for a third of all deaths in England and Wales (Logan, 1950) compared with around one per cent today. However, infectious diseases remain a threat, especially in poorer countries. Worldwide, such diseases account for 13 million deaths, and half of all deaths in developing countries. Tuberculosis, HIV/AIDS, dysentery, measles and cholera are the main killers, accounting for half the deaths in children and young adults worldwide. Infectious diseases also pose a significant risk for the population in industrialized countries (see DoH, 2007b; House of Lords, 2003). Infectious diseases disproportionately affect children, resulting in premature death and a legacy of ill health for some survivors. The cost (both human and economic) of morbidity resulting from infections is significant. Consider food poisoning, which reached 100,000 cases in the UK at the beginning of the new millennium (see Chapter 12). Sexually transmitted diseases are also a major burden on the NHS (see Exhibit 9.2).

Infectious agents may cause more illness and deaths than official statistics suggest. Indeed, a range of diseases have been linked to infectious agents (Parsonnet, 1999), including stomach cancer (Parsonnet et al., 1991), cervical cancer (Schiffman et al., 1993; Brinton et al., 1989; Lehtinen et al., 1996), childhood leukaemia (Kinlen, 1988, 1995; Stiller and Boyle, 1996), Kawasaki disease (a form of heart disease – Taubert and Shulman, 1999), multiple sclerosis (Skegg, 1991) and new variant CJD (see Exhibit 12.1). Furthermore, the threat of epidemics remains, particularly in view of their potentially catastrophic consequences (Krause, 1998; Preston, 1994; Garrett, 1994; Coker et al., 2008). The past contains many examples of large-scale epidemics, such as the influenza epidemic of 1918/19 blamed for 20 million deaths. Although alarmist predictions of a new generation of infectious diseases are probably exaggerated, one should not dismiss genuine concerns about new strains of old infectious diseases (TB, influenza). Some of these are becoming more resistant to drugs. The indiscriminate use of antibiotics has been a key factor here. Antibiotics have often been used inappropriately to treat illnesses for which they have no therapeutic effect. As a result, new drug resistant strains have developed (DoH/SMAC, 1998; House of Lords, 1998a, 2001a; Arason et al., 1996). Although strategies to deal with this have been formulated (DoH/ NHSE, 1999, 2000; DoH, 2003b), the problem remains. Antibiotics are used in animals, to promote growth, despite worries about this practice increasing microbial resistance. It is possible that humans could be infected by drug-resistant strains through the food chain (see MAFF, 1998; DoH/UK Advisory Committee on the Microbiological Safety of Food, 1999; Glynn et al., 1998).

Along with poor hygiene, antibiotic resistance is a factor in the increase in hospital-acquired infections, which each year cost around £1 billion per annum and result in approximately 9000 deaths in the UK. In particular, reported cases of MRSA (*meticillin resistant, staphylococcus aureus*) and *Clostridium difficile* have risen. The government devised a strategy (DoH/ NHSE, 2000; DoH, 2004d) with targets for reducing MRSA and *C. difficile*). Although key targets were met, problems remained, with some trusts struggling to meet minimum standards. Other types of hospital-acquired infection, which together form the majority of infections, were not subject to targets and as a result were neglected (NAO, 2000, 2004b, 2009a).

Environmental factors, such as pollution, the thinning of the ozone layer and global warming, have been linked to increased risks of infectious disease (see Chapter 11). Pollution may increase the potency of infective agents, although the precise mechanism is not known. The ozone layer protects humans and animals from UV rays and any damage to it is likely to lead to greater vulnerability to infection. Climate change, however, poses the greatest threat of all. Hotter temperatures create ideal conditions for outbreaks of infectious disease. Malaria, for example, is likely to become a serious threat in countries not currently affected by the disease. It is also predicted that climate change will bring extreme weather conditions such as hurricanes, floods and other catastrophes, which create conditions for the transmission of infectious diseases.

Other factors include increased trade and greater mobility, which increases the opportunities for the transport of microbes and their vectors. The greater mixing of populations, through new settlement patterns and migration, may also encourage the spread of infectious agents (see Wilson, 1995). Poverty also adds to the risks of infectious disease, not just in developing nations but in industrialized countries too. TB for example is associated with poverty and deprivation (Mangtani et al., 1995; Bhatti et al., 1995).

Media interest in infectious disease – particularly the threat of a large-scale epidemic – is guaranteed (Baggott, 2007; Harrabin et al., 2003). Sometimes this is misplaced, as in the coverage of the so-called 'Flesh Eating Bug' during the 1990s (Gwyn, 1999). The media may exaggerate the threat of infectious disease and produce an overreaction by policymakers. However, the challenge posed by infectious disease is formidable and likely to increase. Governments have begun to respond to this challenge. Following a review of communicable disease strategy (DoH, 2002a), the UK government established a new framework for the control and surveillance of infectious disease and other hazards. The Health Protection Agency (HPA), established in 2003, brought together various organizations in this field, including the Public Health Laboratory Service and the National Radiological Protection Board, to provide a more integrated approach to protection against hazards such as chemicals, poisons, radiation, and infectious agents. There is little evidence on how well these arrangements have performed. There have been concerns about a lack of clarity in the allocation of health protection responsibilities between the HPA and PCTs (Cosford et al., 2006; Hunter et al., 2007b). More specifically, the HPA attracted criticism over its handling of an *E. coli* O157 outbreak in 2009 at a farm open to the public, which affected 93 people, most of whom were young children (Bowcott and Campbell, 2009). An independent inquiry found that the existing regulatory structure for such farms was inadequate and that there was poor leadership and coordination between the various agencies (not just regarding the HPA, whose powers were limited in this case, but other local public health bodies as well) (see *Review of the Major Outbreak of* E. coli *O157 in Surrey, 2009*).

At the time of writing the future of the HPA is in some doubt. The Conservative–Liberal Democrat government has launched a review of health agencies. It also announced an intention to create a new public health service in England, bringing together health protection and health improvement bodies. It is likely that the HPA will be brought into these new arrangements. It should be noted that additional health protection bodies exist in other parts of the UK (Public Health Wales, Health Protection Scotland, and the Northern Ireland Public Health Agency). Meanwhile, at the European level, a new Centre for Disease Prevention and Control was established in 2004 to identify, assess and communicate about the threats of infectious disease.

Vaccination

One of the main weapons against infectious disease is vaccination. It is credited with the decline of devastating childhood diseases such as diphtheria, whooping cough, measles and polio as well as smallpox and TB (although, as discussed in Chapter 3, its role has been challenged). Vaccination has since been extended to other diseases, such as influenza, pneumococcal disease and meningitis C. Some programmes also cover other vulnerable sections of the population, such as influenza vaccination for elderly people and those with chronic conditions.

At the population level the advantages of vaccination appear to outweigh the disadvantages. Although some vaccines are associated with serious adverse reactions, most experts believe these are rare enough to justify mass vaccination. Even so, the evidence base for vaccination has been challenged (see Neustaedter, 2002; Alexander, 2003; Hann and Peckham, 2010; Jefferson et al., 2010). Individuals, moreover, may take a different view of risks. Indeed, as Bedford (2007, p. 340) has pointed out 'for an individual, the safest choice is not to be immunized but to ensure everybody else is.' Immunization raises significant issues of personal liberty, especially where there is an element of compulsion. Indeed, the Victorian era saw well-organized mass campaigns against smallpox vaccination (Chapter 2). Contemporary campaigns (which include organizations such as the Association for Parents of Vaccine Damaged Children and Justice Awareness and Basic Support – JABS) have been formed by parents who believe their children have been harmed by vaccines (Blume, 2006). Their concerns have been taken up by the media, which have fuelled the controversy with allegations of cover up and conflicts of interest among scientific advisors.

In the 1970s, there was controversy about adverse reactions to whooping cough (pertussis) vaccination. This precipitated a crisis in confidence in the programme as well as claims for compensation from parents of vaccine-damaged children. Following media and political pressure, a compensation scheme, much criticized for its parsimony, was introduced (Blume, 2006). Subsequently, in the 1990s there was controversy surrounding an association between MMR vaccination, autism and Crohn's Disease, a chronic bowel condition, following an article published in *The Lancet* (Wakefield et al., 1998). This link was dismissed by government and the medical establishment. Following revelations about the failure of the researchers to declare a perceived conflict of interest, the *Lancet* article was retracted (Horton, 2004). Further studies found no link between the MMR vaccine and autism and bowel disease (Taylor et al., 1999; Kaye et al., 2001; Makela, 2002; Madsen et al., 2002; Dales et al., 2001; DeStefano et al., 2004; Institute of Medicine, 2004; Baird et al. 2008). However, only long-term large-scale studies can fully rule out an association. The issue demonstrated that past decisions had been made on incomplete evidence with an incautious approach to risk. This lack of evidence, coupled with a hostile attitude to those who challenged the orthodox view, seriously undermined rational debate (Horton, 2004; Alexander, 2003).

Scepticism about vaccination has also been fuelled by concerns that it may damage immune systems and cause allergies. As many as 18 million Britons have an allergy (one third of adults and a quarter of children) (Levy et al., 2004) and vaccination is one of several possible causal factors identified, alongside the cleanliness of the environment, central heating systems, pollution, smoking, obesity, and genetic causes (Royal College of Physicians, 2003). Some studies found that lower vaccination rates and higher levels of childhood infections are linked to stronger immunity. Alm et al. (1999) found a lower prevalence of atopy (multiple allergies including asthma, eczema and hay fever) in children with lower vaccination rates and who took fewer antibiotics. Pertussis (whooping cough) vaccination has been associated with atopic disease (Farooqi and Hopkins, 1998). Odent et al. (1994) found that babies immunized against pertussis were nearly six times more likely to have asthma. Another study discovered that children who did not have diphtheria, pertussis, tetanus or polio vaccinations had a much lower risk of asthma or other allergic illnesses (Kemp et al., 1997). However, Nakajima et al. (2007) found no evidence of a link between pertussis, tetanus, polio or smallpox vaccination and asthma. A weak association between diphtheria and asthma was, however, found. This study also discovered a small increased risk of eczema associated with all but smallpox vaccination (and weaker associations between food allergies and all vaccinations except smallpox). No link was found between vaccination and hay fever or with later onset atopic conditions. Other studies did not find significant increases in atopic disease or wheezing illnesses following pertussis vaccination (Nilsson et al., 1998; Henderson et al., 1999). It is difficult to establish clear links between immunization and other medical conditions, partly due to confounding variables (Lewis and Britton, 1998). The evidence base remains weak and there is an absence of good quality, large-scale studies.

Screening

According to Holland and Stewart (2005, p. 6), screening is 'actively seeking to identify a disease or pre-disease condition in people who are presumed and presume themselves to be healthy'. They go on to distinguish two types: *population-based screening*, where entire groups of people at risk from a particular disease are invited for screening; and *opportunistic screening*, where individuals already in contact with clinicians are offered an opportunity to be tested to establish their risk of disease. A wide range of diseases and conditions are subject to screening, including Down's syndrome, sickle cell disease and thalassaemia, cancers (including female breast and cervical cancer) and chlamydia. Screening can be undertaken at different stages of life and may focus on specific sections of the population, such as pregnant women and their unborn children, newborn babies, children, adults, men, women, and older people.

Although screening is not a new intervention, it has become more widespread in recent decades (Holland and Stewart, 2005; Fitzpatrick, 2001; Rose, 1992). Improvements in science and technology have enabled the identification of early signs of disease. In particular, the mapping of the human genome and the availability of genetic tests (discussed below) raise the possibility of screening populations more widely for their predisposition to disease. Screening is seen by the public and by the media as an important means of preventing illness. It is widely assumed that screening enables early identification of disease and quicker treatment thus increasing the chances that lives will be saved. Screening programmes are therefore seen by governments and political parties as a way of reassuring the public and their media critics that they are safeguarding the nation's health. There is also a phalanx of vested interests in favour of screening that includes private commercial organizations (screening technology companies, private health corporations), professional groups (specialists' organizations and clinicians involved in screening programmes), health charities, and health consumers' and patients' organizations.

The Principles and Ethics of Screening

Screening is often presented as unambiguously beneficial. However, like any other intervention, it should only be undertaken on the basis of clear principles and evidence. The key principles of screening are as follows (Charny, 1994; Cuckle and Wald, 1984; Wilson and Jungner, 1968; Holland and Stewart, 1990, 2005; Rose, 1992; NSC, 2000):

- the disease or condition should be an important health problem, whose natural history is understood, and it should have a recognized latent or early symptomatic stage

- the test for the disease should be available, effective, acceptable, and safe and there should be an agreed policy on how to further investigate individuals with a positive test result

- treatment should be available for those identified as having the disease or a premalignant condition

- treatment for the disease at an early stage should be of more benefit than treatment at a later stage and should be acceptable, effective and available to all who need it

- the costs and harms of screening must be outweighed by the benefits and should give value for money in the context of expenditure on medical care as a whole

Screening raises enormous ethical issues. According to Holland and Stewart (2005, p. 146), 'screening may change a healthy individual into one with concerns about some possible illness or abnormality.' Skrabanek (1988) argued that screening healthy people is unethical because of the inherent risks involved. It is true that screening involves considerable risks, either from diagnostic tests or from subsequent treatment (BMA, 2005a). Furthermore, screening systems are not infallible. There will be cases that are not detected by screening (false negatives) and others that will be wrongly identified as at risk (false positives). Indeed, screening services are particularly vulnerable to errors, reflected in the number of 'scandals' highlighted by the media. Obviously quality control is important in order to reduce false positives and false negatives to a minimum. But there also needs to be a greater public understanding of the limitations of screening, and a more balanced portrayal by the media of its costs and benefits (National Screening Committee, 2000).

There are major economic issues to consider. Screening programmes do not necessarily represent value for money. It has been argued (see Chamberlain, 1984; Stewart-Brown and Farmer, 1997) that the potential costs and benefits of screening programmes should be more explicit. Benefits of screening include quicker diagnosis, improved prognosis, the possibility of less radical treatment, resource savings, and reassurance for those with negative results. Costs include a longer period of morbidity for those whose prognosis is unaltered, unnecessary treatment for questionable abnormalities, additional resource costs associated with health needs revealed by screening, misplaced reassurance for those who have received false-negative results, anxiety for those with false-positive results, and finally, the hazards and side effects of the screening process itself.

Another issue is that access to screening is associated with socioeconomic status, in particular ethnicity, deprivation and geographical location (Chui, 2003). If such populations make less use of effective screening programmes, it is possible that health inequalities may widen. However, the link between inequalities in access to screening and inequalities in health outcomes is poorly understood. Furthermore, as some studies have shown, it is possible to design screening programmes in such a way that inequalities between different population groups can be narrowed (Baker and Middleton, 2003).

Exhibit 8.1

_____

Breast Cancer Screening

Breast cancer is the second highest cause of cancer deaths in UK women. Over 40,000 cases of breast cancer are diagnosed each year and there are over 12,000 deaths from the disease (including a small number of men). Treatment has improved, and now over 80 per cent of people with breast cancer survive at least five years after diagnosis. In the UK, the risk of developing breast cancer is higher for affluent than deprived groups (one of the few diseases where the social gradient of illness is reversed). However, among those diagnosed, survival rates are lower among deprived compared with affluent groups. Breast cancer is often portrayed in the media as a primary threat to younger and middle-aged women, although over half the deaths from breast cancer are in women over 70. The incidence of breast cancer is increasing in the UK, the rate escalating by over 50 per cent between 1979 and 2001, partly due to improved detection and diagnosis.

The UK breast cancer screening programme was introduced in 1988. It screens over two million women each year at a cost of around £75 million. Initially the programme invited women aged 50–64 for mammography (x-ray of the breast) every three years. It now covers women aged 50–70, and older women may request the service. From 2012, the service will be extended to cover women aged 47–73. Efforts have been made to improve the quality of the service, through improved quality assurance and audit, and better techniques (such as the use of higher quality images, taking two images of the breast, and double reading mammograms). There has been concern about the number of 'interval cancers' which present between scheduled mammograms (Woodman et al., 1995; Banks et al., 2004). Moreover, there have been several high-profile cases where services have fallen below standard (for example DoH, 1997; White, 2002).

Dixon (2006, p. 499) has stated that 'few topics in medicine have been the subject of so much debate and controversy as breast screening and mammography' (see also Finkel, 2005; Hann, 1996). The main concerns are about the effectiveness of screening and its costs and harms. Initial evaluations of mammography in the USA and Sweden were extremely positive (Shapiro et al., 1982; Tabar et al., 1985), finding that almost a third of breast cancer deaths could be prevented. These studies, however, were subsequently criticized for exaggerating the benefits of screening (Wright, 1986; Skrabanek, 1988; Rodgers, 1990; Watmough et al., 1997). Although several subsequent evaluations found significant mortality reductions (UKTED – UK Trial of Early Detection Cancer Group, 1999; Alexander et al., 1999; Kerlikowske, 1995; Tabar et al., 2001; Olsen et al., 2005; Allgood et al., 2008; Blanks et al., 2000), some did not (Mayor, 1999; Sjonell and Ståhl, 1999; Miller, 1980; Verbeek, et al., 1984; Andersson, 1988; UKTED, 1988). One reason for these contrasting findings was the poor quality of research studies. A meta-analysis found that six of the eight major clinical trials were flawed and that the remaining two found no evidence that screening reduced mortality (Olsen and Gotzsche, 2000), a finding confirmed in a subsequent review (Olsen and Gotzsche, 2001). Both meta-analyses were themselves heavily criticized for applying an unrealistically high standard of evidence (Paci and Duffy, 2005; Woolf, 2000). Indeed, a further review by the International Agency for Research on Cancer (2002a) endorsed breast screening for women aged 50–69 because it reduced breast cancer mortality in this group. A further meta-analysis (Gotzsche and Nielsen, 2006) found a 15–20 per cent reduction in risk from women attending screening, but pointed out that this should be set against the potential harms and costs of such programmes, including false positives and overtreatment. It has been estimated that for every life saved as a result of screening, 2000 women have to be screened for ten years. Ten will be wrongly diagnosed and unnecessarily treated. Overdiagnosis, defined as 'the detection of cases that would never have come to clinical attention without screening' may be as high as half of all cases (Zachrisson, et al., 2006). A 10 per cent overdiagnosis rate is probably nearer the mark (Zachrisson, et al., 2006), although some studies suggest a much lower level, around one per cent of the population screened (Duffy et al., 2005). Overdiagnosis can result from the identification of conditions that may not actually progress to cause mortality. Ductal Carcinoma in Situ (DCIS) now comprises a fifth of cancers identified through screening. It is often treated aggressively (almost a third of cases now result in mastectomy). However, not all DCIS cases become invasive (Evans et al., 2001). There are also false-positive cases that receive further investigation and possibly treatment, even though they do not have cancer. Although in most cases, the all clear will be given at some stage, these women will nonetheless incur unnecessary high levels of anxiety, which may impact on their health and wellbeing (Olsson et al., 1999, Brett and Austoker, 2001).

Other harms include false negatives (Banks et al., 2004). Women may not seek help because they have been falsely given reassurance. The screening process is unpleasant and can be painful (Bruyinckx et al., 1999) – although women may be prepared to experience discomfort in exchange for reassurance. In addition, radiation from mammography may induce cancer (Berrington de Gonzales and Reeves, 2005; Law and Faulkner, 2001) although this appears to be outweighed by the reduced mortality from cancers detected. Costs include staff and equipment and unnecessary diagnostic tests and treatment for those eventually found to be free from disease. Also one must add the opportunity costs of the patients' own time and the loss of benefit from other possible uses of the screening budget. Indeed, critics of breast screening in recent years have included oncologists, concerned that money spent on screening could be put to better use treating those already diagnosed with cancer (Baum, 1999).

Furthermore, some believe that screening diverts attention away from underlying factors that may cause breast cancer (Batt, 1994). These include genetic predisposition, obesity, physical inactivity, alcohol consumption, smoking and exposure to radiation, as well as endogenous oestrogens (Darbre, 2006). The latter can occur as a result of early onset of periods, late menopause, later age of first pregnancy, and not giving birth (Travis and Key, 2003). Breastfeeding, however, is associated with reduced hormone levels and correspondingly lower risk from breast cancer. Increased exposure to oestrogens also occurs from the use of hormone replacement therapy (HRT) and the contraceptive pill – both linked to an increased risk of breast cancer (Beral and Million Women Study Collaborators, 2003; Collaborative Group on Hormonal Factors in Breast Cancer, 1996; Chlebowski et al., 2009). Other hormones, such as progesterone, may also be linked to breast cancer (Travis and Key, 2003). It has also been suggested that certain foods, rich in phyto-oestrogens (such as soya products), might have a protective effect against breast cancer. Such compounds may work by altering oestrogen metabolism in a positive way (Travis and Key, 2003), although current evidence of their effects is inconclusive (see Ingram et al., 1997; dos Santos Silva et al., 2004).

Breast cancer risk may be raised by exposure to certain chemicals, which can disrupt hormonal and endocrine systems (Kortenkamp, 2006). One possible route is antiperspirants (Darbre, 2009), although studies have produced conflicting results (Mirick et al., 2002; McGrath, 2003). Another is contamination by organochlorine pesticides, which persist in the food chain and the environment long after their use has been banned (Epstein, 1992; Watterson, 1995; Potts, 1999). Associations have been found between breast cancer risk and DDT and its metabolite DDE by some studies (Wolff et al., 1993; Dewailly et al., 1994; Romieu, et al., 2000; Hoyer et al., 2000) but not others (Calle et al., 2002; Krieger et al., 1994; Van't Veer, 1997; Hoyer et al., 1998; Lopez-Cervantes et al., 2004; Muscat et al., 2003). Aldrin, Lindane and Dieldrin have also been linked to breast cancer (Westin, 1993; Ibarluzea et al., 2004), as has beta hexachlorocyclohexane (B-HCH) (Zou and Matsumara, 2003; Hoyer et al., 1998). However, in the UK the Committee on the Carcinogenity of Chemicals in Food, Consumer Products and the Environment (2000, 2004), which keeps such matters under review, has maintained that there is no evidence of a link between organochlorine insecticides and breast cancer.

PCBs (polychlorinated biphenyls), used in the past in electrical components, have been identified as possible causes of breast cancer (Falck et al., 1992; Aronson et al., 2000; Dorgan et al., 1999) but this was not found by others (Calle et al., 2002; Hoyer et al., 1998). Another potential culprit is dioxin, produced by incineration of PVC (polyvinyl chloride), PCBs and chlorinated compounds, as well as vehicle exhausts (Brown et al., 1998; Warner et al., 2002; Muscat et al., 2003).

There are major difficulties in establishing an unambiguous link between exposure to chemicals and breast cancer. It is difficult to account for the interplay between endogenous and exogenous oestrogens (Darbre, 2006). Moreover, the impact of chemical compounds may be underestimated when looked at in isolation because of possible synergies (Arnold et al., 1996). In other words, the interaction of these chemicals with humans, their food chain and the environment may have a greater effect than suggested by low-level concentrations of each compound. Indeed, one study, which sought to measure the total burden of organochlorine compounds, found an increased risk for breast cancer (Ibarluzea et al., 2004).

In order to provide a more balanced assessment of the costs and benefits of screening, the National Screening Committee (NSC) was established in 1996. Its task is to advise government on new screening programmes and to review, modify and, if necessary, terminate screening programmes. It is required to base its advice on evidence. The NSC is also responsible for overseeing the introduction and implementation of new screening schemes in the NHS and monitoring effectiveness and quality. Since its establishment, the NSC has improved many aspects of screening, including a more coordinated approach and more effective implementation (Holland and Stewart, 2005). The NSC has brought a more evidence-based approach to new proposals for screening programmes, although it is dependent on the quality of research (which is often weak) and the extent to which the full costs of screening (including, for example, increased anxiety levels, widening health inequalities) are captured. Although the NSC has attempted to introduce greater rationality into the debate, this is not easy given the vested interests involved and the zealotry among both supporters and opponents of screening programmes. Notably, it has not endorsed population-wide prostate cancer screening as current evidence does not support either a national programme or routine testing because of the high risks of overdiagnosis (Schroder et al., 2009). The NSC also initiated a reduction in the coverage of the cervical cancer screening programme (exempting women aged 20–24 and recommending three-yearly smears for younger women). However, this was challenged following the death from cervical cancer of reality-TV star Jade Goody in 2009. The extensive media coverage of the 27-year-old's terminal illness led to pressure for the screening programme to be reopened for younger women, although this campaign was unsuccessful.

The past forty years have seen the development of mass screening, exemplified by programmes for breast and cervical cancer. There has been a shift in favour of 'multiphasic' screening, where individuals are screened for a range of risk factors that might affect their future health (such as heart disease or cancer). This was reflected in the introduction of new NHS health checks (see Cm 6737, 2006; Brown, 2008; DoH, 2008a), despite concerns that programmes may not actually prevent illness (Naish, 2006). Concerns about private health companies offering unnecessary screening to patients led the NSC to issue guidance to GPs (NSC, 2010). A further concern is the marketing of 'whole body' scans to screen for disease. This is a profitable area for private health clinics, yet may cause considerable harm by exposing people to unnecessary radiation (COMARE, 2008).

Genetic Screening

There has been a growing interest in genetic screening (Appleyard, 2000; Nuffield Council on Bioethics, 1993, 2006; BMA, 2007a; Holland and Stewart, 2005; Cunningham-Burley and Amos, 2002; Melzer, 2008). Genetic science has advanced quickly in recent years. The mapping of the human genome was a particularly significant landmark, extending the potential for identifying relationships between genes and diseases (Yates, 1996; Pianezza et al., 1998; Khoury et al., 2000). Further scientific developments raise the prospect of more extensive genetic testing of those at risk of particular diseases, as well as population-wide programmes (BMA, 2005a). Screening for single gene disorders, such as cystic fibrosis, already takes place. With increased knowledge of the susceptibility of individuals to more complex conditions such as cancer, heart disease and neurological illnesses, involving a combination of genes, comes the possibility of extensive screening programmes profiling an individual's risk.

Genetic screening programmes may reassure people that risks are low, reducing anxiety, especially for those with a family history of disease. People at higher risk may benefit from closer surveillance and possibly earlier intervention. In some cases, individuals may make better-informed choices about healthy lifestyles to avoid additional environmental risks. However, they may instead adopt a fatalistic approach, pursuing unhealthy lifestyles once they have learned of their genetic predisposition. Meanwhile, those deemed at low risk may believe they are invincible and may reject healthy lifestyles. A claimed advantage for genetic screening is that new therapies will be developed to enable doctors to treat the genetic causes of disease or to tailor treatments to the individual's genetic profile. However, there is likely to be a long time lag – known as the therapeutic gap (Holtzman and Shapiro, 1998) – between the availability of tests and the introduction of new therapies. One of the main counterarguments is that genetic screening will not necessarily improve outcomes. For many genetic diseases, there is no treatment currently available.

There are doubts about how complex genetic associations with diseases should be interpreted (Colhoun et al., 2003). Questions surround the accuracy of some genetic tests and their ability to predict the onset of disease, particularly where multiple causal factors are involved (Evans et al., 2001; Davey Smith et al., 2005). Furthermore, a range of harms and costs may be associated with screening, such as heightened anxiety about increased risks and an increase in unnecessary treatment. People may opt for radical treatment – for example mastectomy in the case of breast cancer – even though it is not certain that they will develop the disease.

Moreover, genetic screening carries a range of other adverse social implications that need to be carefully examined (see Cunningham-Burley and Amos, 2002; Davison et al., 1994; Vineis et al., 2001; BMA, 2005a; Nuffield Council on Bioethics, 2006). Those deemed at risk could find themselves discriminated against – by employers, and by financial corporations such as banks and insurance companies. There are questions of confidentiality: how will the information be handled and who will be able to access test results? Currently, UK law does not prevent an employer from refusing a job to someone on the basis of a genetic test (Staley, 2003). Most argue against the disclosure of genetic information to insurers (see Ashcroft, 2007). This is mainly because it would lead to discrimination. Others argue that genetic information is no different from other health information and there is no principled reason for excluding it (Holm, 2007). An emphasis on genetic screening could, however, shift attention away from other causes of disease (Melzer and Zimmern, 2002). Many illnesses are associated with environmental and lifestyle factors.

Even when genetic factors are involved, there is interaction with these other elements. Nevertheless, if the importance of genetic screening is exaggerated, there may be less emphasis on collective responses to prevention including tackling powerful commercial interests whose activities are harmful to public health (Clarke, 1995; Willis, 1998).

The key regulatory body in this field is the UK genetic advisory committee on insurance (GAIC). This non-statutory body was established in 1999, following recommendations from several bodies (Human Genetics Advisory Commission, 1997, 2001; Science and Technology Committee, 2001; Nuffield Council on Bioethics, 1993). Its role is to develop criteria on the evaluation of genetic tests, their application and reliability, and to evaluate applications by insurance companies to use tests. It also monitors the insurance industry's compliance with voluntary agreements, including a moratorium (until 2011) on the use of genetic tests for all but the most expensive policies and an approval process for tests applying to such high-value policies. Currently, the scheme has only approved one test (for Huntington's disease) for such policies.

The regulation of genetic science is problematic for governments. The area is fast moving and there are powerful scientific and commercial interests involved. Genetic screening is potentially a lucrative industry and governments have not wished to discourage enterprise in this area, irrespective of the consequences for ordinary people. Only after pressure from Parliament did the British government in 1996 set up an advisory commission – the Human Genetics Advisory Commission (HGAC). This body's brief was to review scientific progress and to report on issues having social, ethical and economic consequences in relation to public health, insurance, patents and employment and to advise on ways to improve public confidence and understanding of the new genetics. However, in 1999, the HGAC, along with two other organizations, the Advisory Committee on Genetic Testing, and the Advisory Committee on Scientific Advances in Genetics, was absorbed into a new body, the Human Genetics Commission (HGC), which reports to ministers on the range of issues covered by the original bodies. Other agencies also have an advisory and regulatory role in this field. The Human Fertilization and Embryology Authority (HFEA), for example, grants licences to fertility clinics allowing them to engage in pre-implantation genetic diagnosis. This technique enables clinics to screen for genetic conditions in in-vitro fertilized embryos, which are then not selected for implantation. Currently this is available for only a few conditions, including Huntington's, cystic fibrosis, beta thalassaemia and familial adenomatous polyposis (an inherited genetic predisposition to colon cancer).

The UK government has supported an expansion of genetics in the NHS, including screening programmes. It has raised the issue of genetic profiling at birth: the identification of genetic risk factors in newborn babies (DoH,

2003c). The HGC and the NSC subsequently reported on this. They rejected genetic profiling and concluded that there were major ethical, social and legal impediments and pointed out problems of stigma and high cost associated with such a scheme (Joint Working Group of the Human Genetics Commission and the UK National Screening Committee, 2005).

Health Education and Health Promotion

The provision of information and advice about health is undertaken by a range of professionals and workers (for example doctors, nurses, health visitors, midwives, teachers and health promotion specialists, community workers and health trainers) and agencies (for example the NHS, local authorities, schools, and voluntary organizations and commercial organizations). Formerly, these activities were grouped under the broad umbrella of 'health education', defined by Downie et al. (1996, p. 28) as 'communication activity aimed at enhancing positive health and preventing or diminishing ill health in individuals and groups through influencing the beliefs, attitudes, and behaviour of those with power and of the community at large'.

Today, health education is viewed as a rather outdated term, and has been superseded by the term 'health promotion' (Naidoo and Wills, 2000a; Green, 2008). As noted in Chapter 1, health promotion is a broad philosophy that encompasses a range of interventions while health education is characterized as a narrowly focused approach, aimed at changing individual behaviour (Weare, 2002). There is some truth in this, health education practice having been dominated in the past by an individualistic, paternalistic and victim-blaming approach. Indeed, it has perhaps been seen as 'a simple matter of telling people what they ought to do to be healthy' (Downie et al., 1996, p. 27). However, such a narrow focus is not necessarily a feature of health education (Green, 2008). Health education can be informed by various models of health promotion, some of which emphasize the importance of social, economic and environmental factors in health and illness (Weare, 2002; Tones and Green, 2004; Wills and Earle, 2007a; Baum, 2002; Rodmell and Watts, 1986). It is not necessarily an individual-focused, victim-blaming approach but it can be radical, challenging structures and cultures that affect health.

The most basic model of health promotion is the health belief model (Becker, 1974), which assumes that individuals make rational decisions about their health based on an evaluation of costs, risks and benefits. This model focuses on how to change individual behaviour by giving information about costs and harms of particular unhealthy activities (such as smoking, for example), the benefits of healthy lifestyles (such as exercise), and by altering perceptions of risk. An alternative model is the theory of reasoned action (Azjen and Fishbein,

1980), which asserts that an individual's intention to behave in a particular way is shaped by their beliefs about health behaviour and how others view them. These factors may reinforce or undermine each other, so that it is possible for someone to fully understand the risks of an activity, such as smoking, but nonetheless persist as a consequence of peer pressure.

A further approach, the 'stages of change' model, assumes that people change their behaviour gradually, at different speeds, and may 'regress' as well as 'progress' (Prochaska and DiClemente, 1983). Changes are not 'once and for all', but part of an ongoing process. Similarly, health promotion efforts must be continuous and not persistent. Moreover, this model suggests that as people vary considerably in their motivation and willingness to change, attempts to influence their behaviour should be tailored accordingly. Finally, the health action model (Tones, 1987), seeks to explain why individuals may act 'irrationally'. It is asserted that individuals have particular beliefs and motivations, which lead them to behave in certain ways. Also, environmental factors, outside the individual's control, exert strong influence on their behaviour. Such factors include poverty and deprivation, which negatively affect individual self-esteem. Self-esteem is a key factor in health behaviour because this motivates people to value health and helps them to cope with challenging situations.

These models support different approaches to health promotion policy. The health belief model supports an individual-focused approach to improve rational decision-making through the provision of information about costs, benefits and risks. The reasoned action and stages of change models place more weight on differences between individuals and social relations between them. These models support approaches that target particular groups or types of people. The health action model goes further in acknowledging the socioeconomic and environmental context within which groups and individuals operate. It supports an approach to health promotion that is centred more on getting people to challenge the underlying determinants of ill health.

Policies for Health Education and Health Promotion

Modern campaigns on diet, exercise, drugs, alcohol and smoking have important precedents. For example, in the Victorian period there were high-profile campaigns by voluntary groups on issues such as alcohol, sanitation and hygiene (Berridge, 2005; Wohl, 1984; Patterson, 1948; Green 2008). These activities became professionalized as local Medical Officers of Health and sanitary inspectors developed a health education role. Local authorities, which acquired responsibilities for public health services such as health visiting, infant welfare centres and the school health service, became involved in health education on issues such as parenting, hygiene, nutrition and alcohol abuse (Berridge, 1989). Central government also undertook health education, particularly in times of national emergency, such as epidemics and wartime.

During the 1920s, the CMO George Newman commented that 'the progress of preventive medicine depends in extraordinary degree upon the enlightenment and education of the people' (quoted in Holland and Stewart, 1998, p. 45). In 1927, a Central Council for Health Education was established for England and Wales (a Scottish Council was created in 1943). It had several functions (Ottewill and Wall, 1990; Webster, 1996): to promote education and research in healthy living; to promote the principles of hygiene and to encourage teaching of these principles; and to assist and coordinate the work of all statutory bodies carrying out public health responsibilities with regard to health education. The interwar period saw an expansion of health education, encouraged further by the granting in 1936 of statutory powers to local authorities to enable them to disseminate health information. Another factor was the growth in mass media, notably cinema, which was used in health education campaigns. During the Second World War period, health consciousness increased. Government education campaigns formed an important part of the war effort, producing memorable slogans, such as 'Coughs and Sneezes Spread Diseases' (Bruce, 1968, p. 300). Other campaigns during this period included headlice prevention and the prevention of venereal disease (Sheard and Donaldson, 2006).

In the postwar period, lifestyle-related illnesses – and in particular smoking – attracted increasing attention from the media and policymakers (Berridge, 2007). Politicians, fearful of offending both commercial interests and the general public, responded with health education initiatives in the form of public information films, posters and leaflets. These efforts were regarded by health campaigners as a minimal response to serious health threats. Yet, as the case of smoking illustrates, even basic health education was opposed by powerful interests and by some government departments and agencies (Sheard and Donaldson, 2006; Webster, 1996; Berridge, 2005, 2007). More generally, there were problems in extending health education (Webster, 1996; Ottewill and Wall, 1990). Local authorities varied in their capacity and willingness to undertake it. Those who practised health education lacked clear professional identity and status. There was a lack of agreement about what constituted effective methods of heath education. Also, health education attracted insufficient resources. Finally, responsibilities for health at national level were not adequately fulfilled, with both health departments and the health education agencies falling short.

To address these problems, a committee of inquiry was established in 1959, chaired by Lord Cohen (Webster, 1996). This eventually reported in 1964, making several recommendations, which included: an expansion of health education; more evaluation of its effectiveness; an increase in expenditure (from public, private and voluntary sources); and the establishment of independent boards at national level to lead campaigns and support local authority health education activities (Ottewill and Wall, 1990). Consequently, the Health Education Council (HEC) was established in 1968 as an independent body. Scotland set up its own new body, the Scottish Health Education Unit. The HEC was given a wide range of responsibilities including advising government on health education priorities, undertaking national campaigns, supporting local health education efforts, promoting training of health educators, and undertaking and commissioning research into the effectiveness of health education. Resources for health education increased, especially during the 1970s, amid heightened awareness of lifestyle-related illness (Webster, 1996). In this period, expansion of health education was backed by several high-profile bodies including a parliamentary committee (House of Commons, 1977) and the Royal Commission on the NHS (Cmnd 7615, 1979).

In 1974, the responsibility for health education was transferred from local authorities to the NHS (Ottewill and Wall, 1990). Area health authorities were given the task of devising health education strategies and coordinating district community health services and professionals. A further reorganization in 1982 abolished AHAs and their responsibilities were reallocated to district health authorities (DHAs). Despite these changes, however, health education continued to face the same old problems: variability, lack of resources, and difficulties in proving its effectiveness. Those who practised health education remained in 'the Cinderella of the community based professions' (Ottewill and Wall, 1990, p. 465) and continued to lack a clear professional identity. In addition, health education was increasingly criticized for blaming the victim and for not taking into account the broader determinants of health (Rodmell and Watt, 1986). It was seen as paternalistic, based on control by experts (Naidoo and Wills, 2000a). Increasingly, those involved in health education rebadged themselves as health promotion specialists, reflecting the broader range of interventions encapsulated by the new public health and WHO's 'health for all' initiative (Bunton and Macdonald, 2002; Green, 2008).

Health education and health promotion came under increasing attack from the political right for advancing the nanny state, undermining individual liberties and curbing the profitability of major industries such as food, alcohol, and tobacco (Anderson, 1985). Health promotion leaders at national level found themselves at loggerheads with powerful political and commercial interests (Sutherland, 1987). The HEC was regarded as an irritant by successive governments, which were reluctant to tackle big business in food, alcohol and tobacco (Webster, 1996; Baggott, 1990; Taylor, 1984). Its position deteriorated further following the election of the Thatcher government in 1979. This government was hostile to the nanny state and protective of health-damaging industries. HEC campaigns on alcohol and tobacco infuriated ministers; its involvement in food policy and health inequalities made them even more irate (Berridge and Blume, 2003). However, the independent status of the HEC made it difficult for the government to entirely control it. In 1987, the Conservative government abolished the HEC, replacing it with the Health Education Authority (HEA). This new body was constituted as a special health authority, making it more directly accountable to ministers than its predecessor. Nonetheless, disputes with government continued. There were significant battles with government on issues such as sex education and tobacco advertising. Ministers considered abolishing the HEA, but instead proposed a contract-based system of funding that reduced its freedom to pursue its own initiatives.

Throughout the 1980s and 90s, however, the Conservative governments provided additional resources for health education, largely for high-profile campaigns on HIV/AIDs, heart disease and illicit drugs. They sanctioned campaigns on alcohol and tobacco, in order to avoid having to adopt more effective interventions (see Chapter 15). As funding shifted towards expensive mass media campaigns, community-based health education began to suffer from under-resourcing (Nettleton and Burrows, 1997). This was countered to some extent by initiatives (for example on heart disease) which stimulated local activity on specific issues. Another feature of this period was the growing interest of some local authorities in health promotion. Although local authorities lost statutory responsibilities for these services in 1974, some, particularly in areas of high levels of deprivation and illness, expanded their health education activities, often in alliance with NHS bodies and the voluntary sector.

The election of a Labour government in 1997 brought further changes in the organization of health education and health promotion at the national level. The HEA was abolished and replaced by the Health Development Agency (HDA). This new body was charged with maintaining a database of research evidence, providing information about the effectiveness of health improvement programmes, setting, implementing and supporting standards of public health work, and acting as a resource to develop the public health workforce (Ewles and Simnett, 2003). The HDA was later merged with NICE, the National Institute for Clinical Excellence (to become the National Institute for Health and Clinical Excellence). Notably, the HDA was not responsible for devising or implementing health education or health promotion programmes, which meant that there was no longer a single agency responsible for national health campaigns, a shortcoming identified by Wanless (2007). The government responded to this criticism by giving overall responsibility for such campaigns to another agency, the National Consumer Council (now part of Consumer Focus).

Wanless also expressed concern about the poor quality of the evidence base for health promotion. This is a long-standing problem. There are difficulties in evaluating health education and health promotion activities, which inhibits the development of an evidence base (MacDowall et al., 2006; Springett, 2001; Naidoo and Wills, 2000a; NICE, 2007). The fundamental problem is that such complex interventions do not take place in a controlled environment. Any improvement in health behaviours cannot be solely attributed to such interventions. An alternative approach is to view health promotion as a process of change rather than a one-off event. This means that processes as well as outcomes must be evaluated. It also implies that evaluation should be a continuous process over a longer period of time than would be the case, say, for a surgical or medical intervention. Another important requirement when undertaking health promotion evaluation is that the target group should not be seen as passive recipients. On the contrary, those whose health is the subject of the programme should participate in evaluation, including its design and implementation. Furthermore, in the context of multi-agency working, evaluation should incorporate the views of other stakeholder agencies with an interest in the issue. This is important because agencies often interpret the effectiveness of programmes in different ways using different criteria.

Exhibit 8.2

Mental Health Promotion

In the past, public health policies have focused on physical illness. This no longer seems sensible given the levels of mental illness in industrialized societies, including the UK. One in six people experience at least one mental health problem at any given time (Singleton et al., 2001). Anxiety and depression is the most common mental disorder, affecting almost a tenth of the population. One in ten children have a mental health disorder (Green et al., 2005). There are inequalities in the experience of mental illness, with women, disadvantaged groups, long-term sick and unemployed people most affected (see Chapter 17). Rates of mental illness are higher among ethnic minority groups (NIMHE, 2003).

There is a connection between mental and physical health. Suicide and attempted suicide are linked to mental health problems. In 2008, over 5700 people in the UK committed suicide (www.nationalstatistics.org.uk, accessed 16.7.10). Every year thousands more attempt to kill themselves. At risk groups include young men, unemployed people, prisoners, young women from the Asian subcontinent, and some occupational groups (farmers, vets, dentists, doctors, pharmacists). Alcohol and drug addiction are also associated with mental health problems. Anxiety and depression can also affect physical health in other ways, for example through self-harm.

Mental health policy and practice have focused exclusively on individual care and treatment. The idea of promoting mental health, both in individuals and in communities, has been neglected (Tudor, 1996; Rogers and Pilgrim, 2001). In recent years, however, mental health promotion has received more attention from policymakers and practitioners (Friedli, 2007, 2009; Handsley, 2007b). There are several reasons for this: the medical model and the dominance of psychiatry in the mental health field has been challenged; the rise of user groups in the mental health field; recognition of the individual and social costs of mental health problems; and increasing acknowledgement of the relationship between mental health promotion and positive health and wellbeing. There is also greater awareness of the ways in which mental health can be protected and promoted by addressing underlying causes (Handsley, 2007b; DoH, 2001d). These include housing problems and homelessness, unemployment, poverty, educational underachievement, family breakdown, drug and alcohol misuse, family history of mental illness, caring roles, and poor physical health. Also, problems can be addressed by strengthening factors that help prevent mental health problems from developing or deteriorating, such as social networks, employment and economic security, and learning opportunities.

In England, the origins of mental health promotion policy were rooted in suicide prevention strategy. The Major government's *Health of the Nation* strategy (Cm 1986, 1992) identified suicide prevention as a priority area and set a target for reducing the suicide rate. The target of the Labour government (Cm 4386, 1999) was to reduce suicide and undetermined injury mortality rates by 20 per cent by 2010 (baseline 1995–7), supported by a national suicide prevention strategy (DoH, 2002b). This set out five goals: to reduce risk in high risk groups, reducing availability and lethality of suicide methods; to improve reporting of suicidal behaviour in the media; to promote research; to improve monitoring of progress on the suicide reduction target; and to promote mental wellbeing in the wider population. A number of groups were identified as targets for mental health promotion, including socially excluded and deprived groups, black and ethnic minorities, people who misuse alcohol and drugs, children and young people and elderly people. Earlier, the government had identified mental health promotion as one of the key areas in its national service framework for mental health (DoH, 1999b; DoH, 2001d). Standard One of the NSF signalled a commitment to mental health for all (not just for those suffering from diagnosed mental illness) and to reduce discrimination experienced by people with mental health problems.

Further impetus came from the government's Social Exclusion Unit (SEU) report into mental health and social exclusion (ODPM, 2004a). This estimated the costs of mental health problems at £77 billion in care, economic losses and premature death. It noted that adults with mental health problems were one of the most socially excluded groups in the country. The SEU set out an action plan to address this issue including: a sustained programme to combat stigma and discrimination, more responsive health and social care services, improving employment opportunities, supporting families, enabling people with mental health problems to participate in their community, improving their access to transport, housing and financial advice.

This was followed by fresh guidance on mental health promotion from the National Institute for Mental Health, responsible for taking forward the NSF (NIHME, 2005). This set out nine key areas for action; marketing mental health, improving access to sources of support for emotional and psychological difficulties; addressing health inequalities in mental health; employment and the workplace; communities; later life; schools; tackling violence and abuse; and parents/early years. The guidance also set out practical steps for individuals to improve their mental health and wellbeing, including moderate drinking, learning new skills, and talking about feelings. Subsequently, the white paper *Our Health, Our Care, Our Say* (Cm 6737, 2006) endorsed the guidance and pledged to include mental health in the government's proposed social marketing strategy.

The suicide rate in the UK fell by a tenth between 2000 and 2007: suicides among young men in England and Wales falling by half in the period 1998–2005 (Biddle et al., 2008). There have been campaigns to combat stigma and discrimination. Around the country, PCTs and other agencies have been revising their mental health promotion strategies. Some innovative projects have been implemented, for example with regard to young men's mental health (NIMHE, 2006). There is also a growing interest in 'social prescribing' for mental health problems, linking people with non-medical sources of support and opportunities in areas such as learning, exercise, arts, mutual support and self-help (Freidli, 2007). In 2009, the government announced an expansion of psychotherapy services in England for people with mental health problems, linked to existing services such as job centres, GP surgeries and NHS Direct. A National Mental Health Development Unit has been established to improve mental health services, including mental health promotion. Even so, mental health promotion remains a low priority for most agencies. Given the limited resources available, projects tend to be piecemeal and short term. Meanwhile, hostile and unhelpful attitudes to mental health remain entrenched, reinforced by media representations, ensuring that stigma and discrimination continue. Despite an acknowledgement of socioeconomic factors that undermine and enhance mental health, little has been done to address these in a systematic way (see Chapter 17).

Other parts of the UK have developed health promotion strategies for mental health. Scotland is at the forefront of mental health promotion (Handsley, 2007b). The Scottish Executive has identified mental health as a key area of health improvement. It has introduced a national anti-stigma campaign ('See Me'), a suicide prevention framework (Scottish Executive 2002b), and has taken steps to raise awareness and promote positive mental health, and to promote and support recovery from mental health problems. There is a national programme for improving mental health and wellbeing (Scottish Executive, 2003c, 2006; Scottish Government, 2009a). This programme focuses on underlying causes of mental health problems and sets out actions in specific areas, including infants, children and young people, work, later life and society. Initiatives include a confidential phone line for people experiencing low mood and depression (Breathing Space), and early intervention for people with mental health problems (Mental First Aid). There has been a clear effort to link mental health with wider policy issues, such as inequality, social justice and discrimination, and other sectors, such as arts and culture, education, housing, employment and transport. Efforts have also been made to integrate mental health promotion within health improvement plans at local level. Other aspects of the programme include: the development of mental health indicators, training opportunities to build capacity, and reviews of the evidence base for interventions.

Wales has an All Wales Mental Health Promotion Network to provide leadership and coordination. It aims to improve public understanding of mental health promotion and to disseminate good practice. The network is led by a board drawn from seven areas of health promotion: children and young people, communities, health and social care, mental health literacy, parenting/early years, workplace and employment. These themes form the basis of an action plan on mental health promotion, which is currently being implemented (Welsh Assembly Government, 2006). The Northern Ireland Health Promotion Agency has acknowledged the importance of mental health promotion (see Health Protection Agency, 1999). More recently Eire and Northern Ireland have worked together on suicide prevention and have cooperated on an all-Ireland mental health promotion campaign.

Finally, mental health promotion is supported by a range of international bodies. The WHO Regional Office for Europe (2005) produced a plan to highlight and address the underlying causes of mental ill health, particularly in sectors outside health (such as housing, for example). The European Commission (2005) proposed that the EU should have a strategy on mental health accompanied by a framework of cooperation between member states. This was followed by a European Pact for mental health and wellbeing (Slovenian Presidency of the EU, 2008) to encourage cooperation between member states and other stakeholders on this issue.

Other countries of the UK have their own health promotion agencies. Scotland, as already noted, has had a separate body for many years. In 2003, the Health Education Board for Scotland (which took over the responsibilities of the Scottish Health Education Unit in 1990) was merged with the Public Health Institute to form a new body, Health Scotland. A Welsh Health Promotion Authority was created in 1987. Following devolution, this responsibility passed to the Welsh Assembly. A range of agencies also developed health promotion responsibilities. Measures to bring these functions together under the auspices of Public Health Wales have now been implemented (see Exhibit 6.1). Meanwhile, in Northern Ireland, a Health Promotion Agency was established in 1990, to provide policy advice on health promotion, to undertake research, to engage in public and professional campaigns, and to support training and professional development in health promotion. This body has now been subsumed within the Northern Ireland Public Health Agency.

Further Developments

Since 2000, policies have endorsed an expansion of health education and health promotion to the public. One strand of this has prioritized the dissemination of advice and information to the public by professionals, lay advisors and voluntary groups. Initiatives include encouraging GPs to promote health and the appointment of 'lay' health trainers to promote lifestyle changes (see

Chapter 6). It might be thought that this would have benefited those who specialize in health promotion, by increasing the demand for their skills and expertise. However, this 'mainstreaming' of health promotion has in effect diluted the specialism. Health advice and information is but one aspect of the health promotion specialist's role, which also encapsulates actions to tackle the socioeconomic and environmental factors that cause illness and impair wellbeing. Health promotion specialists are important not just in producing and disseminating information, but for building capacity for public health interventions, training non-specialists, and encouraging community health development. Unfortunately their contribution has not been fully recognized and as a result they have been marginalized as a professional group (Griffiths and Dark, 2006; Wills et al., 2008).

Another policy relates to mass media techniques aimed at influencing public attitudes and behaviour. The use of mass media, as already noted, has been adopted in the past on issues such as HIV/AIDS, drug abuse, heart disease, smoking and alcohol abuse. As MacDowall et al. (2006) note, mass media techniques have varying degrees of success. They can be successful in putting issues on the agenda, reinforcing local efforts, raising awareness, and conveying simple messages. They are less successful in disseminating complex messages, developing skills, and changing attitudes and behaviour (Boyce et al., 2008). Coupled with other interventions, such as community-based health promotion activities, mass media campaigns can produce benefits (see also Corcoran, 2007; Naidoo and Wills, 2000a). However, there remains a suspicion that mass media techniques are adopted more for their political value than their actual effectiveness in improving health. Politicians find them useful because they are high profile and help convince the public that action is taking place. These measures may be a substitute for stronger and perhaps more effective interventions, such as legislation or fiscal measures, which could upset vested interests. Mass media campaigns may also contribute to victim-blaming if they are not accompanied by measures that address structural and cultural barriers to healthy living.

Nonetheless, there is a world of difference between the health education campaigns of yesteryear and modern campaigns using sophisticated techniques (Berridge, 2007). The world of media and communications has changed. Not only do people have access to television, there are now far more channels. In addition there is now mass communication through the internet and mobile phones. The public has also changed. People are generally less deferential towards and less trustful of authority. They are also influenced by a wider range of social groups, including virtual networks. These factors have led to a search for health promotion techniques which can utilize new information technologies and social networks (Corcoran, 2007).

One approach, which has received much attention in recent years, is social marketing (Hastings and Stead, 2006). Two white papers have backed this approach (Cm 6734, 2004; Cm 6737, 2006). A strategic framework was set out to maximize its use (DoH, 2008c). Social marketing has also been included in strategies on obesity, smoking and alcohol misuse, and has shaped the Change4Life programme introduced by central government and its partners (see Chapters 13 and 15). It has been defined as 'an orientation to health promotion in which programmes are developed to satisfy consumers' needs, strategized to reach the audience(s) in need of the programme, and managed to meet organizational objectives' (Lefebvre, 2002). Social marketing applies commercial marketing techniques to achieving socially desirable goals, such as promoting healthy lifestyles (Donovan and Henley, 2003). The starting point is to understand the motivations of a specific population subgroup, and engage with them as active partners in developing targeted efforts to change behaviour. The emphasis is upon voluntary behaviour change rather than coercion, and on the mutual benefits of intervention (Gordon et al., 2006). Social marketing emphasizes the building of a long-term relationship with the 'consumer', to promote long-term and sustainable changes in behaviour. There is a persuasive logic in copying the kinds of techniques used by 'unhealthy' industries. In one sense, social marketing can be seen as competing with the producers of ill health (such as the alcohol, tobacco and food corporations) to gain advantage (Hastings and Stead, 2006). Furthermore, it raises the possibility of working with responsible companies to share knowledge about consumers to promote health.

There is evidence that social marketing can be effective (National Consumer Council, 2006; Hastings, 2007; Gordon et al., 2006; McDermott, 2005). It can also be seen as a more realistic approach in an era dominated by consumerism, choice individualism and hostility to paternalism and collectivism (French, 2007). But there are also concerns (Corcoran, 2007; MacDonald, 1998). The emphasis on consumerism, inherent in the social marketing approach, can be seen as manipulative, raising ethical issues. By focusing ultimately on individual consumer behaviour (albeit taking into account social and environmental factors that shape individual choices), the social marketing approach may shift attention away from structural factors. Similarly its individualistic consumer focus may undermine those public health interventions based on notions of citizenship. A further problem is that the possible involvement of business organizations (such as the alcohol and food industries) as partners in government social marketing strategies may enable them to exert stronger influence over policy and thus protect themselves from more effective interventions. A further danger is that social marketing may fall short of its own principles, degenerating into tokenistic health education, the main purpose of which is to enable politicians to avoid effective prevention strategies by fooling the public into thinking that something is being done to address health problems.

Conclusion

The public health services discussed in this chapter can make a contribution to the reduction of disease and health improvement. However, they focus strongly on disease prevention in the individual. By emphasizing individual responsibility within a conventional medical model, they divert attention from other socioeconomic and environmental factors that damage health. This is convenient for governments wishing to avoid confrontation with powerful political and economic interests. By expanding public health services, governments can demonstrate their commitment to health and the NHS. This also placates health professionals, especially those directly involved in delivering services, who benefit directly from the investment. Perhaps this explains why the benefits of vaccination, screening and health promotion are often extolled by governments, in preference to structural interventions aimed at altering social, economic and physical environments. Meanwhile, the public and the media remain generally supportive of extending these health services. Even so, scandals and controversies about vaccination and screening, and criticism of 'nannying' health promotion, illustrate an undercurrent of unease about these interventions.

The Health and Wellbeing of Children and Young People

9

The health and wellbeing of children and young people has been at the centre of many policy initiatives in recent years. This chapter begins by exploring why these policy developments occurred. It explores specific initiatives, including Sure Start, Healthy Schools, Every Child Matters, and the Children's Plan. Two special topics – child poverty and sexual health – are examined in Exhibits 9.1 and 9.2 respectively. Although the focus is mainly upon policies in England, developments in Scotland, Wales and Northern Ireland are covered in Exhibit 9.3.

Why Focus on Children and Young People?

In the past, public health interventions have been introduced with the welfare of children and young people in mind. Examples include immunization, school meals, medical inspections, improvements in housing, education reforms, employment restrictions on children, pollution laws and anti-poverty policies. Interventions often came in response to the injustice of children's vulnerability to illness, concern about the exploitation of children, and anxiety about the physical condition of the young generation and the implications for national economic and military strength (see Chapter 3). In modern times, the health and wellbeing of children and young people remains a prominent issue. The ethical reasons for protecting them from harm are still valid (Nuffield Council on Bioethics, 2007, p. xix). Despite the welfare state and rising material standards of living, they are still at risk.

There has also been increasing emphasis upon the rights of children (Roche, 2005). Recent UK legislation has emphasized that the welfare of the child is paramount and that children's interests must be central to policy and practice. The UN Convention on the Rights of the Child (UNICEF, 1989), ratified by the UK in 1991, provides a framework for children's rights (Gelling, 2007). It sets out 42 rights, several of which are health-related. For example, article 6 states that all children have a right to life and that government should ensure that all children survive and develop healthily; article 24 that children have the right to good quality health care, clean water, nutritious food and a clean environment; and article 27 that children have a right to a standard of living that meets their mental and physical needs and government should help families who cannot provide this. Article 31 concerns the right of children to relax and play; article 13 relates to the provision of support services for parents; and article 19 states that government should ensure that children are properly cared for. Other articles seek to protect children from dangerous or harmful work, drugs, sexual abuse, the promotion of harmful material through the media, and from activities that inhibit their development. The Convention also states that, in general, children's best interests should always be served and that they should have a say in decisions affecting them (articles 3 and 12).

There has been particular concern about the safety of children and the need to protect them. This is partly due to anxiety about the vulnerability of children to physical and sexual abuse. But it is also driven by a desire to promote a safer environment for children more broadly.

The health and wellbeing of children and young people has become a major preoccupation. A focus on health needs (Hall and Elliman, 2006) was stimulated by specific issues, including mental health problems among children and adolescents (see Exhibit 8.2), increased levels of childhood obesity (see Chapter 13), sexual health and teenage pregnancy (Exhibit 9.2), alcohol, tobacco and drug use (Chapters 14 and 15), and accidents (Chapter 10). Such concerns were further fuelled by a UNICEF (2007) report that placed the UK at the bottom of the league of industrialized countries for child wellbeing. There was particular disquiet about excessive individualism and commercialization of childhood (The Children's Society, 2009; DCSF, 2009) and about inequalities between affluent and poor children (Bradshaw, 2002; Bradshaw and Mayhew, 2005).

The interest in children and young people's health also has been heightened by the acknowledgement of 'lifecourse approaches', which identify childhood as a key factor in shaping future health status (Barker, 1994; Lundberg, 1993; Barker and Osmond, 1987; Poulton et al., 2002; van de Mheen et al., 1998; Graham and Power, 2004; Kuh and Ben-Schlomo, 2004; Davey Smith, 2003). Although children are relatively healthy compared with adults (Lincoln, 2007; Earle, 2007b), their current lifestyles, environment or economic circumstances may have adverse implications for future adult health. This provides justification for prevention programmes (WHO, 2005b). The prevention of health and other social problems by intervening in the lives of children and families has become a prominent theme in government policy (HM Government, 2007g; DCSF, 2007). This is linked to the notion of a 'social investment state' (see Lister, 2005; Hendrick, 2005), where intervention is justified on the basis of expected improvements in future outcomes (such as better health): reducing costs (for example of the NHS) and creating a better workforce (healthier, for example). However, this approach has been criticized for concentrating too much on children as future adults rather than on their present needs (Lister, 2005; Earle, 2007b).

Sure Start

Sure Start is a cross-departmental initiative to improve the physical, intellectual, social and emotional development of children under five years of age (see Brown and Liddle, 2005; Gustafson and Driver, 2005; Clarke, 2006; Gidley, 2007; Glass, 1999).   It was strongly influenced by the Head Start programme in the US, which sought to intervene in families to prevent future social problems. Sure Start established schemes in deprived areas to strengthen relationships between parents and children, improve parents' understanding of children's needs, and increase access to support services. Its key objectives were to improve social and emotional development, promote healthy development before and after birth, improve children's ability to learn, and strengthen families and communities. Local Sure Start projects included core services: outreach services, parenting and family support, health services, childcare, play, and early learning. They built on current services already provided by the NHS, local authorities and the voluntary sector and on the foundations of existing partnership arrangements (such as health action zones, early years partnerships and regeneration projects). Projects could develop additional services in response to local needs and, indeed, were expected to be innovative, diverse and flexible. They were expected to involve parents and communities in shaping their programmes.

The Sure Start programme began in 1999, initially in England, before extending to other parts of the UK (see Exhibit 9.4). Over the next five years, £3 billion was committed in England to over 500 local projects. Key performance indicators initially included: reducing the proportion of children aged 0–3 years at risk by a fifth; reducing smoking in pregnancy by 10 per cent; reducing by 5 per cent the number of children needing specialist speech and language support by four years of age; and reducing the number of children living in workless households (Clarke, 2006). Subsequent targets included additional indicators relating to personal, social and emotional development and communication, literacy and language skills.

The Impact of Sure Start

The challenges of measuring the impact of Sure Start were formidable. The programme was not introduced in a way that enabled a randomized control trial of the interventions (Kane, 2008). The evaluation programme was based on a quasi-experimental design which meant that only limited conclusions could be drawn. The diversity of local projects made it difficult to evaluate the programme as a whole (Clarke, 2006). Short-term evaluations, while useful to monitor progress, gave little indication of the long-term outcomes (Gidley, 2007). Furthermore, Sure Start coincided with a range of other interventions, making it difficult to distinguish its impact (Gidley, 2007).

Nonetheless, Sure Start can be credited with several achievements, including small but beneficial outcomes for most families and children (Belsky et al., 2006). However, positive effects were found in only 5 of the 14 child health and development outcomes identified (Melhuish et al., 2008) and doubts were expressed that the programme would produce long-term changes in behaviour (Kane, 2008). Some projects demonstrated significant improvements in partnership working between participating agencies (Gidley, 2007; Brown and Liddle, 2005); Sure Start schemes proved popular with many parents and efforts were made to involve them within institutional structures (Gustafson and Driver, 2005; Brown and Liddle, 2005). However, in earlier evaluations, Sure Start failed to help those most in need. The most disadvantaged families living in Sure Start areas (teenage parents, single parents, workless households) were not reached (Belsky et al., 2006; Melhuish et al., 2005). This finding was not, however, replicated in a subsequent evaluation (Melhuish et al., 2008). Sure Start schemes encountered problems in engaging with ethnic minority families (Craig et al., 2007). A further shortcoming was that schemes did not cater for those living outside the designated areas (Gidley, 2007), so poor families living in less deprived areas were neglected. Initiatives to provide similar services in some of these areas were subsequently undertaken, however.

Sure Start schemes were also criticized for not sufficiently engaging with fathers. This was possibly due to the 'maternal' focus of Sure Start and difficulties faced by fathers in accessing services outside 'office hours' (Lloyd et al., 2003; Clarke, 2006). Furthermore, although the programme improved support services for some families, it did not address underlying causes of ill health and social disadvantage (Clarke, 2006). Notwithstanding that family environment is an important factor in children's health and development, it can be outweighed by socioeconomic inequalities and the wider environment (poor housing, local amenities). Sure Start was also criticized for having an authoritarian ethos. Despite considerable diversity and flexibility, schemes were constrained by a centralized performance management framework, underpinned by values that emphasized individualistic and instrumental approaches to combating social exclusion (Clarke, 2006; Gidley, 2007). Parental and community involvement was similarly constrained by national priorities and the power of local experts (Myers et al., 2004; Gustafson and Driver, 2005). Sure Start made limited use of community development approaches to engage with local people, particularly with regard to the involvement of ethnic minorities (Craig et al., 2007).

The impact of Sure Start projects varied, partly due to their diversity and the variable quality of local partnership working. Some projects were better led and managed than others. The national evaluation of Sure Start found that NHS-led projects tended to be the most effective, partly explained by access to records and the use of existing health visitor services as a means of contacting and supporting families (Belsky et al., 2006).

Further Developments

Sure Start Plus was introduced in 2001 to provide support, advice and mentoring for pregnant teenagers and teenage parents (Wiggins et al., 2005). The service was widely perceived as beneficial by service providers, clients and partner agencies. The programme provided crisis support for pregnant young women and young mothers, increased support on emotional issues, improved young women's family relationships and reduced domestic violence, while securing better accommodation and increased educational participation for those under 16. The programme had less effect on specific health objectives (reducing smoking and increasing breastfeeding) and educational participation for those aged 16 and over, and had only limited success in helping young fathers. Subsequently another programme, the family–nurse partnership programme, was developed with similar aims. This programme, which was piloted in 2007, involves specially trained nurses providing structured support for the most vulnerable young mothers and their families with children up to two years of age. The aim is to provide guidance to enable parents to adopt healthier lifestyles for themselves and their children, to provide good care and plan for the future (DoH/DCSF, 2009). An evaluation of the programme found positive outcomes including smoking cessation and breastfeeding. But there were concerns about the sustainability of pilots after initial funding ended and higher than expected drop-out rates (Barnes et al., 2009). It is expected that this programme will be rolled out to other areas. However, as the Audit Commission (2010a) has observed, the extension of the programme could have significant implications for funding and workforce, notably the workload of health visitors.

Sure Start programmes are now being subsumed in children's centres, which aim to improve the life chances of all children, especially disadvantaged children, by improving their future health status, educational achievements, and employment prospects. They seek to integrate services such as childcare, early education, health checks, play sessions, employment advice, speech and language therapy, home visiting services, and pre- and postnatal classes. Providers can be public, private and voluntary services in childcare, social care, family support, employment, training, housing and children services. Children's centres can be based in schools, health centres or in their own dedicated premises. They developed from existing programmes, such as Neighbourhood Nurseries (which provided accessible day care in poor areas), and Early Excellence Centres (which combined early education, day care, social support and adult learning).

Children's centres have been extended beyond the most disadvantaged communities. The Labour government committed to establish 2500 centres by 2008, and to have 3500, in every community, by 2010 (Cm 6374, 2004). Despite the need for high-quality, integrated services, there has been some criticism of this plan. The extension of children's centres to all areas has fuelled fears that resources might become thinly spread and that consequently there might be a shift away from those in greatest need (Health Committee, 2009). An early assessment found that most families were happy with the quality of services and that centres were making efforts to raise the quality and accessibility of services (NAO, 2006). However, there was a failure to target families with high levels of need. There was limited progress too in improving services for fathers, families with disabled children and ethnic minority families (particularly in areas with smaller minority populations), and a lack of awareness by users of the full range of services available. Over half the centres studied reported problems working with local agencies, such as the NHS, and over 10 per cent faced financial problems. Local authorities, which became responsible for children's centres from April 2006, expressed concern about their ability to manage the government's planned roll-out of the scheme. Over half of local authorities were not carrying out any active performance-monitoring of children's centres and there was a lack of data to assess cost-effectiveness. A subsequent report from Ofsted (2008) found that children moving on from children's centres were well prepared for school and that parents valued the variety of childcare options available. However, it also stated that the monitoring and evaluation of the impact of these services could be better. Improvements in coordination and leadership were recommended. Ofsted also found that more could be done to attract families not currently using children centres' services.

In a further development, children's centres were placed on a statutory footing. Ofsted's role was extended beyond inspecting care and education services to cover the full range of activities undertaken by children's centres. It was proposed that every children's centre will have access to a named health visitor, who will oversee the health work of the centre. The aim was to make children's centres a stronger focus for health promotion activities on parental smoking cessation, child obesity and other lifestyle issues. Following the change of government in 2010, the Conservative–Liberal coalition pledged to retain Sure Start and to expand the number of health visitors working on the programme by 4200 (HM Government, 2010c). However, it also stated that Sure Start would concentrate more on the neediest families, reduce outreach services, and involve the voluntary sector more.

The Audit Commission (2010a), in a review of the impact of policies on the under-5 age group, found some evidence of progress. Improvements in infant mortality, low-birthweight babies, breastfeeding rates, obesity and immunizations had occurred. However, the Audit Commission identified considerable room for improvement, including: greater efforts to reduce inequalities (between children in deprived and other areas and between different ethnic groups); greater priority for children's health in local plans and LAAs; more effective targeting and tailoring of provision to those in need; clearer joint priorities and responsibilities at local level; clearer national priorities and less duplication between central government agencies; more monitoring of service usage, quality of services and their impact; and greater sharing of good practice.

Exhibit 9.1

Child Poverty

Child poverty is an important public health issue because of its association with risks of illness and injury (see Chapter 16). The Blair government set a target of reducing child poverty in the UK by half by 2010 and eradicating it by 2020 (Cm 4445, 1999; HM Treasury, 2001). The main measure of child poverty used was children living in house-holds with incomes less than 60 per cent of the median (the middle point of the income distribution) before the deduction of housing costs. It should be noted that when adjustment for housing costs is made, the number of children in poverty is higher. In 2006, it was estimated that 2.8 million children (22 per cent) lived in poverty before housing costs were deducted and 3.8 million (30 per cent) after such costs were taken into account. In 2007, the number of children in poverty rose by 100,000 according to the government's preferred measure. The number of children in poverty is expected to fall to 2.3 million by 2010/11 (Hirsch, 2009).

The Blair government pursued a policy of 'progressive universalism' aimed at supporting all families with children, while targeting additional efforts on the most disadvantaged. Universal child benefit payments were increased alongside a national childcare strategy to enable parents to work and earn additional income. Meanwhile, the minimum wage and tax credits for families with children were aimed at lower-income working families (Sutherland and Piachaud, 2001). Means tested benefits were increased for families with children. Other policies helped to improve the envi-ronment and circumstances of many families (such as Sure Start, regeneration schemes and training and employment opportunities). In addition, the devolved assemblies of the UK pursued additional plans to reduce poverty and inequality in childhood (see, for example, Welsh Assembly Government, 2005b, 2005c; Scottish Executive, 2000b).

These policies had some success in raising families out of poverty, although problems with the administration of tax credits caused some hardship (Treasury Committee, 2006). In 1998, the UK had the highest level of child poverty in Europe (Paxton and

Dixon, 2004). In the years that followed, 600,000 children were removed from poverty (Sharma, 2007). Nonetheless, the target of reducing child poverty by a half by 2010 is unlikely to be met (Hirsch, 2009). Child poverty in the UK remains high compared with other similar countries (UNICEF, 2005, 2007). Furthermore, researchers have found that children from deprived backgrounds lack facilities and skills that might enable them to move out of poverty (Palmer et al., 2007; Prince's Trust, 2007).

The Work and Pensions Committee (2004) identified child poverty as a persistent and major problem. It called for greater access to affordable childcare, the mainstreaming of anti-poverty strategies across all and not just the poorest geographical areas, and concerted action to help disabled parents, parents with disabled children, minority ethnic parents and lone parents to move into employment. It also called for more financial help for poor families. The committee stated that child poverty must have a higher profile in the context of a fairer society with a stronger cross-departmental approach. It argued that the anti-poverty strategy should move beyond raising incomes and address the human dimensions of poverty and raising children's life chances. In a further report, the committee agreed that although work was the best route out of poverty for families with children, this did not guarantee that children would be lifted out of poverty. Indeed, by taking jobs parents could be worse off financially, despite government claims to the contrary. The committee called for a long-term strategy on benefit income for those families where parents could not work (Work and Pensions Committee, 2008). Others have called for more effort to reduce child poverty. Sharma (2007) called for a £3.8 billion investment in benefits and tax credits to meet interim child poverty targets. This report also argued for greater efforts to tackle the roots of child poverty, such as barriers to work, low pay, childcare, and low social mobility as well as specific measures to address poverty in the school holidays, fuel poverty and debt. Meanwhile, Hirsh (2006) estimated that a further £28 billion would be needed to fund current policies on benefits and tax credits to eliminate child poverty by 2020. His report urged greater redistribution towards low-income groups, improved education and training for disadvantaged groups, better access to childcare, and equal pay for women.

The Brown government subsequently established a joint child poverty unit, drawn from the Department of Work and Pensions and DCSF, to improve coordination. The 2008 budget placed a higher priority on reducing child poverty by increasing child benefit and tax credits (see HM Treasury et al., 2008). In 2010, a Child Poverty Act was passed, setting statutory targets. These were: to reduce by 2020 the percentage of children living in households in relative poverty to less than 10 per cent, those in absolute poverty to less than 5 per cent and those in low-income households living in material deprivation to less than 5 per cent. A further target, to reduce persistent poverty, was also endorsed but not specified at this stage. Under the terms of the Child Poverty Act, the government must publish a national child poverty strategy, revising it every three years, and report to Parliament annually on progress towards the targets. A child poverty commission will be established to advise the government and new duties placed on local authorities to undertake needs assessment, devise local strategies and work with partners, such as the NHS. The Cameron government, which inherited the legislation, endorsed the commitment to eradicate child poverty by 2020.

Health Services for Children and Young People

The NHS has provided services for children and young people since its inception, including immunization, child health surveillance, screening, health education, specialist care and treatment services. Nonetheless, these services have often attracted criticism for poor coordination, overemphasizing disease rather than health promotion, and failing to meet the needs of children and their families. There have also been concerns about the under-resourcing of community-based services and a lack of capacity in the children's health workforce (Cmnd 6684, 1976; Hall and Elliman, 2002).

An important landmark was the national service framework (NSF) for children, young people and maternity services introduced in England in 2004 (other parts of the UK have their own frameworks – see Exhibit 9.3). The NSF aims to improve the quality and equity of services through national standards for health and social care. It is a ten-year plan linked to *Every Child Matters*; a broad programme of action across health, education, welfare and other services, discussed later in this chapter.

The NSF set out eleven standards, accompanied by specific interventions. The standards relate to:

- promoting health and wellbeing

- supporting parenting

- child-, young people- and family-centred services

- supporting young people as they grow into adulthood

- safeguarding and promoting the welfare of children and young people

- providing advice and services for children and young people who are ill or injured

- services for children and young people in hospital

- services for disabled children and young people and those with complex health needs

- services for children and young people with mental health problems

- safe and effective medicines for children and young people

- maternity services

NHS bodies are expected to work closely with local authorities, other public agencies and the voluntary and private sectors to promote the health and wellbeing of children and young people. Service providers are required to give children, young people and parents more information and choice and involve them in planning; promote physical and mental health and emotional wellbeing through healthy lifestyles; intervene early to prevent problems; assess needs in a timely and comprehensive way; improve access to services according to needs; tackle health inequalities; and promote and safeguard children's welfare in situations where staff have concerns. The NSF requires services to ensure that pregnant women receive high-quality care and are involved in decisions about childbirth. It also introduced an evidence-based Child Health Promotion Programme (CHPP, since renamed the Healthy Child Programme – HCP), setting out health promotion services offered to pregnant women and children (DoH and DCSF, 2008).

The role of nurses, midwives and health visitors in children's health and welfare has been highlighted. The Chief Nursing Officer (DoH, 2004b) issued best practice guidance to address the gaps in current services. This recommended that services should be organized on the basis of needs rather than professional roles or titles. Greater co-location of nurses, midwives and health visitors in integrated children's teams was envisaged. The guidance underlined the importance of the leadership role of these professionals for children and families with health and development needs. It stated that professionals working with vulnerable children and young people needed core competences and specialist skills, and that training should be commissioned to strengthen them. Other recommendations included: a learning and career framework for nurses working with children; integrated workforce planning for children and young people's services across health, social care and education; measures to ensure adequate workforce capacity (such as recruitment and retention of staff); a stronger emphasis on prevention in the work of health visitors; an expanded role for practice nurses in health promotion.

In the light of the Children's Plan of 2007 (discussed later in this chapter), a review of children's health services took place. This led to prioritization of children's health in the NHS operating plan (DoH, 2008a), new guidance on commissioning children's health services (DoH, 2009d), and a strategy for children and young people's health, which set out plans for universal, specialist and targeted services for this group (DCSF and DoH, 2009). This strategy heralded changes to inter-agency working arrangements (discussed in a later section). It promised to strengthen the child health workforce through assessment of capacity and an expansion of training. One of the key themes of the strategy was that parents should get more information about services. Another theme was the importance of support for parents during pregnancy and in the early years of children's lives. Further development of the health visitor workforce was promised, to enable it to lead the HCP. A new antenatal and preparation for parenthood programme was proposed along with an expansion of the family–nurse partnership scheme, mentioned earlier. Children's centres were given a bigger role in health promotion programmes, working closely with health visitors, who would oversee this. The strategy also highlighted the importance of the health of school-age children. It promised an improved HCP for this age group alongside a stronger healthy schools programme (discussed below), while reiterating commitments to make personal, social and health education (PSHE) statutory within the curriculum, increase the take-up of healthy school meals, and increase physical education (PE) and sporting opportunities. School health teams were to be established in every local area to provide the range of services required by schoolchildren. The strategy set out a number of proposals to give young people aged 16–19 healthier opportunities including sport and PE, access to user-friendly health services and a new campaign to increase knowledge of contraceptive methods. A further issue was the specific requirements of children with acute health needs. The strategy promised individual care plans for children with complex health needs and funding for support services for families with disabled or terminally ill children.

Healthy Schools

According to DeBell (2007, p. 124), 'the school is an opportune location for health promotion work because it is where children and young people gather; where they spend the greatest part of their growing up years outside the home environment; and it is effectively their workplace.' The importance of the school as a setting for health improvement interventions has long been recognized (see Chapter 3). However, the school health service subsequently declined and lost its distinctive identity long before being absorbed into the NHS in 1974. On a more positive note, health education in schools expanded from the 1960s onwards (Beattie, 2002; Denman, 1999; Lewis, cited by Naidoo and Wills, 2000b). But these initiatives were piecemeal, and focused on specific lifestyle risks such as smoking and drugs. They did not form part of a holistic approach to improving the health of children and young people. Nor were they embedded in the philosophy and practice of schools, which increasingly focused on narrow academic achievement and preparation for employment. The worlds of health and education remained distinct, both in policy and in practice.

In 1992, however, the Major government identified schools as one of several settings where 'healthy alliances' between the NHS and other bodies should flourish. This did encourage some local alliance building between health and education bodies. Meanwhile, the WHO regional office established a network of health promoting schools in Europe, including the UK. The key aim of a health promoting school was defined as 'achieving healthy lifestyles for the total school population by developing supportive environments conducive to the promotion of health' (WHO Regional Office for Europe,

1993b). This encouraged a 'whole school' perspective on health promotion (Denman, 1999; Beattie, 2002). This required substantial investment in health education alongside a stronger physical and social environment, to enable children to develop skills and make healthy choices. The school ethos was identified as a crucial factor in building self-esteem and developing healthy life skills (West et al., 2004; Bonell et al., 2007).

Studies found that health promoting schools could contribute to improved pupil self-esteem, reduced levels of bullying, and possibly dietary intake and fitness. Improvements were evident in the social and physical environment in terms of school lunch provision, exercise and social atmosphere (Moon et al., 1999; NFER, 1998; Denham, 1999; Lister-Sharp et al., 1999; Stewart-Brown, 2006). Some studies also indicated a reduction in use of alcohol, tobacco and other substances (see NFER, 1998; Moon et al., 1999), although specific school-based programmes on substance abuse were regarded as relatively ineffective (see Chapter 14). The importance of key interventions and activities was highlighted (Denman, 1999), including: a school-based review as a first step to facilitate change; a designated coordinator with status and leadership skills; a school policy and action plan; adequate resources; strong management and staff support and involvement; effective management and communication structures; consultation with staff, parents and pupils, clear arrangements with outside agencies providing support; training and support for staff; coordination of activities throughout the school and the community; and a health education curriculum of high status.

The National Healthy Schools Programme

The Blair government introduced a National Healthy Schools Programme (NHSP) in 1999 (DFEE, 1999; Wicklander, 2006). National healthy school standards (NHSS) were introduced for local programmes (Sinkler and Toft, 2000) to improve partnership working and programme management. Coordinators were appointed to advise and support schools seeking to improve the health of pupils. Schools could participate at different levels: at level 1 (the lowest level) the school would simply be informed about the programme; at level 2 it would be involved with healthy school projects; at level 3, the school would be involved in target setting, audit and action planning. To achieve the highest level, a school had to demonstrate its commitment to social inclusion and reducing inequalities, evaluate the effect of continuing professional development on healthy school activities, deliver the requirements of statutory and non-statutory guidance and the NHSS criteria, and reflect the views of all pupils in school activities.

The NHSP achieved its target that all English local education authorities (LEAs) must join an accredited healthy school partnership by 2002. By

January 2002, 90 per cent of schools had achieved at least level 1, with a third attaining the highest level (HDA, 2002). Subsequently, the *Choosing Health* white paper (Cm 6734, 2004) decreed that half of all schools would be healthy schools by 2006. Additional milestones were set, including that 75 per cent of schools must attain healthy school status by the summer of 2009. In the meantime, however, the criteria for healthy school status were altered. By December 2008, 80 per cent of schools had attained the healthy school status under the new regime (www.healthyschools.gov.uk). It should be mentioned that the devolved assemblies, which also pursued healthy school policies, adopted different targets and implementation strategies (see Exhibit 9.3).

The new regime meant that schools must meet criteria across all themes of the programme: PSHE, healthy eating, physical activity, and emotional health and wellbeing (DoH and DfES, 2005). They must demonstrate that they are using a whole school approach, reaching the entire school community. The application process is self-validated, with a minority of applications moderated by local healthy school teams or regional assessors. Schools that have healthy school status may adopt an enhancement model, to help them plan for improvements in health and wellbeing (DoH/DCSF, 2009). This involves working closely with other partners in local government, the NHS and the voluntary sector and an annual review process to maintain progress.

In 2007, a statutory duty was imposed on schools to promote the wellbeing of their pupils. Ofsted inspections now involve an integrated approach that incorporates health and wellbeing. New metrics are being developed in order to measure the effectiveness of school health and wellbeing strategies. These include surveys of parents and pupil perceptions and school-level outcome indicators (such as take-up of school lunches, participation in sport and PE). Schools received further guidance on improving health and wellbeing. In a further move to raise the status of the subject, the Brown government decided to make PSHE a statutory requirement. However, this legislation did not pass before the 2010 general election and PSHE remains for the time being a non-statutory subject.

The Impact of the Healthy Schools Programme

Studies of the pre-2005 healthy schools programme found some impact on school effectiveness and improvement (Thorpe et al., 2002). After controlling for deprivation, schools working at level 3 of the healthy schools standard had better results at some assessment stages, although not at GCSE level. Level 3 schools in the primary sector showed slightly higher rates of improvement than other schools (although this was closely linked to eligibility for free school meals, associated strongly with level 3 status). Schools with level 3 status in the secondary sector, however, did not show higher rates of improvement. The report did not draw any firm conclusions about the link between participation in NHSS and school performance. The evaluation by Blenkinsop et al. (2004), however, found that schools valued NHSS and that the status of health-related work in schools had risen as a result. The study found only a few significant differences in outcomes between schools having level 3 healthy school status and other schools. For example, level 3 schools had better Ofsted ratings in PSHE provision and pupil enthusiasm. The study's authors believed that the NHSS was beginning to have an influence, particularly in areas related to social inclusion. They warned, however, that more active participation of children and young people in the programme was essential to its success. Wicklander (2006) found that the programme was not consistently implemented and argued that there was no way of bringing deficient schools up to standard. Furthermore, the success of the programme was dependent on cultural factors, in particular recognition of the importance of the health dimension in school settings. Much depended on the role of the head teacher in acknowledging health issues and securing the active involvement of the school in the programme.

Although an Ofsted (2006) report was broadly positive about the impact of the healthy schools programme, it also found shortcomings. PSHE played a positive role, but there was a lack of effective assessment and little use was made of assessment guidance. A minority of schools focused insufficiently on drugs, smoking and alcohol. A minority were restricted in their promotion of physical activity by the lack of outdoor facilities. Ofsted found that where food was not produced on the premises, there was continuing poor nutritional value in school meals. It was disappointed that mental health issues were not tackled sufficiently across the PSHE curriculum. Ofsted identified consultation with parents and pupils as a key factor in effective health promotion and noted this was underdeveloped in some schools. Its report was critical of the failure of some secondary schools to build on the foundation provided by primary schools, and to make links across the curriculum. This led to fragmentation and limited the impact of health promotion activity. In a subsequent report, Ofsted (2007a) evaluated the PSHE curriculum. It found that pupils' knowledge and understanding had improved over the previous five years. Leadership and management of the subject was rated as good in nine out of ten schools, although weaknesses remained in monitoring and evaluation. The quality of teaching had also improved but there were shortcomings identified in teaching by non-specialist tutors. There was also evidence of poor lesson planning and weaknesses in assessment. Ofsted found that although considerable progress had been made in reviewing and developing the curriculum, pupils' needs were not always identified clearly. However, the NHSP was acknowledged as a stimulus for improvements in the planning and provision of PSHE. Others have raised similar issues. For example, the limited involvement of parents and the community in school health promotion has been noted (DeBell, 2007; Denman, 1999). Another common complaint has been the marginalization of health promotion in the school curriculum and the failure to integrate key themes (DeBell, 2007; Naidoo and Wills, 2000b; Denman, 1999). A key criticism was that PSHE was a non-statutory subject and lacked priority (De Bell, 2007), although this was not universal (see Ofsted, 2007a).

An evaluation of the post-2005 national healthy schools programme is currently being undertaken. An interim report (Barnard et al., 2009) found much variation in the implementation of the programme. Responsibility for the programme varied. Some schools gave responsibility for implementation to junior staff, while others demonstrated clear support and leadership from senior management. Where NHSP had impact, it influenced a move towards a more structured delivery of PSHE, a review of topic coverage, increased pupil consultation and the development of evaluation and assessment tools. NHSP was a factor in raising schools' awareness of their physical activity provision and encouraging reviews of policies on emotional health and wellbeing. NHSP also had a positive impact on healthy eating policies. Research undertaken as part of this evaluation programme found a small but significant relationship between achieving and working towards NHSS and Ofsted ratings. Healthy school status was also associated with lower absence rates, higher contextual value added (CVA) scores (a measure of pupils' progress taking into account their socioeconomic background), and higher levels of pupil participation in PE and sport, but these associations were small and not consistent.

Other initiatives have affected school health policies and practice in recent years. These include child welfare policies such as *Every Child Matters* (discussed in detail below). Specific programmes such as Extended Schools, which emphasizes the broader role of schools in providing access to a wide range of education, childcare, health, welfare and other support services especially in deprived areas, are also relevant (HM Government, 2005a). It is intended that the healthy school approach will be extended into others parts of the education system, such as nursery education and pupil referral units. The government has introduced school initiatives on obesity, physical exercise and sport, healthy eating and school meals (see Chapter 13) and, school travel plans (Chapter 12). Schools have also been a focus for addressing health issues such as smoking, alcohol and drug abuse among children and young people (Chapters 14 and 15) and sexual health (Exhibit 9.2). There have been specific initiatives to strengthen school nursing (see Chapter 6), although the number of school nurses remains low. In 2008, only a quarter of secondary schools had a full time school nurse.

Exhibit 9.2

Sexual Health and Teenage Pregnancy

The Health Committee (2003b) identified a national crisis in sexual health, attributing this to a lack of political leadership and pressure, inadequate resources, and an absence of performance management. Policy responses have been inhibited by moral issues and taboos surrounding sexual health issues. They have also been constrained by a preoccupation with a disease model and a failure to take into account the wider aspects of sexual health. Indeed, as Weyman and Davey (2007, p. 158) have argued, 'sexual health is not just about the absence of ill heath, rather it is about enabling people to have fulfilling relationships, which are good for their physical mental and social wellbeing.'

Sexual health has risen up the political agenda in recent times. In the 1980s, fears of an HIV/AIDS epidemic forced the Thatcher government into adopting policies at odds with majority public opinion and its own ideological position (Day and Klein, 1989; Berridge, 1996; Garfield, 1994b). The absence of effective treatment for the disease and the unpredictable nature of the threat to public health led to a reliance on expert advice, resulting in a high-profile programme of health promotion. This was restricted, however, in ways that reflected the government's ideology and its proximity to right-wing moral pressure groups (Durham, 1991). The content of health education materials was toned down, restrictions placed on health education about homosexuality and a large-scale survey of sexual lifestyles was refused government funding.

Subsequently, sexual health was included in the Major government's *Health of the Nation* strategy in 1992. Targets were set for a reduction in the incidence of gonorrhoea by at least a fifth between 1990 and 1995, as an indicator of HIV/AIDS trends. Also, reflecting concern about teenage pregnancy, the government set a target of reducing by half the conception rate among under-16s between 1989 and 2000. Although the gonorrhoea target was achieved ahead of time, critics argued that it was a poor indicator of behaviour change with regard to sexually transmitted disease generally and HIV/AIDS in particular (Adler, 1997). Teenage pregnancy levels fell, but the target reduction was not achieved. The gap between the UK and other comparable countries continued to widen, leaving it in the unenviable position of having the highest teenage pregnancy in Western Europe.

Under the Blair government, sexual health policy was reinforced by concerns about health inequalities and social exclusion. The Acheson inquiry on health inequalities (see Chapter 17) endorsed policies to promote sexual health and reduce unwanted teenage pregnancy. Meanwhile, the government's Social Exclusion Unit (1999) developed a teenage pregnancy strategy. This set a target to reduce teenage pregnancy (defined as conceptions in girls under 18) by half between 2000 and 2010, as well as reducing conceptions in under-16s. The strategy established a central government unit to coordinate policy and implementation, a system of performance management holding local councils and other agencies to account for their efforts in this area, local multi-agency partnerships, regional coordinators and additional funds for implementation. Efforts were made to link this initiative with other policies and programmes aimed at improving the health and welfare of children and young people, such as Sure Start, Connexions, Healthy Schools, and Every Child Matters. In addition, national and local campaigns discouraged teenage pregnancy and warned of the dangers of sexually transmitted infections. Funding for a national helpline (Sexwise) was also provided. New guidance on sex and relationship education in schools was produced in 2000 and an expansion in training for teachers. Efforts were made to improve contraception services in clinics, general practice and schools. Although the under-18 pregnancy rate for England subsequently fell by around 10 per cent between 1998 and 2008 this was less than needed to achieve the target (Wilkinson et al., 2006). Although the under-16 conception rate is also lower than in 1998, it has actually increased in recent years (Family Planning Association, 2009). British teenagers remain the most sexually active in Europe, with almost four out of ten 15-year-old girls in England and Wales (and 34 per cent in Scotland) reporting having had sexual intercourse (Godeau et al., 2008).

The other main driver of sexual health policy was the rise in sexually transmitted infections (Weyman and Davey, 2007; Evans, 2006). HIV/AIDS is still a major issue. By the end of 2005, an estimated 83,000 people in the UK were living with HIV/AIDS, around a quarter of whom had not been diagnosed (Health Protection Agency, 2009). Improvements in therapy in the late 1990s reduced death rates and improved the quality of life for people with HIV/AIDS. However, any optimism was balanced by the increase in the annual number of newly diagnosed individuals (over 7000, almost double that in 2000) and concerns about resistance to drug therapies. There has also been alarm about a large increase in other sexually transmitted infections, diagnoses of which rose by 63 per cent in the UK between 1997 and 2006, reaching a total of 376,508. Syphilis cases rose by over 1600 per cent (to 2766) in this period, chlamydia by 166 per cent (to 113,585), gonorrhoea by 46 per cent (to 19,007), herpes by 31 per cent (to 21,698) and genital warts by 22 per cent (to 83,745) (Health Protection Agency, 2007a).

The Blair government introduced a sexual health strategy in 2001 (DoH, 2001e, 2002c). This initiative set out targets for reducing infections, standards for sexual health services and chlamydia screening, and launched new education campaigns and advisory services (see above). Additional funding was provided, but this was regarded as too little (Kinghorn, 2001; Evans, 2006). The report of the health committee, mentioned above, created further pressure and sexual health was identified as a one of the main public health priorities of the government in the *Choosing Health* white paper (Cm 6374, 2004), and it subsequently became one of the six top priorities for the NHS. Extra funding (£300 million) was announced for the modernization of sexual health services and high-profile prevention campaigns. The government also committed itself to achieving a 48-hour maximum waiting time for those wishing to attend a GUM (genito urinary medicine) clinic by 2008. In addition, the white paper accelerated plans to introduce the chlamydia screening programme

The impact of the sexual health strategy and its prioritization in *Choosing Health* was limited (Evans, 2006). Many PCTs did not prioritize sexual health in their local plans, and only half stated that their spending in this area had increased (Terrence Higgins Trust et al., 2006). A disconnection between national strategy and local action was evident, with two-thirds of clinicians reporting insufficient prioritization at local level (Terence Higgins Trust et al., 2006, 2007). Under two-thirds of PCTs indicated that money allocated for improvements in sexual health services had been diverted to other purposes (Terence Higgins Trust et al., 2006). Diversion of resources was also a concern of the Independent Advisory Group (IAG) on Sexual Health and HIV (2006), which expressed anxiety that changes in the NHS, with regard to commissioning, contracts and reconfiguration of health authority boundaries could place sexual health services and, in particular, contraception services in jeopardy. Although access to GUM clinics gradually improved (by August 2007, 72 per cent of clients had been seen within 48 hours, compared with 57 per cent in August 2006 and less than 40 per cent in 2004), it remained short of the government's target (Health Protection Agency, 2007b). Moreover, some of this apparent increase may reflect cosmetic changes aimed at restricting the availability of appointments rather than actual improvements in accessibility (Terence Higgins Trust et al., 2006). The Healthcare Commission (2007a) found that over half of PCTs had achieved their own plans to provide 48-hour access, while 8 per cent underachieved and 33 per cent failed. In contrast, over 90 per cent of PCTs performed well on reducing teenage pregnancy, perhaps because of the additional resources allocated to this programme. Meanwhile, the promised high-profile campaign on sexual health was delayed and there were fears about possible cuts in its budget (Boseley, 2006). In the event, a publicity campaign was undertaken across TV, cinema, radio, press and the internet. The chlamydia screening programme was implemented, although questions were raised about its effectiveness and value for money (Low, 2007; PAC, 2010). Government backed the vaccination of teenage girls against HPV (human papillomavirus), which has been linked to cervical cancer. Research found that over a fifth of women aged 10–29 had signs of infection by at least one strain of HIV (Jit et al., 2007).

Sexual health policy, relating both to teenage pregnancy and sexually transmitted disease, remains flawed both in design and implementation. Studies of the impact of sex education programmes cast doubt on their effectiveness (see DiCenso et al., 2002; Henderson et al., 2006; Tucker et al., 2006). There is little evidence on the impact of mass media campaigns. More generally, policies in the UK suffer from inconsistency and are contradictory, giving out mixed messages (Lewis and Kijn, 2002). There is often a lack of coordination across government and different policy sectors. Religious and right-wing groups still exert considerable influence and are able to block policies and programmes that might be effective (Weyman and Davey, 2007; Lewis and Kijn, 2002). For example, sex education in schools is still controversial in the UK. In the past parents have been able to withdraw children from classes if they so wish. The Brown government decided that PSHE – which includes sex and relationships education – should be a statutory part of the curriculum. However, this measure was enacted before the 2010 general election and so provision remains non-statutory.

Ironically, a belief in the innocence of youth contrasts with a culture that largely ignores the sexualization of children by the media and commercial advertisers. Particularly powerful is the media obsession with celebrity culture, which is itself highly sexualised (Evans and Hesmondhalgh, 2005; Cashmore, 2006). Perhaps there should be a closer link between sexual health policy and policies on media regulation (The Children's Society, 2009). Moreover, a holistic approach to risk is needed, which does not look at sexual health behaviour in isolation but links it to other risks. For example, the link between alcohol, drugs and sexual activity, although often acknowledged, has been neglected by researchers and policymakers and it is only fairly recently that good evidence about these connections has come to light (see Independent Advisory Group on Sexual Health and HIV, 2007; Standerwick et al., 2007). Finally, sexual health policy is still detached from policies affecting social and economic contexts. As several studies have pointed out, programmes aimed at preventing teenage pregnancies and sexually transmitted diseases must not ignore socioeconomic factors such as poverty, deprivation and social exclusion (Evans, 2006; Wilkinson et al., 2006; Henderson et al., 2006).

The government has since updated its sexual health and HIV strategy (DoH, 2009c). This was informed by a report commissioned by the DoH from the Independent Advisory Group on Sexual Health and HIV and the Medical Foundation for AIDS and Sexual Health (2008). Its recommendations included a requirement for PCTs to undertake comprehensive needs assessments in this field, and clearer responsibilities for sexual health at board level. It also recommended a new set of indicators to monitor progress at national and local level (including guaranteed access to all sexual health services not just GUM clinics within 48 hours, abortion rates, under-18 conception rates). The report called for more joint commissioning of services, improved partnership working between PCTs, local government and other agencies, improved workforce planning and training, and greater incentives to provide services (reflected in the GP quality and outcomes framework and NHS tariffs).

Other parts of the UK have their own plans and strategies for sexual health and teenage pregnancy (DHSSPS, 2002b; NAfW, 2000a; Scottish Executive, 2005c). Wales and Scotland face similarly high levels of teenage pregnancy and sexually transmitted infections. Northern Ireland's situation is different as there is less data on the extent of the problems (accurate teenage conception data is not available in the province because of lack of data on abortions) and until recently a great reluctance, due to religious and moral attitudes, to address them. The approaches taken in other parts of the UK are similar to those pursued in England, although targets differ (Scotland, for example, aims to reduce the under-16 pregnancy rate by 20 per cent between 1995 and 2010), there are differences in emphasis (Scotland and Wales make stronger links to socioeconomic factors and other risk factors such as alcohol and drugs; and both have gone further in emphasizing the importance of sexual health and wellbeing), and there are variations in strategy and planning mechanisms: for example, there is an All Wales Sexual Health Network, while Scotland has created mechanisms for strengthening the coordination of policy across government and at NHS board level. In addition, some parts of the UK have devised their own projects (for example in Scotland, the Healthy Respect project, which promoted sexual health among young people) and provided additional funding for sexual health services.

Protecting Children and Young People

The Blair government introduced a number of initiatives to help children and young people in need and to protect those at greatest risk of harm. Quality Protects, introduced in 1998, aimed to improve children's social services in an effort to safeguard and promote children's welfare. The Children's Fund, launched in 2000, sought to tackle disadvantage among children and young people and prevent future problems through early intervention by partnerships of statutory and voluntary agencies (Edwards et al., 2006). Measures were also introduced to improve the health of young people leaving care. Nonetheless, continuing disquiet about the lack of policy coherence at national level and problems with inter-agency working at local level came to a head following the abuse and murder of a little girl, Victoria Climbié, by her aunt and her aunt's partner. The Climbié inquiry, chaired by Lord Laming, like many previous inquiries into child abuse, told a tragic story of poor coordination between agencies, a failure to share vital information, weak accountability, poor management, lack of staff capacity, staff shortages and inadequate training (Cm 5730, 2003).

The government initiated a reform programme, 'Every Child Matters' (ECM), bringing together policy and services on children's health and welfare (Cm 5860, 2003; DfES, 2004a, 2004b). ECM sought to establish integrated provision of services to improve five key outcomes for children and young people: to be healthy; stay safe; enjoy life and achieve; make a positive contribution to society; and to overcome socioeconomic disadvantages to achieve full potential. It heralded, at national level, the creation of a minister for Children, Young People and Families within the Department for Education and Skills (DfES), to provide strategic direction and to coordinate policy. Following the lead of other parts of the UK (see Exhibit 9.3), a Children's Commissioner was established in England, to act as an independent champion.

'Top tier' and unitary local authorities were required to appoint a director of children's services to head new children's services authorities (CSAs), responsible for both education and social services. These local authorities also designated a lead council member responsible for this area. The CSAs were charged with promoting cooperation between local partner agencies (see DfES, 2005). These included district councils, police authorities, probation boards, youth offending teams, strategic health authorities and PCTs, which in turn were required by law to cooperate with such arrangements. In addition, duties were placed on these and other authorities, including NHS trusts, foundation trusts and special health authorities, to ensure that they safeguarded and promoted the welfare of children. CSAs were empowered to establish pooled budgets, to promote inter-agency cooperation, and were required to draw up children and young people's plans (CYPPs). They also had to establish local Safeguarding Children Boards for their areas. Additional proposals concerned the sharing of information about children at risk between agencies.

The drive to promote joined-up working led to a common framework for inspecting children's services (Ofsted, 2005a, 2007b). The framework was established to support new joint area reviews (JARs). The purpose of JARs was to evaluate the extent to which local children's services had improved the wellbeing of children and young people, and how the various partner agencies worked together. They operated under arrangements made by Ofsted, and included the key inspection bodies concerned with children and young people's services (such as the Audit Commission and the Care Quality Commission). In 2009, JARs were replaced by the comprehensive area assessment (CAA) (see Chapter 7).

Legislation was introduced in the form of the Children Act 2004. Although there was widespread acceptance of change, concerns were expressed about some aspects of the policy, including data protection issues surrounding child databases, the failure to require some agencies (notably GP practices and schools) to cooperate with local partnership arrangements, and a lack of resources needed to implement the new policies (Education and Skills Committee, 2005). There was also scepticism about the prospect of getting local agencies with a long history of poor joint working into partnership (Hudson, 2006).

Children's Trusts

A central element of the new policy was the creation of children's trusts. Initially, the government envisaged new integrated structures but decided to allow local bodies to determine their own precise arrangements. This was reflected in the omission of a statutory duty to form children's trusts. Nonetheless, central government expected all areas to have children's trust arrangements by 2008. Thirty-five pathfinder children's trusts were launched in 2004 to develop new models of working and share their experience with others.

The evaluation of these pathfinders (University of East Anglia/National Children's Bureau, 2007) found they were a catalyst for integrating children's services. Early indications of positive outcomes for children and young people were also reported. The evaluation found that pathfinder trusts had enabled joined-up approaches to training and facilitated new occupational roles that operated across traditional professional and organizational boundaries. Less positively, they sometimes found it difficult to engage partners in key sectors, notably in the context of funding difficulties or where accountability frameworks were complex. All pathfinders had published CYPPs by 2006. Education, social services, health and the voluntary sector were usually involved in joint planning, other partners less so (University of East Anglia/National Children's Bureau, 2007). However, there was a concern that the relationship between the CYPP and the local area agreement (LAA) (which underpins partnership working at local level – see Chapter 7) needed clarification. It was pointed out that plans needed to demonstrate a clearer link between targets and actions.

The evaluation of pathfinders found that the pooling or alignment of budgets across agencies providing children's services was rare. The proportion of services using pooled budgets was highest in the health sector, where budgetary flexibilities had been introduced earlier. Some pathfinders faced problems as a result of disagreement between partners about the legal status of pooled budgets and a lack of expertise in this area. Half the pathfinders had joint commissioning strategies and new services had been developed to meet needs. However, greater mutual understanding of joint commissioning by commissioners, providers and users at local level was needed. More meaningful ways of involving service users were also required.

The pathfinder evaluation also found that the majority of pathfinders had adopted written protocols for sharing information across agencies and around half were piloting information-sharing databases. However, the sharing of child-level data was described as uneven and patchy. All children's trusts studied were piloting common approaches to the assessment of needs. A national common assessment framework (CAF) had been introduced, initially on a pilot basis. This was used by half the pathfinders, with the remainder using a local format. However, a low number of assessments were actually completed. The need for integrated IT systems was identified as a key issue in the report. In addition, joint cross-sector training on information sharing and assessments was identified as a priority.

The Audit Commission (2008) produced a critical report on children's trusts. It found little evidence of improvement in outcomes. The study reported that too much time and energy was spent on structures and processes. There was too much central direction, which impeded local efforts to promote collaboration. The relationship between children's trusts and other local partnerships was unclear. Children's trusts were uncertain about their role, particularly whether they should be more concerned with strategic planning or the details of service delivery. The Audit Commission also found that children's trusts had little oversight of budgets and there was little evidence of value for money. It recommended more flexibility in local collaboration, greater involvement by children and young people in service design, stronger participation in partnerships by GPs, skills agencies, and schools and better integration of children's trusts with other partnerships.

A further round of reform was prompted by more cases of child abuse, in particular that of 'Baby Peter' which came to light in 2008. Despite extensive contact between the family and local agencies, this child suffered horrific neglect and physical abuse, culminating in his death from multiple injuries. Haringey Council, the local authority responsible for children's services, was later found to have misled regulators about its performance. This case raised questions not only about the standard of children's services and the new partnership arrangements, but about the role of regulatory agencies, particularly Ofsted.

A fresh inquiry was launched, also undertaken by Lord Laming (2009). His report found continuing problems in partnership working, including a failure to share information about children at risk. He recommended new statutory targets and performance indicators for child protection, and a new national delivery unit to ensure the implementation of changes. Other important recommendations included:

- that government departments create a comprehensive approach to children through national strategies

- that directors of children's services who lack a background in child protection must appoint a senior manager within their team with such expertise

- stronger performance management of PCTs' role in child protection

- that children's trusts should regularly review the needs of all children and young people in their area

- that schools' role in child protection should be more explicitly recognized in inspection and improvement regimes

- that a national integrated system of child protection should be considered

- stronger inter-agency working, including sharing of information

- clarification of the relationship between children's trusts and local safeguarding children boards

- improvements in the children's services workforce and better training (including leadership training for councillors and managers)

- improved systems of referral where there are concerns about child safety (in police services and A&E departments for example)

Laming recommended that all referrals to children's services from other professionals lead to an initial assessment and engagement and feedback to the referring professional. He also called for core group meetings, reviews and casework decisions to include all professionals involved with the child. Another recommendation was that Ofsted inspectors responsible for child protection must have direct experience of this field of work.

The government accepted Laming's recommendations. It also proposed that children's trust boards should be a statutory requirement. Schools and colleges (and Job Centre Plus) were brought within the scope of the duty to cooperate with children's trusts. A similar duty was not imposed on GPs, although it recommended in guidance that a lead GP should be a member of the children's trust board. A further change was that the CYPP became the responsibility of the children's trust board rather than the local authority.

Other developments, already underway, included a children and young people's workforce strategy (DCSF, 2008a). This included additional spending on social work training, a review of social work practice, a development programme for senior staff and a national partnership to advise on the delivery of the national workforce policy. Another was the establishment of the national children's database (Contact Point). This had been delayed by fears about access, confidentiality and security. The roll-out of the database began in one region of England in 2009. Concessions were made to the opponents of the policy. For example, details of abuse would not be recorded on the database and restrictions were imposed on its access and use. On taking office in 2010, the Cameron government announced it would abolish the Contact Point database.

The Children's Plan

A policy review by HM Treasury and DfES (2007) identified areas where more could be done to help children: securing more active participation by young people in 'positive' pursuits; help for disabled children; and support for families caught in a cycle of low achievement. This fed into the Brown government's public service targets published in autumn 2007. Children's health and wellbeing was identified as a key priority for government, and was subject to a public service delivery agreement (HM Government, 2007g). The delivery agreement specified several indicators: increasing breastfeeding at 6–8 weeks; increasing take-up of school lunches; reducing the proportion of children who are obese; improving the emotional health and wellbeing of children; and improving the services used by disabled young people and their parents.

In 2007, a new ministry was established to focus on the needs of children. The Department for Children, Schools and Families (DCSF) (taking over from the DfES) became the key department for children's welfare, with the Department of Health as its key partner in coordinating efforts across government to achieve the PSA targets. The DCSF was charged with producing a comprehensive plan for children, young people and families. This was duly published in 2007 (DCSF, 2007). It set out five key principles: support for parents and families; maximizing the potential of all children; the need for children to enjoy their childhood as well as being prepared for adult life; the need for services responsive to children, young people and families; and the need to prevent failure. The plan comprised targets for improving child development, literacy and numeracy, and academic achievement, and for reducing child poverty, obesity and youth crime. It outlined new and continuing policies to achieve these aims including an expansion of parent support and advisory services; personal progress records on children's development; an expansion of children's centres and the improvement of outreach services and intensive support for the neediest families; and a children's workforce plan. It also promised a child health strategy, already discussed.

In response to concerns that children lacked facilities to play safely outside, a programme of playground building and refurbishment was announced. New strategies on play and on child safety were promised. A new joint unit was established by DCSF and the Department for Work and Pensions to coordinate preventive action on child poverty across government, including poor housing, where an action plan was promised. Other proposals included reviews of potential risks to children of exposure to inappropriate internet content, video games and commercialization, and encouraging 20 mph zones to reduce child pedestrian deaths.

The Plan set out reforms to improve education and early years care. This included measures to encourage parental involvement in schools, free early education and childcare to two-year-olds in the most disadvantaged communities; intensive support to children in primary schools at risk of falling behind; a review of the primary school curriculum; and improvements in the teaching of children with special needs. In addition, a range of measures to improve the early years and school teaching workforce were proposed including more continuing professional development and higher level qualifications for staff. Underachievement by school children was also addressed, aimed at improving outcomes for those children who behave badly, are excluded, or who do not attend school, and those who are unable to attend a mainstream school. Other educational reforms included raising the 'participation age' for education to 17 by 2013 and 18 by 2015 and measures to re-engage those aged 16 not in education, employment or training (known as 'Neets').

Following an earlier announcement, additional funding was allocated to youth facilities. An entitlement for young people to participate in 'positive activities' was also promised. These were accompanied by extending measures to prevent antisocial behaviour and crime by young people. A youth alcohol action plan was promised alongside a new drugs strategy (see Chapter 15). A review of sex and relationships education was also announced (see Exhibit 9.2.).

Exhibit 9.3

Children's Policies in Other Parts of the UK

Policies on child health and welfare are similar across all four countries of the UK. Indeed, many policies are UK-wide, such as Sure Start, the National Childcare Strategy, the Child Poverty Strategy, and tax/benefit policies affecting families. Nonetheless, there are important variations both in policy and implementation.

Each country of the UK has a Children's Commissioner, beginning with Wales in 2001, followed by Northern Ireland (2003), Scotland (2004), and England (2005). Although their roles and powers are similar, the Welsh, Northern Irish and Scottish commissioners are more explicitly described in terms of promoting and safeguarding rights. The English commissioner's role is described in terms of promoting awareness of the views and interests of children (although the commissioner must have regard to the UN convention on children's rights, as interpreted by the UK government). The English commissioner has jurisdiction over other parts of the UK on matters not within the remit of devolved governments and may launch inquiries on issues of UK-wide significance.

Other parts of the UK have their own plans on child health and wellbeing. Although broadly similar to those in England, there are some differences in emphasis and detail (see Welsh Assembly Government 2000, 2002b, 2004; Scottish Executive, 2001b, 2005b, 2007; Office of the First Minister and Deputy First Minister, 2006, 2007a, 2008; DHSSPS, 2006a). Northern Ireland's policy aims are that children should be healthy, enjoying learning and achieving, living in safety and with stability, experiencing economic and environmental wellbeing, contributing positively to community and society, and living in a society that respects their rights. The aims of the Scottish strategy are that children should be nurtured, safe, active, healthy, engaged in learning, achieving, included, respected and responsible. The Welsh strategy sets out seven core aims to give every child and young person in Wales: a 'flying start' in life; a comprehensive range of education and learning opportunities; the best possible health and freedom from abuse, victimization and exploitation; and access to play, leisure, sporting and cultural activities. It also seeks to ensure that children and young people are listened to, treated with respect and have their race and cultural identity recognized; have a safe home and community supporting physical and emotional wellbeing; and are not disadvantaged by poverty. Devolved governments have set their own targets to improve child health and wellbeing, some of which reflect UK-wide goals (for example child poverty) and others that reflect specific national priorities.

As in England, devolved governments have appointed ministers with specific responsibilities for children and young people. They have similarly established coordinating mechanisms to promote cross-departmental cooperation and integration of services at the local level. In 2004, Scotland introduced integrated children services plans within each local authority area to identify needs, develop services, monitor and evaluate impact on the basis of collaborative inter-agency working. Scottish ministers subsequently proposed new duties on agencies to cooperate with each other and share information, although planned legislation has not yet been introduced. In Wales, local multi-agency framework partnerships were established to produce plans for children and young people. The Children Act 2004 (which made separate provision for Wales) provided a statutory basis for partnership arrangements, including duties on agencies to safeguard and promote welfare of children; duties of cooperation; and pooled budgets. Local authorities were required to appoint lead directors of children and young people's services. However, unlike England, there was no requirement to merge education and social services for children and no expectation that children's trusts would be established. Northern Ireland also sought to improve joint planning and inter-agency collaboration on children's services, although the picture here is complicated by the fundamental reforms of public administration in the Province (see Chapter 4).

Other parts of the UK have reformed child protection arrangements, and have introduced health service reforms and frameworks that identify the specific needs of children. In addition, the devolved governments have pursued specific priorities in a number of areas. For example, Wales has invested in early years provision for children (the 0–3 age group) in areas of deprivation, under the 'Flying Start' initiative (Welsh Assembly Government, 2005c). This builds on pre-existing programmes including Sure Start, the National Childcare Strategy and Cymorth (a fund for supporting children and young people, administered through local partnerships). Flying Start seeks to provide a comprehensive service that includes free childcare, increased health visitor support, learning and play, parenting programmes and inter-professional working delivered primarily through integrated centres or community-focused schools. It aims to improve children's development in language, cognitive skills, social and emotional development, physical health and to identify high needs at an early stage.

Early years policy has also been a priority in Scotland. The Scottish Executive (2003d) introduced an early years strategy which sought to ensure that vulnerable children under five received an integrated package of health, care, and education support, targeting deprived families with children aged 0–3 years. This strategy was reviewed in 2008 (Scottish Executive/COSLA, 2008), with a re-emphasis on integrated working, capacity building and early intervention. These initiatives built on previous programmes including Sure Start, the National Childcare Strategy and Starting Well. The latter was a demonstration project, which aimed to pilot and disseminate the lessons learned from innovative integrated, multidisciplinary and multi-agency approaches to care and support of vulnerable families and children (Mackenzie et al., 2004; Mackenzie, 2008). Meanwhile in Northern Ireland, an expansion and enhancement of Sure Start has been planned, with new programmes for two-year-olds and an extension of services to more local areas.

Devolved governments have also promoted healthy schools. Scotland's policy appears to be the most advanced (Scottish Executive, 2003a). The Scottish Executive set an ambitious healthy schools target and strengthened the system of accreditation and support, by creating a Scottish health promoting schools unit. Health promotion is enshrined in education policies, notably integrated community schools, which aim to integrate educational, health, social work and other services in and around schools. Schools are required to contribute to integrated children's service plans. Moreover, health promotion is identified as one of the key areas in the Scottish education curriculum. Furthermore, legislation passed in 2007 (the Schools Health Promotion and Nutrition Act) placed specific duties on the Scottish Executive, local education authorities and schools to ensure that schools promote health. Education authorities are required to include efforts to improve health promotion in their annual statements of educational improvement.

Conclusion

This chapter has shown that a wide range of policies have been introduced in an effort to improve child health and wellbeing. It is, however, too early to draw firm conclusions about the impact of these initiatives, as their full benefits can only be gauged in the longer term. Optimistically, the emphasis upon child- and family-centred policies and on integrated approaches to policy, planning and service delivery augurs well. New programmes have been developed, some of which have shown early benefits. Even so, there is considerable scope for further improvement. In particular, it is vital that those in most need are targeted. Problems of joint working across agencies also remain and need to be addressed. Moreover, these initiatives will not succeed if there is a failure to deal adequately with underlying structural factors that harm children's health and wellbeing, such as poverty, inequality, poor housing, obesity, addictions, accidents, pollution and transport. These issues are discussed in more detail in the chapters that follow.

Health and the Environment: Pollution and Accidents

10

Environmental health has been defined as 'those aspects of human health, including quality of life, that are determined by physical, chemical, biological, social and psychosocial factors in the environment. It also refers to the theory and practice of assessing, correcting and preventing those factors in the environment that can potentially affect adversely the health of present and future generations' (MacArthur and Bonnefoy, 1998, cited in Burke et al., 2002). It is estimated that 23 per cent of deaths worldwide, and 17 per cent of deaths in developed countries, can be attributed to environmental factors (Prüss-Üstün and Corvalan, 2006). The potential health risks of the environment include physical agents (radiation, noise, fire); chemical agents (toxic substances); biological agents (fungi, bacteria, viruses); natural forces (tidal waves, floods, extreme weather); hazards from social conflict (violence, riots, terrorism, war) and complex hazards arising from new technologies (GM food, nanotechnology) (IRGC, 2005, cited by Ball, 2006). In practice, however, it is difficult to attribute injury and illness to a single factor. Moreover, a particular aspect of the environment, such as the transport system, for example (see Exhibit 11.1), can have multiple consequences for health.

The list of environmental health risks is long. Rather than analysing every single issue, this chapter focuses on two specific areas: pollution and accidents. In the following chapter, the broader challenges of sustainability and climate change are explored. Food, which can be regarded as an environmental issue, is considered in Chapter 12. Housing and regeneration, which have an important impact on people's immediate living environment, are considered in Exhibits 16.2 and 17.1.

Pollution

Some chemicals, notably lead and asbestos, are clearly associated with specific diseases (Alloway and Ayres, 1997). Although large-scale exposure to toxic chemicals, as a result of industrial accidents, for example, is hazardous to health, it is more difficult to assess the impact of long-term low-level contamination through multiple channels (air, water, food). People are exposed to a 'cocktail' of chemical agents throughout their lives. Multiple exposure could play a part in the onset of neurodevelopmental disorders such as autism, mental retardation and ADHD (Grandjean and Landrigan, 2006) and a range of cancers (Knox, 2005; Newby and Howard, 2005; Clapp et al., 2006), although this is difficult to prove. For example, persistent organic pollutants (POPs), which include organochlorine compounds (such as DDT, aldrin and lindane), polychlorinated biphenyls (PCBs), dioxins and furans, are produced by industrial processes and accumulate in the environment and in the food chain (Baldwin, 1997; Friends of the Earth, 2001). Some believe that they damage hormone and immune systems, and may cause cancer (Newby and Howard, 2006; McGregor et al., 1998), notably breast (see Exhibit 8.1) and testicular cancer. These chemicals have also been linked to poor brain development in children (Walkowaik et al., 2001; Jacobson and Jacobson, 1997), low fertility rates and problems in pregnancy (Baldwin, 1997). Another chemical, phthalates, found in paints, plastics and deodorants, has been linked to low-birthweight babies (Zhang et al., 2009).

Air Pollution

Many airborne chemicals are harmful to human health (Walters, 2009). These include sulphur dioxide (SO_2) and nitrogen oxides (NOx), which affect the lungs and also cause 'acid rain' that damages buildings, crops and forests. Others include volatile organic compounds (VOCs) from solvents, pesticides and carbon combustion. VOCs such as benzene and polycyclic aromatic hydrocarbons (PAHs) are linked to cancer (Thompson and Anthony, 2005). Low-level ozone, formed by the photochemical effects of sunlight on NOx and VOCs, can cause respiratory problems and trigger asthma attacks. It also increases the chances of dying from lung diseases, such as pneumonia, bronchitis and emphysema by up to 30 per cent (Jerrett et al., 2009). Fine airborne particles or 'particulates' have been identified as possible causes of ill health (COMEAP, 2007; WHO Regional Office for Europe, 2006a). Such particles are graded by size (PM2.5 are very fine particles of 2.5 micrometres and PM10 are particles of up to 10 micrometres). They can contain many harmful substances, including compounds from traffic fumes, construction and incineration, and compounds produced from chemical reactions between pollutants as well as biological material such as spores, bacteria and pollen.

Air pollution can affect lung development (Gauderman et al., 2007), cause lung irritation and trigger respiratory illnesses, such as asthma and bronchitis (Venn et al., 2001; Kunzli et al., 2000). Airborne particles have been linked to a range of diseases including childhood cancer (Knox, 2005), lung cancer (Pope et al., 2002; COMEAP, 2007), heart defects in babies (Ritz et al., 2002) and heart attacks and strokes (COMEAP, 2006, 2007; Peters et al., 2004; Pope et al., 2002; Sunyer et al., 2003; Miller et al., 2007). Exposure to particulate and SO_2 pollution has been associated with excess risks of mortality (Elliott et al., 2007). Exposure of pregnant women to air pollution has been linked to the risk of low-birthweight babies (Rich et al., 2008). According to some estimates, up to 24,000 UK residents may die prematurely as a result of air pollution (COMEAP, 1998). Actual deaths could be as high as 50,000 (EAC, 2010a) according to more recent estimates. Air pollution has been identified as the cause of 6 per cent of total annual mortality in Europe, half of this attributed to motorized traffic (Kunzli et al., 2000). It has also been associated with a reduced life expectancy of 8.6 years across the European Union (WHO Regional Office for Europe, 2006a).

Hazardous Waste

The transport, disposal and processing of waste has implications for health. Although most attention has focused on the most harmful detritus, even 'non-hazardous' waste can cause health problems, through air and water pollution, and indirectly through its contribution to global warming and climate change (see Chapter 11). Proximity to hazardous waste landfill sites has been associated with higher risks of birth defects in children (Dolk et al., 1998; Elliott et al., 2001; Palmer et al., 2005; Vrijheid et al., 2002). Waste incinerators have been linked to cancers and birth defects (Dummer et al., 2003; Elliott et al., 1996a, 2000) and may affect immune systems and heart disease (Thompson and Anthony, 2005). However, given the range of other possible factors that might be involved, it is difficult to prove a causal relationship.

Radiation

Some forms of radiation (ionizing and ultraviolet) have been linked to cancer. These can occur naturally (for example radon gas, solar rays) as well as being 'man-made' (x-rays, nuclear power). Nuclear installations are feared because of their potential for catastrophic accidents, such as the Chernobyl disaster of 1986. Adverse health consequences can also result from low-level contamination from nuclear power stations and waste processing facilities. No conclusive link between nuclear installations and cancer has ever been proved, despite the existence of 'clusters' of cases nearby (COMARE, 2005). There is disquiet about the carcinogenity of other forms of radiation, such as electricity pylons and mobile phones (Interdepartmental Expert Group on Mobile Phones, 2000; Draper et al., 2005; NRPB, 2001) but as yet no conclusive link has been found.

Noise Pollution

Noise is believed to affect health adversely. Findings from one study indicated that 3 per cent of heart attacks and strokes (approximately 3000 deaths in England each year) might be triggered by noise pollution (Coghlan, 2007). Specifically, night-time aircraft and road traffic have been linked to excess risks of hypertension (Jarup et al., 2008). Antisocial neighbourhood noise, complaints about which have increased in recent years (a fivefold increase between 1984 and 2004 – Social Trends, 2007), is also believed to damage health through stress and sleep deprivation.

Exhibit 10.1

Drinking Water and Health

Drinking water quality appears to have improved across the UK, with sharp reductions in nitrate levels (3 per cent of samples failed to meet the standard in 1990, compared with less than 0.1 per cent now). Iron, lead and other contaminants have also been reduced (Drinking Water Inspectorate, 2007). Today, less than 0.1 per cent of samples fail to meet standards in England and Wales (compared with 0.6 per cent in Scotland and Northern Ireland). However, concerns remain about risks to health, notably from nitrates and microbial agents, such as campylobacter and crytosporidium, both linked to outbreaks of gastroenteritis (Drinking Water Inspectorate, 2008). Standards for drinking water have been set by WHO since the 1980s (latest version: WHO, 2006a). The EU has introduced directives on drinking water and quality standards in rivers, lakes and coastal areas. The drinking water directives specify limits for chemical and biological agents, including pesticides, lead, nitrates and bacteria (see Council of the European Communities, 1980, 1998). The EU requires member states to implement procedures for monitoring, regulating water quality and for taking action to prevent and ameliorate breaches of standards. The body responsible for regulation in England and Wales is the Drinking Water Inspectorate (Scotland and Northern Ireland have their own agencies).

One of the most controversial issues in this field is fluoridation. Fluoride in water supplies reduces tooth decay in children and reduces inequalities in dental health (MRC Working Group, 2002; McDonagh et al., 2000). Even so, research evidence is of poor quality and there has been misrepresentation of findings (Nuffield Council on Bioethics, 2007). Opponents of fluoridation claim it is linked to bone fractures, problems of brain development, birth defects, disorders of the immune system, cancer, and discolouration of the teeth (Bryson, 2004). They also argue that fluoridation raises civil liberty issues because it is 'enforced medication'. Some water supplies contain fluoride naturally (in East Anglia, for example), while in others (West Midlands, Tyneside) it is added. Legal changes in 1985 to encourage fluoridation had little effect, because of the anti-fluoridation campaigns and anxiety among water companies about legal liability. Following the Acheson report on health inequalities (see Chapter 17) which recommended fluoridation, legislation was introduced in

England and Wales in 2003 to empower health authorities to engage in public consultation, to compel local water companies to fluoridate water supplies while indemnifying them from legal action, and to provide additional resources to encourage fluoridation. In Scotland, however, the Executive's initial backing for a similar plan was shelved following public consultation.

Pollution Policy

Historically, policies addressed the most visible and the most dangerous forms of pollution in isolation. Separate bodies were established to regulate air, water and waste. During the late 1980s an attempt was made to create a more comprehensive and systematic approach to pollution control with the creation of Her Majesty's Inspectorate of Pollution (HMIP) from an amalgamation of agencies. This was superseded in 1996, when the Environment Agency for England and Wales was established. The new agency acquired comprehensive powers and responsibilities for environmental regulation coupled with a responsibility to 'champion the environment'. Local authorities retained some regulatory roles in relation to the environment (see below and Chapter 11). Scotland and Northern Ireland have their own Environment Agencies. Although there are differences in institutional structures in different parts of the UK, on most environmental policy issues there is a UK-wide approach.

The Environment Agency struggled with its wide brief. There was an apparent lack of leadership and vision, a low public profile, continuing problems of staff morale, lack of accountability and poor decision-making (Environment, Transport and Regional Affairs Committee, 2000). Business interests criticized the agency for being too confrontational and beholden to the environmental lobby, while environmental pressure groups thought it too close to industry (Bell and Gray, 2002). Later, there were signs of improvement, notably with regard to the timeliness and consistency of regulatory and enforcement functions (EFRAC, 2006). Even so, concerns remained about the agency's ability to manage a wide range of responsibilities, recruit specialist staff and combine the roles of regulator and environmental champion.

Integrated Pollution Control

Integrated pollution control (IPC), introduced in 1990, required an integrated assessment of impact on air, water and land (O'Riordan and Weale, 1989). Sites (for example industrial plants, factories) were required to use the 'best available technology not entailing excessive cost' (BATNEEC) to reduce emissions. Those producing several different forms of pollution had to use the 'best practicable environmental option' (BPEO) to minimize overall harm. Two further principles underpinned this policy: the 'precautionary principle', that pollution hazards should be assessed in advance and steps taken to prevent or minimize harm (O'Riordan and Cameron, 1994); and the 'polluter pays' principle, that the costs of regulating and reducing environmental harms should be met by producers.

A new prior authorization process was introduced in the 1990s, following the European directive on integrated pollution prevention and control (IPPC) (Official Journal of the European Communities, 1996). Polluters now had to demonstrate use of 'best available techniques' (BAT) in reducing pollution. However, as cost considerations were an aspect of availability, this was not much different in practice from the previous regime. IPPC was, however, wider in scope, covering more environmental issues including noise, light, heat, vibration, accidents, and energy efficiency. More activities were covered, such as food and drink factories, waste sites and some farms. The regime also related to the lifetime of an installation, including decommissioning. IPPC focused on entire installations rather than specific industrial processes, increasing the scope for integrated pollution control.

It was intended that IPPC would strengthen the role of health advice in decisions about pollution control, but this did not happen. Many applications under IPPC regulations did not elicit substantive comments from PCTs (which have a statutory right to consultation). There was a lack of capacity and capability in responding to such applications (Lanser and Pless-Mulloli, 2003). Other weaknesses were also evident. Only half the installations in Europe meant to be covered by IPPC actually received a permit (Europa, 2007). A further directive on industrial emissions was agreed in 2008, to promote greater consistency in regulation across Europe by setting new inspection and monitoring standards (Official Journal of the European Union, 2008). The system was amended again in 2008 when new environmental permitting (EP) regulations came into force in England and Wales, combining pollution prevention and control with waste management licensing. This was done to reduce the regulatory burden on business, while strengthening the link between the pollution control and waste management.

The Role of the EU and Other Agencies

Domestic policy has been shaped by EU initiatives. The expansion of EU activity in environmental policy is well documented (see Jordan, 2005; Hildebrand, 2005; Carter, 2007). Although the 1957 Treaty of Rome did not specifi cally mention the environment, measures were introduced under existing powers to protect the safety of workers and citizens and to remove internal barriers to trade. However, it was not until 1973 that the European Community adopted its first environmental programme. Further landmarks were the Single European Act of 1987, which strengthened the legal basis of environmental policy, and the establishment of the European Environment Agency in 1990. The EU's environmental policy was strengthened by the subsequent treaties of Maastricht and Amsterdam; the latter requiring that environmental protection be enshrined in all EU policies. Decisions by the European Court of Justice on environmental matters further expanded the EU's influence. There are now over 500 pieces of EU environmental legislation.

During the 1990s, the relationship between environment and health became a significant theme in Europe. The European Commission, along with the WHO Regional Office, and other bodies (notably the European Environment and Health Committee, which brings together health ministers, environment ministers, international agencies and non-government organizations) developed an environment and health strategy (Commission of the European Communities, 2003). This called for an integrated approach to environmental health to reduce the disease burden, prevent new health threats, and strengthen policymaking capacity. This was followed by an action plan for 2004–2010 (Commission of the European Communities, 2004a) with three main themes: improving information about the links between sources of pollution and health (by developing environmental health indicators, for example); strengthening research and addressing emerging issues (by targeting research on diseases and exposures); and reviewing policies and improving communication (by improving organizational capacity).

This strategy built on the work of the WHO Regional Office, which had earlier produced a charter on environment and health (WHO Regional Office for Europe, 1990, p. 4) setting out the entitlement of individuals to 'an environment conducive to the highest attainable level of health and wellbeing.' This document emphasized the importance of prevention and evidence-based action. A European Environmental Health Action Plan followed (WHO Regional Office for Europe, 1994), which sought to: promote the development of national action plans; encourage a wider range of actors to participate in securing environmental health objectives; ensure joint participation of environmental and public health agencies; share responsibility among all economic sectors (such as energy and transport); improve policy tools; and promote international cooperation. Subsequently 'a healthier and safer physical environment' became a key priority in the European Region's revised health strategy (WHO Regional Office for Europe, 1999c). The Children's Environment and Health Action Plan was also adopted by European ministers (WHO Regional Office for Europe, 2004). This identified four priorities to improve child health: improve access to safe and affordable water and sanitation; reduce health consequences of accidents, injuries and lack of physical activity by promoting safe, secure and supportive environments; prevent and reduce respiratory disease due to indoor and outdoor pollution and reduce asthma attacks; and reduce exposure to dangerous chemicals, excessive noise, biological agents and hazardous working environments during pregnancy, childhood and adolescence. In a further development, in 2010, health and environment ministers from the WHO European region signed a new declaration on environmental health. Known as the Parma declaration, this committed member states to a new European environment and health planning process. This will monitor progress on targets, including a 2015 deadline for providing clean air for children and protecting them from harmful substances (WHO Regional Office for Europe, 2010).

The Regional Office's approach lay within a global framework. Acknowledgement of environmental factors was reflected in WHO's Health for All strategy (WHO, 1981) and its successor, Health 21 (WHO, 1998a), which included commitments to reduce accidents and injuries and to protect people from pollution, contamination and other hazards. WHO (1991) also sought to promote environmental health by emphasizing sustainable development (see Chapter 11).

The Regulation of Chemicals

Chemicals regulation in the UK is shaped by international agreements and EU legislation (Cm 5827, 2003; Elliott, 2004; Selin and Eckley, 2003). International agreements include the Geneva Convention on long-range transboundary pollution, which sought to limit airborne pollution (discussed further below). The Rotterdam Convention of 1998, ratified by the UK in 2004, established a process of 'prior informed consent' when importing certain hazardous chemicals. The Stockholm Convention on persistent organic pollutants (POPs) of 2004, ratified by the UK in 2005, restricts the production, use and trade of a group of chemicals known as the 'dirty dozen', including organochloride pesticides, industrial chemicals and dioxins. Although POPs are now banned in the UK, they remain a problem. Traces of pesticides covered by the Stockholm Convention are still found in water, and dioxin levels in soil remain significant (DEFRA et al., 2007). However, large falls (at least 60 per cent) have occurred in dioxin and PCB emissions in air, in dioxins and PCBs in food, and in PCB levels in soil.

Other international bodies have a role in regulation. The OECD has promoted voluntary agreements on the classification of substances and labelling, and has sought to harmonize risk assessment and testing procedures. The EU also has a regulatory role (Warhurst, 2005; Cm 5827, 2003). During the 1960s, efforts to eliminate trade barriers between member states led to regulations on the classification, packaging and labelling of chemicals. In the 1970s, occupational health and safety considerations (see Exhibit 10.2) influenced restrictions on the marketing and use of chemicals. Regulations on pesticides, veterinary medicines, pharmaceutical products and radioactive substances were also introduced. In the 1980s, a European system of notification and assessment of new chemicals was introduced, followed in the 1990s by limited measures covering products already in use.

Despite this, EU regulation has been regarded as ineffective and piecemeal. Only a small proportion of high-production volume chemicals had satisfactory data on safety, and regulators had insufficient capacity to assess risks (Warhurst, 2005). Moreover, there was criticism of a two-tier system in the regulation of new and existing chemicals (Cm 5827, 2003). The strengthening of the EU's competences in environmental policy led to a more robust approach. A new system called REACH (Registration, Evaluation, Authorization and Restriction of Chemicals) is being introduced (European Commission, 2007). This seeks to establish a comprehensive and systematic approach covering all chemicals, new and old. Manufacturers will be required to collect data on the safety of products, recorded on a central database under the auspices of a new European Chemicals Agency. It is intended that this will provide more information on hazards and risks along the entire supply chain. Regulation will target high-risk chemicals, under an authorization process. New processes will be created to regulate manufacture, sale and use. Introducing this system is a huge task and therefore it will not be fully implemented until 2019. The new regime was subjected to intense lobbying from industry and diluted as a result (Carter, 2007), raising doubts about its effectiveness (Hansen et al., 2007).

Action on Air Pollution

A number of international agreements set the framework for reducing airborne pollution (Elliott, 2004). The Geneva Convention of 1979, adopted by industrialized countries in Europe and North America, recognized the problem of airborne pollution but did not force countries to cut emissions. The Helsinki protocol of 1985, however, did set targets for reducing sulphur emissions. Unfortunately, this did not come into force until 1991 and even then excluded the biggest producers of sulphur dioxide (UK, USA and Poland). A new protocol, setting out sulphur emission targets, was agreed at Oslo in 1994. Other related agreements include the Sofia protocol of 1988, which sought to restrict NOx levels, an agreement in 1991 to reduce the emission of VOCs and the Gothenburg protocol of 1999, which set emission limits for sulphur, VOCs, NOx and ammonia across European countries, the USA and Canada. WHO (2006b) has also been active in this field, setting global standards for pollutants, including particulates, ozone, NOx and sulphur dioxide, with targets for reducing them.

The WHO Regional Office for Europe (1987, 2000a) has produced air quality guidelines for some years. The EU has tried to improve air quality through its pollution control regime, discussed above, which covers all emissions, and by introducing air quality directives. From the 1990s, member states were required to develop air quality strategies. Further impetus was added by a new air quality programme in 2001, 'Clean Air for Europe'. National emission ceilings were set for sulphur dioxide, NOx, VOCs and ammonia, which each member state must achieve by 2010. There are also targets for other pollutants, including benzene, carbon monoxide, lead and ozone. In 2008, the EU introduced a new directive on air quality, setting standards for the reduction of fine particles (PM2.5). Member states are required to reduce levels by a fifth between 2010 and 2020. However, the directive also gave EU countries more flexibility in meeting targets for the reduction of coarse (PM10) particles, as well as nitrogen dioxide and benzene, by extending deadlines for compliance. The EU has attempted to reduce emissions from specific sectors, such as large combustion plants, transport (see Chapter 11), and waste incineration (see below). Even so, a number of EU countries, including the UK, have failed to meet air quality targets and face legal action from the European Commission if they do not improve.

UK air quality policy operates within these global and European frameworks. The Major government produced an air quality strategy (DoE, 1996) that set standards for the most dangerous pollutants. Environmental campaigners were critical of this for failing to address the main causes of pollution, such as waste incineration and road traffic. The Blair government revised the air quality strategy, setting standards and targets for levels of benzene, carbon monoxide, butadiene, NOx, sulphur dioxide, particulates, ozone and lead (Cm 4548, 2000). This was later altered, strengthening the standards for particulates, benzene, carbon monoxide, and a new standard for PAHs. Subsequently, new targets for ozone reduction and for PM2.5 were proposed. In 2007, the Labour government produced a further air quality strategy (Cm 7169, 2007). It endorsed some fairly modest measures, but shied away from a radical plan to address major sources of air pollution such as road traffic and industry. Interestingly, the Cameron government identified air quality as a key issue and stated that it would work towards full compliance with European standards (HM Government, 2010c).

Local authorities have a significant role in regulating air pollution. Since 1997, they have been required to assess air quality against national standards. Where standards are not met, local councils must designate an air quality management area (AQMA). A plan is then devised to improve air quality, which may include improvements in traffic management or controls on industrial emissions. By 2008, over 200 local authorities had created AQMAs. In practice, plans tend to focus on short term measures (targeting high-polluting vehicles) rather than long-term structural changes (such as major changes to transport infrastructure). More recently, local authorities have been encouraged by central government to integrate air quality plans with other local plans (for example on transport). London, which has very high levels of air pollution, has devolved powers and responsibilities for air quality. The London mayor is responsible for air quality strategy and works with other agencies including local authorities to achieve improvements. The mayor cannot hold local authorities to account for improving air quality but does have powers with regard to transport that can help to achieve these objectives through structural changes (see Exhibit 11.1).

As already noted, the UK is unlikely to meet all its air quality targets (DEFRA, 2008a; NAO, 2009c; EAC, 2010a). Levels of particulates, ozone and nitrogen oxides are likely to exceed the 2010 targets. However, official figures indicate some improvement. Sulphur dioxide emissions fell over 80 per cent between 1990 and 2006 and NOx by over 40 per cent in the same period. VOCs (excluding methane, largely arising from natural sources) are now at less than half their 1990 levels. PM10 particulate levels declined significantly (by 50 per cent since 1990), although increased slightly in 2006. Carbon monoxide, benzene, butadiene, PAHs and lead levels have all fallen dramatically. For example, airborne lead fell by 96 per cent between 1990 and 2006, largely from the introduction of unleaded petrol (DEFRA, 2008a).

Improvements have occurred from deindustrialization, improved pollution controls, regulation of road vehicles and fuels, and changes in the energy industry, notably, a reduction in coal-based electricity generation. Nonetheless, there is criticism that the planning and regulatory framework is not adequate to the scale of the problem (Walters, 2009; EAC, 2010a). In particular, critics point out that enforcement is weak and under-resourced. They also note that much more must be done to address the underlying causes of air pollution, notably transport (see Exhibit 11.1).

Waste

Waste is another area where international action has set a framework for domestic policies (Elliott, 2004). The 1987 Cairo Guidelines on the management of hazardous waste, and the Basel Convention on transboundary movements of hazardous waste and its disposal (which came into force in 1992) were both significant developments. The EU has also introduced a number of directives on waste. Europe's first comprehensive strategy, introduced in 1989, aimed to improve production technologies and recycling. The strategy was renewed in 1996, with greater emphasis on reducing the movement of waste. Waste recycling was identified as a priority in the Sixth Environmental Programme, covering the period 2001–11. In addition, the EU introduced directives on issues such as waste oil, disposal of batteries and electrical products, packaging waste, PCBs, and motor vehicles. Directives on landfill and incineration were also introduced, discussed below. In addition, the IPCC directive and air quality directives, discussed above, had implications for waste disposal.

The UK has introduced regulations in line with international obligations and EU legislation. With regard to hazardous waste, measures were introduced in 2005 requiring waste producers to register with the Environment Agency. Subsequently waste management was integrated with IPPC under 'environmental permitting', mentioned earlier. Meanwhile the definition of hazardous waste was extended to cover more substances and products. To promote a more consistent approach, there is now a European-wide catalogue of hazardous waste. Other changes include rules on the separation of hazardous and non-hazardous waste introduced in 2004. Nonetheless, there are grounds for believing that controls are ineffective. In 2005, it was estimated that 700,000 tonnes of hazardous waste was unaccounted for (EFRAC, 2005a).

In recent years, waste management sites have been subject to greater regulation. Waste can only be accepted by a landfill site if it meets the criteria for that type of site. Particular wastes are now banned from landfill including liquid waste, tyres and dangerous substances such as clinical waste and explosive or corrosive materials. Municipal waste incinerators have been gradually subjected to tougher EU standards, leading to the closure of some older incinerators. An EU directive of 2000 set stricter standards on emissions, notably with regard to dioxins. Even so, concerns about incinerators remain. Only a small proportion of pollutants emanating from incinerators are measured and the risks of pollution from such installations may be underestimated (Thompson and Anthony, 2005).

The management of waste is shaped by the 1999 EU landfill directive, which led to a national strategy for reducing landfill and encouraging recycling (Cm 4693, 2000). The main aims behind this were to promote sustainable development and reduce greenhouse gas emissions and thereby global warming (see Chapter 11). New schemes were introduced to minimize waste and encourage recycling, and targets set for local authorities. A system of tradeable landfill allowances was implemented. A landfill tax was introduced, later increased following criticism that it was too low (EAC, 2003a; EFRAC, 2005a). The imposition of a 'tax escalator' (built-in increases in tax rates in future years) meant that the landfill tax would double between 2007 and 2011 (DEFRA, 2007). An aggregates tax was imposed in 2002 to reduce the extraction of sand, gravel or rock and to encourage recycling. Although the use of 'green taxes' was broadly welcomed, doubts were raised about implementation. Indeed, it was argued that poor enforcement, coupled with the increasing costs of landfill, had encouraged fly tipping' (EFRAC, 2005a).

The waste strategy for England was revised (DEFRA, 2007), setting out a range of policies to meet the requirements of the landfill directive and encourage more recycling. It established higher than previous targets for recycling (including a target to increase recycling to 50 per cent by 2020) and recovery of municipal waste (75 per cent by 2020). It promised a new target for the reduction of commercial and industrial waste going to landfill. The strategy set out key policies for achieving these objectives, such as the afore-mentioned increases in landfill tax, incentives for waste reduction and recycling households, further action on illegal dumping of waste, targeting specific sectors to reduce waste (such as food and paper industries), working with producers to reduce excess packaging, more segregation of waste at source, more investment in energy recovery from waste, and improvements in regional and local planning in waste management. In an effort to improve coordination, powers were granted to create Joint Waste Authorities to take on the functions of local authorities. Despite these revisions, criticism of government policy persists (House of Lords, 2008a). Concerns remain about poor quality data on waste, inappropriate targets for local authorities, and poor coordination by local authorities of waste services as well as the need for measures to promote sustainable product design and consumption and to reduce overall waste. A shortage of recycling plants has been observed (NAO, 2009b) and councils are continuing to dispose of recyclable waste in landfill (Hope and Neville, 2008). There is also a shortage of incineration capacity to take up the shortfall caused by tougher rules on landfill disposal. As a result the UK recycles a relatively low proportion of its waste, around a third of the total, and it is unlikely that it will meet EU targets. Meanwhile, at the time of writing, the EU is revising its framework directive on waste, which is likely to bring further changes.

Accidents and Violence

Like pollution, accidents and violence are major public health issues. Every year around 20,000 people a year die from injury in the UK, two-thirds from unintentional injuries. There are many others who survive serious or minor injuries. Six million A&E visits each year are due to non-fatal injuries. Accidental injury is the leading cause of child death and a major cause of disability in children and older people.

Accidents and violence can be prevented by altering the environment. Unlike, say, the prevention of cancer or heart disease, the benefits of accident and violence prevention emerge quickly in terms of falling death and injury rates. However, the potential for 'quick gains' in this field has not ensured action. Although some issues, such as road safety, have featured among government priorities, accidents and violence generally have had low political status. Furthermore, even when identified as priorities, these areas have often suffered from poor implementation and insufficient resources (Watson and White, 2001). This is partly because the public health consequences of accidents and violence are spread across different sectors such as health services, the criminal justice system, transport, schools, the workplace, and the home. This creates difficulties in formulating coherent policy responses, as cooperation is required from multiple agencies. On top of this, data on accidents, violence and health consequences is of poor quality (Watson and White, 2001), as no single body has overall responsibility for data collection. Research evidence about interventions is weak, partly due to inadequate funding and also because of the difficulty of designing studies of multiple causality. Furthermore, even when good quality evidence is available, this does not guarantee action, as prevention is often opposed by powerful industrial and economic interests.

Accident Prevention Strategies

At the international level there have been efforts to raise the profile of accidents and violence as health issues. WHO and UNICEF (2008), focusing specifically on children, estimated that 830,000 worldwide died each year in accidents. Their report expressed concern about the lack of information on the cost-effectiveness of accident prevention and highlighted over 20 proven interventions including the use of seatbelts in cars, helmets for cycling, regulations on hot water, separate cycle lanes, and redesign of play equipment and toys to improve safety. Deliberate injury is also a major global public health problem. It has been estimated that 1.6 million deaths worldwide can be attributed to violence (Krug et al., 2002). This includes suicides, murder and deaths in armed conflict.

The WHO European Region has highlighted the need to reduce injuries, disabilities and death from accidents and violence (WHO Regional Office for Europe, 1985, 1999c). It has focused particularly on children's safety and the prevention of road accidents. The EU also took steps to prevent accidents and injuries, mainly through directives on product safety and occupational health. In 1999, it introduced an injury prevention programme. Specific actions include the establishment of an injury database across several member states and encouraging member states to take steps to prevent injuries in 'priority areas' (children and adolescents, vulnerable road users and elderly people) and to reduce self-harm, suicide and violence. In 2007, the EU adopted a revised policy, encouraging all member states to establish a national policy for injury prevention, to develop a national injury surveillance system, and to ensure that injury prevention and safety promotion are included in the training of health professionals. The European Commission has been tasked with supporting a community-wide injury surveillance system, the establishment of a system for exchanging information between relevant stakeholders, encouraging changes to professional training and supporting the development of good practice in accident and injury prevention. Seven priority areas were identified: the safety of children and adolescents, elderly citizens, vulnerable road users, and the prevention of injuries caused by products and services, sports, self-harm, and interpersonal violence.

UK health strategies have identified accidents as a priority area. The Major government's *Health of the Nation* strategy (Cm 1986, 1992) aimed to reduce death rates from accidents between 1990 and 2005, among children under 15 by at least a third, among young people aged 15–24 by at least a quarter, and among elderly people by a third. The strategy tried to promote a holistic approach to accident prevention by bringing together health authorities, police, fire brigades, ambulance trusts, schools and local authorities into local alliances, sharing information and pursuing joint strategies on accident prevention. Although good examples of local action emerged, much depended on the willingness of local agencies to collaborate. The Blair government set two overall targets: to reduce the death rate from accidents by at least a fifth and serious accidental injury by 10 per cent between 1996 and 2010 (Cm 4386, 1999). It built on the previous government's approach by encouraging local partnerships. However, the BMA (2001) noted that fragmentation of agencies in accident prevention had continued. It called for a new national agency to coordinate matters, more research into injury prevention, and surveillance centres in each part of the UK to collate, interpret and disseminate injury statistics. Subsequently, a DoH (2002d) task force rejected a national agency, but recommended a more integrated approach to accident prevention at all levels, better data collection and access, more structured professional training, and dissemination of good practice.

It proved difficult to achieve government targets. The death rate from accidents actually rose by one per cent by 2004 and the serious injury rate by 4 per cent (Audit Commission and Healthcare Commission, 2007). Additional targets were introduced to be achieved by 2010: to reduce the number of accidental fire-related deaths in the home by 20 per cent; to reduce the number of people killed or seriously injured on the roads by 40 per cent, and the number of children killed or seriously injured in road accidents by half. The government declared a commitment to reduce the higher incidence of accidents in disadvantaged communities. Targets were also introduced for workplace accidents (see Exhibit 10.2). In the meantime, the overall number of accidental deaths rose from 10,794 to 12,231 in England and Wales between 2000 and 2008. Accidental deaths increased both as a proportion of total deaths (2–2.4 per cent) and as a proportion of the population (from 20.3 to 22.5 per 100,000 population) in the same period (source of data: ONS, 2002, 2009c).

In *Choosing Health* (Cm 6374, 2004), the Blair government restated its commitment to reducing accidents, but did not identify accident prevention among its top priorities. No major programme was launched, but some actions were undertaken including an accreditation scheme for multi-agency safety centres, which offer advice, education, information and training. Specific initiatives in areas such as road safety, falls in elderly people and child accidents were introduced, discussed in more detail below. These were stimulated as much by concerns about the health inequalities agenda and children's health as by the accident prevention agenda (see Chapters 9 and 17). The risk of accidents is disproportionately high among disadvantaged people, and especially their children. Accidental death rates are 13 times higher among children whose parents are long-term unemployed or who have never worked, compared with children born into professional or managerial families (Edwards, 2006). Some local NHS bodies and local authorities have targeted accident prevention as a means of reducing health inequalities. Even so, there remains a lack of central direction in accidental injury prevention. In particular, there is 'no single, clear, cross-government statement which draws together what has to be done to reduce unintentional injury' (Audit Commission and Healthcare Commission, 2007, p. 6). Despite examples of good practice, prevention of accidents and violence has lost impetus at local level.

Meanwhile, on a more positive note, different parts of the UK have developed their own initiatives on accident prevention. Scotland, Wales and Northern Ireland have safety strategies, and have established their own child safety and elderly falls-prevention initiatives. Some have adopted innovative approaches. For example, Wales pioneered an accident surveillance system, collating data from A&E departments and using this to monitor and prevent accidents. It also established a collaboration for accident prevention and injury control (CAPIC) to bring together agencies and professionals to support injury prevention.

UK government policy on non-industrial accidents has focused on three areas: children and young people, older people and road accidents. Unintentional injuries are the main cause of death in children and are the main cause of hospitalization in this age group (Audit Commission and Healthcare Commission, 2007). Some local areas have developed more coherent approaches to accident prevention in children, including multi-agency working and improved systems of data collection (Audit Commission and Healthcare Commission, 2007). Central government provided a stronger lead with an action plan on children's safety (DCSF, 2008c). This set out a wide range of measures, including accident prevention. These included communication and information campaigns, implementation of a new road safety strategy for children (see below), a new home safety equipment scheme targeted at deprived families, and a review of local accident prevention schemes. A new national indicator to reduce hospital admissions for child injuries was also introduced.

The prevention of injuries, in particular falls, in older people is an important public health issue. The impact of a fall for an elderly person can be devastating for the individual and their family. It also adds to the costs of health and social care: 40 per cent of 'fallers' aged over 65 end up in long-term care (Henry, 2005). Population-based prevention strategies (which involve a range of activities such as educational advice, home visits and the removal of hazards), usually involving multiple agencies, can reduce fall-related injuries by up to a third (McClure et al., 2008). The NSF for older people aimed to establish integrated falls services to prevent falls and reduce their impact, but these were slow to develop. NICE (2004) produced guidance on the assessment and prevention of falls to improve practice in this field. There have been many local projects, including those participating in the Healthy Communities Collaborative, a government-backed project (HDA, 2003). National campaigns have been used, such as the DTI's 'avoiding slips, trips and broken hips' campaign in 2002 and the National Falls Awareness Day, which began in 2005. Voluntary groups such as Help the Aged and Age Concern (now merged as Age UK) also play an important role in falls prevention by providing resources and information.

Every year in the UK around 3000 people are killed on the roads with a further 30,000 seriously injured. Almost a quarter of a million people receive slight injuries as a result of road accidents and around 3000 children are killed or seriously injured. Although the UK has a low level of road deaths and injuries compared with other European countries, it has a higher than average number of child fatalities (PAC, 2009b). There are also concerns that current systems of recording accidents underestimate the problem (Transport Committee, 2008a). Official figures, however, show that the number of fatalities on the roads has fallen in the UK, by over half in the past forty years and by 10 per cent in the past decade. Child deaths and serious injuries also halved in this period. This is to some extent due to successive governments giving higher priority to prevention. Over the years there have been publicity campaigns on road safety (such as the long-running THINK! campaign) alongside legislation (such as drink-driving laws, seat belt legislation, and penalties for speeding and dangerous driving). Also, road safety has been given a high priority in policing and enforcement (although not high enough according to some – see Transport Committee, 2008a). Specific initiatives have been aimed at reducing speed, such as fixed and mobile cameras (Pilkington and Kinra, 2005) and lower speed limits in residential areas (Webster and Mackie, 1996; Grundy et al., 2009). Furthermore, road safety interventions have long been part of an overall strategy with outcome-based targets. For example, the 2000 strategy (DETR, 2000a) set targets for reducing fatal and serious accidents and these were incorporated in the performance objectives of the Department of Transport and other public bodies. The Road Safety Act 2006 introduced new penalties for speeding and new offences for careless driving. It also extended the government's powers to make grants to local authorities and other bodies to promote road safety. There have been specific strategies and targets to reduce accidents involving children. A new children's road safety strategy was introduced in 2007 (DfT, 2007), setting out plans for improved education of child pedestrians, encouraging local partnerships to deliver coordinated road safety activities, encouraging 20 mph zones and coordinating road safety and school travel activities. Despite all this, calls continue for better coordination, more research, stronger measures and tougher enforcement (Independent Inquiry into Inequalities in Health, 1998; Roberts et al., 2002; Breen, 2002; Transport, Local Government and Regions Committee 2002; Transport Committee 2006, 2008a; PAC, 2009b). Governments have been accused of being preoccupied with the reaction of the roads lobby and blaming the victim by focusing too much on changing the behaviour of cyclists and pedestrians. A more fundamental criticism is that road safety is shaped strongly by transport policy, which prioritizes the roads at the expense of safer (and more environmentally friendly) forms of transport (see Exhibit 11.1). The change of government in 2010 is unlikely to lead to a reversal of this approach. Indeed, the new government seemed to be responding strongly to the motoring lobby with a commitment to reduce funding for speed cameras.

There are international pressures to reduce road accidents. The EU adopted a road safety policy in the 1980s. In 2001, it set an ambitious target to halve road accident deaths by 2010 as part of its transport strategy. It has taken steps to prevent and reduce deaths and injuries from road accidents, largely through harmonization of laws and improved motor vehicle safety technologies, although with limited success. The World Bank and WHO (2004) have highlighted the need for public health intervention to improve road safety. However, the motor industry is a powerful multinational lobby and is able to counter measures both internationally and within particular countries that reduce its markets or impose additional costs.

Violence

Policies have been introduced to reduce violent deaths and injuries. In the UK, violence is an important cause of premature mortality and morbidity, largely because it disproportionately affects younger age groups. It also impacts significantly on health inequities. In England, for example, people living in the North West region are three times more likely to be admitted to hospital due to violence than in the South East (Sivarajasingam et al., 2002). Ethnic minorities and unemployed people living in poverty are also likely to suffer higher than average levels of violence (ESRC, 2008). The public health implications of violence have been acknowledged (Keithley and Robinson,

2000). This has been partly due to research about the extent and impact of violence on health (Sivarajasingam et al., 2002; Shepherd et al., 2000) and by greater social awareness of particular aspects of violence, such as domestic violence. A public health approach to violence has been recommended (Shepherd and Farrington, 1993; Krug et al., 2002; Independent Inquiry into Inequalities in Health, 1998). This addresses individual and social manifestations of violent behaviour and redesigning the environment to reduce aggression and access to weapons. It also involves research into the causes of violence, and the relationship between violence and ill health and multiagency working between health bodies, local government, voluntary sectors and the police and criminal justice system. In the UK, plans have developed along these lines. In England and Wales, for example, local crime prevention and safety partnerships bring together a range of local agencies including the NHS. Initiatives include the use of accident and emergency data to help identify problem areas, an approach pioneered in Wales (Home Office, 1999; Shepherd et al., 2000). A partnership approach has also been pursued in Scotland, where an explicit public health approach to violence has been adopted. A national violence reduction unit was created to spread best practice. Violence reduction was declared a national priority and a strategic plan adopted (Violence Reduction Unit, 2007). In addition, UK governments have taken steps to prevent violent crime in a range of measures including domestic and child abuse, as well as further restrictions and increased penalties for possession of weapons. Policies on alcohol and drugs (see Chapter 14 and 15) have implications for violence and health. Furthermore, recent governments have adopted policies on suicide prevention, with targets to reduce the number of deaths (see Exhibit 8.2).

Exhibit 10.2

Health and Work

Hazards associated with particular occupations have been known since Greek and Roman times (Rosen, 1993). The industrial revolution brought fresh evidence about occupational health risks, giving rise to legislation in the nineteenth and twentieth centuries protecting workers from longer hours, harmful working conditions and hazardous substances (see Chapter 2). There have been visible improvements. In 1938, 2668 people died in industrial accidents in Britain. This more than halved by 1961 and the decline has continued to the present day. Even so, around 250 workers are killed in their workplace each year, with a further 90 members of the public fatally injured. The downward trend in fatalities is due largely to the decline of dangerous industries, such as mining, and improvements in regulation. The Health and Safety at Work Act 1974, which resulted from high-profile regulatory failures, created a more integrated regulatory regime under the auspices of the Health and Safety Executive (HSE), accountable to an independent Health and Safety Commission (HSC). Local authorities, however, retained a role in regulation through their responsibilities for health and safety in offices and shops. Following the establishment of the new regime, fatal injuries to employees fell by three-quarters, and non-fatal injuries declined by a similar proportion.

The EU has shaped workplace regulation. A framework directive in the late 1980s placed responsibilities on employers to safeguard the health and safety of workers and set out key principles of risk management in the workplace. Employers were required to monitor and assess a much wider range of hazards and risks. Europe has set out measures on health surveillance, training and information, and has specified standards on issues such as pregnant women in the workplace, the control of hazardous substances, safety signage, and the use of computer equipment. A European Agency for Safety and Health at Work was created in the 1990s to promote improvements by disseminating information about reducing workplace health risks.

Despite this activity, there is much room for improvement. Over two million people in Britain suffer from illnesses related to work and 36 million working days are lost due to work-related illness and injury. There are over 140,000 officially reported injuries annually with even more (275,000) self-reported (HSE, 2008). Although most industrial diseases have declined, their grim legacy persists. For example, there are around 3000 deaths from asbestos-related disease each year, arising from past contamination. Alongside such long-standing industrial diseases is the new 'epidemic' of work-related stress (see Wainwright and Calnan, 2002). Although a complex phenomenon, subject to different interpretations and explanations, stress is undoubtedly seen as a major problem. The HSE (2007) has estimated that stress-related absenteeism costs over £500 million per annum. Others believe that as much as 10 per cent of the UK's national income could be lost due to work-related stress (MIND, 2005). Poor conditions at work, including heavy demands, imbalance between effort and reward, little autonomy, and low levels of support, have been linked to a range of illnesses including anxiety, depression and heart disease (Bosma et al., 1997; Chandola et al., 2008; MIND, 2005; Stansfield et al., 1999). Long working hours have been associated with stress, injury and illness (Dembe et al., 2005; Kivimaki et al., 2002). This is worrying given that UK full-time employees work the longest hours in Europe. Over a quarter of UK employees work over 48 hours a week, the second highest proportion among industrialized countries (ILO, 2007).

Some believe that government and the HSE fail to take a tough stance on organizations that damage their employees' health. Critics point to falling numbers of convictions, prosecutions and enforcement notices (Mathiason, 2008). There has been criticism of the level of resources allocated to the HSE (Work and Pensions Committee, 2008). The reduction in inspectors means that an employer can expect an inspection once every 14.5 years on average. The level of penalties for breaches of the law is regarded as inadequate (Work and Pensions Committee, 2008). It is argued that, despite efforts to promote health and safety, the work environment is adversely affected by broader trends such as deregulation, job insecurity, poor job design and inappropriate performance management systems. Critics maintain that the extent of work-related illness is understated. For example, exposure to harmful substances is often underestimated and work-related cancers are a much larger problem than currently acknowledged by the authorities (File on 4, 2007; Watterson and O'Neill, 2007). Furthermore, it is argued that there is too much emphasis on preventing accidents and injuries and not enough on promoting positive health in the workplace, such as encouraging workers to adopt healthy lifestyles and persuading employers to invest in health promotion initiatives (Dugdill and Springett, 1994; PricewaterhouseCoopers, 2008).

In recent years, the health of the working-age population has risen up the political agenda. A key factor has been the desire by government to get people off welfare and into work, while seeking to maximize the productivity of current workers and ensuring they continue in employment. In 2001, NHS Plus was established as a network of NHS occupational health departments providing support and advice to employers. Subsequently, the *Choosing Health* white paper (Cm 6374, 2004) set out key objectives: to increase employment, improve working conditions, promote health in the workplace, and use the public sector to lead by example. This was followed by a strategy for health and wellbeing of working-age people, which emphasized the importance of engaging stakeholders (such as employers and trade unions), improving working lives, and improving coordination between agencies on this issue (HM Government, 2005b). Subsequently, a review from the government's newly appointed national director for health and work (Black, 2008), advanced several proposals including: the replacement of sick notes with 'fitness notes', a new 'Fit for Work' service to support sick workers, and the provision of greater advice, support and encouragement for employers to get them to invest in workplace health initiatives. The national director recommended bringing occupational health into mainstream health services. Occupational health was excluded from the NHS at the outset and many now believe that this has inhibited efforts to integrate prevention, treatment and rehabilitation of illness and injuries in people of working age (Harling, 2007). Subsequently the Darzi review (Cm 7432, 2008) emphasized the importance of services to enable people to stay healthy at work. NICE (2009a) introduced guidance on reducing sickness absence at work, which called on GPs to exercise greater caution in issuing sick notes and for employers to engage with workers on sick leave to encourage them to return to work. The government has also backed specific schemes and projects to improve workplace health, such as the 'well@work' programme led by the British Heart Foundation. This pilot project operated across over 30 workplaces and tested workplace initiatives such as pedometers, cycling to work, encouraging stair use, health checks and healthy eating. It was found that the scheme led to increases in the level of exercise and intake of fruit and vegetables as well as improvements in staff morale (Loughborough University, 2008). NICE (2008b, 2009b) has also introduced guidance to employers on promoting mental wellbeing and physical activity in the workplace.

Another measure to safeguard the welfare of employees, and the wider public, is the Corporate Manslaughter and Corporate Homicide Act 2007. This Act, which came into force in 2008, was a much-delayed response to problems encountered in prosecuting large companies for fatal accidents. In a number of cases, senior management was able to evade responsibility because it proved impossible to attribute deaths directly to a senior individual in the organization (a 'directing mind'). To secure a conviction under the new legislation, it must be proved that the organization has grossly breached its duty of care to the deceased and that this is attributable to poor management. The organization rather than managers will face prosecution under the Act, although individuals may still be prosecuted under other health and safety legislation. There is currently no limit to the fine that can be imposed on an organization found guilty of corporate manslaughter (or its equivalent 'corporate homicide' in Scotland).

Conclusion

Interventions to protect public health through environmental regulation are justified on grounds that people cannot individually escape from hazards. There are also strong arguments for using the environment as a means of promoting health, for example in the workplace. The chapter has shown that governments at all levels have acknowledged and responded to specific environmental health risks. There is evidence of progress, both in terms of adoption of strategies and reduced risks to the population. However, the chapter has also shown that efforts to deal with environmental health problems have often suffered from low priority, poor coordination and inadequate implementation and have been delayed and diluted by powerful economic lobbies. Government responses have been undermined by fragmentation of responsibility between different agencies. In some areas there is a lack of good quality data and research evidence on the links between environment and health, which leads to disputes about the extent of threats to health and how best to address them. Similar themes are also found in relation to the systemic environmental risks posed by climate change, discussed in the next chapter.

Climate Change and Sustainable Development

11

In the past, environmental health interventions have concentrated on the polluting effects of specific industrial and technological production processes and significant causes of accidents and injuries. Although these remain important problems, attention has now shifted towards global environmental threats, such as ozone layer depletion, global warming and climate change (Landon, 2006). This chapter explores these issues in the context of policies to promote sustainable development.

Global Environmental Threats

Ozone Layer Depletion

Ozone layer depletion, initially found over Antarctica but since spreading over populated areas, is a serious problem. It is attributed to chloroflourocarbons (CFCs), by-products of industrial processes, refrigerators, and aerosol sprays. Ozone depletion exposes humans to higher levels of ultraviolet light, with adverse implications for health. It has been estimated that a 10 per cent drop in ozone levels in the stratosphere could lead to 300,000 extra cases of skin cancers worldwide (UNEP, 1992). Ozone depletion also damages immune systems. Ultraviolet (UV) radiation is associated with increased susceptibility to infections (Godlee, 1992). Cataracts have been linked to ultraviolet light, a particular problem in ageing populations. Eyes and skin can be damaged in the short term by overexposure to UV light, increasing conditions such as erythema (inflammation of the skin) and keratitis (inflammation of the cornea). In addition, plants and animals may be damaged by UV exposure, although some are more resistant than others (Landon, 2006). The net indirect effect on ecological systems, crop yields, food systems and human health is therefore difficult to estimate.

Global Warming and Climate Change

Since the 1980s, much attention has been given to the rise in global temperatures and associated climatic changes known as global warming. Global
warming has been attributed to the 'greenhouse effect' produced by increased
levels of carbon dioxide and other gases, such as methane and nitrogen
oxides, in the atmosphere. The production of carbon dioxide from fossil fuel
combustion has been identified as the chief cause of the greenhouse effect
(Mann et al., 1998; Hansen, 2004). Carbon dioxide levels have increased by
over a third since the pre-industrial period. Deforestation, among other
factors, exacerbates the problem, as trees absorb carbon dioxide. The dominant scientific view is that human pollution, and in particular carbon dioxide
emissions, is the main cause of global warming. Global temperatures have
increased by almost 0.8°C over the past century, with eleven of the twelve
warmest years occurring between 1995 and 2006 (IPCC, 2007). Other evidence
includes: an increase in night-time temperatures over land; fewer cold spells;
more intense rainfall; a decrease in mountain glaciers and ice; rising sea levels
(3mm a year, 1993–2003) and a decrease in arctic sea ice (2.7 per cent reduction since 1978) (IPCC, 2007). It is predicted that temperatures will rise
between 1.1° and 6.4°C above 1990 levels by 2100 (IPCC, 2007). This is likely
to cause higher sea levels, more extreme weather (such as floods, droughts,
forest fires, and heat waves), and to have an impact on agriculture. With
regard to the UK, central England temperatures have risen by about a degree
Celsius since the 1970s, with temperatures in Scotland and Northern Ireland
rising by 0.8°C since 1980. The sea level around the UK is rising at a faster rate
than the average for the twentieth century. There have been more severe
windstorms in recent years and all regions have seen an increase in heavy
precipitation events (Jenkins et al., 2008). This is, however, a contentious area.
Climate change sceptics dispute the evidence that CO_2 levels have caused
global warming (Booker and North, 2007; Booker, 2009a). They argue that
temperature fluctuations are due wholly or mainly to natural phenomena
rather than man's activities. Changes in climate, they argue, are due to factors
such as the activities of the sun, cloud cover and ocean currents. Climate
change sceptics attack the findings of those who believe global warming has
increased rapidly by historical standards and argue that their findings are
flawed or fabricated. Sceptics have identified errors in reports from climate
change bodies and researchers. In 2009, the IPCC was forced to admit that
some of its predictions, notably regarding the melting of Himalayan glaciers,
were based on flawed evidence, although it maintained that the overall findings were robust. There was also controversy about email correspondence
stolen from UK climate researchers at the University of East Anglia, which
critics believed supported allegations that researchers refused to share data
and manipulated results (Booker, 2009b). An independent inquiry into these

allegations concluded that although there had been a consistent pattern of failing to display the proper degree of openness, the rigour and honesty of the scientists was not in doubt (Russell, 2010). The fightback by climate change sceptics has sown the seeds of doubt. The public are somewhat confused. However, the dominant scientific view is that global warming is a major threat to human life and that the threat is largely man-made. Recent evidence (Scott et al., 2010) appears to confirm this.

Exhibit 11.1

Transport and Health

Transport has wide-ranging implications for health, including accidental deaths and injuries, noise and air pollution (Rutter, 2007). It contributes to the production of greenhouse gases and climate change. Transport systems also have implications for social interaction, quality of life and people's ability to access services.

Road traffic has particularly adverse effects on health (Kunzli et al., 2000). Proximity to main roads and motorways is linked to impaired lung function in children and increased risks of respiratory illness (Venn et al., 2001; Gaudermann et al., 2007). Exposure to road traffic is associated with heart attacks in adults (Peters et al., 2004). Road traffic accounts for almost two-fifths of accidental deaths and is a key source of noise pollution. It also contributes disproportionately to air pollution, being responsible for over half the level of nitrogen oxide, a quarter of PM10, and 67 per cent of benzene (Faculty of Public Health Medicine, undated). Road traffic is responsible for a quarter of CO_2 emissions. Overall levels from this source have increased since 1990. The reliance on road transport has an adverse effect on health by reducing physical activity (see Chapter 13) and impacts adversely on communities and social capital (Rutter, 2007). Aviation is a major source of noise pollution and a significant emitter of CO_2.

A report by the Royal Commission on Environmental Pollution (RCEP) (Cm 2674, 1994) called on government to adopt targets to reduce carbon dioxide levels. It recommended increasing the proportion of journeys on public transport to 30 per cent of the total by 2020; increasing the fuel efficiency of cars by 40 per cent; doubling the cost of petrol and diesel in real terms by 2005; and reducing spending on roads while increasing subsidies for rail, public transport and cycle routes. The Major government called for a debate on the issue (Cm 3234, 1996), but was reluctant to adopt policies that offended the motoring lobby. Its commitment to transport privatization inhibited the adoption of integrated approaches to public transport. Even so, it did introduce a cycling strategy and a 'fuel duty escalator', which imposed above-inflation taxes year on year. The Blair government, initially at least, emphasized the integration of transport strategy with other objectives, such as environmental sustainability and health; promoting walking and cycling; promoting public transport and reducing the impact of road traffic (Cm 3950, 1998; DETR 2000b, 2000c; Docherty and Shaw, 2008). The government signed up to a European charter (WHO Regional Office for Europe, 1999b), which pledged action on the health implications of transport by reducing the need for motorized transport, shifting transport towards environmentally sound and health-promoting modes, and reducing transport emissions. New government targets were set to encourage cycling and public transport use, and to reduce traffic congestion. Meanwhile, the other countries of the UK, stimulated by the devolution agenda of the Labour government, began to devise their own transport strategies. These differed from English policies in emphasis and detail, for example greater weight placed on integrated transport, sustainable development, public transport and specific schemes to encourage cycling and walking. Nonetheless, implementation of these policy aims was limited and there was in practice a high degree of policy convergence (Docherty and Shaw, 2008).

In England, transport authorities were required to draw up local transport plans (LTPs), consistent with national guidance and regional strategies. These plans set out how local authorities intended to deliver safe, integrated, efficient and economic transport. A local innovations fund was created, to develop new approaches, such as road pricing or public transport schemes. A review of LTPs (Atkins Transport Planning et al., 2006) found that local authorities supported the underlying principles; that the profile of transport issues had risen among council members and chief officers; that LTPs were well integrated with national policies and increasingly consistent with regional objectives and priorities. However, there was poor delivery against national targets, particularly with regard to increasing public transport use and cycling. Progress on local targets was better, but still weak on environmental objectives, such as air quality and climate change. According to the RCEP (Cm 7009, 2007), LTPs must be strengthened by the inclusion of statutory targets for reducing urban traffic, focusing particularly on 'hot spots' of traffic pollution. The main problem is that local authorities have few powers over transport and even these have been diminished through deregulation and privatization of bus and rail travel. The Local Transport Act 2008 was paraded by government as restoring some local authority influence over bus services, but its provisions lacked teeth.

Other initiatives to stimulate local action in England include the Sustainable Travel Towns initiative, a pilot scheme aimed at encouraging walking and cycling. Specific interventions include 20 mph zones, park and ride schemes, improvement of cycle routes and public transport. Efforts were also made to address congestion caused by the 'school run': the Blair government introduced school travel plans (STPs) in England in 1999 (DETR et al., 1999). It established a School Travel Advisory Group (2000), which called for a reduction in the proportion of children taken to primary school by car from 37 per cent to 20 per cent by 2010. In 2003, the 'Travelling to School Initiative' was introduced. This provided funding for local authorities to appoint travel advisors to help schools develop STPs. Funding was made available to enable schools to develop new initiatives to reduce car use, such as safe travel routes and walking to school schemes. Although by 2008 seven out of ten schools had travel plans, the majority did not experience a significant reduction in car use (DfT, 2005; Transport Committee, 2008b).

Road pricing and congestion charges have been explored as a means of discouraging motor vehicle use. Road pricing, charging for the use of roads at rates that may vary by time of day and by place, is a possibility (Glaister et al., 2006). The UK government has examined the feasibility of a national scheme, but there is stiff opposition from the roads lobby and the media. Congestion charging is a more limited scheme aimed at deterring drivers from using busy roads in city and town centres. Although controversial, it is more acceptable than a comprehensive system of road pricing. The lessons of the London congestion charge in 2003 show what can be achieved (Glaister et al., 2006): a 30 per cent reduction in congestion, 40 per cent fall in accidents, a 12 per cent fall in emissions, and an 18 per cent reduction in traffic levels. Bus journeys and cycling increased, and there was no adverse impact on the London Underground (source: www.lcc.org.uk).

Although there have been some improvements, transport strategy made little headway in encouraging environmentally sound and healthy forms of travel (Commission for Integrated Transport, 2002, 2007; Docherty and Shaw, 2008). And while there have been increases in both bus and rail travel in recent years, car usage and air travel have continued to increase (National Statistics and DfT, 2007, 2010). Meanwhile, cycle use has declined. The motor car remains the most important mode of passenger transport, accounting for over 80 per cent of distance travelled. Governments could have done more to encourage modes of transport that are better for health and the environment. They have allowed schemes such as new and expanded airports, new housing developments that are distant from local services and workplaces, and out of town shopping development. Better planning could contribute to closer integration of transport schemes (road and rail) and could be used to require planning authorities to reduce car use (EAC, 2006a). Also, successive governments have allowed car and air travel to remain relatively cheap compared with other forms of transport. Since 1980, bus and rail travel have become more expensive in real terms, while the cost of motoring and air travel has fallen. These trends have continued over the last decade (National Statistics and DfT, 2007, 2010). This reflected the power of the motoring lobby. The fuel duty escalator, which raised the costs of motoring, was abandoned by the Labour government, following protests against high fuel prices. However, more recently the costs of motoring have increased due to the rise in oil prices worldwide and changes to vehicle taxation (see below).

The Labour government failed to introduce a national walking strategy for England, which it had earlier promised. There was also a lack of progress on cycling, which was the subject of a national strategy. Although additional funding was allocated to promote cycling through demonstration projects ('cycling towns') and the development of national cycling routes, this was no substitute for large infrastructure investment to make cycling an easier and safer option (EAC, 2006a). There is also a role for targeted change behaviour programmes, which can produce a shift of around 5 per cent of trips in motivated subgroups in the population (Ogilvie et al., 2004).

The Labour government produced a further strategy, which continued earlier themes (Cm 6234, 2004; Docherty and Shaw, 2008) – increase usage of buses and public transport, improve travel to school and work, and make walking and cycling more attractive. Sustainable development was mentioned, but transport is only loosely connected to this agenda (EAC, 2006a). A specific target for reducing carbon emissions from transport was eventually introduced. Road user charging has been explored, but this is beset with technical and political difficulties. Congestion charging was left to devolved governments and local authorities to decide. Although an attempt was made to relate vehicle taxation to CO_2 emissions, more could be done to tax vehicles that emit the highest levels (EAC, 2006a, 2008b). Air travel was favourably treated by the Exchequer, with no VAT on international tickets, no tax on aviation fuel and only a relatively small levy on air passengers.

Towards the end of its tenure, the Labour government was influenced by the Eddington (2006) inquiry which emphasized the importance of transport infrastructure for business and the economy. This was reflected in the PSA agreement on transport (HM Government, 2007b). The combination of environmental, health and economic considerations may yet produce more radical transport policies. Notably, the Conservative–Liberal coalition government has committed to policies that might move us in this direction. These include sustainable travel initiatives, a new system of HGV road user charging, fair pricing for rail travel, a review of air travel taxation, and a national recharging network for electric and hybrid vehicles. The government also pledged to reform the way in which decisions were made about transport projects in order to fully recognize their environmental benefits, particularly with regard to low carbon proposals. However, the political obstacles to radical change in this field remain formidable.

Finally, it should be noted that the EU sets the framework for domestic transport policies. However, the environmental aspects of EU transport policy were slow to develop (Glaister et al., 2006). The EU has stated its intention to reduce CO_2 emissions from transport, largely through voluntary agreements with manufacturers to improve vehicle fuel efficiency and reduce emissions. But these agreements have had limited impact, and the UK is lagging behind other countries in implementing them (EAC, 2006a).

The Health Effects of Climate Change

The potential health impacts of climate change are as follows (DoH and Health Protection Agency, 2008; Haines et al., 2006; Lancet / UHL Commission on Climate Change, 2009). Hot weather exacerbates chronic conditions such as heart and respiratory diseases, disproportionately affecting the elderly and vulnerable. It was estimated that the August 2003 heatwave caused over 35,000 deaths across Europe. Global warming is likely to compound respiratory problems related to air pollution. For example, it may encourage the formation of harmful low-level ozone (see Chapter 10). In addition, warmer temperatures affect the production of pollen and spores leading to an increase in allergic reactions. Skin cancer levels are likely to increase because of exposure to warmer weather. There could also be more injuries, infections and deaths arising from extreme weather events, such as floods. Such devastating events can have a major impact on mental health and material wellbeing, as illustrated by the 2007 floods in the UK. Other effects include the spread of vector-borne diseases, such as malaria. It is also likely that communicable diseases, particularly food-related or water-related infectious diseases would be transmitted more easily in a warmer climate. Human health may also suffer as a result of damage to ecological and agriculture systems worldwide: for example, food production may be adversely affected by warmer and more extreme weather conditions (Battisti and Naylor, 2009). Rising sea levels, another consequence of global warming, could severely affect the health and welfare of populations in coastal and low lying areas. Poorer countries are less well-equipped to deal with the consequences of global warming and this might have further knock-on effects such as an increase in world poverty and migration, generating further health consequences (see Lambert, 2002). More generally, it is accepted that inequalities will be exacerbated by climate change (*Lancet*/UHL Commission, 2009).

Although the challenges posed by global warming are enormous and greater than previously predicted (see UNEP, 2007; IPCC, 2007; Baer and Mastrandrea, 2006), there may be some benefits (Haines et al., 2006). In the UK, for example, cold-related deaths and injuries are likely to fall. It is also possible that nutrition may benefit from higher farming yields in temperate regions. Moreover, as temperatures continue to rise, adaptation to the new climatic conditions may be undertaken. Improved systems of public health surveillance and environmental management may develop, and technological advances could minimize the adverse consequences of global warming (see Haines et al., 2006; *Lancet*/UHL Commission, 2009). However, there is no room for complacency. Global warming poses a serious threat to human health, possibly even to the future of humanity. This suggests that efforts to address the root causes of the problem must be undertaken.

Promoting Sustainability

The 1972 UN Conference on Human Environment held in Stockholm set the future agenda for sustainable development (Elliott, 2004). It laid the foundations for the UN Environmental Programme (UNEP), which has since been a catalyst for global interventions on pollution and climate change. Another landmark was the inquiry by the UN World Commission on Environment and Development (1987). This defined sustainable development as 'development that meets the needs of the present without compromising the ability of future generations to meet their own needs' (p. 43). Chaired by Gro Harlem Brundtland, the Commission's report stated that 'environmental protection and sustainable development must be an integral part of the mandates of all agencies of governments, of international organizations, and of major private sector institutions' (p. 313). It recommended that the UN introduce a convention on environmental protection and sustainable development.

The Brundtland report emerged during heightened anxiety about global environment issues, such as ozone depletion and global warming. Progress on ozone depletion demonstrated what could be achieved by international cooperation (Doyle and McEachern, 2001; Elliott, 2004). Following evidence of harm caused by ozone-depleting chemicals, an international framework convention to protect the ozone layer was adopted in Vienna in 1985, followed by an implementation protocol agreed in Montreal in 1987. The major industrialized countries agreed to reduce production of the most damaging CFCs by half by 1999 (from a 1986 baseline) and to freeze output of less harmful products at 1986 levels by 1992. Some countries, including the EU, took unilateral action to phase out these products even more quickly. Subsequent agreements between 1990 and 1999 entailed a complete cessation of CFC production by 2000 and a stricter timetable for phasing out other harmful products. Despite the iconic status of the CFC agreements, they did have shortcomings (Elliott, 2004). CFCs persist for long periods in the atmosphere and the benefits of discontinuing them will only be realized in the longer term. Moreover, the agreements contain loopholes and exclusions that limit progress. For example, developing countries were given a ten-year period to comply with the protocols. CFCs are still produced and used and it is difficult to prevent their being traded illegally. Furthermore, some CFC substitutes add to ozone depletion, although to a lesser extent, while some contribute to global warming.

During the 1980s, as agreements to reduce CFCs were being formulated, global warming attracted increasing attention (Elliott, 2004). Calls to reduce greenhouse gases arose from a series of conferences during this decade. In 1988, the UNEP and the World Meteorological Organization established a new expert body, the Intergovernmental Panel on Climate Change (IPCC), which documented the trends in global warming, possible causes and consequences and how the process might be stabilized or reversed (see above). The next milestone was the United Nations Conference on Environment and Development (known as the 'Earth Summit'), which took place at Rio de Janeiro in 1992. This produced two international conventions – on biodiversity and climate change – signed by 150 countries (Grubb et al., 1993). It also produced three further non-binding agreements: the Rio Declaration comprising 27 principles for action; the forest principles, which arose out of a failed attempt to produce a convention; and Agenda 21, a plan of action on sustainable development (Elliott, 2004).

The Agenda 21 document covered environmental and development issues, including: economic development; natural resources and fragile ecosystems; participation of major groups in the strategy, and means of implementation. Although Agenda 21 was criticized, not least for stating the obvious, it set guidelines and benchmarks against which national policies and programmes could be appraised. It was also credited with prompting action by communities through Local Agenda 21 (LA21), discussed later in this chapter. The major limitation of Agenda 21 was that it was not enforceable. Much depended on the willingness of individual states, business and other interests to comply with its aims and principles. The Earth Summit's achievements were limited by the opposition of the United States and multinational business organizations (Doyle and McEachern, 2001; Carter, 2007).

Kyoto

At the Kyoto convention on climate change in 1997, industrialized nations agreed to adopt legally binding targets to reduce emissions of greenhouse gases (carbon dioxide, methane, nitrous oxide, halofluorocarbons, perfluoro-carbons, and sulphur hexafluoride) by an average of 5.2 per cent (from 1990 levels) by 2008–12. Each country was set a specific target to reduce emissions. Kyoto also introduced 'flexibility mechanisms': an emissions trading system whereby countries could meet their targets by purchasing 'emissions credits' from others; joint implementation, which gave credits to countries for imple-menting emission reduction schemes in other developed countries; and a clean development mechanism, which allowed developed countries to acquire credits for implementing emission reduction programmes in developing coun-tries. Although the Kyoto agreement was a major achievement, implementa-tion has been too slow and the proposed reductions in greenhouse gases will be insufficient to avert global warming (Haines et al., 2006; UNEP, 2007; Baer and Mastrandrea, 2006; Pielke et al., 2008). There are significant gaps in the agreement, such as the exclusion of emissions from international aviation and shipping. Furthermore, reservations have been expressed about the emissions trading system, which enables countries to pay for continuing high levels of greenhouse gas emissions (Damro and Mendez, 2003). Although most indus-trialized countries ratified Kyoto, the largest single polluting country, the USA, refused to comply. Moreover, newly industrializing countries (such as Brazil, China and India) were not subject to limits on greenhouse gas emis-sions, despite their increasing contribution to global warming. A further problem was contradiction between the Kyoto protocol and trade agreements, which did not prioritize environmental considerations (Hornsby et al., 2007; Juniper, 1999).

Since Kyoto, international efforts to promote sustainable development and tackle climate change have continued. Environmental sustainability was chosen as one of the Millennium Development Goals (UN General Assembly, 2000). Subsequently, a world summit on sustainable development was held in Johan-nesburg in 2002 (UN, 2002; Hens and Nath, 2003; EAC, 2003b). This pledged to accelerate sustainable patterns of production and consumption and increase renewable energy. It also gave support for initiatives to ensure sustainable fisheries, maintain biodiversity, protect forests and develop a strategic approach to international chemicals management. Additional commitments were made regarding access to sanitation and water, education for sustainable develop-ment, and corporate accountability. The summit endorsed a stronger institu-tional framework for sustainable development, including the creation of partnerships between government and society. Although these commitments were broadly welcomed, few were linked to explicit targets. There was disap-pointment in some quarters that actions and timetables for implementation were not clearly specified. It was also believed that relationships between trade, environment and development should have been addressed.

Growing concern that the Kyoto targets would not avert global warming led to calls for a tougher approach (Baer and Mastrandrea, 2006; UNEP, 2007; Stern,

2006; Stockholm Network, 2008; EAC, 2008f). The G8 summit of 2008 produced a statement that countries should aim to cut greenhouse gas emissions by at least 50 per cent by 2050, although there was a lack of detail about how and when this would be implemented (Pendleton, 2008). A further UN summit to discuss action on climate change was held in December 2009, in Copenhagen.

Despite hopes of a successor to Kyoto, countries failed to produce a legally binding agreement. Instead, an accord was negotiated by five large polluters (USA, India, China, Brazil, and South Africa) and signed by 49 countries. This represented an acknowledgement that the future rise in global temperatures must be kept below 2°C. However, no mandatory targets on greenhouse gases were set, there was no clear timetable for implementation and only limited resources were available to help poorer countries prevent and mitigate the effects of climate change.

The EU, Sustainable Development and Climate Change

The EU adopted sustainable development as an overarching objective in the 1997 Treaty of Amsterdam. In 2001, following proposals from the European Commission (Commission of the European Communities, 2001), the European Council agreed to introduce a sustainable development strategy (known as the Gothenburg strategy), which identified four main priorities: climate change; public health; natural resources; and transport (Gothenburg European Council, 2001). The Gothenburg strategy called on member states to develop their own national sustainability strategies. It sought greater integration of economic, social and environmental policymaking, with greater use of impact assessment (see Exhibit 11.2). The strategy was revised following the enlargement of the EU (Council of the European Union, 2006). The priority areas were now: climate change and clean energy; sustainable transport; sustainable consumption and production; conservation and management of natural resources; public health; social inclusion, demography and migration; global poverty and sustainable development. The revised strategy outlined key actions, including: meeting Kyoto commitments, improving energy efficiency, a sustainable consumption and production plan, and the introduction of a new system of chemical regulation; it also reiterated the importance of impact assessment. Although mainly a summary of existing and previously planned developments, the new strategy did identify the multiple, interlinked challenges of sustainable development across several policy areas.

With regard to climate change, the EU has sought a global leadership role (Elliott, 2004). It has led by example, agreeing to unilateral reductions in greenhouse gases and setting a strategic framework for member states. In 1991, the EU developed a strategy aimed at reducing CO_2 emissions and improving energy efficiency. It has promoted international agreements, including the Kyoto protocol. Under the protocol, it agreed to reduce overall emissions by 8 per cent in the then 15 member states. It later introduced a European climate change programme, to implement its Kyoto commitments, which included efforts to increase renewable energy sources, improve energy efficiency, address transport issues, and promote public awareness. An EU emissions trading scheme (ETS) was introduced in 2005, covering around 45 per cent of CO_2 emissions.

The EU climate change programme was renewed in 2005, followed by further commitments to unilaterally reduce greenhouse gases by 20 per cent by 2020 and to press for an international agreement reducing greenhouse gases by developed countries. The EU also pledged to increase energy efficiency by a fifth and the share of renewable energy sources to 20 per cent by 2020. Other elements of the programme included the possible extension of ETS to other areas, including aviation, the reduction of car emissions by using tax and other instruments, and measures to improve energy efficiency of buildings. The EU has since stated that it will cut greenhouse gases by 30 per cent by 2020 (1990 baseline), subject to other comparable countries making similar commitments as part of an international agreement. It has also proposed changes to ETS to include aviation emissions within the EU area.

By 2007, the EU as a whole had reduced greenhouse gas emissions by 9.3 per cent since 1990, more than its Kyoto target (European Environment Agency, 2009). However, the decline in emissions among the 15 member states that were party to the original EU target was only 4.3 per cent. Six of these countries had already met their individual target (UK, Sweden, Greece, Germany, France and Belgium). The European Environment Agency reported that all but three countries (Spain, Italy and Denmark) were on course to meet their commitments under Kyoto.

EU strategy has, however, been hampered by disagreements between states, some of which are less supportive of action on climate change than others. The ETS, although acknowledged as a cornerstone of policy, has flaws (House of Lords, 2008c; EAC, 2010b). It has not placed a tough enough limit on emissions, meaning that carbon allowances are overallocated. This has not placed sufficient pressure on emitters to invest in reducing carbon emissions. The scheme excludes over half of greenhouse gas emissions, including industries such as agriculture, forestry, road transport and shipping. It has, however been extended to aviation and there are plans to include shipping. In addition, there are problems of enforcement and compliance. Further criticism of EU policy highlights tensions with other aspects of its reform agenda. Indeed, the Lisbon Agenda (Lisbon European Council, 2000), which emphasizes the importance of free markets, competitiveness and economic growth, overshadows environmental concerns. Moreover, the EU has failed to fully integrate concerns about sustainability and climate change in key policies and programmes, such as transport, energy and the Common Agricultural Policy (see Chapter 12).

Sustainable Development and Climate Change Policy in the UK

The Major government introduced a UK-wide strategy on sustainable development (Cm 2426, 1994). However, it was heavily criticized for failing to prioritize sustainable development across all sectors of decision-making. Reforms introduced by the Blair government sought to address this. A new Department of the Environment, Transport and Regions (DETR) was created to improve coordination of policy. A Cabinet committee on environmental issues was established to coordinate policies on sustainable development. This was accompanied by clarification of the responsibilities of ministers for Green issues across Whitehall. Further guidance on environmental policy appraisal was issued by DETR. In addition a new parliamentary committee, the Environmental Audit Committee (EAC), was established to scrutinize environmental policy across government.

The Blair government reformed the sustainable development strategy (Cm 4345, 1999), to accommodate health, quality of life, social and economic context, and physical environment. Indicators were used to measure progress, including healthy life expectancy, the quality of housing stock, crime rates, and measures of social exclusion and inequality. The Sustainable Development Commission (SDC) was established in 2000 to monitor progress and build consensus about future action. The new strategy proposed changes in the planning system. It was envisaged that the planning of economic development, regeneration and transport would be more closely integrated. Regional development agencies were given responsibilities for sustainable development alongside economic development and regeneration. These bodies were expected to produce coherent plans that reflected sustainable development priorities. It was proposed that regional plans should be subject to environmental impact assessment (see Exhibit 11.2). The strategy also emphasized the importance of local authorities. Guidance from DETR was issued on how to enshrine sustainable development within the planning process and in local development plans. The government continued to endorse local action within the context of Local Agenda 21, setting a target that all local authorities should have an LA21 strategy by the year 2000.

The revitalized sustainable development strategy was applauded for seeking to galvanize a holistic, cross-government approach to sustainable development. However, it had little impact (EAC, 2004a). The chosen indicators failed to provide a clear picture of sustainability. There was a failure to address the challenges of sustainable production, consumption and lifestyles. There was a lack of environmental appraisal of policies. Poor coordination within government remained a problem. This was not helped by the abolition of DETR (established, remember, to improve coordination). Doubts about current policies were reinforced by a study that placed the UK's performance on sustainable development 65th out of 146 countries (Yale Center for Environmental Law and Policy/Center for International Earth Science Information Network, Columbia University, 2005).

The sustainable development strategy was again revised (Cm 6467, 2005). There were now four priorities: sustainable production and consumption; climate change; natural resource protection; and sustainable communities. 'Living within environmental limits' was included as a guiding principle of policy alongside 'achieving a sustainable economy', 'ensuring a strong healthy and just society', 'promoting good governance', and 'using sound science responsibly'. Each government department was now required to produce an action plan. The Department for Food, Environment and Rural Affairs (DEFRA) was designated as the lead department for sustainable development. The strategy also set out a number of commitments including: a new programme of community engagement; sustainable procurement in the public sector; placing sustainable development at the centre of land use planning; and new powers for local authorities to improve their local environment. To monitor progress, a new indicator set was formulated, with a greater emphasis on measurable outcomes. In addition, the SDC became an independent watchdog, reporting to ministers at Westminster as well as the devolved governments. Other parts of the UK developed their own sustainable development strategies, based on the same principles as the English strategy.

Climate Change

The UK government's Chief Scientist, Sir David King (2004), stated that climate change is 'the most severe problem that we are facing today – more serious even than the threat of terrorism'. Since then further work has been done on the implications of climate change for the UK (see www.ukclimate-projections.defra.gov.uk). This suggests that by 2080 all areas of the UK will have increased temperatures, but some regions will be affected more than others. Mean daily maximum temperatures in the south could rise by as much as 5.4°C. Winters will be less cold, particularly in the south of England. There is likely to be increased rainfall in the west in winter (up to a third higher). Parts of the far south are likely to have much less (up to 40 per cent) rainfall in summer. Sea levels are likely to rise, again particularly in the south.

The UK government developed policies on climate change from the early 1990s. The Major government pledged to reduce CO_2 emissions and introduced policies such as the 'fuel escalator' (see Exhibit 11.1) and a landfill tax (landfill waste, which produces methane, a greenhouse gas, is also a cause of water and ground pollution – see Chapter 10). It also imposed VAT on domestic gas and electricity in 1994, although at lower than the standard rate. This was further reduced by the Blair government. Following the Kyoto protocol, under which the UK was required to reduce greenhouse gases by 12.5 per cent between 1990 and 2008–12, the Blair government made an additional pledge to reduce CO_2 emissions by a fifth by 2010. Following a recommendation from the RCEP (Cm 4749, 2000), the UK government set a further target of reducing CO_2 by 60 per cent by 2050, with an interim target of a 26 per cent cut by 2030. Further impetus was provided by the Stern review, established by the Treasury to examine the economic aspects of climate change (Stern, 2006). The review argued that early action to reduce greenhouse gases and mitigate climate change should be regarded as an investment and that a failure to act now risked serious, irreversible damage. It estimated that action to reduce emissions would cost around one per cent of GDP by 2050, much less than the costs of inaction, which could be as high as a fifth of national income.

The Blair government's first climate change programme, introduced in 2000 (Cm 4913, 2000) was relaunched (Cm 6764, 2006). The main components of this programme were as follows:

- *Energy.* The Blair government introduced a climate change levy (CCL) on large users of energy from 2001. Discounts were given to energy-intensive sectors, which agreed to improve efficiency under climate change agreements (CCAs). The Carbon Trust, a body funded by CCL revenues, was established to advise business and public sector organizations on how to reduce dependence on fossil fuels. Specific schemes were introduced for public sector bodies to encourage investment in energy efficiency. In addition, renewable energy sources and combined heat and power schemes were exempted from the CCL, and investment allowances given to companies using energy efficient technologies. A target of increasing renewable energy sources (such as wind and wave power) to 10 per cent of total electricity supply by 2010 was set, subsequently increased to 15 per cent by 2015, and 30 per cent by 2020. This is likely to increase in the light of further EU commitments on renewables. Electricity suppliers are required to source specific percentages of their output from renewable sources (known as the 'renewables obligation'). In an attempt to encourage energy efficiency in the residential sector, new homes and apartments that met standards were granted exemption from stamp duty land tax. New building regulations strengthened energy efficiency requirements. Home insulation and energy efficiency schemes were also launched. In addition, measures were introduced to improve energy efficiency of domestic appliances. However, the Blair government refused to reverse its decision to reduce VAT on domestic gas and electricity. It announced a shift in energy policy in favour of coal-fired power stations and against nuclear power, which many regarded as retrograde steps. However, in later policy statements the Labour government indicated support for a greater role for nuclear power (Cm 7124, 2007; Cm 7296, 2008).

- *Emissions Trading*. The UK introduced a voluntary scheme in 2002 under which businesses were allowed to emit a certain amount of greenhouse gases, but could buy permission to release excess emissions or sell unused allowances. This was followed by an EU-wide scheme, mentioned earlier, which began its first phase in 2005. Following the Stern review's support for 'carbon pricing' (measures to ensure that the cost of using fossil fuels is fully reflected in costs and prices), the government began to use 'shadow carbon prices' in cost–benefit analysis for investment decisions (Willis, 2008). In a further move, the carbon reduction commitment will apply emission limits to large commercial and public sector organizations. The government is exploring a new technology known as carbon capture and storage (CCS), which involves storing greenhouse gas emissions underground (for example in disused oil and gas fields) (see EAC, 2008a). Carbon offsetting schemes may also be used to absorb CO_2 from the atmosphere by, for example, planting new forests.

- *Transport*. Initially, the Blair government imposed higher taxes on petrol and diesel in accordance with the fuel duty escalator introduced by its predecessor. However, following rises in the price of fuel in 2000, which led to widespread protests from farmers, road hauliers and motorists, this was abandoned. A big rise in oil prices in 2007–8 led to pressure on government to cut fuel taxes. A duty increase planned for 2008 was deferred. The government promoted congestion charging and road pricing as a means of reducing traffic pollution. Changes based on fuel efficiency have been made to the tax regime for vehicles, including changes to the company car taxation. Vehicle excise duty has been raised on the most polluting cars and reduced on low carbon vehicles. Measures to increase the use of biofuels by motor vehicles have also been implemented (although biofuels are themselves contentious – see EAC, 2008c). An air passenger duty introduced in 1997 was doubled in 2007. It was raised again in 2009, with larger increases for longer distance flights.

- *Other measures* include efforts to reduce methane emissions by improved farming methods and by increasing recycling (see Chapter 11). Landfill tax was increased substantially. In 2007 a plastic bag tax was proposed (not just to reduce the use of carbon, but to protect wildlife, and reduce pollution and litter), should voluntary efforts by retailers prove ineffective. Following concerns that the public were not engaging with the imperatives of climate change (see Ereaut and Segnit, 2008), new publicity campaigns on energy efficiency and recycling were launched. The government also funded schemes to encourage energy efficiency, including a community energy efficiency programme. Some have suggested introducing personal carbon allowances, extending emissions trading to individuals (see Sustainable Development Commission, 2005; Bird and Lockwood, 2009).

- *PSA agreements* included commitments on climate change. In 2006, an Office of Climate Change was established within DEFRA to strengthen coordination across Whitehall. In 2007, two new cross-cutting PSA delivery agreements were introduced on the natural environment and on climate change to promote more effective cross-governmental action (HM Government, 2007c, 2007d). In addition, accountability was strengthened in 2006 by a new requirement on government to report annually to Parliament on climate change.

These measures had a limited impact. Environmental taxes represented a lower share of taxation in 2007 compared with 1997, a reduction from 9.4 per cent to 7.3 per cent in 2007 (Friends of the Earth, 2008). Tax changes have been piecemeal and unlikely to affect behaviour on a large scale. Road transport taxes are controversial and government has lacked the courage to alter the balance of costs between private motoring and public transport (see Exhibit 11.1). The CCL and CCAs, however, appear to have had some positive impact on reducing emissions. It was estimated that the CCL would reduce energy demand by almost 3 per cent by 2010. Reductions in energy use have also been attributed to CCAs (HM Treasury, 2006a; EAC, 2008d). Although these measures have had an effect, they are insufficient to achieve the cuts required (Bowyer et al., 2005). Moreover, the CCL has not worked as originally planned, notably with regard to small and medium size businesses and less energy intensive firms (EAC, 2008d).

The general picture is one of mixed success. One study found that of 66 climate change targets set by government, 25 (38 per cent) were not met or were unlikely to be met (Singh and Sweetman, 2008). CO_2 levels began to rise in 2003 and although the UK is on course to meet its Kyoto target, it is less likely to meet its self-imposed CO_2 target for 2010 (DEFRA, 2009). At the time of writing, the UK had cut emissions by 17.4 per cent (European Environment Agency, 2009). Moreover, using alternative measures, which take into account greenhouse gases associated with UK consumption of goods and services (rather than production), its contribution to global warming internationally actually increased by a fifth since 1990 (Helm et al., 2007). This has occurred as a result of the UK consuming carbon-intensive products manufactured overseas. Other criticisms of climate change strategy include a failure to address road transport and aviation issues, as well as the need to strengthen measures to improve energy efficiency and to increase the contribution of renewable energy sources (EAC, 2006b; EFRAC, 2005b, 2007; PAC, 2009a). Tellingly, the

Business and Enterprise Committee (2008, p. 21) of the House of Commons observed that 'the government needs to take action to ensure the credibility of its claims that climate change forms as important a part of the UK's energy policy as security of supply'. In particular, there has been poor progress on renewable energy sources: by 2007 these contributed only 2 per cent of electricity generated. The UK has a relatively poor record in this field compared with other countries (Frankl, 2008; NAO, 2010b).

The institutional framework of policymaking has been criticized. EFRAC (2005b, p. 49) expressed its frustration at 'the absence of a clear central direction to the Government's work on climate change' and recommended a minister for climate change or a stronger coordinating role for the Secretary of State for Environment Food and Rural Affairs. This was echoed by the EAC (2007a), which recommended a climate change cabinet minister with a cross-departmental brief and a new Climate Change and Energy Secretariat located in the Cabinet Office. The Labour government responded in 2008 by establishing a new Department for Energy and Climate Change to take over the leadership and coordination role for this area of policy.

Further Developments

In 2008, the UK Parliament passed a Climate Change Act (EAC, 2007b). This set new targets for reducing carbon dioxide emissions and other greenhouse gases by at least 80 per cent by 2050 with at least a 26 per cent cut by 2020 (baseline 1990). The 2050 target included emissions from aviation and shipping. In a further move, prompted by its advisors, the government pledged to reduce greenhouse gas emissions by 34 per cent by 2020. The Climate Change Act includes a requirement on government to set five-year carbon budgets with binding targets beginning with the period 2008 to 2012. Although international shipping and aviation were not initially included in these budgets, they will have to be by 2012 or an explanation provided to Parliament for their continued exclusion. Moreover, in the meantime projected emissions from these sources must be taken into account when decisions on carbon budgets are being made. An independent statutory Committee on Climate Change (CCC) (to advise on carbon budgets) was also established. This reports annually to Parliament on progress of the carbon reduction strategy. A subcommittee was also established to provide advice and scrutiny of government plans on adaptation to climate change.

The CCC, reporting in 2008, stated that a range of technologies are available or could be adapted to reduce emissions and that this would cost between 1 and 2 per cent of GDP 2050 (Committee on Climate Change, 2008). It identified decarbonization of the power sector as the key to meeting targets, including greater emphasis on renewable energy sources and nuclear power. It also placed faith in energy efficiency and carbon capture and storage technology.

Transport was identified as a key area where emissions could be cut. Again the emphasis was upon new technologies, such as improved fuel efficiency and alternative fuels. Although the committee was right to identify technology as an important contributor to reducing greenhouse gases, much will also depend on changing modern lifestyles, infrastructure and environment to reduce the demand for energy (*Lancet*/UHL Commission, 2009). The CCC recommended that international aviation and shipping should not for the time being be included in the forthcoming carbon budgets, although it did call for clear strategies to achieve emissions reductions in these areas and that annual reports on progress should be accompanied by reports on aviation and shipping.

In 2009, the Labour government announced its Low Carbon Transition Plan (HM Government, 2009a). This planned to cut emissions by 18 per cent between 2008 and 2020. All major government departments were set a carbon budget and expected to draw up their own plans. The government reiterated its aim to increase the share of renewables in electricity, while piloting carbon capture and storage schemes and facilitating the building of new nuclear power stations. An expansion in energy efficiency programmes was announced. The government also planned to cut transport emissions by encouraging new technologies. Each sector was given a specific target to reduce emissions. Power and heavy industry were set a target of 22 per cent; homes, 29 per cent; workplaces, 13 per cent; transport, 14 per cent; farming and waste, 6 per cent. The EAC (2010c), while acknowledging the UK government's actions in this field, made several recommendations for improvement. It stated that the government should aim for a 42 per cent reduction in greenhouse gases by 2020, should ensure that all parts of government understood the importance of reducing cumulative emissions, and in particular make clear the impact of emissions from aviation and shipping on progress towards the targets. The committee also urged the government to shape and inform public opinion on climate change, to reduce emissions further. Other recommendations included increasing the price of carbon, strengthening policy on energy efficiency and improving the measurement of greenhouse gases.

It is important that policy doesn't lose sight of the broader objective of sustainable development. As the New Economics Foundation (NEF) (2010) has noted, for example, too much emphasis has been placed on economic growth as a solution to societies' problems, in particular poverty. Climate change is not the only limit to orthodox economic growth and more must be done to address its impact on the finite nature of earth's resources. On a practical level, the Sustainable Development Commission (2009) identified 19 'breakthrough ideas' to improve sustainability. These include: free bicycles, initiatives to produce local food, a sustainability bank to invest in projects, energy efficiency measures, personal carbon budgets and low carbon zones.

Further developments in national policy on sustainability and climate change will occur as a result of the change of government in 2010. The

Cameron government's programme (HM Government, 2010c) highlighted the importance of sustainable development, stating that it would create a presumption in favour of sustainable development in the planning system and would increase the proportion of tax revenue raised by environmental taxes. It pledged to work towards a zero waste economy with incentives for recycling. The new government's programme endorsed the policy of a low-carbon and eco-friendly economy, stating that it would support an increase in the EU's emission reduction target to 30 per cent by 2020 and would press for an ambitious global climate deal. It endorsed new energy efficiency measures, and stated that it would seek to increase the target for energy from renewable sources (subject to advice from the Climate Change Committee). Measures to encourage marine energy, and to substantially increase energy from waste schemes were promised. The Cameron government also said that it would press for changes in carbon trading, such as a minimum price for carbon and full auctioning of ETS permits. It delighted environmental campaigners by cancelling the proposed third runway at Heathrow airport, refusing permission for additional runways at Gatwick and Stansted airports, and proposing the replacement of air passenger duty with a per flight duty. A promise to create a Green investment bank was also positively received in these quarters. However, other proposals were less welcome from an environmental perspective, such as the abolition of the Sustainable Development Commission and the Royal Commission on Environmental Pollution, which had done much to keep environmental issues on the agenda. Finally, and to the further chagrin of environmentalists, the programme heralded the replacement of nuclear power stations (despite Liberal Democrat opposition to this). It also backed investment in CCS, which would allow an expansion of coal-fired power stations subject to certain safeguards on emissions standards.

Sustainable Development and Climate Change at the Subnational Level

So far the discussion has been mainly about international and national policies on climate change and sustainable development. However, it is important to examine the role of subnational government, for several reasons. Subnational governments, such as devolved governments, regional bodies and local authorities, can ensure that top-down policies are implemented, while tailoring them to local circumstances. They can also help to coordinate different policies developed by higher-tier governments. Furthermore, lower-tier governments, particularly local government, can play a valuable part in developing new approaches to problem-solving from the 'bottom up' by working with local communities and practitioners.

Local Government

According to the Local Government Association's Climate Change Commission (LGA Climate Change Commission, 2007), local government is uniquely placed to tackle climate change. It has a democratic mandate, close proximity to citizens through its services, and a strategic role to lead and collaborate with other public authorities, the voluntary sector and business. Local authorities are responsible for planning and service delivery across a range of issues having important implications for sustainable development and climate change, such as housing, transport, education, waste management, regeneration and economic development. Local authorities are large users of energy and could directly contribute to sustainable development by changing their practices (EAC, 2008e).

The role of local authorities in sustainable development was recognized at the Rio Summit in 1992. As noted earlier, Local Agenda 21 (LA21) was championed to encourage local authorities to think holistically about their activities and in particular about how different sectors such as transport, waste disposal, and planning impact upon the environment. LA21 was embraced by local authorities across the UK and is credited with promoting innovative working across different sectors (Young, 1996). However, implementation was patchy. In most councils, LA21 was not a priority (Littlewood and While, 1997). LA21 lost impetus but its spirit survived through other initiatives aimed at getting local authorities to adopt a more holistic approach towards improving their local environment. As noted in Chapter 7, local authorities have powers to promote the economic, social and environmental wellbeing of their areas. They also have a duty to prepare a community strategy for their area. To reflect the importance of climate change and sustainable development, these were later renamed 'sustainable community strategies' (SCS).

Other important developments have since taken place with regard to local authorities' role in promoting sustainable development. Legislative changes include the Climate Change and Sustainable Energy Act 2006, under which local authorities must have regard to the government's annual report on energy efficiency and climate change. Under the Sustainable Communities Act 2008, local authorities were given a role in developing and facilitating sustainable development projects put forward by local communities. Larger local authorities are required to participate in the government's carbon reduction commitment, discussed above.

Local authorities are subject to a range of central government planning and guidance on sustainable development issues such as housing, transport, and energy efficiency. They also receive central guidance on their planning role, which has in recent years emphasized the importance of sustainable development and climate change (ODPM, 2005b; DCLG, 2007a). Guidance has also been issued on specific planning issues such as renewable energy, flood risk and waste management. In relation to this, important changes to the planning system were introduced in 2004, requiring local authorities to produce local development frameworks consistent with regional strategies. They are expected to take account of sustainability and climate change policy and report annually on how these objectives are being achieved. Further changes in the planning system are being introduced at the time of writing, which simplify the planning process and take the planning of major infrastructure developments out of local hands (Barker, 2006). This may be seen as a retrograde step as it reduces community involvement, which some regard as an essential element in building support and social capital to bring about adaptation to climate change (*Lancet*/UHL Commission, 2009). Moreover, there is much greater scope for a planning system that protects and promotes health through environmental change. For example, the Health Committee (2009) has recommended that the government issue a planning policy statement which requires planners to create a built environment that encourages healthy lifestyles (for example through transport plans, plans for recreational amenities, and regulation of food outlets). It recommended that PCTs should be statutory consultees on local planning decisions.

Local authorities operate within a formal system of planning and performance management. Changes in this framework have emphasized the importance of sustainable development and climate change. The development of local strategic partnerships and local area agreements (see Chapter 7) may strengthen planning across agencies at local level on issues such as sustainable development. Sustainable development and climate change were identified as priorities in Labour government PSA agreements, which shaped the context for the performance management of lower-tier authorities (HM Government, 2007c, 2007d). These issues were also subject to local authority performance indicators. In addition, local authorities demonstrating innovative and excellent performance in the field of sustainable development were recognized through the Beacon Council scheme, which rewarded and disseminates best practice in service delivery.

Nonetheless, local authorities vary in their commitment to action on climate change and sustainable development (LGA, 2007; EAC, 2008e; Cm 7009, 2007). Not all give these issues the priority that many believe is deserved. Currently, climate change and sustainable development issues are covered by the national performance indicator set (for example: indicator 186 relates to per capita CO_2 emissions; 188 to planning to adapt to climate change; 185 to CO_2 reduction in local authority operations). However, local authorities and their partners are expected to focus on a subset of 35 priority indicators which are subject to targets agreed in LAAs between themselves and government regional offices (see Chapter 7). These targets do not have to include sustainable development indicators. However, in 2008, 90 per cent of LAAs did include at least one target for indicators 185, 186 and 190 (www.energysav-ingtrust.org.uk). Two-thirds had a target for reducing per capita CO_2 emissions, 37 per cent for planning adaptation and 23 per cent for CO_2 reduction in local authority operations.

Local authorities and their partners face conflicting national priorities, chiefly between economic development, housing, transport and energy policies on the one hand and sustainable development and climate change policies on the other. It is also argued that local authorities lack necessary support and skills to develop appropriate responses to sustainable development and climate change. Moves to galvanize local authority efforts in this field were stimulated by the Nottingham declaration of 2000 (www.energysavingtrust. org.uk). So far, 300 councils have signed this declaration, which commits them to increase their efforts in this area.

Other recommendations have been made to strengthen the local authority contribution to sustainable development and action on climate change. The EAC (2008e) called on central government to minimize inconsistencies between policies and implement a joined-up approach that integrates environmental and economic policy. Related to this, the LGA Commission urged for the new economic development duty imposed on local authorities to be clarified as sustainable economic development (LGA, 2007). It also urged for national carbon reduction targets to be a material consideration in planning laws. The RCEP (Cm 7009, 2007) has also called for clearer central guidance, including new planning guidance on climate change requiring all new developments of a certain size to have a strategic approach to energy.

Some believe that a higher priority would be given to sustainable development and climate change if performance indicators were compulsory. Both EAC and the LGA Commission argued that all LAAs should be required to include climate change indicators and plans to adapt to climate change. More broadly, the RCEP called for a new system of environmental performance assessment based on three criteria: minimum standards, aspirational objectives and innovative action. There are mixed views on whether additional statutory duties should be imposed. The LGA Commission supported statutory duties to tackle climate change being given to all public bodies, including local authorities. Meanwhile, the RCEP recommended that local authority discretionary powers on wellbeing should be upgraded to a statutory duty to protect and enhance the environment. Other important recommendations have been to make environmental impact assessment compulsory (Exhibit 11.2), either in terms of climate change (LGA, 2007) or with regard to effects on environment and health (Cm 7009, 2007). A review of support and skills available to councils to help them respond to the demands of sustainable development and climate change has also been recommended (EAC, 2008e; LGA, 2007).

Exhibit 11.2

Environmental and Health Impact Assessment

One way of building environmental considerations into decisions about policy, planning or projects is to undertake systematic assessments of their environmental impact. Strategic environmental assessment (SEA) relates to the impact of policies, plans or programmes, while environmental impact assessment (EIA) is concerned with the assessment of specific projects and developments. Both SEA and EIA have a statutory basis in European law, which specifies areas where assessment is required. For SEA, these include policy areas with significant environmental effects (for example agriculture, energy and transport). For EIA, they include power stations and large transport projects. There are also 'discretionary' areas where environmental assessment may be applied (such as wind farms and theme parks). Even so, there have been calls to extend both SEA and EIA (see, for example, Cm 7009, 2007).

The UK is expected to apply European law and has carried out SEA and EIA under these obligations. However, assessments may fail to take into account the full environmental implications and can be biased and of poor quality (Watson, 2003). The UK government also carries out regulatory impact assessments, which attempt to evaluate the costs and benefits of a proposed measure. Although focused primarily on the financial costs and benefits of regulation, these are now expected to incorporate sustainable development and climate change criteria. The LGA (2007) Climate Change Commission went further and recommended that all major policy, planning, investment and spending decisions should be subject to a carbon impact assessment.

Health impact assessment (HIA) is defined as 'a combination of procedures, methods, and tools that systematically judges the potential and sometimes the unintended consequences of a policy, plan, programme or project on the health of a population, and the distribution of those effects within the population' (Quigley et al., 2006). Although it can be considered as part of SEA or EIA, health has not carried sufficient weight in these processes (BMA, 1998; Cm 7009, 2007; Lock and McKee, 2005). This is partly because HIA lacks a statutory footing in all but a few countries. There are also methodological difficulties (Kemm et al., 2004). It is difficult to provide accurate assessments of the health impact of many environmental risks, their costs, and the benefits of reducing them. Moreover, there is little evidence about how HIA affects decision-making and improves health (Quigley and Taylor, 2004). It is also poorly integrated within the decision-making processes (Lock and McKee, 2005).

Nonetheless, there is a growing interest in HIA, both as part of SEA or as a free-standing tool (Lock and McKee, 2005; Metcalfe and Higgins, 2009). HIA has been endorsed by the WHO Regional Office for Europe (1999a), EU institutions (European Commission, 2007; UK governments (Cm 4386, 1999; Cm 6374, 2004; Cm 4269, 1999; NAfW, 1999b; Scottish Executive, 2000a; Cm 3992, 1998; DHSSNI, 1997; DHSSPS, 2002a) and official reports (Independent Inquiry into Inequalities in Health, 1998; Cm 7009, 2007). It has been used in national policymaking (for example the national alcohol strategy for England – see Chapter 15). HIA is increasingly being employed at local and regional level. Liverpool's housing programme, the Manchester Airport extension and Edinburgh's transport policy have all been subject to HIA (see Gorman et al., 2003). The London mayor has also used HIA in formulating strategies on waste, transport and economic development. In addition, there has been increasing pressure to incorporate health inequalities within health impact asessments (see Chapter 17).

Regional Government

Regional structures have had an important role in developing plans on sustainable development and climate change (EAC, 2008e). Government regional offices (GORs) were tasked with ensuring that national priorities, including those for sustainable development and climate change, would be reflected in regional strategies and programmes and at local level. Regional development agencies and regional assemblies also had important strategic planning roles with regard to the environment, sustainable development, housing, transport, infrastructure, and waste. However, there was criticism that insufficient attention was given to sustainable development in regional plans (EAC, 2008e). At the time of writing, regional development agencies and regional assemblies are in the process of being abolished. It is expected that their roles will be devolved to local government. GORs also face an uncertain future (see Chapter 7).

London has special arrangements, being the only English 'region' to have devolved government arrangements. The London mayor has duties and powers that include environmental protection and sustainable development. London has its own sustainable development plan (Mayor of London and London Sustainable Development Commission, 2003), has integrated sustainable development issues in its overall development plan for the capital (Mayor of London, 2004) and has taken steps to address the environmental problems arising from the transport system, for example (see Exhibit 11.1). Under new powers and roles granted in 2007, the mayor will have more influence over local development planning, waste and recycling. The mayor is also required to write a climate change and energy strategy for London and an adaptation strategy covering how the capital should adapt to climate change.

Scotland, Wales and Northern Ireland

The devolved administrations have their own strategies on sustainable development and climate change (Scottish Government, 2008; Welsh Assembly Government, 2009a; Northern Ireland Office, 2006). These reflect the different powers and responsibilities of each part of the UK as well as different priorities and circumstances. It should be noted that some devolved governments have set different targets to England. Scotland for example has a different interim target, aiming to reduce greenhouse gas emissions by 42 per cent by 2020. It also seeks to increase renewables to 31 per cent of electricity demand by 2011 (and half by 2050). Scotland has its own climate change legislation – The Climate Change (Scotland) Act 2009 – and has taken steps to formulate an adaptation framework to deal with the unavoidable consequences of climate change. Meanwhile, Wales has adopted a target of annual carbon reductions of 3 per cent per annum by 2011 in areas of devolved competence.

Conclusion

This chapter has shown the magnitude of potential challenges posed by climate change. Although the future is uncertain and some doubts remain, policymakers cannot simply watch and wait while further evidence accumulates. There are signs that climate change is now being taken more seriously, with stronger policy commitments to reduce greenhouse gases. However, there are still major gaps between the level of action required and what governments are prepared to do in terms of policy, particularly with regard to energy use and transport. There is a major task of coordination to be undertaken to ensure that international bodies, national and subnational government, businesses and civil society all play their part in averting the effects of climate change and adapting to changes that cannot be prevented. One must also be aware of the challenges of sustainable development, over and above the global warming challenge. The limits of conventional economic growth must be addressed. Also required is a much stronger link between environment and health, which weakened during the second half of the twentieth century (Hume Hall, 1990; Environmental Health Commission, 1997). Health consequences strengthen the case for tougher environmental policies to combat climate change and other environmental problems discussed in the previous chapter (*Lancet*/UHL Commission, 2009). Environmental interventions should be regarded as key instruments of health policy (Stone, 2006).

Food Safety, Security and Sustainability   12

According to Tansey and Worsley (1995, p. 49) 'sufficient, safe, nutritious food is an essential ingredient for good health'. No one would seriously challenge the assertion that food is essential for health. However, the relationship between food and health is complex. In this and the following chapter, the specific health issues relating to food are explored in some detail. This chapter focuses upon food safety, security and sustainability; the next on diet, nutrition and obesity.

Food Security and Sustainability

Historically, food policy in the UK has been overwhelmingly focused upon 'food security' – the need to protect the state from the political and military implications of food shortages (Mills, 1992). During the First World War, anxiety about food security led the government to plan on an unprecedented scale. A Ministry of Food regulated food production and supply, and a formal system of food rationing was later introduced. Although a nutritional dimension to food policy existed, it was not the primary factor (Mills, 1992, p. 76). Food controls were dismantled after the war but restored when hostilities broke out again in 1939 (Hammond, 1951). The resurrection of the Ministry of Food and a rationing system in the Second World War ensured that all individuals received an adequate supply of food. Rationing contributed to better nutrition, along with initiatives such as the National Milk Scheme, which ensured that supplies reached priority cases, for example pregnant women and children. According to Hammond (1951, p. 369) 'the diet theoretically available to the British civilian was not only maintained but actually improved during the war'. During the 1930s, hunger and malnutrition had been common among poor and unemployed people. A third of the population had diets deficient in protein and fats, and a tenth were deficient in all nutritional aspects (Boyd Orr, 1936).

The Postwar Period

The key policy objective after the Second World War was to ensure adequate food supplies by maintaining farming incomes within a stable market (Lang et al., 2009). This was implemented through a complex regime of subsidies and guaranteed prices, underpinned by a close working relationship between farmers' representatives, in the form of the National Farmers' Union (NFU), and the Ministry of Agriculture, Fisheries and Food (MAFF) (Self and Storing, 1962; Body, 1991). Consequently the interests of producers prevailed, while others, such as doctors, nutritionists and consumers, were marginalized. Medical advice on diet was located in the Ministry of Health, at arms-length from key decisions about food policy. By the 1970s, health and nutrition policies were divorced from food and agriculture (Centre for Agricultural Strategy, 1979). Relationships between the health departments and MAFF were such that health considerations had little impact on policy except in extreme circumstances, such as serious outbreaks of food poisoning. Interdepartmental relations became even more strained in the years ahead, as concerns about healthy diets and food safety intensified.

The UK and the European Union

From 1973, domestic agriculture and food policy was strongly influenced by membership of the EEC. The UK was now subject to the Common Agricultural Policy (CAP). The CAP placed great emphasis on assuring availability of food supplies by increasing agricultural production through market intervention. This was achieved principally by subsidies and import duties, which ensured that commodity prices exceeded market prices. This encouraged production and market stability and supported agricultural communities by providing higher incomes than would have been the case in a free market. As unease about food security subsided, pressures to reform CAP grew (see EFRAC, 2002, 2007; House of Lords, 2008b; Booker and North, 2005). Countries like the UK, net food importers with small and relatively efficient farming sectors, pressed for change. More broadly, there was criticism of the cost and inefficiency of CAP, manifested in production surpluses (such as the infamous 'butter mountain' and 'wine lake'). There was disquiet that the model of agriculture supported by CAP was unsustainable both economically (by supporting unviable farms) and environmentally (by promoting intensive agriculture that caused pollution and damaged ecosystems).

Efforts have been made to reform CAP. Production quotas were introduced in the 1980s. In the early 1990s, the McSharry reforms sought to link subsidies more closely to structural reform (such as the closure of inefficient farms) and environmental objectives (such as reduced pollution) by shifting the emphasis away from price support to direct payments. A further round of changes were heralded by 'Agenda 2000'. These reforms continued the shift from subsidized prices and production towards maintaining farmers, encouraging rural development and promoting environmental objectives. They brought rural development and environmental funds under a single CAP regulation, known as 'Pillar 2'. The Fischler reform of 2003 represented a fresh effort to break the link between subsidies and production. It introduced a single payment scheme for farmers that combined various funding streams. This reform, described as a radical shift in the EU's agricultural policy (House of Lords, 2008b), ushered in a new review mechanism (the so-called 'health check'). This mechanism, coupled with reviews of the CAP budget, could lead to more radical changes in the future.

Food Crises and Shortages

At a global level, starvation, malnutrition and undernourishment are major health problems. Indeed, 11 per cent of the global disease burden has been attributed to undernutrition (Black et al., 2008). These problems are concentrated in poorer countries and those beset by war and civil strife. Even so, it has been estimated that over two billion people worldwide suffer from inadequate nutrition (Lang and Heasman, 2004, p. 61). More recently, population growth, changing patterns of consumption and problems associated with supplies mean that food shortages and higher prices could pose a problem for industrialized countries as well (Chatham House, 2008a, 2008b; Midgely, 2009; EFRAC, 2009). Food prices globally rose by 75 per cent between January 2006 and July 2008 (Lock et al., 2009). These trends may return us to an era when Western governments were preoccupied with fears about food scarcity and malnutrition. However, for some sections of the population these issues have never gone away. The level of poverty and deprivation in the UK (see Chapters 16 and 17) has meant that some have faced persistent problems in accessing nutritious food (Food Commission, 2004a). Indeed, it is believed that the UK has a higher level of food poverty than other EU countries (Lang and Heasman, 2004, p. 95). There are problems in getting access to food in some socially deprived areas (Hitchman et al., 2002). Some communities have been identified as 'food deserts', where local provision is overwhelmingly from 'fast food' outlets. Although the existence of food deserts has been challenged (Cummins and Macintyre, 2002), recent studies have confirmed their existence (see, for example, the Canadian study by Larsen and Gilliland, 2008). Food poverty was recognized by the Acheson report on health inequalities (see Chapter 17). This report called for measures to 'increase the availability and accessibility of foodstuffs to supply an adequate and affordable diet', including policies to ensure adequate retail provision and policies that improve the health and nutrition of women of childbearing age and their children (Independent Inquiry into Inequalities in Health, 1998). The Labour government did reform the welfare food scheme (now named 'Healthy Start' in 2006), aimed at the poorest families, to extend access to fruit and vegetables. The Acheson report also called for a comprehensive review of CAP on health and inequalities in health and a strengthening of its surplus food scheme to improve nutrition in the less well-off.

Sustainability and the Environment

Concern about environmental damage caused by modern food and agriculture systems has raised sustainability and ecological issues (Lang et al., 2001, 2009; EFRAC, 2009; HM Government, 2010a). Agriculture is a major source of pollution (Environment Agency, 2002). It has had an adverse impact on biodiversity (there has been a 40 per cent reduction in farmland birds since the mid-1970s – Council for the Protection of Rural England, cited in EFRAC, 2002). Food and agriculture systems are a major contributor to global warming and climate change, responsible for over a fifth of greenhouse gases in the UK (Garnett, 2008; Friel et al., 2009). Meat and dairy production, for example, are highly resource intensive and produce high levels of greenhouse gases. Food and agriculture can also provide a solution to these problems (House of Lords, 2008b; Sustainable Development Commission, 2009; EFRAC, 2009). Agriculture could reduce the impact of environmental problems through reforestation and the production of renewable fuels. Indeed, over the past two decades a number of schemes have emerged, such as 'environmentally sensitive areas' (ESAs), which cover 10 per cent of farmland in the UK, and the countryside stewardship scheme. These are based on agreements between government and farmers, which pay the latter to protect, conserve and enhance the environment (DEFRA, 2002). Food distribution systems are also harmful to the environment. Road transport of food, for example, causes pollution and greenhouse gases. Added to this is the cost of driving to 'out of town' supermarkets. Food packaging has environmental costs, in terms of both the resources to produce it and the costs associated with its disposal. Moreover, food waste is a major problem. It is estimated that the real cost per capita of the UK food budget would be over 10 per cent higher if external environmental costs were taken into account (Pretty et al., 2005).

A number of suggestions have been made to create a more sustainable food system (Policy Commission on the Future of Farming and Food, 2002; International Commission on the Future of Food and Agriculture, 2003). Organic farming, which builds on biodiversity and seeks to minimize adverse effects on natural resources, has become more popular (Soil Association, 2000; European Union, 2002). Cultivation of organic food has increased dramatically since the 1980s, although it still represents a small share of both production (around 3 per cent of agricultural land is devoted to organic farming) and consumption (around 2 per cent of food sales). Both EU and UK policies have promoted organic food (Stolze and Lampkin, 2009; Reed, 2009). It has been estimated that a switch to organic production could save over £1 billion per annum in environmental costs (Pretty et al., 2005). However, it should be noted that organic food has environmental consequences – there are transport costs as 70 per cent of organic food is imported. Organic food is more expensive and therefore less affordable for poorer people. Research has also shown that organic food is not necessarily more nutritious than conventional farm produce, although it may be healthier due to the lack of pesticides (Dangour et al., 2009). More research into the impact of organic farming on environmental and health is needed (Hole et al., 2005).

Some have called for lower consumption of meat and dairy production and food of little nutritional value (Garnett, 2008; Friel et al., 2009). Another proposal is to reduce 'food miles' and the transport costs of food by encouraging more local sourcing of food. The Sustainable Development Commission (2009) has also backed a number of ideas including promoting locally produced food and growing vegetables on public land. Efforts to cut food packaging have been made to reduce environmental impact. A voluntary agreement was drawn up between major UK food companies and WRAP (Waste Reduction Action Programme – a government sponsored body that promotes waste reduction and recycling) to reduce food and packaging waste by 2010. In addition the Food and Drink Federation, which represents the largest companies in this sector, has set targets to reduce CO_2 emissions, improve energy efficiency in factories, reduce food waste, improve water efficiency and promote 'green' food transport.

Following the foot-and-mouth disease epidemic of 2001, which caused severe problems for the farming industry and rural areas, the UK government established an independent policy commission on farming and food (Policy Commission on the Future of Farming and Food, 2002). The Commission declared that 'the situation in England's farming and food industry today is unsustainable, in every sense of that term. It is serving nobody well' (p.109). It argued that the food chain underperformed economically (with low profit levels in agriculture); environmentally (the damaging effect of emissions, waste and pollution); and socially (with regard to diet and health, tourism and the wider rural community). The Commission called upon the whole of the food chain to reconnect with customers, the global economy, the countryside and environment. Its many recommendations included: substantial reform of CAP; more opportunities for local sourcing of food products; a comprehensive animal health strategy, a more systematic approach to meeting environmental and social objectives, with stronger incentives and more coherent regulation; ongoing support for organic farming; a re-examination by supermarkets of their food supply routes in the light of environmental concerns; a strategy to encourage healthy eating; and continued efforts to reduce risks from pesticides and antibiotics.

The government broadly accepted the commission's recommendations and set out a strategy for England (DEFRA, 2002 – other parts of the UK developed their own approach see, for example, Scottish Government, 2005). This included: an action plan for organic farming; measures to increase local sourcing; the establishment of a centre to identify and tackle inefficiencies, measures to promote collaboration within farming and between farmers and other parts of the food chain; more funding for agricultural schemes that benefit the environment, rewards for good environment practice, and a more comprehensive approach to managing the impact of farms on the environment. Subsequently, DEFRA introduced a food and health action plan (discussed in the next chapter). It also introduced a food industry sustainability strategy (FISS), with five work streams: energy use and climate change; ethical trading; food transport; waste; and water (DEFRA, 2006a; Lang et al., 2009).

Although such efforts have been welcomed, efforts to improve the sustainability of the food system require a holistic and comprehensive approach backed with legislative and fiscal powers (Garnett, 2008; International Commission on the Future of Food and Agriculture, 2003). They also require government to tackle vested interests and consumer behaviour in ways that may be politically unpopular. The Labour government set out a strategy linking key issues such as healthy diet, a profitable and competitive food system, increasing sustainability, reducing greenhouse gases, reducing waste and increasing the impact of skills, knowledge research and technology (HM Government, 2010a). However, this placed great faith in markets, technology and voluntary efforts to solve these problems. Moreover, UK policy is constrained by EU membership, particularly CAP.

The introduction of the second pillar of CAP, promoting rural development and environmental schemes, has already been mentioned. This now accounts for just under a quarter of total CAP expenditure (EFRAC, 2007). Member states are now compelled to make small transfers (5 per cent) from Pillar 1 budgets (subsidies for farmers) to Pillar 2. They are also permitted to voluntarily transfer up to 20 per cent of the Pillar 1 budget to the second pillar (currently only Portugal and the UK have opted to do this). Moreover, Pillar 1 of CAP now has an environmental dimension. Farms receiving support from this source must demonstrate compliance with environmental and animal welfare standards (House of Lords, 2008b). However, much more could be done to increase the contribution of CAP to the environment, sustainable development and public health. There have been calls for CAP to be reoriented to meet environmental, climate change and rural development objectives (DEFRA, 2002, 2007; House of Lords, 2008b). Some have called for agriculture to be integrated more fully into climate change policy, by including it in emissions trading (DEFRA; 2002; House of Lords, 2008b). From a wider public health perspective, CAP has failed to promote health in other ways, which need to be addressed. For example, it has inflated the prices of healthy products (fruit and vegetables) while encouraging the production of products that can damage health (tobacco, alcohol and saturated fats) (see Elinder et al., 2003).

Food Safety

There are three main types of food safety issue: the acute effects of a poisoning incident; the long-term effects of such an incident (such as organ damage and disability); and the long-term effects of prolonged exposure to a particular chemical, biological or physical agent. Such concerns are not new. There was much public agitation in Victorian times following revelations about the adulteration of bread, tea, milk and other food products (Smith, 1979). Even by historical standards, however, food safety is a prominent issue today. Since the early 1980s, it has been constantly on the agenda, fuelled by periodic health scares arising from high-profile outbreaks of salmonella, Escherichia coli (notably E. coli O157), listeria, and new variant CJD (Creutzfeldt-Jakob disease). There has also been unease about food technologies, including genetically modified foods, food irradiation, pesticides, antibiotics and additives.

Microbiological Agents and Food Poisoning

Reported incidents of food poisoning in the UK rose dramatically in the 1980s. Some of this increase was attributed to a greater willingness (possibly due to increased media coverage of food poisoning) to seek treatment and report cases. Eating, arguably, has become riskier as people eat out more, consume more takeaway and barbecued food, and shop less frequently for groceries (increasing the likelihood of consuming spoiled or out of date food). Consumers now eat more pre-prepared food, which can be harmful if not stored or heated properly. Another possible explanation is that people have become less hygienic in preparing food. Food poisoning risks may also have increased as a result of the expansion of overseas travel and the globalization of food markets.

Outbreaks of food poisoning attract attention, especially when there are fatalities, or where the victims are vulnerable (for example children, elderly people, patients). Indeed, the high-profile food poisoning outbreaks of the 1980s are still remembered (see Pennington, 2003; Booker and North, 2007):

the outbreak of salmonella at the Stanley Royd hospital in Wakefield, where 19 people died (Cmnd, 9716, 1986); the salmonella in eggs crisis (Agriculture Committee, 1989); and the 'hysteria' about listeria in cheeses and pâtés (Health Committee, 1990). The 1980s also saw the emergence of E. coli O157, which has since been implicated in other incidents, including an outbreak in central Scotland in 1996 that affected 500 people, 20 of whom subsequently died (Scottish Office, 1997; Pennington, 2003) and another in South Wales in 2005 where 156 people, mainly children, became ill and one child died as a result (Pennington, 2009). Infection by E. coli O157 can occur from eating meat products not properly cooked, as well as from direct contact with farm animals (as occurred in an outbreak in England during 2009, which affected a number of children). It can have particularly severe consequences, including bloody diarrhoea, organ failure and brain damage, and is particularly dangerous to older people, children and those already in poor health (Pennington, 2003).

The other major food scare of recent times was bovine spongiform encephalopathy (BSE) or 'mad cow disease', with its potential threat to humans in the form of a degenerative brain disease, CJD. This issue, examined in Exhibit 12.1, did much to destroy public trust in the system of food regulation in the UK and led to significant reforms discussed later in this chapter.

Exhibit 12.1

Mad Cow Disease

One of the major food crises of modern times was associated with so-called 'mad cow disease' (Booker and North, 2007; Ratzan, 1998; Hodgett, 1998; Baggott, 1998; van Zwanenberg and Millstone, 2003). During the late 1980s, a small but increasing number of people were diagnosed with a degenerative and fatal brain disease called Creutzfeldt-Jakob disease (CJD). Normally this disease was rare and affected mainly elderly people. However, a growing number of cases were found in younger people. Some scientists believed that a new variant of the disease had emerged and that this was acquired by eating beef from cattle infected with bovine spongiform encephalopathy (BSE), itself a newly documented disease. They further believed that cattle had acquired the disease from sheep infected with a similar and long-recognized disease called scrapie. Suspicion fell on the practices of the animal feed industry, which was accused of including material from sheep in cattle feed and, in the context of deregulation, using inadequate production processes that failed to destroy infectious agents. Although recycling of animal proteins in feed was identified as the main probable cause of BSE/CJD, this remains an area of great uncertainty (Pennington, 2003).

Initially, the UK government denied a link between these diseases. It did, however, establish a scientific committee in the late 1980s. This body recommended a series of precautionary measures, including a ruminant feed ban (cattle, sheep and deer were not allowed protein derived from other animals), a ban on specified bovine offal

(SBO) from cattle aged six months and over (brains, spinal cord, thymus, spleen, intestines, tonsils) in human food, and a compensation scheme that gave farmers half the market price for keeping BSE-infected cattle out of the food chain. These measures were criticized. Some argued that the SBO ban should apply to all cattle, not just those aged six months and over. The compensation scheme was ungenerous and provided little incentive to keep sick animals out of the food chain. Calls for a computerized tracking system, to identify the movement of healthy and unhealthy animals, were rejected. However, such a scheme was introduced in Northern Ireland and has since been extended across the UK. Further criticism was levelled at the agriculture ministry's control of the research process, which blocked or delayed projects that might have revealed earlier the full extent of the problem and how best to deal with it.

In 1990, the agriculture minister, John Gummer, famously fed a beefburger to his young daughter, under the full gaze of the media. This, and other efforts to reassure the public, failed miserably. As other countries became increasingly worried about the safety of British beef, the EU sought to impose additional restrictions. Revelations about poor enforcement of the UK government's BSE regulations added further pressure. In March 1996, the UK government eventually admitted that a new variant of CJD had been identified in young people and this had probably been acquired by eating BSE-infected beef. This was followed by stricter controls on beef and a programme of slaughtering older cattle to keep them out of the food chain. The European Union immediately banned the export of British beef, which left the industry in a state of near-collapse.

A public inquiry into the handling of the BSE crisis, established by the Blair government, illustrated the breathtaking complacency of ministers and officials (Independent Inquiry on BSE, 2000). The inquiry, chaired by Lord Phillips, found that insufficient weight had been given to the risks to public health. Although effective measures had been introduced, these were often delayed and not adequately implemented or enforced. The report criticized government for seeking to reassure the public. However, it did not accuse ministers and officials of a deliberate 'cover up'. The report called for more openness about risk assessments with a stronger emphasis on reasonable precautionary measures, even when health risks seemed remote. Relationships between the Department of Health and the Ministry of Agriculture were found to be poor, with the latter introspective and secretive in its handling of the crisis. In particular, there was a failure to consult with the Chief Medical Officer (CMO) on the public health implications of BSE/CJD.

Other inquiries showed the European Commission in a poor light. Although it had been seen as the defender of public health on this particular issue, it transpired that the Commission had mishandled the crisis by thwarting research into the BSE–CJD link, yielding to pressure from the UK Ministry of Agriculture, and generally downplaying the health risks to avoid disruption to the beef market (European Parliament, 1997). Subsequently the European Commission reorganized its responsibilities for food safety, bringing scientific committees on issues such as pesticides, animal and plant health, and food safety under the Health and Consumer Protection portfolio, and establishing an independent European Food Safety Agency.

Around 500 people a year die from the effects of food poisoning in the UK. The number of reported cases of food poisoning fell 20 per cent between 2000 and 2005, but remains a significant problem with around 80,000 reported cases every year in the UK. Moreover, reported cases are only a fraction of those who actually suffer from food poisoning. A number of factors suggest that food poisoning rates may increase in future. Climate change, for example, is likely to raise food poisoning risks. A one per cent rise in temperature is associated with a 5 per cent increase in food poisoning cases (Bentham and Langford, 1994). In addition, some of the trends described earlier, which have contributed to increases in food poisoning in the past, particularly the globalization of food production and the increase in international travel, are likely to continue.

Chemical Contamination

Over 500 chemicals are added to food as colourings, flavourings, and preservatives. Some are synthetic while others occur naturally, in plants for example. It has been estimated that each person eats 6.5kg of additives every year (Food Commission, 2004b). While some additives may make food more palatable or, in the case of preservatives, may even protect the consumer from food poisoning, they can damage health. The colouring tartrazine, for example, has been associated with allergic reactions and behavioural problems (Neuman et al., 1978; Freedman, 1977; Bateman et al., 2004). Tartrazine and other food colourings – sunset yellow, quinoline yellow, allura red, carmoisine and ponceau – and the preservative sodium benzoate have been linked to hyperactivity in children (McCann et al., 2007). The effects of longer term exposure to additives is more difficult to measure, although some, such as the sweetener saccharin, and the colouring allura red, have been associated with cancer in laboratory experiments.

Chemical contamination can also occur as a result of pesticide use. As noted in Chapter 10, some pesticides are extremely harmful to the environment. They persist for long periods in the food chain and cause long-term damage to animal and human health. Pesticides have been linked to cancer and neurological diseases (Bassil et al., 2007; Tanner et al., 2009). More research is needed, especially on the cumulative effects of exposure to a cocktail of pesticides (Committee on Toxicity, 2002; Axelrad et al., 2002). Regular analysis of food samples has revealed that over a third of food products tested contained traces of pesticide and around 2 per cent exceeded maximum revenue levels (Pesticide Residue Committee, 2007). These figures are higher than in the previous decade (MAFF/HSE, 1999). Ironically, free fruit given to children to promote healthy eating (see Chapter 13) was more likely to contain traces of pesticide than fruit and vegetables bought in the shops, although less likely to exceed maximum permitted levels (Pesticide Residue Committee, 2007).

People are exposed to chemicals through other agricultural practices, such as the routine use of veterinary medicines and growth-promoting drugs. Although antibiotics can improve animal health, there are problems when used primarily to promote growth and productivity. Overuse of antibiotics has implications for antibiotic resistance in both animals and humans (House of Lords, 1998a, 2001a; Advisory Committee on the Microbiological Safety of Food, 1999). This could be linked to antibiotic-resistant strains of *E. coli* and *staphylococcus aureus*, found in some animals, which could spread to workers and consumers. A related issue is the use of growth-promoting hormones in livestock, which may cause cancer in humans and damage immune systems.

Harmful chemicals can enter the food chain through industrial and other forms of pollution. Dioxins and PCBs, discussed in Chapter 10, have been linked to cancers, damage to immune systems and harm to reproductive systems. Although measures to reduce these pollutants have been successful, they persist for long periods in the environment. Analyses of food samples indicate that dioxin and PCB levels are low, and below regulatory limits set by the EU (FSA, 2007), although unease remains about cumulative exposure over long periods.

New Technologies

Further concerns about food safety arise from new food production technologies. Ionizing radiation can be used to kill bacteria and pests, and delay the ripening of fruit (Food Commission, 2002). Its supporters argue that it protects against food poisoning. However, the process is principally a means of increasing shelf life and reducing spoilage, so reducing food industry costs. Irradiation may even reduce incentives to improve hygiene. Notably, irradiation does not guarantee that food is safe, as some pathogens (notably the bacteria that cause botulism) can survive the process. Moreover, irradiation can reduce the nutritional value of food by destroying vitamins. There may be additional health risks from the by-products of irradiation, such as hydrocarbons (linked to allergies and cancer, although these risks are not proven). As we shall see later, food irradiation is tightly restricted, although in some cases consumers have been unwittingly exposed to it (FSA, 2002).

Genetically modified (GM) food has been a controversial issue for over a decade. GM crops are opposed for their wider environmental implications, such as harm to wildlife, loss of biodiversity and adverse impact on agriculture. There is also disquiet about possible health consequences for the consumer, although no evidence yet shows that GM food causes health problems (Donaldson and May, 1999). It could harm health in a number of ways – by promoting greater antibiotic resistance in both animals and humans, and greater resistance to pesticides in crops. It is also possible that GM food may have a direct impact on gastrointestinal conditions and food allergies. However, these effects are unknown and it is acknowledged that more research is needed, particularly on the possible impact of GM technologies on vulnerable groups such as children, pregnant women, elderly and chronically ill people (Royal Society, 2002). The CMO and chief scientific advisor (Donaldson and May, 1999) both called for a system of health surveillance and the FSA has since commissioned research. But this will only identify problems after they have materialized. Defenders of GM food say that there are potential health advantages, such as increased crop yields (to reduce price and availability of food). Interestingly, concerns about food security and shortages have bolstered arguments for exploring GM food technologies (EFRAC, 2009; Royal Society, 2009). GM food could be grown to improve the nutritional value of food, by boosting levels of vitamins and other nutrients. Genetic modification is also seen as a way of reducing infestation and pesticide use, which again may have health benefits.

Genetic technologies can be applied to livestock. Although selective breeding is not new, there is great alarm about livestock genetic technologies. Cloning of animals has attracted particular concern. Recent cases in the UK have exposed shortcomings in regulation (Sample, 2007; BBC, 2010a). There are worries that cloning and other genetic modification techniques may have unforeseen consequences for environment, biodiversity and human health (Agriculture and Environment Biotechnology Commission, 2002). Food from cloned animals is classified as 'novel food', subject to special regulation discussed later in this chapter. Other novel foods include those produced by nanotechnology, which may also present new risks (House of Lords, 2010).

Other Food Safety Issues

Other food safety issues also deserve mention. One is contamination of food with 'foreign bodies' (including insects, rodents, pieces of metal and wood, and so on) of which there are around 2000 reported cases every year (BBC, 2002). Another worry is the deliberate contamination of food and water supplies by terrorists. Criminal activity, such as fraud, has been behind a number of food safety incidents. In one case in 2001, a man (labelled by the media as 'Maggott Pete') was convicted of supplying condemned meat to caterers. The food was distributed to schools, old people's homes, shops and restaurants. In view of the potential threat to food safety of this kind of actvity, a food fraud task force was established in 2006. This recommended: that food fraud should have higher priority in food enforcement; better training for food enforcement officers; sharing of intelligence between regulatory authorities in the UK in Europe and globally; improvements in the registration of food businesses; better coordination between enforcement authorities; and a rapid response food fraud investigation team. Despite this, however, food fraud remains a relatively low priority.

Food Safety Regulation

Given the range and diversity of food safety issues, it is not surprising that the regulatory framework is complex. Regulation occurs at global, European and UK levels.

Global Level

The main institutions at global level are the Food and Agriculture Organization (FAO) and WHO. In recent years, food safety has risen up the international agenda. In 2002, the World Food Summit held under the auspices of FAO, reaffirmed 'the right of everyone to have access to safe and nutritious food' (FAO, 2002). Meanwhile, WHO (2002) devised a global food safety strategy and prioritized this issue within its work programme. The strategy aimed to 'reduce the health and social burden of foodborne disease', by 'advocating and supporting the development of risk-based, sustainable, integrated food safety systems'; 'devising science-based measures along the entire food production chain' to prevent exposure to harmful agents in food; and 'assessing and managing foodborne risks and communicating information' in cooperation with other bodies (WHO, 2002, pp. 1–2).

Another international body, the Codex Alimentarius Commission (known as Codex), created by FAO and WHO in 1963, has an important role. It sets standards on issues such as the labelling of food products, product composition, food safety standards (including maximum permitted levels of additives, pesticides, contaminants, and veterinary drug residues), guidelines on processes and procedures of food hygiene. Since 1994, Codex standards have had a vital role in relation to trade agreements (see Chapter 5), providing a basis for WTO judgements on the legitimacy of trade barriers. If health standards are lowered, countries with higher domestic standards of food safety would face a competitive disadvantage from countries with lower standards and their markets would be open to food imports harmful to health. It has been argued that Codex is too close to commercial interests and subject to their influence (Tansey and Worsley, 1995; Millstone and van Zwanenberg, 2002). A common complaint is that consumers and environmental and public health interests are underrepresented in its processes. Although Codex does have consumer representation, these lack resources, political contacts and economic leverage.

Critics argue that trade agreements, and by implication Codex standards, have not protected health standards (Lee and Koivusalo, 2005). One of the classic cases is that of hormone-treated beef. The EU banned animal growth hormones in 1989 citing health reasons. Imports of hormone-treated beef from countries such as Canada and the USA were consequently banned. They took their case to the WTO, which ruled in their favour, maintaining there was insufficient evidence of risk to human health. The EU refused to comply with the WTO judgement. The issue remains contentious, with the EU accused of protectionism. Irrespective of the ban's impact on trade, it has been argued that the precautionary principle should prevail, given the level of uncertainty about the effect on consumer health. The EU has since brought forward further scientific evidence on the effects of some hormones while seeking a provisional prohibition on others where the evidence is less clear.

Codex has also been criticized for not fully acknowledging the potential impact of food technologies on the health of consumers on other issues, such as irradiated food and GM food. The importance of international standards in both consumer protection and public health has been acknowledged in an evaluation of Codex and food standards (FAO/WHO, 2002). This report recommended greater speed in Codex decision-making and expert advice; increased inclusiveness of developing countries in the development of standards; more effective capacity building for development of national food control systems; and standards that are more timely and relevant to countries' needs. It also called for clearer prioritization in Codex work; greater independence; and that its system of expert advice should be strengthened and better resourced.

The European Union

The original Treaty of Rome gave the EU powers to intervene in a wide range of food and agricultural issues. This role was strengthened by the development of a European-wide environmental policy and the extension of the EU's role in promoting public health (see Chapter 5). The BSE crisis was a particularly important stimulus for action. Early areas of EU intervention included pesticide control, veterinary medicines and food additives. Regulation was later extended to food hygiene procedures and standards, the regulation of GM and novel foods, and the microbiological safety of food. Efforts to strengthen food safety across Europe were brought together in a white paper (Commission of the European Communities, 2000), setting out plans for a European-wide food authority. In 2002, the European Food Safety Authority (EFSA) was established, with three main tasks: the provision of independent scientific advice, EU-wide monitoring, and the establishment of a food safety network across Europe. Although this further extended the EU's authority in assessing and communicating risk in this area, the main aim was to restore market confidence without threatening powerful food businesses or the autonomy of member states (Taylor and Millar, 2004). Some argue that EFSA does not have the resources to carry out full risk assessments and that it depends too heavily on industry for sources of information. The EU has also established an early warning system for food safety issues and has shown a greater willingness to tackle food safety through the courts by introducing bans and prosecuting member states for regulatory failures.

The UK

UK food safety policy is shaped by international and EU regulation. Regulation of pesticides, food hygiene and food additives has been influenced by developments at the EU level. Nevertheless, the UK has also been an important driver of food safety, largely because some of the most serious incidents have occurred here. The response of UK policymakers has provided lessons for the rest of the EU. Following a spate of food safety incidents, the Food Safety Act of 1990 was passed. This established a new committee to advise on the microbiological safety of food, new powers for environmental health officers (EHOs), such as the power to close outlets immediately on public health grounds, and a code of practice to guide enforcement. Offences with regard to food safety were clarified. A system of registration of food outlets was introduced along with compulsory training for food handlers. Although the new legislation was seen as a step forward in some quarters (see Pennington, 2003), it was argued that the legal provisions could have gone further in deterring poor practice and depended on under-resourced EHO departments to enforce the law (Audit Commission, 1990). Amid continuing concerns about food safety, further changes came in during the 1990s, inspired mainly by EU initiatives, including the creation of a national meat hygiene service and stricter regulation of slaughterhouses. In 1995, new general hygiene regulations were introduced, requiring food businesses to assess and control potential hazards. Businesses were encouraged to use a system called HACCP (hazard analysis critical control point), identifying hazards at each stage of the food production and handling process, assessing risks and identifying the stages at which controls are needed to ensure safety, the listing of preventive measures, and effective monitoring. HACCP has been endorsed by Codex, the EU and WHO.

The BSE crisis and the Scottish outbreak of E. coli O157 added to the pressure to create a more robust system of food safety. Inquiries into these incidents produced authoritative reports that endorsed a precautionary approach to food safety, and the need for a more open, independent and transparent system of regulation (Independent Inquiry on BSE, 2000; Scottish Office, 1997). Following a change of government, a national Food Standards Agency

(FSA) was established (Cm 3830, 1998). This was constituted as a statutory non-departmental public body accountable to Parliament via the Secretary of State for Health, and to the devolved administrations of Scotland, Wales and Northern Ireland. It was given powers over food safety, nutrition and labelling, taking over responsibilities of the DoH and MAFF. However, the DoH retained responsibilities for nutritional policy, while MAFF remained in control of pesticides regulation and animal health. Although the agency has not escaped criticism, this has been of a much lower level and intensity than in the pre-FSA era. Surveys undertaken on behalf of the FSA indicate a high level of public support for its work and a declining level of public concern about food safety issues (FSA, 2008a). Reported cases of food poisoning have fallen significantly since 2000, as already noted.

The Health Protection Agency (HPA) was also given an important role in relation to food safety. The HPA took over the responsibilities of the Public Health Laboratory Service (PHLS) for monitoring food poisoning in 2003. There was concern that this takeover, coupled with the transfer of microbiology labs to local NHS trusts, would lead to a downgrading of foodborne disease surveillance as a priority. However, the change brought opportunities for the HPA to enforce new national quality standards for all laboratories undertaking microbiological analysis of food. The HPA was also charged with giving advice at national, regional and local level on how to prevent and deal with outbreaks of foodborne disease.

At the time of writing, both the FSA and the HPA face an uncertain future. In 2010, the Cameron government, as part of a review of 'arms-length' agencies, stated its intention to abolish the HPA and subsume its functions within a new public health service. Meanwhile, stories appeared in the media that the FSA would also be abolished, its functions transferred to the Department of Health and DEFRA. At the time of writing, no final decision has been made on the future of the FSA.

Although the FSA and HPA acquired responsibilities for foodborne disease and food safety across the UK, devolved governments also have an important role. Governments in Scotland, Wales and Northern Ireland have their own approach to food safety and have worked closely with their devolved section of the FSA. Meanwhile, at local level, food safety laws are enforced by EHOs. It has been recognized that environmental health departments are under-resourced. In particular, the expansion of food businesses has added to their workload. In 2006/7, around two-thirds of UK establishments were inspected. Just under half of these were found to have committed an infringement leading to formal action by enforcement authorities, usually a written warning (FSA, 2008b). Fewer than 500 establishments were prosecuted, the majority successfully. It has been estimated that around 6 per cent of UK food establishments pose a risk to public health (FSA, 2008c). Enforcement varies between different local authorities. The FSA reviewed enforcement and has drawn up plans to give local authorities greater flexibility in improving food hygiene standards. In future, they will be expected to concentrate on high-risk premises. They are also expected to build more effective partnership working with businesses to improve compliance. Another long-standing problem has been the limited powers of EHOs, although there have been some improvements in recent years. EHOs now have more power to name and shame food businesses with poor standards of hygiene. Fines for breaches of hygiene laws and regulations include jail sentences and unlimited fines. However, most cases are dealt with in magistrates' courts, which impose smaller penalties. Although the maximum penalty imposed by a crown court is two years in prison, an unlimited fine or both, even this does not reflect the severity of the most serious cases. Some cases, however, have been success-fully tried under fraud legislation, which carries more severe sentences than food safety infringements (as in the 'Maggott Pete' case mentioned earlier). Hygiene of food businesses was identified as one of the priority areas of local authority regulation (Rogers, 2007), which some hoped would lead to an increase in resources in the future.

Since 2000, a range of measures have been introduced to improve food safety. Some are broad, while others address specific problems. General measures include the licensing of all butchers, introduced in 2000 following the recommendations of the Pennington inquiry (Scottish Office, 1997). HACCP, also endorsed by Pennington, was extended to all businesses except farms. EU regulations, introduced in 2006, provided impetus for the extension of HACCP. All food business operators, except farmers and growers, must implement a permanent procedure for maintaining food hygiene, based on HACCP principles. Other aspects of the EU food hygiene legislation include a requirement that food business, including farms, must be registered with a competent authority (in most cases, the local authority). The EU also revised and extended criteria for levels of contamination by micro-organisms per unit of food, setting standards both for products on the market and in processing. Other measures include FSA advertising campaigns to address poor personal hygiene. Campaigns have targeted catering businesses and staff as well as the public. The FSA attempted to improve staff training, by providing training materials direct to food busin-esses and funding local authorities to provide training programmes.

New schemes have been introduced for informing the public about inspec-tion reports. Some councils have adopted a 'SmileSafe' ratings scheme. This indicates the outcome of inspections using a smiley face symbol, its expres-sion reflecting the hygiene rating of the establishment. Information and summary reports have been made available online. Outlets are encouraged, but not compelled, to display their 'SmileSafe' rating on their premises. A similar scheme, 'Scores on the Doors', adopted by around 90 councils, produces publicly available hygiene star ratings for food businesses.

Food Additives

A number of measures have also been introduced to deal with concerns about food additives. Some harmful additives have been prohibited, such as the colouring E105 ('Fast yellow'). Others have been voluntarily withdrawn by the food industry. For example, some confectionery manufacturers removed additives linked to child behavioural problems. Food additives are subject to EU regulation. A system of additive labelling, using the E number system, was introduced in the 1980s. In the 1990s, a common list of additives was approved across the EU. The EU introduced a new system of food additive regulation in 2009, with a common authorization procedure under which additives will only be permitted if they are safe, necessary and have benefits for the consumer. The regulations allow approved maximum levels for additives to be set where appropriate. They also establish a re-evaluation system which means that eventually all additives currently in use will be assessed by the EFSA. Enforcement of these new rules will be of paramount importance. Despite regulation, the public has still been exposed to dangerous additives. For example in 2005, Sudan I, a food dye linked to cancer and banned in the UK, was found in imported chilli powder. The powder was used in the making of Worcestershire Sauce, an ingredient in over 400 different food products, including pasta dishes, shepherd's pie, hot pot, sauces and dressings. Although these products were recalled, it is likely that many people had already been exposed.

Pesticides and Other Chemicals

Pesticides are regulated at both the EU and UK level. Some, such as DDT, have been banned for many years. At the UK level, the Pesticides Safety Directorate (part of the HSE) is responsible for registration and approval of pesticides in Britain (Northern Ireland has its own system). The UK government pursued a voluntary approach to pesticide regulation, to encourage the agriculture and chemical industries to minimize the impact of pesticides on the environment and food chain. Some producers have voluntarily stopped using particular pesticides, while some retailers have refused to sell products that contain these substances. This approach was criticized for not prioritizing pesticide issues and in particular for not having a strategic approach to the sustainable use of pesticides (EAC, 2005). A pesticide strategy was eventually introduced after some delay (DEFRA, 2006b).

An EU directive of 1991, implemented four years later in the UK, established a review programme to examine the safety of pesticides. Substances associated with unacceptable risk to people or the environment must be phased out. In 2005, the EU set new maximum residue levels for pesticides, which led to some being restricted or withdrawn from use. In 2006, a new thematic strategy was proposed, including a new directive on the sustainable use of pesticides. The aim was to ensure that less harmful pesticides and safer non-chemical alternatives are substituted for more dangerous ones. At the time of writing, this was set to be finally approved by EU institutions. The new regulations entail the establishment of a new list of approved substances at the EU level. Highly toxic chemicals will be banned unless in very small concentrations. There will be processes for substituting harmful substances with safer alternatives within a specific time frame. However, current pesticides can be used until their existing authorization expires and there are provisions for authorizing pesticides in situations where there are serious threats to plant health. Other measures include: encouragement of non-chemical forms of pest control, and restrictions on use of pesticides near drinking water sources, residential areas, parks and schools. However, campaigners argue that much more needs to be done, and quickly, to protect health and the environment. One suggestion is a pesticides tax, to incentivize a shift towards less harmful pesticides and non-chemical alternatives.

Other measures to reduce harmful chemicals in food include EU restrictions on antibiotics in animal feed. An EU-wide ban on antibiotics for use as growth promoters was introduced in 2006. This followed earlier restrictions imposed on specific antibiotics. However, antibiotics are still permitted for therapeutic purposes, for example to prevent or treat disease in animals, and they are heavily used. Indeed, almost half the total consumption of antibiotics in Europe is by animals (Follett, 2000).

Food Technologies and GM

Food technologies are also subject to regulation. Food irradiation, for example, although not a new technology, has been a controversial issue in recent years (Food Commission, 2002). Irradiated food can be sold in the UK, but only for certain product categories (fruit, vegetables, cereals, bulbs and tubers, spices and condiments, fish and shellfish and poultry). All foods that contain irradiated ingredients must be appropriately labelled. Under EU rules, each country can decide which products it will allow. Any such product can be internally produced or imported from any other member state provided that it is irradiated at an authorized plant and correctly labelled. Currently, only herbs or spices can be legally sold across all EU countries, and imported from outside the EU. The EU sets limits on the levels of radiation used in the process. However, there is pressure on the EU from the WTO to deregulate food irradiation. Such a move is opposed by most of the EU food industry as well as consumer organizations. In addition to deregulatory pressures, there are problems of enforcement. The European Commission found that 3 per cent of food samples tested across EU member states were illegally irradiated or not labelled as such. The UK had a higher than average rate (11 per cent) of illegal irradiation (Commission of the European Communities, 2009).

There is also regulation of GM food technologies (Toke, 2002). Following the imposition of a de facto ban on GM products in 1998, the EU introduced new regulations in 2003 permitting commercialized GM food or animal feed (Lieberman and Gray, 2006). An important change was that companies could no longer argue that a full safety assessment was unnecessary because the GM product was substantially equivalent to the conventional product. The new process meant that applications for authorization could be made to any single member state. EFSA then gives an opinion. Following a period of public consultation, the European Commission makes a final decision. The EU currently permits 10 GM crops for use in animal feed, including herbicide- and insecticide-resistant maizes, herbicide-resistant soya bean and herbicide-resistant sugar beet. Only two GM crops (both maize) have been licensed for commercial cultivation within the EU.

The EU introduced mandatory GM labelling in the late 1990s, for food products containing over one per cent of authorized GM ingredients. New rules on traceability and labelling were introduced in 2003. Labelling requirements were extended to catering and restaurant suppliers. Producers were required to establish an audit trail to identify the source of genetically modified organisms (GMOs). The threshold required for labelling GM ingredients was reduced to 0.9 per cent. Moreover, products containing up to this level of GMOs were only allowed where contamination was technically unavoidable or unintentional. Specific requirements for labelling GMOs in animal feed were introduced, but this excluded products made from animals fed on GM products (meat, eggs, milk) or those produced by GM technology but not containing GM (for example cheese).

Three GM foods were licensed for sale in the UK in the 1990s, although none were actually grown here. Permission has been granted for the cultivation of GM maize for fodder under certain conditions, but so far no producer has met them. No food crops are currently grown commercially in the UK. Following the election of the Blair government, which strongly supported the biotechnology industry and commercial planting of GM crops, the momentum for commercial exploitation of GM crops increased. But public and media opposition was strong. GM was also opposed by parts of the food industry, notably organic farmers and the large supermarkets. The government agreed to farm trials of GM crops prior to commercial planting, but even this was controversial (EAC, 2004b). Sceptics agreed that the long-term impact on health and the environment would not be properly evaluated. Even so, field trials found that GM crops had adverse implications for farmland biodiversity, (although in one case, GM maize, there was evidence of some beneficial effect) (Royal Society, 2002; ACRE, 2004, 2005). Some believe that the trials will lead to an irrevocable spread of GM crops causing damage, in particular, to organic farms. Pollen from GM crops has been found several miles from the trial sites (Toke, 2002). There have been other contamination incidents: for example one case in 2000, where GM oilseed rape seed not cleared for commercial planting was accidentally sown. In general, the scientific basis for allowing GM is weak and little is known about the longer term impact of these technologies on the environment and health (GM Science Review Panel, 2003, 2004). A cautious approach is therefore warranted.

GM food is unpopular with the UK public. A national consultation exercise produced an extremely negative response. People were uneasy about GM and the more they engaged in GM issues, the more hostile they became. The majority of people were against GM. Around half were implacably opposed; a further third less strongly opposed. There was little support for commercialization of GM crops, with most people either opposed or cautious about the technology and wanting to see further tests and safeguards. The consultation revealed widespread mistrust of government and multinational corporations (Steering Board of the Public Debate on GM and GM Crops, 2003). Public hostility has meant that retailers are reluctant to stock GM labelled products. The main use of GM crops is therefore in animal feed. The UK imports an unknown quantity of animal feed from countries that grow GM crops. Although the feed must be labelled according to EU rules, the final product, as noted above, does not require labelling and therefore the consumer is unaware that their meat, eggs, and so on have been produced with the help of GM organisms.

International regulators, pressured by the USA and other countries where GM food technologies are extensively used, have adopted a weak approach. An FAO/WHO (2000) report approved procedures to assess the safety of GM foods, but noted that it would be difficult to identify long-term effects on animal and human health. The USA has sought to use WTO processes to break into markets that are hostile to GM food. Codex, which in 2003 introduced new standards on GM food, including safety evaluations, product tracing and surveillance, has been lobbied by the USA to dilute proposals for stricter labelling requirements and other rules on GM food. The USA and other GM-food producing countries argue that EU regulations are simply trade barriers. Proponents of GM have also used concerns about food security (see above) to strengthen their case. Meanwhile, environmentalists, consumer groups and organic farmers are campaigning to maintain and extend restrictions on GM food, highlighting potential effects on health, biodiversity and organic producers, and calling for more rigorous scientific assessments, monitoring of the impact of GM and tighter restrictions such as a lower threshold for compulsory labelling of GM products.

Conclusion

The food scares of the 1980s and 90s have had an important legacy. They increased awareness of food safety issues and led to new regulations and institutions. According to some perspectives, this has gone too far and we are now exaggerating risks and being overcautious (Booker and North, 2007). For others, there is a need for greater vigilance and extended regulation, particularly with regard to emerging technologies such as GM (Lang and Heasman, 2004). From this perspective, clearer and more independent scientific advice is needed, with decisions based explicitly on the precautionary principle. Critics also point out that in spite of increased regulation, rules are often poorly enforced, with the result that illegal additives and foodstuffs enter the food chain. From this perspective, regulatory authorities should be given more power and resources, and fines and penalties for breaking the law should be increased.

Food safety, security and sustainability – and issues relating to diet and nutrition, the subject of the next chapter – are often treated as separate issues. In reality, they are connected. Many of the problems of food safety and sustainability, for example, have a common root – the dominance of intensive food producers and 'fast food' corporations, supported by governments within economic and political systems that are not geared to protecting health and the environment. This also plays a role in the dietary and nutrition problems discussed in the next chapter.

Diet, Nutrition and Obesity

13

Food safety, security, and sustainability raise important public health issues. But what we eat – the amount and balance of nutrients in our diet – is equally crucial. This chapter examines the role of diet and nutrition in public health. The first part examines evidence about the impact of diet on particular conditions and diseases, such as cancer, heart disease and obesity. The second explores the response of policymakers and others to the extent of diet-related illness.

Diet and Disease

Fat, Fruit and Fibre

Dietary fat has been identified as a risk factor for cardiovascular disease, including coronary heart disease (CHD) and stroke (Keys, 1980; Key et al., 1996). Even so, some studies have not found an association between dietary fat and stroke (He et al., 2003). The link between fat and heart disease has also been questioned (Skrabanek, 1994; Atrens, 1994). Some fats are more harmful to health than others. Saturated fats, found mainly in food derived from animals, can increase the risk of cardiovascular disease (Hu et al., 1997), although not all studies confirm this (Fehily et al., 1993; Gillman et al., 1997). Processed meat, which often contains high levels of saturated fat and salt, is associated with increased risks of CHD and diabetes mellitus (Micha et al., 2010). Unsaturated fats (mono- and polyunsaturates), found mainly in fruit, vegetables, nuts, and oily fish, are regarded as healthier. For example, it is believed that Omega 3 unsaturated fats (found in fish, plant oils and nuts) are particularly beneficial in protecting against coronary heart disease. A systematic review, however, found that they had no clear effect on mortality, cancer, and cardiovascular events (Hooper et al., 2006). Transfatty acids (known as transfats, transunsaturated fat, hydrogenated fat), although unsaturated, are strongly associated with CHD, more so than conventional saturated fats (Hu et al., 1997). Most transfats are manufactured from vegetable oils and are found in spreads, biscuits, snacks, baked and fried foods.

High fat diets, particularly those high in saturated fat and transfats, increase risks of cardiovascular disease by raising blood cholesterol. Low-density lipoprotein (LDL – known as 'bad cholesterol') has been identified as a key factor. Put simply, higher LDL is associated with deposits of cholesterol in the arteries, increasing the chances of cardiovascular problems. Meanwhile, high-density lipoprotein (HDL or 'good cholesterol') is associated with lower cholesterol deposits (Tall, 1990). Although some argue that cholesterol is a 'red herring' in cardiovascular disease (Ramsey et al., 1994; Verschuren et al., 1995), the dominant scientific view is that HDL should be increased and LDL reduced. This can be achieved through diet (Hooper et al., 2001) and physical activity (see Exhibit 13.2). Cholesterol can also be reduced by drugs known as statins. Statins also reduce blood pressure, a known risk factor for CHD and stroke (Strazullo et al., 2007; Golomb et al., 2008). Most studies support their use in people who have had a heart attack or have a substantial risk of cardiovascular disease (defined by NICE, 2006a, 2008c, as a 20 per cent risk in the next 10 years). Although statin therapy has been associated with a 30 per cent reduction in the risk of coronary events and a 19 per cent reduction in stroke (Brugts et al., 2009), their effectiveness is disputed (Abramson and Wright, 2007). It has been suggested that statins may be harmful (Newman and Hulley, 1996; Ravnskov et al., 2006); possible side effects including heart failure, cancer, muscle fatigue, and neurological symptoms. Lower cholesterol levels have been linked to depression and suicide in some studies (Jacobs et al., 1992; Gallerani et al., 1995), but not others (Law et al., 1994; Wannamethee et al., 1995). There is a clear association between fruit, vegetable and fibre consumption and lower risks of CHD (Key et al., 1996; Wolk et al., 1999; Hung et al., 2004; Jansen, et al., 1999). Frequent consumption of nuts reduces the CHD risk (Hu et al., 1998). Cereals and fruits, rather than vegetables, may provide the greatest protection (Pereira et al., 2004). Fruit and vegetable consumption is linked to lower risk of stroke (He et al., 2006), with people eating five or more portions of fruit and vegetables a day having a 25 per cent lower risk of stroke than those eating fewer than three servings.

Almost a third of cancers in developed countries are related to diet (Key et al., 2002; WCRF, 2007; Thiebaut et al., 2007; Bingham et al., 2003). High levels of meat consumption (particularly processed and red meat) are associated with bowel cancer (Giovannucci, 2003) and breast cancer (Taylor et al., 2007). Fruit, vegetable and other sources of dietary fibre are linked to lower cancer risk, including breast, colon, and pancreatic cancer (Platz et al., 1997; Key et al., 2002; WCRF, 2007; Bingham et al., 2003). Fruit intake in childhood is associated with a lower risk of cancer in adulthood (Maynard et al., 2003). Later studies, however, suggest that preventive effects of fruit, vegetable and fibre consumption may be weaker than initially thought (Fuchs et al., 1999; Hung et al., 2004; Boffeta et al., 2010).

Salt and Sugar

High salt consumption is clearly associated with high blood pressure and cardiovascular disease (Intersalt Cooperatives Research Group, 1988; Elliott et al., 1996b), as well as stomach cancer and osteoporosis (Joosens et al., 1996; Devine et al., 1995). Processed foods contain high levels of salt and therefore carry greater risk. Sugar has also been linked to disease and illness (Yudkin, 1972), including dental caries (Rugg-Gunn and Edgar, 1984). However, suggestions of a link between sugar consumption and cancer, notably bowel cancer (Slattery et al., 1997) and breast cancer (Potischman et al., 2002), have been challenged (Burley, 1997, 1998). Sugar may have a role in obesity, however, by contributing significantly to energy intake. Excessive consumption leads to weight gain, if energy is not expended. Added sugar may encourage consumption by making food more palatable. More specifically, sugar-sweetened drinks have been identified as a factor in weight gain and obesity (Malik et al., 2006). Nevertheless, evidence from animal experiments suggests that the replacement of added sugar with artificial sweeteners may increase calorific intake and weight gain (Swithers and Davidson, 2008). Although obese people derive a lower proportion of energy from sugar than people of normal weight (Gibson, 1997), total sugar consumption is positively related to body mass index (Bingham et al., 2007).

The Impact of Dietary Changes and Lifestyle Factors

Although specific dietary changes don't always reduce health risks (Howard et al., 2006; Beresford et al., 2006), there is strong evidence that take-up of a Mediterranean diet (high consumption of fruit and vegetables, oily fish, legumes, olives and olive oil, whole grain bread and pasta, green salad, nuts; moderate consumption of alcohol) is associated with significant reductions in overall cardiovascular mortality of around 9 per cent, and a 6 per cent reduction in cancer incidence and mortality (Sofi et al., 2008). Researchers found that by making only two changes to people's diet towards the adoption of a Mediterranean diet, the risk of cancer could be reduced by 12 per cent (Benetou et al., 2008). Such diets have also been associated with a reduction in the risk of stroke (Fung et al., 2004). Changes to diet that contribute most to reduced mortality are moderate alcohol consumption, low meat consumption, high consumption of fruit, vegetables, nuts, legumes and olive oil (Trichopolou et al., 2009).

Other lifestyle factors compound the effects of unhealthy diets. A US study of middle-aged women found that five factors (smoking, overweight, little physical activity, low diet quality – that is, high in fat, low in fruit and vegetables and with no moderate alcohol consumption) increased the risk of cancer mortality by over three times; cardiovascular mortality eightfold and all causes of death by a factor of four (van Dam et al., 2008). Low-quality diet alone was associated with 9 per cent increased risk of cancer deaths and an 18 per cent increase in the risk of death from cardiovascular diseases. A British study discovered that men and women aged 45 and over had four times the risk of mortality if they did not consume at least five fruit and vegetable servings a day, were physically inactive, did not consume alcohol moderately and smoked tobacco (Khaw et al., 2008). A study of older people in Europe identified a greater than 50 per cent reduction in all causes of mortality (including cancer and coronary heart disease) over a 12-year period among people who had a Mediterranean diet, didn't smoke, took exercise and consumed alcohol in moderation (Knoops et al., 2004).

Adherence to a Mediterranean diet has been associated with a reduction in the incidence and mortality from Parkinson's disease and Alzheimer's disease (Sofi et al., 2008). Meanwhile, diets high in sugars and saturated fats have been linked to mental health problems such as depression, attention deficit disorder and schizophrenia (Mental Health Foundation and Sustain, 2006). Particular attention has alighted on a possible link between deficiency of essential fatty acids (in particular Omega 3), and depression (Tanskanen et al., 2001; Hibbeln, 2002). Vitamin and mineral deficiencies may also cause mental health problems. Interventions using dietary supplements have been tested on people with symptoms of mental health problems and other vulnerable groups with positive results, notably in children with ADHD symptoms and young offenders (Mental Health Foundation and Sustain, 2006). In addition, there is emerging evidence that improvements in school meals (see Exhibit 13.1) may have a positive effect on educational performance (Belot and James, 2009).

Obesity and Overweight People

It is estimated that there are one billion overweight people worldwide, of which 300 million are obese (WHO, 2002). This has been described as a 'global epidemic.' In the UK, the Chief Medical Officer described obesity as 'a health time bomb' (DoH, 2003d, p. 44). In adults, overweight and obesity are usually defined in relation to body mass index (BMI), calculated by dividing a person's weight in kilogrammes by their height in metres squared. An adult with a BMI of 30 and above is classified as obese, whereas a BMI of between 25 and 29.9 is considered overweight. A BMI of between 18.5 and 24.9 is regarded as normal, below 18.5 as underweight.

In England in 1980, only 6 per cent of men and 8 per cent of women were obese. By 2005 this had risen to almost a quarter of adults (NHS Information Centre, 2009a). In England, obesity rates are higher in the north and lower in the south (Moon et al., 2007). Obesity is more prevalent in deprived communities, in social class V, and among certain ethnic groups (Black African, Black Caribbean, Pakistani and Bangladeshi populations). Within the UK, Scotland has the highest obesity rates. Although all European countries face similar trends, the UK has one of the highest obesity rates. The proportion of people who are overweight has also increased. Currently, over four out of ten men and a third of women in England are overweight, meaning that approximately 60 per cent of adults are either obese or overweight.

There is much concern about the continuation of present trends. Obese adults could make up almost a third of the population by 2012 (Zaninotto et al., 2009). It is possible that 60 per cent of men and 50 per cent of women could be obese by 2050 (Foresight, 2007, 2009). The combined proportion of obese and overweight people is expected to rise, meaning that a small minority (10 per cent of men and 15 per cent of women) could have 'healthy weight'. The overall costs of obesity were estimated at least £3.3 billion per annum (Health Committee, 2004), forecast to rise to almost £50 billion by 2050 (Foresight, 2009). This includes cost to the NHS and wider social costs such as loss of earnings, state benefits and reduced productivity.

Why is a Rising Obese and Overweight Population a Problem?

Obesity and overweight populations have higher risks of disease and death. It is estimated that being overweight or obese increases the risk of death from all causes by 14 per cent, death from cardiovascular disease by over 30 per cent and cancer by 8 per cent (van Dam et al., 2008). People who are obese or overweight are more at risk from diabetes and cardiovascular diseases. Around half of cases of type 2 diabetes are linked to obesity (NAO, 2001). Such cases have increased and affect younger people more than in the past. Most cases of hypertension are linked to being overweight or obese. Obese people are also more at risk from strokes (Hu et al., 2007; Zhou et al., 2008).

There is an association between higher BMI and cancer (WCRF, 2007). Among UK postmenopausal women, 5 per cent of cancers are attributed to being obese or overweight (Reeves et al., 2007). The percentage of cancer cases in the EU due to overweight or obesity is estimated at 6 per cent for women and 3 per cent for men (Bergstrom et al., 2001; McMillan et al., 2006). In the USA, as many as 14 per cent of male and 20 per cent of female cancers could be due to overweight or obesity (Calle et al., 2003). Overweight and obesity have been linked to cancers of the breast, colon, prostate, kidney, gallbladder, thyroid, oesophagus and endometrium (Calle et al., 2003; Berrington de Gonzalez et al., 2003; Bergstrom et al., 2001; Renehan et al., 2008; Lin et al., 2004). Obese people have a 75 per cent increased risk (and overweight people a 35 per cent increased risk) of developing dementia (Whitmer et al., 2005). They face higher risks of arthritis, largely due to excess weight on joints, although there is also a possible link between metabolism and arthritis (Coggon et al., 2001; Cooper et al., 2001; Eaton, 2004). Obesity has been linked to other conditions, including infertility (Zacharia and Acharya, 2008).

Usually the health risks of being obese or overweight are measured by BMI. But the location rather than amount of excess weight is also regarded as an important factor. People who are 'apple shaped' (whose excess weight is concentrated in their abdomen) may be more at risk than 'pear shaped people' (who have excess weight on their hips and buttocks). High 'waist to hip' ratios, which indicate a more central distribution of fat, are linked to risk of heart attack (Yusef et al., 2005) and early signs of cardiovascular disease (See et al., 2007). Increases in waist circumference have been linked to the risk of premature death (Pischon et al., 2008). Furthermore, measures of central obesity are associated with an increased risk of breast cancer (Harvie et al., 2003).

Child Obesity

Obesity and overweight is now believed to be more common among children and young people (Royal College of Physicians et al., 2004). The measurement of child obesity is not straightforward, however, as weight gain in children is part of the natural growing process. Furthermore, increases in weight may constitute a longer term trend in human development towards taller and heavier people. To complicate matters further, there are different measures of childhood obesity (see Social Issues Research Centre, 2005; Kipping et al., 2008). The International Obesity Task Force (IOTF) measures obesity and overweight status with reference to an international classification system based on height and weight distributions in several countries. The UK national measure calculates obesity and overweight with regard to age–weight distribution curves (a child is defined as obese if they are above the 95th percentile for their age, and overweight if between the 85th and 95th percentile).

Although different approaches produce contrasting estimates of obesity, the overall trend is similar (Social Issues Research Centre, 2005). Using IOTF methodology, Foresight (2007) found that in 2004 among boys, 10 per cent of 6–10 year olds and 5 per cent of 11–15 year olds were classified as obese. Among girls, 10 per cent of 6–10 year olds and 11 per cent of 11–15 year olds were obese. It was predicted that by 2050 these percentages would more than double in both sexes. Using the UK methodology, however, the problem looks even worse. The National Child Measurement Programme in England, which uses the UK national measure to calculate obesity, began measuring children's weight in 2005 (NHS Information Centre, 2008a). In the 2007/8 school year, 13 per cent of children in reception classes (aged 4–5 years) were overweight and a further 10 per cent were obese. In year 6 (10–11 years), 14 per cent were overweight and a further 18 per cent obese. These figures may not present the full picture, however. Obesity and overweight levels may be even higher if, as suspected, children with higher BMI scores do not participate in measurements. Other studies using the UK methodology also found high proportions of obese and overweight children. The Health Survey for England found that in 2007 around one in six children aged 2–15 were obese, and three out of ten were overweight or obese (NHS Information Centre, 2009a).

A range of problems are associated with child obesity (see Reilly and Wilson, 2006; Kipping et al., 2008), including poor psychosocial health resulting from bullying and low self-esteem, diabetes, asthma, liver disease and orthopaedic problems. Paediatric obesity may have consequences for adult health, such as cardiovascular disease, diabetes, arthritis, and depression. There appears to be a link between child obesity and cancer in adulthood (Jeffreys et al., 2004). Being overweight or obese in late adolescence increases the overall risk of adult mortality (Neovius et al., 2009). However, some studies have found that obesity in childhood is not necessarily a predictor of obesity in adulthood (Funatogawa et al., 2008).

Is Obesity Really a Problem?

Despite the evidence on obesity, there are dissonant voices. The food industry, especially producers of fatty and sugary foods, is keen to play down the obesity problem. Those adopting a libertarian standpoint see the 'war' on obesity as an assault on the pleasures of ordinary citizens by the nanny state (Bennett and Di Lorenzo, 1999). Some believe that it is a form of oppression against 'larger' people, as well as, more specifically, ethnic minorities and women (Orbach, 1978, 2009), although men, too, face victimization (Monaghan, 2008a). At the very least, the social and sociological aspects of obesity require further analysis (Crossley, 2004). Action on obesity can be seen as an exercise in social regulation and victim-blaming, shifting attention away from external causes of illness and politically contentious issues such as food poverty (Gard and Wright, 2005; Townend, 2009; Monaghan, 2008a). From these perspectives, concern about obesity is driven by political and cultural issues rather than threats to public health, and may reflect negative attitudes towards poor people and ethnic minorities (who are more likely to be overweight and obese) (Campos et al., 2006). Some go further, arguing that emphasis on 'normal' weight and dieting can be extremely damaging to health. It may add to contemporary pressures to be slim, leading to eating disorders such as anorexia and bulimia (Lawrence, 1987), and variation in body weight over time (through 'yo-yo' dieting), which has adverse implications for health (Blair et al., 1993)

Critical perspectives contend that obesity has been exaggerated and is now a 'moral panic'. As Monaghan (2008a, p. 20) has noted: 'The war on obesity is a holy war and conscientious objectors risk excommunication.' The imagery of crisis, stimulated by the official terminology of 'epidemic', 'timebomb', 'war', is reinforced by the media, which portray the problem in particular ways (that is, lazy, fat people must change their habits) and selectively report evidence on the dietary causes of ill health to maintain the dominant narrative (see Gard and Wright, 2005). Critics of policy on obesity support their arguments by challenging the evidence. They point out that average adult weights have increased only slightly (Social Issues Research Centre, 2005). The increase in obesity has not been uniform and some groups (for example men aged 16–24) show a slight decline. They also point to research that indicates that obesity is confined to a minority of children. The average child is no heavier than 25 years ago, according to some researchers (EarlyBird, 2010). Critics also argue that evidence linking obesity and overweight to ill health is flawed and uncertain. Being obese and overweight is not necessarily harmful to health (Gard and Wright, 2005; Noppa et al., 1980). Obese people do not always have specific risk factors for diabetes and cardiovascular disease, including insulin resistance, low levels of HDL cholesterol and high blood pressure, while some people of normal weight do have them (Stefan et al., 2008; Wildman et al., 2008). Obese and overweight people who maintain fitness levels can remain relatively healthy (Lee et al., 1999; Sui et al., 2007). Being overweight (rather than obese) does not increase overall mortality. Indeed, overweight people have lower risks of mortality than obese and underweight people (Flegal et al., 2005). They may be healthier than people of normal weight, according to some researchers (Orpana et al., 2009).

What Causes Obesity?

There are many theories of obesity (see Foresight, 2007, 2009; WHO, 2000b: Lang and Heasman, 2004). In simple terms, obesity is an imbalance between energy intake and expenditure; in reality the situation is more complicated. There appears to be a link between specific genes and obesity (see Foresight, 2007; Roberts and Greenberg, 1996; Nagle et al., 1999; Loos and Bouchard, 2003). Some affect the stimulation of hormones affecting energy intake and storage. For example, leptin, found in fat cells, regulates food intake (Baskin et al., 1998; Wang et al., 1999; Havel, 2002), ghrelin, found in the gut, stimulates food intake (Druce et al., 2004), while peptide YY (also located in the gut) is believed to affect appetite suppression (Batterham et al., 2003). Other recent research has identified the contribution of particular genes to obesity (Fischer et al., 2009; Yen et al., 2009; Wardle et al., 2009).

There is much enthusiasm for future drug therapies based on such studies, as well as surgical treatments, such as gastric bands. However, an ecological model, incorporating biological, social and environmental factors, may be more fruitful both in explaining obesity and providing a rationale for policy and intervention (Foresight, 2007, 2009). Egger and Swinburn (1997) coined the term 'obesogenic environment', for the 'sum of influences that the surroundings, opportunities, or conditions of life have on promoting obesity in individuals and populations.' Possible factors include easier access to cheap energy-dense food and drink as well as cultural or economic factors that encourage excessive eating and 'fast food' (Pereira et al., 2005; Prentice and Jebb, 2007). Other factors relate to the expenditure of energy. Exercise levels appear to have fallen (see Exhibit 13.2). We live in a society where people have greater access to labour-saving technologies and where planning, production and transport systems reduce the opportunities for physical activity. There is some dispute over whether diet or lack of exercise is primarily to blame for the rise in obesity (Prentice and Jebb, 1995; Weinser et al., 1998). The broad consensus, however, is that a primary prevention strategy combining energy intake reduction and increasing physical activity is the best approach, with appropriate medical and surgical treatment for those who cannot lose weight through diet and exercise.

Diet and Nutrition Policy

UK food policies cannot be developed in isolation from the rest of Europe. The UK government is restricted by the Common Agricultural Policy (CAP), which continues to undermine nutritional health by promoting the production of meat and dairy products and destruction of fruit surpluses (Elinder, 2003). Although the EU has enormous potential influence over nutrition, it has been reluctant to use this, largely because of the power of agriculture and food industry interests. The EU has been weak on issues such as the marketing of food and nutritional labelling, preferring a voluntary approach, working with the food industry to promote self-regulation rather than direct regulation.

Following its expanded remit for public health, the EU took more interest in diet and nutrition. In 2005, the European Commission published a green paper on the prevention of overweight, obesity and chronic disease (Commission of the European Communities, 2005) as a basis for consultation on these issues. It also established a 'platform for action' on diet, physical activity and health, to provide a forum for partnership among interested parties (such as industry, researchers, consumer and public health groups). Subsequently, a white paper was published (Commission of the European Communities, 2007a), which proposed a further review of nutrition labelling, and the development of codes of conduct on advertising and marketing of food, particularly in relation to children, as well as education and information campaigns to raise awareness. The Commission declared that CAP would be used to promote public health goals, including, for example, the distribution of surplus fruit and vegetables to educational institutions.

UK and EU policy must be examined in the context of global governance frameworks. WHO and other UN agencies have long been involved in food and nutrition policy. Initially their focus was upon malnutrition and food security. During the 1990s, there was a shift in focus towards unhealthy diets and overnutrition. A WHO study group recommended concerted action to prevent chronic disease related to diet (WHO, 1990). During the 1990s, the WHO nutrition programme included among its priorities the need to tackle obesity and diet-related disease. In 1997, WHO, in conjunction with the newly formed IOTF, undertook an expert consultation. The IOTF (which interestingly derives funding from the drugs industry – Moynihan, 2006) aimed to raise awareness and promote action on obesity, forging close links with WHO. The expert consultation produced an interim report (WHO, 1998c) and then a final report (WHO, 2000b), setting out the evidence base. Subsequently, a joint FAO/WHO (2003) expert consultation recommended population nutrient intake goals: no more than 30 per cent of energy from total fat; less than 10 per cent of energy intake from saturated fatty acids; less than one per cent from transfats; less than 10 per cent from added sugars, at least 400g of fruit and vegetables a day; and no more than 5g a day of salt. WHO (2004a) subsequently proposed a resolution on global strategy on diet, physical activity and health, endorsing the FAO/WHO guidelines for reducing fat, salt and sugar, and encouraging consumption of fruit and vegetables and other sources of fibre, alongside recommendations for increasing physical activity. WHO backed efforts to improve public awareness of the relationship between diet, physical activity and health, to limit the marketing of unhealthy foods, especially to children, and to improve standards of nutritional labelling. Governments were urged to consider policies consistent with a healthy diet, including fiscal policies. Corporate and national interests lobbied strongly against WHO's approach, particularly the USA and the large multinational food corporations (Boseley, 2004).

The WHO Regional Office for Europe (1988, 1998) has devised strategies for preventing diet-related illness and monitors member states' policies. It introduced a food and nutrition action plan, a framework for member states to develop their national plans (WHO Regional Office for Europe, 2000b). This has since been updated (WHO Regional Office for Europe, 2008b). The new plan identified specific priorities, including: improving the availability and affordability of fruit and vegetables; improving the nutritional quality of food served in public institutions; ensuring commercial provision of food is consistent with dietary guidelines; introducing food-based dietary guidelines; conducting public information campaigns; and ensuring appropriate marketing practices and appropriate food labelling. In addition, the WHO European Region established a charter on counteracting obesity in 2006, which included commitments to reduce fat, sugar and salt and ensure adequate nutrition labelling, as well as improved nutritional guidelines and measures to promote exercise (WHO Regional Office for Europe, 2006b).

UK Policies

The UK government was initially sluggish in responding to evidence on diet and nutrition (see Cannon, 1987; Mills, 1992). Others, notably the Nordic countries, were much more active in promoting changes in diet, and reducing consumption of fat (particularly saturated fat), salt and sugar while increasing fruit and vegetable consumption. For example, Finland, which had a high level of cardiovascular disease, introduced a comprehensive programme in the 1970s to prevent illness through dietary change (Pekka et al., 2002). The programme did reduce CHD, but not obesity (Vartiainen et al., 1994). In the UK, the government's scientific advisors, the Committee on the Medical Aspects of Food, recommended changes to diet, but without explicit targets (COMA, 1974). A National Advisory Committee on Nutritional Education (NACNE) was later established, but proved controversial amid disagreement between health, consumer and industry interests. NACNE (1983) set out nutritional guidelines (recommending reductions in fat, salt and sugar consumption and an increase in fibre) alongside recommendations for action (such as improvements in food labelling and food supply). Its advice was not welcomed by the government, especially the departments working closely with the food industry (such as the Ministry of Agriculture Fisheries and Food and the Department of Trade). NACNE's recommendations were strongly opposed by the industry, particularly the purveyors of meat and dairy products, and the manufacturers of soft drinks and snacks. These were strongly represented in business trade associations, government and Parliament, and mobilized effectively against policy developments that affected their interests. NACNE was subsequently abolished. A further report from the Committee on Medical Aspects of Food and Nutrition Policy (COMA) (1984) maintained the pressure on government to act, but policy continued to reflect the industry's position, producing a voluntary labelling scheme and some nutritional guidance for the public (Mills, 1992).

The Major Government

The *Health of the Nation* strategy (Cm 1986, 1992), established targets for reducing mortality from diseases related to diet, such as cancer, heart disease and stroke. It set risk factor targets to reduce dietary fat, saturated fat, blood pressure levels, alcohol consumption, and obesity. A Nutrition Task Force (NTF), including the food industry, consumer groups, health and nutrition experts and other stakeholders, was charged with producing an action plan. The food industry again blocked interventions, such as targets for reducing dietary fat, clearer nutritional labelling, and tough restrictions on advertising. It successfully opposed high profile media campaigns on healthy eating.

However, minor changes in broadcast advertising codes were implemented and new guidelines to improve hospital and school meals introduced. The NTF irritated government and the industry by calling for a nutritional strategy for people on low incomes (DOH/NTF, 1996) and a large reduction in dietary fat (DoH/NTF/PATF, 1995). Unsurprisingly, it was abolished in 1996. Meanwhile, COMA (1994) continued to make recommendations about reducing fat and salt content and increasing fruit and fibre. It recommended there be no rise in dietary cholesterol and set maximum levels for: saturated fat (no more than 10 per cent of energy); total fat (35 per cent of energy); sugars (10 per cent of energy); and salt (6g per day). It also recommended that complex carbohydrates be increased to 50 per cent of energy and an increase in dietary fibre to 18g per day. As national policy stalled, the focus moved to the local level. With encouragement from the DoH, 'healthy eating partnerships' were formed by local authorities, NHS organizations and non-governmental organizations (NGOs). These sought to improve diet through practical and low-key steps, such as providing professional training to improve dietary advice to the public and giving information and support to local people to encourage changes in their diet.

The Blair Government

The Blair government came to office with promises of reform in diet and nutrition policy. It created the Food Standards Agency (FSA) (see Chapter 11), seen as a progressive step towards improving the safety of food and nutritional standards (Barling and Lang, 2003). But while food safety policy continued to have a high profile, diet and nutrition policy did not. A flaw in the new government's policy was the abandonment of diet, nutrition and obesity risk factor targets set by its predecessor. It appeared as unwilling as the Conservatives to take on the food industry on nutritional matters. When COMA (1997) recommended that people cut their meat intake, its advice was toned down by the government. Ministers denied it was due to lobbying from the meat industry.

Slowly, however, initiatives on diet and nutrition emerged. The NHS Plan for England (Cm 4818, 2000) promised a new national scheme to provide free fruit and vegetables daily to children at nursery and infant school; a 'Five a Day programme' to encourage fruit and vegetables consumption for everyone; local action to tackle obesity, informed by evidence; and work with the food industry to increase access to fruit and vegetables and improve the overall balance of the diet with regard to salt, fat and sugars. Even so, the impact was modest. The free fruit and vegetables for schoolchildren, initially funded from the National Lottery, had some success. The percentage of children in the scheme consuming the recommended five pieces of fruit and vegetables a day rose from 32 per cent in 2004 to 44 per cent in 2006, with average consumption increasing from 3.6 to 4.4 pieces per day. Other factors, such as improved school meals, also contributed to increased fruit and vegetable consumption (Blenkinsop et al., 2007).

For all children aged 5–15, not just those covered by the free fruit and vegetable scheme, consumption rose from 2.4 units in 2001 for boys to 3.3 in 2007 (NHS Information Centre, 2008a). For girls, it increased from 2.6 to 3.4. The proportion of children eating the recommended level of fruit and vegetables doubled from 10 per cent to 21 per cent between 2001 and 2007. However, four out of five children still eat less than recommended daily levels. In 2008, the mean number of portions of fruit and vegetables consumed by boys and girls fell slightly, as did the percentage of children meeting the 'five a day' guidelines (NHS Information Centre, 2010). For adults, fruit and vegetable consumption was 13 per cent higher in 2007 than in 2000, but, at an average of 3.9 portions of fruit and vegetables a day, fell short of recommended levels (DEFRA, 2008b). Those eating at least 'five a day' rose from 25 per cent to 31 per cent of women between 2001 and 2007, and from 22 per cent to 27 per cent in men (NHS Information Centre, 2009a). As with children, fruit and vegetable consumption among adults fell in 2008, and the proportion meeting 'five a day' guidelines was reduced to 25 per cent of men and 29 per cent of women (NHS Information Centre, 2010). In addition, the amount of fibre in the adult diet has remained stable since 2001 at around 15g per person per day and remains below the 18g level recommended by government (DEFRA, 2008b).

The Labour government encouraged local action to improve diet, by PCTs, local authorities and voluntary and private sector organizations, building on projects fostered by the previous government. The Health Development Agency produced advice on interventions to prevent and treat obesity (Mulvihill and Quigley, 2003). GPs were encouraged to identify patients needing help with weight loss. Some PCTs received additional funds (from the National Lottery) to encourage fruit and vegetable consumption through community initiatives. Activities included work with school-age children, cook and eat activities, and media campaigns. Although fruit and vegetable consumption increased in areas receiving interventions, they did not show any greater improvement than elsewhere. Even so, some PCTs were innovative and successful in building local partnerships. A number of these initiatives have now developed into broader programmes to encourage healthy eating and exercise at the local level.

The Food Industry

The Labour government sought to work with the food industry to improve access to healthy food and to help people eat a balanced diet. Supermarkets were urged to increase access to fruit and vegetables. Food manufacturers were encouraged to voluntarily reduce the salt, sugar and fat content of their products. The food industry was expected to develop clearer nutritional labelling and to act responsibly in marketing its products.

The food industry – and its allies in advertising and marketing – is economically and politically powerful. Its motives are primarily economic – increasing profitability and market share. The industry has opposed policies aimed at improving diet and health in the UK, other countries and internationally (Schlosser, 2002; Lang and Heasman, 2004; Nestle, 2003). However, it is not always united against such initiatives. Indeed, some parts of the food industry – organic producers, for example – have benefited from trends towards healthy eating. Some retailers have sought competitive advantage by promoting healthier food lines or providing better information about nutritional content (Seth and Randall, 2001). Moreover, some changes, such as reduction in portion size, can increase profits.

The industry is dominated by large global food producers and food service corporations. Most of these have adopted corporate social responsibility (CSR) policies and commitments to improve their products, by for example reducing fat, salt and sugar (FSS) levels. Some have adopted a self-regulatory approach to marketing, particularly to children. A number, including Pepsico, Cadbury's, Coca-Cola, and Nestlé, have explicitly endorsed initiatives to reduce obesity. Nonetheless, many large corporations, even those with CSR statements, are not seriously engaged with the public health agenda (Lang et al., 2006a; Lewin et al., 2006). There is also considerable suspicion about some CSR activities. For example, in 2010, McDonald's was condemned by nutritionists and obesity campaigners for its deal with Weightwatchers in New Zealand. Weightwatchers agreed to promote certain items on the McDonald's menu and allow its logo to be used by the company. McDonald's responded by claiming that it was promoting healthier choices. Its critics saw it as a marketing ploy to lure consumers into its restaurants (*Guardian*, 2010).

Food retailers have actively promoted improvements in food quality and diet (Seth and Randall, 2001; Lang and Heasman, 2004). In the UK, the grocery market is dominated by four companies (Tesco, Asda/Walmart, Morrisons and Sainsbury's), which together control three-quarters of food sales. Their positive contributions include making organic food more widely available, improving nutritional labelling and reducing the FSS content of their products. However, the role of the large supermarkets is ambiguous. They promoted the expansion of ready meals, many of which are high in FSS (Yates, 2008). The supermarkets' record is mixed in other respects. They have contributed to improved food safety and have been 'consumer champions' on issues such as food irradiation and GM (see Chapter 12; Seth and Randall, 2001). However, their record on sustainability has not been good, given their promotion of out of town stores and reliance on air and road transport.

Supermarket chains are now trying to address some of these issues by creating more local stores and reducing reliance on fossil fuels (although this is driven more by business than environmental reasons, to increase market share and reduce costs).

In seeking to work with industry, government's main priority has been to reduce the salt content of food. In 2003, the FSA set new targets. By 2007, salt in UK ready meals had fallen to almost half the level in 2003 (CASH, 2007). Between 2001 and 2008, daily salt consumption fell from 9.5g to 8.6g per person. Even so, this still exceeds the WHO maximum recommended level and that recommended by the UK government's scientific advisors. Moreover, some products continue to contain high levels of salt. This is particularly a problem for children, as their maximum daily recommended levels are lower than adults. The FSA has set voluntary targets across food categories. In 2008, stricter targets were introduced for some foods, including meat products, cheeses spreads, and snacks. In addition, a publicity campaign ('Full of It') was introduced in 2009 to persuade people to reduce their salt consumption.

Government has tried to encourage the industry to reduce fat and sugar content. Some manufacturers have cut these levels. However, the average contribution of fat, saturated fat and sugars in the diet remained at about the same level between 2001 and 2007 (DEFRA, 2008b). In 2007, saturated fat was 14.5 per cent of total dietary energy compared with the government's maximum limit of 11 per cent, while total fat was 38.3 per cent (compared with 35 per cent maximum recommended contribution). Added sugars were 14 per cent (compared with the government's maximum recommended level of 11 per cent). In 2008, the FSA placed greater emphasis on getting industry to reduce saturated fats, total energy intake and sugar content. Food campaigners were disappointed that more was not done to reduce transfats. Although these contribute a much smaller proportion of the British diet than saturated fats, they are regarded as more harmful. Bans on transfats have been introduced in several countries (including Denmark and some US states). In the UK, the target is to reduce transfats to 2 per cent of energy intake through voluntary action by industry.

Choosing Health

Disquiet about nutrition and obesity increased after the millennium. Stronger action was supported by an increasingly vociferous and well-organized lobby, which included health and consumer organizations, and coordinated by bodies such as the National Heart Forum and the National Obesity Forum. Action on obesity was given added impetus by several reports during this period (DoH, 2003d; Wanless, 2004; NAO, 2001; PAC, 2001; Health Committee, 2004; Royal College of Physicians et al., 2004; Policy Commission on the

Future of Farming and Food, 2002). Recommendations from these sources included: a wide-ranging and long-term programme to reduce obesity; stronger partnership working between the NHS and other local organizations; a review of food advertising regulation for children; improved food labelling; a health promotion campaign; school policies on obesity; continued efforts to improve the nutritional content of food; greater efforts by NHS organizations and professionals to identify, support and treat people with weight problems; more resources for obesity treatment and services; and more opportunities for physical exercise for both children and adults.

Obesity was a key theme of the *Choosing Health* white paper (Cm 6374, 2004; DoH, 2005a). This proposed: a new cross government strategy to raise awareness of the risks of obesity; improvements in nutrition labelling, including a signposting system of labelling for consumers to indicate the nutrient content of food; continued efforts to work with industry to increase the availability of healthy food, reverse the trend towards larger portion sizes, and produce clear and consistent labelling; further restrictions on the advertising and promotion of HFSS (high in fat, salt and sugar) foods to children; evidence-based improvements in obesity prevention and treatment services; priority and planning guidance for PCTs; and improvements in nutrition in schools (see Exhibit 13.1). Another key theme was the promotion of physical activity, explored further in Exhibit 13.2. The white paper also called for improvements in partnership working between the NHS, local authorities, voluntary organizations and the private sector.

The Labour government established a PSA target, jointly owned by the Departments of Health, Culture, Media and Sport, and the Department for Education and Skills (later the Department for Children, Schools and Families) 'to halt the year on year rise in obesity in children under 11 years of age by 2010'. In addition, a food and health action plan was introduced (DoH, 2005d), to improve coordination and establish partnerships to improve nutrition and reduce obesity. The government's approach emphasized social marketing, labelling, restrictions on marketing to children, specific actions by the NHS and partnerships. These aspects are now examined in more detail.

Social Marketing and Labelling

Great emphasis was placed on helping people to make healthier choices. This was evident in campaigns such as the '5 a day' message, discussed above. Another example was the 'Small Change, Big Difference' campaign, launched in 2006, which encouraged small lifestyle changes that could have large effects cumulatively. In addition, attempts were made to improve the flow of information to individuals about healthy eating and exercise. NHS organizations and professionals were expected to do more in this regard. The FSA had a significant role here too, launching its 'Eatwell' website in 2004, containing tips on healthy eating, food labels, shopping, cooking and food safety.

Choosing Health and the Food and Health Action Plan signalled a more comprehensive and coherent approach. A cross-government obesity social marketing campaign was announced. The government promised to work with the food industry, creative media, consumers, health professionals and others to develop such a programme. Industry personnel and advertising agencies, previously involved in food and drink marketing, were recruited to advise on the campaign. Eventually, 'Change4Life' was launched in England in 2009, at a cost of almost £75 million of public funds with additional funding of £200 million in services and support from food and advertising companies. The campaign, also backed by health charities, involved TV advertising, a website, and other materials (posters, leaflets and videos). The initial focus was to persuade families with children to change their lifestyles by eating healthily and doing more exercise. This was later extended to people aged 45–65. In 2010, Change4Life was launched in Wales.

A further set of measures related to the quality of food information. Nutrition labelling is not mandatory in the UK, except with regard to positive health claims and warnings about allergies. For other aspects, the UK has adopted a voluntary approach, working with the industry to improve details of nutritional content. UK governments are restricted by the framework of food labelling legislation set by the EU, which has in the past rejected mandatory nutrition labelling. The European Commission has since reviewed its approach. In 2008, it proposed a mandatory approach that will cover, among other things: legibility of labels, nutrition labelling with regard to energy, fats, saturates, carbohydrates (with specific reference to sugars and salts). The proposals cover pre-packed foods as well as foods supplied by caterers and restaurants. They also extend the rules on the labelling of allergens to non-pre-packed foods. However, the new rules will not extend other aspects of nutrition labelling to non-pre-packed foods. So restaurants will not have to give information about the nutritional value of their menus, a requirement in parts of the USA, for example (see McColl, 2008). However, the Labour government called for a voluntary approach to nutritional information on food eaten outside the home (HM Government, 2010a), a policy which looks set to be continued by the current government.

Meanwhile, following recommendations from the Health Committee (2004), the FSA introduced a 'traffic light' system for food manufacturers and retailers, using highly visible colour-coded information to inform consumers about nutritional content. The traffic light system displayed a colour for each nutrient (fat, saturated fats, calories, salt and sugar), red denoting a high level, amber for medium, and green for a low level. Some food companies adopted this system or variations of it (including Waitrose, Marks & Spencer, the Co-op and Sainsbury's). A larger group (including Tesco, Morrisons,

Unilever, Kellogg's, Coca-Cola) devised their own systems based on recommended guideline daily amounts (GDAs) of salt, sugar and fats. The Health Committee (2009) later expressed its frustration that the traffic light system had not been fully introduced, and recommended that it be statutory and extended to takeaway outlets and restaurants. However, at the time of writing, the European Commission and the European Parliament have rejected a traffic light system and endorsed GDAs. Following extensive lobbying by opponents of the traffic light system, the FSA decided not to force the industry to adopt it. Furthermore, as the Cameron government has now rejected this approach, its future looks bleak, particularly as its main sponsor, the FSA, is itself faced with possible abolition.

Codex Alimentarius, the international food standards body discussed in the previous chapter, has an important role in relation to labelling. Since the 1980s, Codex has issued guidelines on food nutritional labelling. These are mandatory only where nutritional claims are made (that is, where it is being claimed that the food has particular nutritional properties). Otherwise declaration is voluntary, although, if this is done, further Codex guidelines apply (concerning the listing, calculation and presentation of nutrients). Codex does not preclude 'additional means of presentation' (such as traffic light or other indicators). Interestingly, Codex has not sought to promote nutritional information as a means of shaping healthier food choices (Lang and Heasman, 2004). Indeed its guidelines expressly state that exact quantitative recommendations about the balance of nutrients for individuals should not be used in labelling. Codex has been criticized for not doing more to ensure that international food labelling standards reflect WHO recommendations on nutrition, diet and obesity (for example FAO/WHO, 2003).

Advertising and Promotion

There is growing evidence that advertising adversely influences children's food and drink preferences (Hastings et al., 2003; OFCOM, 2004; Dixon et al., 2007; Committee on Food Marketing and the Diets of Children and Youth, 2006; Veerman et al., 2009). In the light of pressure to act (see Health Committee, 2004; www.sustainweb.org/childrensfoodcampaign/), restrictions have been imposed on HFSS food and drink advertising and promotion. In 2007, OFCOM, the UK media regulator, imposed new restrictions on television advertisements, identified by a nutrient profiling scheme developed by the FSA. The initial proposal was to ban all advertisements of HFSS products around programmes appealing to children under nine years of age, later extended to cover children under 16. This meant a ban on advertising HFSS products around all preschool programmes, cable and satellite children's channels; programmes in children's airtime; and youth-oriented programmes. In addition, further restrictions were placed on the content of advertisements. A ban was imposed on TV advertisements targeted at primary school children using celebrities or characters licensed from third parties. There was to be no promotional activity such as free gifts in TV advertisements targeted at primary school children. Advertisers were barred from making nutritional or health claims to this audience. The new regulations were phased in from 2007.

A number of consumer and health organizations, along with the FSA, pressed for a ban on all HFSS food advertisements before 9pm and were disappointed with these measures. They pointed out that the new regulations contained loopholes. For example, corporations with HFSS foods in their portfolio were permitted to market their corporate brand images (for example Cadbury's, McDonald's) without restriction. They could evade the rules on celebrities and characters in advertisements by directly owning the rights rather than licensing them from third parties. Astonishingly, advertising of HFSS foods was permitted around programmes seen by large numbers of children, providing they did not constitute a high proportion of the total audience. The industry was also unhappy with the new regime. It criticized the nutrient profiling scheme for not taking into account the frequency of consumption or the positive nutrient content of foods. The adverse impact of the rules on foods regarded as healthy when eaten in moderation, such as marmite and cheese, was particularly highlighted.

In parallel with the TV regulations, changes were made to the radio advertising code. The non-broadcast code of advertising practice (the CAP code), which covers posters, press, cinema, text and internet, was also revised. These new codes related to children under 16, although some provisions covered preschool and primary school children only. The CAP rules did not target HFSS foods, were not based on FSA nutrient profiling, and did not impose additional restrictions on media particularly aimed at children. It should be noted that with the exception of cinema advertising, non-broadcast advertising is subject to a weaker regulatory regime than TV and radio advertisements.

Taken together, advertising regulations are fragmented and fail to address the comprehensive and cumulative exposure of children to marketing messages (Lewis and National Children's Bureau, 2006; DCSF, 2009). Many areas of marketing remain unregulated (such as mobile phone and some online promotions). Increasingly marketing is done on websites and social networking forums, not covered by the rules. The advertising industry is currently discussing ways of extending the CAP code to more aspects of online marketing. But much depends on food and advertising firms acting responsibly. In 2007, a voluntary agreement was drawn up by 11 large food corporations, responsible for over half the total food advertising in Europe, under the auspices of the European Platform on Diet, Physical Activity and Health. They pledged that by the end of 2008 they would not advertise HFSS products in media (including TV, press and internet) where at least half the audience was under 12 and would not undertake commercial communications in primary schools. Although this reinforced the socially responsible image of these corporations, it will not prevent children's exposure to the marketing of foods high in fat, salt and sugar.

Research into the impact of regulation found that although overall child-themed advertising expenditure fell by 41 per cent between 2003 and 2007, this masked substantial increases in some non-TV advertising categories (DoH, 2008d). Press advertising, for example, increased 42 per cent over the same period. Children saw a third less advertising of food and drink overall and two-thirds less 'children-themed' advertising in 2007 compared with 2003. A review by OFCOM (2008) found a reduction in children's exposure to licensed characters and brand characters, but an increase in exposure to celebrities.

Campaigners continued to argue for greater restrictions, including a total ban on food advertising to children on TV. It should be noted that only a few countries or states have done this, as part of a policy prohibiting all TV advertisements to children (Sweden, Norway and Quebec). Many other governments, however, have imposed restrictions on TV food advertising to children with regard to content, timing or the use of techniques (for example Finland, Denmark, Germany and Australia). The UK government is currently reviewing whether further action is required. Pressure is also building at an international level. In 2006, the WHO European Charter on Counteracting Obesity recommended the adoption of regulations to reduce commercial promotion of energy-dense foods and the development of international approaches, such as a code on marketing (WHO Regional Office for Europe, 2006b). In 2007, member states at the World Health Assembly in 2007 called on WHO to develop recommendations on marketing of food and non-alcohol drinks to children. Subsequently, the International Obesity Task Force, Consumers International and the International Association for the Study of Obesity (2008) drafted an international code to protect children from internet and TV marketing of food and drink. This included: recommendations that there should be no marketing of energy-dense, nutrient-poor HFSS foods to children and that restrictions on broadcast advertisements should be based on absolute numbers watching or listening rather than simply the proportion of the audience that are children; a more comprehensive approach to non-broadcast marketing; that settings where children are gathered should be free from commercial inducements to consume such foods; and that there should be restrictions on marketing such foods to adults with caring responsibilities for children. WHO (2009a) issued its own recommendations, which called for a reduction in children's exposure to marketing of foods high in fats (saturated and transfats), sugars and salt. It also recommended that settings where children gather should be free from the marketing of such foods, and that government should provide leadership and set a clear policy framework to reduce the impact of food marketing on children.

NHS Services and Partnerships

Policies introduced by Labour governments since 1997 have included measures to improve NHS services for overweight and obese people. Changes to the QoF scheme for general practice, introduced in 2006, rewarded practices for keeping registers of obese patients. It was hoped that this would make it easier to identify and treat such patients. However, GPs have been reluctant to refer obese patients for treatment (Dr Foster, 2008). More generally, primary care services for obese people have been patchy and poorly coordinated (Epstein and Ogden, 2005; Lewis, 2003). The government sought to raise the profile of obesity on local NHS agendas by requiring PCTs to set targets on childhood obesity. Additional resources (£55 million) were allocated to PCTs between 2006 and 2008, specifically for action on diet, physical activity and obesity. They were also encouraged to bid for funds under other programmes (such as Healthy Communities) to undertake pilot schemes in obesity prevention.

PCTs and health professionals are expected to follow guidance produced by NICE (2006b) on the prevention, identification and management of overweight and obesity in adults and children. This integrated clinical and public health guidance was directed at local authorities and other partners as well as the NHS. It identified key priorities for public health intervention, including: to prioritize obesity and allocate resources; partnership working between agencies to create safe spaces for physical activity; encourage active play and healthy food for children in preschool settings; all school policies to ensure that children and young people maintain a healthy weight; workplaces to provide opportunities to eat a healthy diet and be physically active; PCTs and local authorities to recommend self-help, commercial and community weight management programmes providing that they follow best practice. The guidance outlined clinical care recommendations, including: the need for interventions that combine several components; childhood interventions to address lifestyle within family and social settings; that drug treatment must be given with appropriate counselling, information and support; and that bariatric surgery must be regarded as a first-line option only in cases of extreme obesity, although may be given to those who have unsuccessfully tried all appropriate non-surgical measures.

To measure the scale of the obesity problem in schoolchildren, and to monitor progress against national and local targets, a national child measurement programme was introduced in 2005. This involved children in reception classes (4–5 year olds) and Year 6 (10–11 year olds). Parents could refuse permission for their children to be involved and the children themselves could decide not to participate. The early surveys under this scheme produced large non-response rates, although this has gradually improved. Parents and children have the right to opt out, but parents of children who were measured from 2008 to 2009 will receive feedback on their measurements, unless they specifically request otherwise.

The Blair government emphasized that the prevention of obesity was not just a task for the Department of Health and the NHS. At national level, improved coordination was promised between government departments and agencies, and partnership between government, charities and the food industry. At the local level, obesity was chosen as a key area of partnership working between the NHS and other statutory agencies, such as local authorities. Local strategic partnerships and local area agreements were identified as key vehicles for securing agreement between the NHS and its partners. Many local area agreements now include obesity targets. Government regional offices were expected to help coordinate action with other regional bodies (such as SHAs and regional PHOs) providing support.

Following *Choosing Health*, pressure for action on obesity intensified. There was no visible progress on reducing the proportion of obese and overweight people. Moreover, as noted earlier, nutrient targets for fruit and vegetables, fibre, sugars, fat and saturated fat remained elusive. There was some progress in reducing the level of salt consumed, although this still exceeded the target.

Exhibit 13.1

School Meals and Obesity

Schools meals have become a prominent public health issue (Gustafson, 2002; Morgan, 2006). Nutritional standards declined during the 1980s and 90s, as a result of deregulation, budget cuts and the popularity of packed lunches. In 2001, minimum standards were reintroduced in England, but had little impact (Nelson et al., 2006). They were difficult to achieve due to a lack of investment in school meal services, low budgets for ingredients, and a system of competitive contracting geared to low-cost, low-quality provision. Another important factor was the pressure on children, reinforced by marketing, to consume HFSS foods and drink.

In 2005, a media campaign by the celebrity chef Jamie Oliver took the issue to the top of the political agenda. His Channel 4 TV series, *Jamie's School Dinners*, highlighted the state of the school meals service and the task facing those seeking to improve the diets of schoolchildren. There was a huge public reaction to the series and the 'Feed Me Better Campaign' that it inspired. The Blair government commissioned a review (School Meals Review Panel, 2005) and introduced a three-year funding package for school meals costing £280 million, partly funded by the National Lottery. New mandatory food and nutrient standards for school meals were introduced to reduce fried food, crisps, chocolate and fizzy drinks, to cut salt, fat and sugar levels and increase the consumption of high-quality meat and fish, fruit and vegetables and essential nutrients. Vending machines and 'tuck shops' were included in this regime, and were expected to promote sales of healthy snacks and drinks and end the provision of fizzy drinks, confectionery and junk food. Many schools developed food policies (Blenkinsop et al., 2007) covering all aspects of food and nutrition (Barnard et al., 2009). Action on food and diet was increasingly integrated with physical activity strategies as part of a whole school approach to obesity (see Exhibit 13.2). An independent School Food Trust was established to promote higher standards in school meals. School inspections were extended to cover diet and nutrition. Subsequently, in 2008, the government stated that it would introduce compulsory cooking classes for 11–14 year olds.

There has been considerable improvement in the nutrition quality of school meals. In primary schools there has been reduced consumption of fats, sugar and salt and increased consumption of fruit, vegetables and starchy foods not cooked in fat (School Food Trust, 2009). However, many schools are not yet compliant with the new standards and there is considerable room for improvement in the implementation of school food policies (Ofsted, 2010). Indeed, following the strengthened nutritional standards, demand for school meals fell (Ofsted, 2007c). Uptake has since risen, although currently less than half of primary and secondary pupils eat school meals. Packed lunches provided by parents contain higher levels of sugar, salt and fat (Rees et al., 2008). Currently, there are no national regulations covering food brought from home. Despite advertising restrictions and the provision of free fruit and vegetables in primary schools, children remain subject to marketing messages and peer group pressure (Ludvigsen and Sharma, 2004). Mobile fast food outlets and shops near schools can counteract the impact of a school's food policy (Sinclair and Winkler, 2008). One possibility, explored by the Labour government, would be to encourage local authorities to use their planning powers to prevent a proliferation of outlets near schools.

Other parts of the UK have also sought to improve school nutrition (see Welsh Assembly Government 2007, 2008a; Department of Education for Northern Ireland, 2008). For example, Scotland's pioneering 'Hungry for Success' programme (Scottish Executive, 2003e) set out a whole school approach to school meals, with new standards, and measures to improve take-up of healthy school meals. The Scottish Executive subsequently introduced free school meals for all 5–8 year olds, beginning with primary schoolchildren in deprived areas. This universal policy, also adopted by some English local authorities (notably Hull City Council), was also piloted south of the border.

Further Developments

One of the main criticisms of government policy was the pace of implementation. For example, the social marketing initiative mentioned in *Choosing Health* was not introduced until 2009. It took three years to introduce new advertising restrictions. Labelling initiatives and product modification were also slow to develop. The government's decision to work in partnership with industry was a major cause of delay. The need to consult and involve businesses, although useful for building consensus and voluntary action, presented them with opportunities to dilute and delay policies. Another reason for poor implementation was the low priority given to diet, nutrition and obesity by the NHS and partners at a local level. National, regional and local coordination remained weak (NAO et al., 2006).

The limitations of the Labour government's strategy were exposed by further reports on obesity and public health (BMA, 2005b; PAC, 2007; Health-care Commission and Audit Commission, 2008; Foresight, 2007, 2009; Wanless, 2007). Recommendations were made for clearer and stronger leadership within a coherent policy and service framework. Meanwhile, the anti-obesity lobby pressed for radical policies such as: further restrictions on HFSS food and drink advertising; higher taxation for HFSS food and drinks products and subsidies for fruit and vegetables; mandatory traffic light labelling; statutory targets for the reduction of HFSS products; and restrictions on the location of fast food outlets. There is increasing evidence to support such interventions. Researchers have found that localities with higher concentrations of fast food restaurants and convenience stores have higher rates of obesity (Spence et al., 2009). Other studies have found that taxes on less healthy foods can reduce consumption of these goods (Smed et al., 2007) and health problems linked to diet (Mytton et al., 2007). Some countries, such as Denmark for example, have used taxation to raise the price of HFSS foods. However, such taxes can disproportionately affect the real incomes of the poor, leaving them less able to afford a healthy diet. This could be mitigated through subsidies for healthy foods, however.

Evidence from intervention studies on diet and health (and physical activity – see Exhibit 13.2) collated by WHO (2009b) identifies measures likely to be effective in reducing obesity and related health problems, including:

- regulatory policies to support healthier composition of foods

- pricing and fiscal policies

- high-intensity school-based interventions (that are comprehensive, multi-component, include a curriculum taught by trained teachers, in a supportive school environment, and with healthy food options available)

- multi-component workplace programmes to improve diet

- community diet education targeting high risk groups, which are multi-component involving community development activities and group-based programmes

- targeted primary care interventions aimed at groups at high risk of developing chronic diseases

More specifically with regard to cancer, the WCRF (World Cancer Research Fund) and the American Institute of Cancer Research (AICR) (2009) drew up policy recommendations to improve diet and physical exercise, which also impinge on obesity. Those concerning diet include: the protection of public health in international agreements, such as trade, food and environment;

national governments to encourage healthy foods and discourage unhealthy foods (including restrictions on the advertising of fast and processed food and sugary drinks); the requirement of schools to provide meals of high nutritional standard; voluntary action by the food industry to ensure that healthy foods are available and affordable and to stop advertising unhealthy foods and sugary drinks to children, and ensure that information is available, accurate, and uniform in product marketing and labelling. It was also recommended that schools incorporate food and nutrition in the mandatory core curriculum, ensure teaching materials are free from commercial bias, provide healthy meals, withdraw unhealthy food and drinks from sale and do not allow vending machines that offer unhealthy products. Workplaces were called on to incentivize healthy eating, make available healthy food and drinks, withdraw unhealthy products and not to allow vending machines offering fast food and sugary drinks. Recommendations were also made to encourage civil society organizations, health professionals, the media and people generally to support moves to improve diet and health.

A further contribution to the debate came from the Nuffield Council on Bioethics (2007) report on public health. It maintained that on ethical grounds a long-term strategy for preventing obesity in schools, including the weighing and measuring of children to monitor progress, was justified. The Council also argued that the industry had an ethical duty to help people to make healthy food choices. Where the market failed, government was right to intervene. For example, if industry would not accept effective labelling schemes, a legislative approach should be pursued.

Exhibit 13.2

Physical Activity, Obesity and Health

Increasing physical activity levels can prevent obesity (FAO/WHO, 2003; DoH, 2004e; Foresight, 2007, 2009). Physical exercise can also prevent a range of specific diseases and medical conditions, including cancer of the colon and breast, heart disease, stroke, diabetes, depression, dementia and osteoporosis (DoH, 2004e; Suzuki et al., 2008; Laukkanen et al., 2009; Leitzmann et al., 2008; McTiernan et al., 2003; Wolin et al., 2009; WCRF/AICR, 2009; WHO, 2009b). Being physically active also has a positive effect on cognitive functioning and academic achievement (Erickson and Kramer, 2008; Castelli et al., 2007) and may even retard the ageing process (Blackwell, 2007).

In England, the average distance walked per person fell by over a fifth between the mid-1970s and 2003, the distance cycled fell by a third and car use increased by 10 per cent (Foresight, 2007). For most people, modern technology has made physical life less strenuous. Sedentary leisure activities, such as TV and computer games, have contributed to low levels of physical activity, obesity and health problems (Elliath et al., 2002; Grund et al., 2001; Hardy et al., 2009). According to some, children are less active than in previous generations and this may be partly responsible for rising levels of obesity. However, the relationship between diet, exercise and obesity is complex. Inactivity may be a cause and a consequence of obesity (Wilkin et al., 2005; EarlyBird, 2009). It is easy to blame single factors such as the decline of PE in schools and the 'school run' for reducing activity levels. However, overall levels of physical activity are not necessarily determined by school PE opportunities (Mallam et al., 2003). Being driven to school does not reduce physical activity (Metcalf et al., 2004) nor do better recreational opportunities necessarily produce more activity (EarlyBird, 2010).

It is recommended that adults undertake 30 minutes or more of moderate or vigorous exercise at least five days per week (DoH, 2004e; FAO/WHO, 2003), although some adults may need 45–60 minutes to prevent obesity (FAO/WHO, 2003). Moderate exercise such as walking, housework, swimming and gardening have positive health benefits (Hamer and Chida, 2008). Vigorous sport can have health benefits, although it has higher risks of adverse incidents, such as injuries, (Blackwell, 2007). In 2008, only 39 per cent of men and 29 per cent of women in England attained these recommended levels of exercise, although this represented an increase from 32 per cent of men and 21 per cent of women in 1996 (NHS Information Centre, 2009a). The recommendation for children is at least 60 minutes of at least moderate physical activity every day (DoH, 2004e). However, only 32 per cent of boys and 24 per cent of girls in England achieve these recommended levels (NHS Information Centre, 2010).

Reviews of evidence (Kahn et al., 2002; Hillsdon et al., 2005; NICE, 2006c, 2009c; WHO, 2009b) indicate that the following interventions can be effective in promoting physical activity:

- point-of-decision prompts to motivate use of stairs
- community-wide campaigns
- school-based PE
- social support in community settings
- individually based health behaviour change programmes
- enhanced access to physical activity facilities and spaces
- brief advice from a health professional
- referral to an exercise specialist based in the community

In addition, changes to the built environment and to transport systems may encourage cycling and walking (Association of Directors of Public Health et al., 2008; Frank et al., 2007; Handy et al., 2002; NICE, 2008d; WHO, 2009b; Health Committee, 2009; Nuffield Council on Bioethics, 2007). However, cultural factors, including the perceptions of safety and feasibility of healthier forms of transport, are also important (Panter and Jones, 2008).

Other interventions used in isolation are regarded as ineffective, or as having limited, short-term or doubtful effectiveness. These include: mass media campaigns, classroom-based health education; school-based education to reducing TV/video games; exercise referral, use of pedometers and community-based walking and cycling schemes; and family-based social support. However, there is a lack of good research evidence about some interventions (for example community exercise projects and exercise referral).

Further studies may shed light on the effectiveness of these approaches. Furthermore, it appears that the most effective approach is a combination of interventions to improve exercise levels rather than isolated initiatives (van Sluijs et al., 2007; Kriemler et al., 2010; Gonzalez-Suarez et al., 2009). For example, with regard to children's health, the evidence supports the use of sustained, multi-level campaigns, integrated with other strategies to encourage play, sport and reduce obesity (NICE, 2009c).

Policies in England have focused strongly on improving children's physical activity. In 2002, less than half (25 per cent) received two hours of PE each week. The Labour government set targets to increase participation in high-quality PE and school sport: 75 per cent of pupils to be engaged in at least two hours per week by 2006 and 85 per cent by 2008. The latter target was met in 2007, but was superseded by a new target of five hours of PE and sport per week (two hours in the curriculum and three hours in the community or after school). The government also set a goal that 70 per cent of adults would participate in 30 minutes of moderate physical activity at least five times a week by 2020.

Physical activity levels have been the subject of several strategies (The Prime Minister's Strategy Unit, 2002; DoH, 2005c; HM Government, 2009b), including sport and PE strategies (DfES and DCMS, 2003; DCSF and DCMS, 2008), and a children's play strategy (DCSF, 2008b). Specific interventions include: GP referral schemes for exercise; walking and cycling schemes using the workplace to promote physical activity; incentives for gym membership; and free swimming for children and elderly people. The NHS was also issued with guidance to improve commissioning of physical activity at local level (DoH, 2009e). The Labour government backed local projects, some of which are supported through national health promotion pilot programmes such as Communities for Health and the Healthy Towns initiative. In addition, LEAPS (local exercise action pilots) were introduced in 2004 to test new ways of promoting exercise. Located in 10 deprived areas, the pilots explored a range of interventions including exercise referral, exercise classes and groups, motivational interviewing, peer mentoring, campaigns, outdoor exercise schemes and transport training for leaders and coordinators. Although providing a useful test bed, these schemes had little impact on physical activity at the community level (Carnegie Research Institute, 2007). Other local schemes include over 200 projects under the auspices of the Active England programme (funded by the National Lottery and Sport England), aimed to encourage innovative projects to improving exercise levels and participation in sport from 2004. These schemes, engaging an estimated 800,000 people by 2008, included projects to improve sport infrastructure, build capacity among organizations promoting physical activity, undertake outreach programmes to involve disadvantaged groups, and encourage outdoor exercise. An interesting initiative emerging in recent years is the 'green gym', which encourages people to engage in physical activities such as planting, harvesting, and improving green spaces. There is evidence that natural open spaces may have positive effects on both physical and mental health (see Curtis, 2004; English Nature, 2003; Mitchell and Popham, 2008).

There has been criticism that these policies do not go far enough (Health Committee, 2009). Many local projects are short term and there is often poor coordination. Moreover, other policies undermine or inhibit the effectiveness of physical activity strategies. For example, the sale of school fields continued, despite new rules introduced by Labour, to supposedly protect them. Notably, the Cameron government has pledged to protect school playing fields. The closure of swimming pools and other facilities occurred against the grain of the government's physical activity strategy (PAC, 2007). Furthermore, sports policy continues to be elitist rather than participatory. The hosting of the Olympics in

London in 2012, although perhaps inspiring a new generation of athletes, will inevitably divert resources away from community-based physical activity programmes.

Other parts of the UK have also pursued strategies to improve physical activity (see Health Promotion Agency for Northern Ireland, 1996b; DHSSPS, 2004b, 2006b; Welsh Assembly Government, 2006b; Scottish Executive, 2003f) which vary in detail. For example, Scotland is aiming that by 2022 half the adult population should participate in 30 minutes of moderate exercise five times a week and that 80 per cent of children should engage in a hour of physical activity a day. The Scottish Physical Activity and Health Council, chaired by a minister, is taking forward the strategy. The Scottish Physical Activity Alliance seeks to assist the implementation of the strategy by disseminating and sharing evidence, knowledge, policy and practice among practitioners, and building capacity. National physical activity strategies increasingly operate in a European context. The European Commission produced a white paper on sport, which recommended closer cooperation between sport, health and education sectors in the context of action to counteract obesity and promised new physical activity guidelines for member states (Commission of the European Communities, 2007b).

A New Obesity Strategy

The Labour government under Gordon Brown revised the PSA target on obesity to 'reduce the proportion of overweight and obese children to 2000 levels' by 2020 (HM Government, 2007a). A new obesity strategy (HM Government, 2008b) subsequently identified five priority areas: children's health; promoting healthier food choices; building physical activity into people's lives; creating incentives for better health; and personalized advice and support.

- With regard to *children's health,* plans included: the identification of at risk families and the promotion of breastfeeding as the norm for mothers; making cooking a compulsory part of the curriculum for 11–14 year olds; promoting healthy lunch box policies in schools; improving cycling infrastructure; and introducing a social marketing programme.

- *Healthy food choices* involved: the production of a Healthy Food code of good practice for the industry aimed at reducing consumption of saturated fat, salt and sugar; encouraging local authorities to use planning regulations to manage the proliferation of fast food outlets; and further reviews of TV advertising of unhealthy foods.

- *Building physical activity into our lives* involved: a campaign to promote walking; a new scheme, 'Healthy Towns', to introduce pilot schemes based on 'whole-town' approaches to reducing obesity and increasing exercise; and a review of physical activity strategy.

- *Creating incentives for better health* included: plans for pilot schemes promoting health in the workplace; and the use of incentive schemes to encourage people to lose weight, eat healthily and be active.

- *Personalized advice and support* included: developing the NHS Choices website to give personalized advice on diet and activity; and supporting the commissioning of weight management services.

The Labour government pledged more support for research into obesity. To strengthen implementation, additional funds were allocated for the obesity programme. Obesity was included as a national priority in the NHS operating framework – which required PCTs to develop plans to tackle obesity. It was also a priority in the children and young people's health strategy (see Chapter 9). However, there was no compulsion for PCTs and local authorities to include obesity in their LAA targets. Instead, central government promised support and guidance for local organizations seeking to develop local strategies, including a national obesity support team. A new cross-departmental obesity unit was established, based in the DoH, but led jointly with DCSF. The unit was charged with leading the strategy and developing further proposals, as well as managing the interface between government, industry and other stakeholders.

Critics pointed out that although some of these initiatives were new, others repeated, reiterated or recycled earlier commitments. The new strategy did not propose any radical policies, such as legal regulation and fiscal policies, but persisted with a voluntary approach, working with industry. The commitment to a more coherent approach across central government was welcomed, but there were doubts about the ability of the new central unit to coordinate departments with close ties to food industry, advertising and media interests. The focus on child obesity, while understandable as a means of achieving medium and long-term goals, was criticized for downplaying the importance of adult obesity (although the PSA target was set 'in the context of reducing obesity across the population' and many of the measures in the strategy addressed adults as well as children). Some of the commitments set out in the new obesity strategy were reiterated in the Labour government's food strategy in 2010 (HM Government, 2010a). Additional proposals included making land available for growing community food, a greater role for the food industry in educating children about food, and plans to help families at most risk from poor nutrition to improve their cooking skills.

Other parts of the UK pursued their own approaches to diet, nutrition and obesity. In Scotland, a national diet action plan with targets was introduced in the 1990s (Scottish Office, 1994, 1996). This plan included building consumer skills and capacities; improvements in the supply of food; and better information about food and nutrition. It was strengthened in 2004 with a new strategic framework 'Eating for Health', which established a Food and Health Council (to provide leadership, expert advice and coordination) and a Food and Health Alliance, a network for implementation that included the NHS, local government, community and voluntary sector, research bodies and business. Lang et al. (2006b) found that the Scottish plan was a timely intervention with laudable goals. Substantial progress was made, including the appointment of a national-level food and health coordinator to lead implementation and encourage government coordination; the creation of food and health alliances; efforts to support community level food initiatives (via a Scottish Community Diet campaign); the development of whole school approaches to healthy eating, catering and supply ('Hungry for Success', see Exhibit 13.1); improvement in breastfeeding rates; and the development of new campaigns on healthy eating (the 'Healthyliving' campaign – a multimedia and multi-agency communication and education campaign on healthy eating and physical activity). However, little progress was made towards the dietary targets, the only positive outcome being a small reduction in fat consumption. The reasons for these shortcomings are complex but include: underestimation of the impact of inequalities; failure to link actions to the narrow range of food and nutrient targets; resources and initiatives being too thinly spread; uneven implementation at the regional level; and failure to engage fully with the supply chain (Lang et al., 2006b). The consensual approach to working with the food industry may have led to a failure to confront trends and activities that undermined health messages and policies. There was a reluctance to adopt regulatory and legislative powers. The Scottish government (2009b) has since adopted a new national food policy, which aims to encapsulate all aspects of the food chain and incorporate a range of issues, including sustainability and health.

In Wales, efforts to prevent diet-related illness began during the 1980s with a strategy on heart disease prevention. Since devolution, the Welsh government has adopted a nutrition strategy with targets (Welsh Assembly Government, 2003b). Initiatives include a scheme to develop young people's cooking skills and measures to increase access to fruit and vegetables through the establishment of local food cooperatives. As in Scotland, there has been a focus on improving the diet of children in school settings (Welsh Assembly Government, 2006b, 2007). A review of the Welsh strategy on nutrition found that the profile of these issues had been raised and there was a stronger commitment to action in this field alongside new structures, mechanisms and resources (Davis et al., 2007). However, the review also revealed unevenness in take-up of ideas across Wales, both geographically and with regard to some groups, notably older people. Other problems included: short-term project funding, which undermined continuity; and a lack of systematic evaluation, which inhibited the development of an evidence base. The review called for a more joined-up, holistic and strategic approach, including the supply chain and incorporating sustainable development issues.

Northern Ireland introduced nutritional targets in the 1990s, as part of a food and nutrition strategy (Health Promotion Agency for Northern Ireland, 1996a). Since then the focus has been mainly on child obesity, with a new strategy 'Fit Futures' introduced in 2006, identifying a multi-agency approach to halve child obesity rates by 2025 (DHSSPS, 2006b). Activities are targeted at improving diet and physical activity levels, and include a social marketing campaign and school-based and community-based initiatives.

The Cameron Government

The Conservative–Liberal coalition, while acknowledging that obesity and chronic illness were linked to diet, argued that the previous government had not been successful in improving the situation. The Secretary of State for Health, Andrew Lansley, appeared to reject as ineffective the 'Jamie Oliver' approach (see Exhibit 13.1) to improve school meals, although later acknowledged that his efforts were well-intentioned and should be applauded (BBC, 2010b; Lansley, 2010b). The new government's approach placed emphasis on voluntary activity (by business, communities and individuals) rather than state intervention. It announced that funding for the Change4Life programme would be reduced, with charities, business and local authorities expected to fill the gap. Under a 'responsibility deal', food businesses would be expected to be more responsible in marketing food and developing healthier products. Although further regulation in some areas was not ruled out, notably with regard to advertising and marketing to children, the presumption was that business would voluntarily change its practices to improve the nation's diet and nutrition. To the delight of some of the largest and most powerful companies in the food industry, the government rejected the traffic light approach to food labelling. Meanwhile the FSA, which promoted this scheme, faced an uncertain future. 'Government sources', reported in the media, suggested that it would be abolished and its functions transferred to the Department of Health and DEFRA. At the time of writing, the Cameron government's food and nutrition policy is still developing. There is criticism, even from the government's supporters, that its approach is naive and playing into the hands of the food industry. It remains to be seen whether this will force the government into adopting a more robust regulatory approach.

Conclusion

It is clear from this and the previous chapter that food and diet have wide-ranging implications for health. In the past, health was marginalized in debates about food and farming (Lang and Heasman, 2004; Lang et al.,

2009). Policy was dominated by a productionist approach, which attached little weight to the wider costs imposed by food and agriculture systems. Apart from high-profile cases of food poisoning and contamination, responsibilities for health were seen almost wholly as a matter for the individual, rather than the government. Moreover, the various health-related policy issues – safety, environmental protection, sustainability, poverty and nutrition – were treated separately with no regard for the links between them. Now there is a realization that a more integrated approach is necessary (Policy Commission on the Future of Food and Farming, 2002; Prime Minister's Strategy Unit, 2008a; Lang and Rayner, 2007; Lang and Heasman, 2004; Lang et al., 2009; HM Government, 2010a). The logic of an ecological approach, where 'the key purpose of food and farming is – or should be – to advance the health and wellbeing of the population' (Lang and Rayner, 2002), is powerful, although this must encompass not only food and farming, but other policies that have a bearing on these issues, such as planning, transport, waste, rural development, regeneration and food and farming policies. Moreover, strategies and interventions cannot simply be at local, regional or national levels, important as these may be. The framework for many aspects of farming, food and health is determined at the international and European level. Therefore a multilevel approach, involving global and European regional institutions and powers, is crucial.

The greater awareness of food and health issues, and acknowledgement of the need to act in an integrated way, has not occurred by chance. The growing strength and coherence of the health and consumer lobby on food issues, coupled with the sustained interest of the media in these matters, has been a major factor. Another explanation for the emergence of these issues lies in the fracturing of the food industry (Lang and Heasman, 2004) which, although remaining a powerful commercial interest, is increasingly divided. Indeed, parts of the industry – because of genuine CSR commitments or for strategic commercial reasons, or both – have broken ranks and openly endorsed moves to improve safety, sustainability and diet. There are also important differences between different sections of the industry (organic vs industrial farming; retailers vs producers; snack food vs fruit/ vegetable producers). Nonetheless, the food industry remains a powerful interest group and, through partnership working arrangements and wider political networks, is able for the time being at least to neuter attempts to introduce more radical policy options.

Illicit Drugs

14

The use of illicit drugs for recreational purposes is widespread and linked to a range of health and social problems. This chapter examines the public health implications of illegal addictions, possible interventions to reduce harm, and the reasons why particular policies are pursued. In the next chapter, the problem of legal addictions, alcohol and tobacco, is explored.

Illicit Drugs

Why should illicit drugs be regarded as a public health problem? The first and most obvious reason is that they are associated with a significant number of deaths. Nonetheless, the calculation of drug-related mortality is complex (ACMD, 2000). Drug poisoning kills around 2500 people in England and Wales each year (O'Dowd, 2008). These figures include mortality from legal drugs such as antidepressants and painkillers, but exclude alcohol and tobacco. Drugs also contribute to an unknown number of deaths from accidents, cancers and other diseases. The second reason is that they are associated with significant morbidity. Over 38,000 hospital admissions in England involve a diagnosis of drug-related mental health disorder (NHS Information Centre, 2008b). A further 10,000 admissions relate to drug poisoning. Around 200,000 people a year are in contact with structured drug treatment services. It is estimated that there are 280,000 heroin and crack users, the majority of whom are not receiving treatment (Prime Minister's Strategy Unit, 2003a), while the overall number of problem drug users is thought to be over 320,000 (NHS Information Centre, 2008b).

Health problems are linked to particular drugs (Reuter and Stevens, 2007; Devlin and Henry, 2008). Cocaine is associated with cardiovascular problems, such as stroke and cardiac arrest (Egred and Davis, 2005). Cannabis is related to cancers of the lung, larynx and mouth and throat (WHO, 1997c). It is also linked to mental illnesses including anxiety, depression, psychosis and schizophrenia (Fergusson et al., 2005; Di Forti et al., 2009; Henquet et al., 2005;

Moore et al., 2007; Patton, 2002; van Os et al., 2002), although lifetime risks are small (ACMD, 2006b). Ecstasy is associated with a range of conditions (ACMD, 2009) including: long-term cognitive functioning and memory problems (Morgan, 2000; Schilt et al., 2008), depression (Guillot and Greenway, 2006) and acute dehydration (Rogers et al., 2009). Amphetamine, cocaine and crack use are all linked to psychosis (Farrell et al., 2002).

Many health problems result from drug administration, side effects and contamination. Excessive water intake associated with ecstasy can lead to water intoxication and death. Repeated injection of drugs damages veins while needle sharing causes infections. Harm may occur when drugs are mixed with other substances. For example, cannabis is usually smoked with tobacco, while heroin and cocaine are 'cut' with other, sometimes harmful, substances. Solely in terms of harm to health, safely administered illicit drugs taken in a controlled environment are less dangerous than commonly supposed. However, the rationale for taking action on drugs is based on wider social consequences such as crime, violence and disorder associated with drug lifestyles and the drugs trade, which have important implications for public health and wellbeing.

Measuring drug prevalence is difficult (Newcombe, 2007). Heavy users of illegal drugs (such as prisoners, homeless people, sex workers) are underrepresented in surveys. Furthermore, respondents to social surveys may exaggerate or understate their consumption. Bearing this in mind, over a third of the adult population (16–59) in England stated they had taken illegal drugs at some time in their lives, a tenth in the previous year, and just under 6 per cent in the previous month (NHS Information Centre, 2008b). The most popular drug was cannabis (30 per cent of adults reported having tried this drug at least once), followed by amphetamines (12 per cent), cocaine (8 per cent) and ecstasy (7 per cent). Under one per cent admitted to heroin use. Drug use was higher among younger adults than other age groups. The proportion of 16–24 year olds reporting lifetime, past-year and past-month use was 45 per cent, 24 per cent, and 14 per cent respectively.

The use of illegal drugs among children and young people is perceived as a particularly serious problem because of their greater vulnerability. A tenth of pupils aged 11–15 in England claimed to have taken illicit drugs in the past month; 17 per cent in the past year. A quarter reported having taken drugs at least once in their lifetime (NHS Information Centre, 2008b). As with adults, the most common drug taken is cannabis (used by 9 per cent in the past year). Four per cent of secondary school pupils claimed to have tried class A drugs in the past year.

So-called soft drugs, particularly cannabis, are often seen as 'gateways' to harder drugs, such as heroin and cocaine. Although soft drug use typically precedes the use of hard drugs, there is no evidence that individuals move in a linear fashion from the former to the latter (Golub and Johnson, 2001;

van Ours, 2003; Hall and Lynskey, 2005). Other factors such as pre-existing traits and contextual factors (such as peer group pressure, socialization into subcultures and settings that promote hard drugs) shape future drug use. In reality, drug choices made by children and young people are complex, involving both illegal and legal drugs. Illegal drugs have become normalized, are no longer a symbol of crime and deviance among the young but an essential part of their lifestyles (Parker et al., 1998). The normalization thesis has been used by governments and the media to universalize the drug threat and this may have contributed to moral panic about drugs (Blackman, 2007; RSA Commission, 2007). Others argue that the level of drug use among children and young people has been exaggerated (Shiner and Newburn, 1997). Indeed, it is true that most do not try drugs and only a minority engage in long-term use.

Another reason for concern about drugs is crime (Bennett and Holloway, 2005; McSweeney et al., 2007). Although crime is associated with drug use, there is disagreement about how much is drug-related. By definition, people are committing a crime when supplying or possessing illegal drugs. However, the link with other offences is more complex Although prostitution, robbery, assault, homicides, fraud, burglary and theft are all associated with drug taking and supply, it is difficult to prove direct causation. Crime may be a cause or a consequence of drug use. Alternatively, both crime and drug use may be caused by other factors like deprivation. Arrestees and offenders are more likely than the general population to have a drug habit (Bennett and Holloway, 2005; McSweeney et al., 2007). Those involved in crime acknowledge drug abuse as a reason for offending (Bennett and Holloway, 2005; Hearnden and Magill, 2004). A drug habit not only creates the need for income but is likely to impair the ability to earn it through legitimate means. Heroin and crack/cocaine users have an annual average illegal income of approximately £17,000 a year (Bennett and Holloway, 2005). A small number of addicts commit a disproportionate number of crimes, mainly related to theft. In one study, 1100 drug addicts committed over 70,000 crimes over a two-year period (DoH, 1996). Although the level of crime committed by drug users is disproportionately high (Dorn et al., 1994; Bennett and Holloway, 2005), they often have other legitimate sources of income (Hammersley et al., 1989). Those who need large incomes to maintain their habit – chiefly heroin and crack/cocaine users – are a minority and their contribution to overall crime levels is small, perhaps as little as one per cent of property crime (Dorn et al., 1994). Although illicit drug users are more likely to commit crime than non-users, the majority do not commit non-drug offences.

The criminalization of drugs unavoidably adds to the costs of the criminal justice system. The punitive approach to drugs, discussed below, has been held responsible for increasing offending. The number of drug offences committed in the 1950s was less than 300. By 1998 this reached 131,000, most for cannabis possession (Newcombe, 2007). The increase was partly due to new offences and stricter law enforcement. One must also consider the broader costs of drug misuse and its impact on social welfare and public health. The total cost of class A drug misuse in the UK for 2003/4 was estimated at over £15 billion (NHS Information Centre, 2008b). This includes costs of drug-related crime (90 per cent of the costs), deaths, and health and social care services. Other costs are less measurable, but nevertheless important, such as family breakdown and child neglect. Given the key role of the family in maintaining health, preventing illness and nurturing children, this has obvious implications for the health of the community as a whole.

Has the problem of illicit drugs deteriorated? As already noted, the number of drug offences has increased substantially. The numbers in treatment and the percentage of the population admitting to lifetime and recent use of drugs has also increased (Newcombe, 2007). In the mid-1960s only one per cent of adults admitted to having used drugs and the number of registered addicts was under a thousand. The UK has a high level of drug use and problems, having the fourth highest rate of drug-related deaths among industrialized countries and the second highest level of problem drug use (Reuter and Stevens, 2007). It has relatively high rates of cannabis, cocaine, heroin, amphetamine and ecstasy use (EMCDDA, 2008; UNODC, 2008). In the European 'league tables' for drug abuse, the UK has the third highest rates of opiate use. England and Wales is second in the table for cocaine and ecstasy use, seventh for cannabis and top of the league for amphetamines. Although time series and comparative statistics are alarming, it should be noted that growth has been partly due to changes in policy, such as tougher laws and enforcement policies which have revealed more use and abuse. Changes in the way in which statistics are collected and recorded also had an effect, notably on the number of drug users and drug-related deaths identified. Statistics have been affected by cultural changes, such as a greater willingness to admit to previous drug misuse and to identify drug abuse as a cause of death.

Drug Policies

Opiates were widely available in Victorian times (Stimson and Oppenheimer, 1982; Berridge and Edwards, 1981). Unease about their misuse led to increased regulation during the late nineteenth century. The first three decades of the twentieth century saw international agreements to control the drug trade and control policies in individual countries. In Britain, although new laws were passed to criminalize the drugs trade, the problem of drug addiction was medicalized. Doctors could prescribe addictive drugs if they believed patients could live an otherwise stable life. By the late 1950s, however, this so-called 'British system' was under strain (Strang and Gossop, 1994). Concerns about drug taking among young people led to the Brain committee of inquiry, which reported that no fundamental changes in regulation were necessary (Interdepartmental Committee on Drug Addiction, 1961). Shortly afterwards the number of known addicts rose and the Brain committee was reconvened, deciding that regulation must be tightened (Interdepartmental Committee on Drug Addiction, 1965).

Following the second Brain committee report, the British government introduced a system of central registration for drug addicts. It encouraged the development of specialized drug treatment services in the form of drug dependence units while limiting the role of GPs. Meanwhile, law enforcement powers were increased in the late 1960s. The law was consolidated in the form of the 1971 Misuse of Drugs Act, which remains in force today. The 1971 Act controls drugs in three classes (A, B and C). Offences related to drugs in the higher classifications attract greater maximum penalties than the lower categories (see Table 14.1).

Table 14.1 UK Classification of Drugs under the Misuse of Drugs Act 1971

Class	
A	ecstasy, LSD, heroin, cocaine, crack, magic mushrooms, methadone, amphetamines (for injection)
B	amphetamines, cannabis, ritalin, pholcodine, naphyrone, mephedrone
C	tranquillisers, ketamine, GHB (gamma hydroxybutyrate), anabolic steroids, some painkillers

Drug Policies under Thatcher and Major

Concerns about rising levels of heroin misuse in the 1980s led to a national drugs strategy. This aimed to reduce supply from abroad; improve enforcement; maintain deterrents and controls; develop prevention; and improve treatment and rehabilitation (Home Office, 1985). Specific measures included reclassification of drugs, increased penalties for breaking the law and powers to confiscate the assets of drug traffickers. There was a shift towards community-based approaches to treatment with the establishment of community drug teams to coordinate local prevention and treatment services. There was also an endorsement of drugs education, aimed particularly at children, young people and their parents. In 1985, a high-profile £2 million anti-heroin campaign was launched. Funding was allocated to enable local education authorities to employ drug and health education coordinators and to expand drug education training for teachers. A drugs prevention initiative was set up in the late 1980s to promote new prevention projects.

An emerging theme in this period was harm minimization, 'to limit the potential injury associated with drug use' (Bayer, 1993, p. 15). This became more prominent largely due to the emergence of HIV and AIDS (Berridge, 1998). Concerns about the transmission of the disease through unhygienic drug-taking practices such as needle sharing led to the establishment of needle-exchange schemes, health promotion campaigns based on harm minimization rather than total abstinence, and safe sex campaigns aimed specifically at high risk drug-using populations (notably prostitutes). HIV and AIDS helped to promote a more enlightened approach towards drug users, an approach credited with minimizing infections. The UK has a relatively low level of HIV/AIDS infection related to injecting drug use, currently less than 6 per cent (Reuter and Stevens, 2007). However, there has been a large rise in hepatitis C cases linked to injecting drug use. The harm-reduction philosophy spread to other areas of drug use unconnected with HIV/AIDS. For example, ecstasy users were given information and advice on how to use the drug safely.

The Major government's strategy *Tackling Drugs Together* (Cm 2846, 1995) represented a shift in emphasis towards reducing demand. However, supply-side policies remained a key element. The strategy aimed to improve the coherence of policy at national level through better interdepartmental coordination. To improve local coordination, drug action teams (DATs) were established throughout England, incorporating representatives from health authorities, local authorities, the police, and probation service. These now include PCTs, Youth Offending Teams and the Connexions service. Similar bodies were established in other parts of the UK. Additional resources were promised, although these were not regarded as sufficient for the task (Newburn and Elliot, 1998). The government continued to place its faith in drugs education becoming part of the national curriculum for schools.

The Blair Government's Drug Policy

The Blair government set out its policies in a white paper, *Tackling Drugs to Build a Better Britain* (Cm 3945, 1998). This reiterated the need to improve coordination at all levels. A national drugs czar was appointed (significantly, a former police chief constable). At local level, new partnerships were proposed to combat drug abuse, alongside other social problems such as crime, poor education, ill health and deprivation. DATs were retained, but subjected to greater monitoring and performance assessment. The Blair government continued the shift in emphasis towards prevention and reducing the demand for drugs. A drugs prevention advisory service was established in 1999 to provide evidence on strategies and to promote good practice, superseding the drugs prevention initiative. An expansion of school-based drugs education was launched, discussed below. Treatment was a key element in the government's plans, closely linked to the criminal justice system. New drug treatment and testing orders were introduced for offenders in 1998. Building on an earlier initiative requiring certain offenders to attend drug treatment, these orders enabled community sentences to include conditions requiring tests and treatment. Other initiatives included arrest referral schemes, offering treatment to drug misusers at point of arrest, allowing access to treatment at an earlier stage (Crowther-Dowey, 2007).

The Blair government set out a range of quantitative performance targets for its strategy, which included:

- reducing the level of repeat offending among drug misusing offenders (by a quarter by 2005 and by half by 2008)

- increasing the number of problem drug users in treatment programmes (by two-thirds by 2005 and by 100 per cent by 2008)

- reducing the proportion of young people under 25 reporting drug use (for example, reduce heroin and cocaine users by a quarter by 2005 and by half by 2008)

- reducing access to all drugs among under 25s significantly (including reducing access to heroin and cocaine users by a quarter by 2005 and by half by 2008)

These targets were incorporated into public service agreements between the Treasury and relevant government departments, such as the Department of Health and the Home Office. Additional resources were promised, funded partly by seizures of drug dealers' assets that would require further legislation.

Further revisions followed. A report from ACMD (2000), calling for a new integrated approach to the prevention of drug misuse deaths, led to an action plan to cut deaths by a fifth by 2004. In addition, PCTs were required to invest in drug prevention while giving greater support to schools in delivering health education about drugs. In 2001, new measures to require drug testing of offenders were introduced. In the same year, the National Treatment Agency for Substance Misuse (NTA) was created to improve the availability, effectiveness and capacity of drug treatment services in England.

In 2002, the government again revised its strategy. This followed criticism from a number of sources, including a report from the Police Foundation (2000) which argued that a revision of the legal framework of drug control was long overdue. In addition, the Home Affairs Committee (2002) recommended a stronger focus on harm reduction and a public health target for drug misuse. Meanwhile the drug czar resigned and the responsibility for the strategy moved from the Cabinet Office back to the Home Office. The new strategy aimed to expand and improve drug education in schools. It included a new communications campaign on class A drugs (HM Government, 2002). Guidance later emphasized a whole school approach to drugs (DFES, 2004c). All schools were expected to have a drugs policy and an education programme. As noted, drug education was already in the national curriculum. There was a statutory requirement to provide drug education as part of the science curriculum. Drug education was also provided as part of citizenship studies, a statutory subject for older pupils. However, much drug education was provided under PSHE, a non-statutory subject (see Chapter 9).

The 2002 strategy led to a new campaign (the Frank campaign) to raise awareness about drugs. This campaign uses the internet as well as conventional media such as press, radio and TV to educate and inform young people. It has a telephone helpline, to offer advice and support, and where appropriate to refer to other services. The Frank campaign cost over £8 million between 2003 and 2006 (Hansard 21/3/06, column 262w). Other initiatives included the Blueprint programme, introduced in 2004. This multicomponent drugs education programme was tested in over 20 secondary schools. The key features of the school-based part of the programme include a two-year curriculum, training for teachers, interactive lessons and high-quality teaching materials. Other components included parental involvement and information, coordination with other agencies' activities (such as PCTs and DATs), a health policy component (to raise awareness of drug education among health professionals and link with local enforcement strategies on underage sales of alcohol and volatile substances) and relationships with local media to raise wider awareness of the initiative in the community. The Blueprint programme was viewed positively by parents and children and appeared to increase knowledge about drugs (Home Office, 2009). However, pupil drug use (and smoking and drinking) increased with age in participating schools. Unfortunately, the design of the programme did not allow for effective assessment, as it failed to allow for an accurate comparison of participating and non-participating schools. Another programme, Positive Futures, was introduced as a means of reducing antisocial behaviour, crime and drug abuse among young people in areas worst affected by these problems. The programme funded over 100 projects that provide sport and leisure activities, delivered by charities, clubs and local authorities. These projects are credited with preventing problems among marginalized young people (Crabbe, 2006).

With regard to enforcement, the Labour government downgraded the classification of cannabis to a class C drug (a decision later reversed – see below) while increasing penalties for drug dealers. The focus on supply was maintained by commitments to maintain and extend enforcement, particularly with regard to recovering drug-related assets, disrupting local supply and international cooperation to prevent production and trafficking. In 2004, police acquired new powers to close so-called 'crack houses' – premises used to produce and supply class A drugs, causing nuisance and disorder to local neighbourhoods.

The new strategy heralded further developments in the treatment of offenders. The drug interventions programme was introduced in England and Wales in 2003 bringing together police, courts, prison service, probation service, treatment providers and DATs to improve rehabilitation and reintegration of offenders. As noted, drug testing and assessment was introduced for some offenders. New powers were introduced to impose drug abstinence requirements, drug rehabilitation requirements and bail restrictions in order to promote compliance with treatment. For less serious cases, offenders would now receive a conditional caution, requiring them to attend sessions with drug workers as an alternative to prosecution. Another innovation was specialized drug courts, piloted in some areas, which deal with offenders who have problems and can give sentences requiring treatment and rehabilitation.

The new strategy led to changes in targets (see Exhibit 14.1). Ten key targets were identified, covering similar areas as before, but with less emphasis on quantitative measures. Notably, an ambitious target to halve heroin and cocaine use among young people by 2008 was dropped. The targets were altered again in 2004 and in 2006. A key change was the introduction of a drug harm index to integrate various targets in one measure. Although this explicitly gave weight to harm reduction, by including a range of indicators relating to crime and health, it did not capture all adverse effects of drugs, only those that the government wished to include (MacDonald et al., 2005). The index excluded important areas of impact such as work productivity, parenting/family, homelessness, and unemployment. This index was contentious because it relied on estimates, such as the amount of crime related to drugs, that depended on certain assumptions. A further element of subjectivity related to the weightings of each element in the index, which reflected value judgements about the relative importance of different harms and social costs (Mowoombe, 2000).

Exhibit 14.1

Drug Policy Targets (2006)

1 To reduce the harm caused by illegal drugs as measured by the drug harm index by 2007/8 (from 2002 baseline) including to substantially increase the number of drug-misusing offenders entering treatment through the criminal justice system (from a 2004 baseline of 700).

2 To increase the participation of problem drug users in drug treatment programmes by 100 per cent (by 2008) from 1998/9 baseline of 100,000) and increase year on year the proportion of users successfully sustaining or completing treatment programmes.

3 To reduce the use of class A drugs among the under-25s (from a baseline of 8.6 per cent of 16–24s in 1998 and 2.4 per cent of 11–15s), and reduce frequent use of illicit drugs among all under-25s (2002 baseline) and 'vulnerable' under-25s (2003/4 baseline).

In 2007, a new PSA delivery agreement was introduced. Of the five indicators identified, three related to drugs:

● the number of drug users recorded as being in effective treatment

● the rate of drug-related offending

● the percentage of the public who perceive drug use or dealing as a problem in their area

---

A further ten-year drug strategy was subsequently introduced by the Brown government (HM Government, 2008c). This aimed to protect communities through enforcement to tackle supply, drug-related crime and antisocial behaviour; prevent harm to children, young people and families; and deliver new approaches to drug treatment and social reintegration. The strategy championed a family-centred approach, in an effort to break the cycle of drug use and other problems passing between generations. It emphasized early prevention, focusing on children and families before problems arose. The role of other addictions, such as alcohol and volatile substances, was acknowledged. The strategy echoed earlier policies by encouraging joined-up working between relevant agencies, including improvements in information sharing. It continued to support public information campaigns and education about drugs. The strategy emphasized targeting resources where benefits would be maximized – by concentrating on effective interventions and those most at risk. A new theme was that users must take more responsibility to engage in treatment. If necessary, the welfare benefits system should be used to incentivize drug users into treatment. The strategy promised proposals to create personalized support for people undergoing and completing drug treatment, including pilot schemes for individual budgets for those successfully completing treatment, enabling them to access housing, education and training.

The drug strategy dovetailed with other initiatives, notably the Children's Plan (see Chapter 9). The Children's Plan contained a commitment to review the effectiveness of drug and alcohol education. This review recommended increasing parents' and carers' knowledge and skills about drug and alcohol education so that they were better able to inform and protect their children; improve the quality of drug and alcohol education by making PSHE a statutory subject under the national curriculum; to improve training for teachers; and improve identification and support for young people who are vulnerable to drug misuse (Advisory Group on Drug and Alcohol Education, 2008).

Drug Policies in Other Parts of the UK

Devolution enabled each part of the UK to develop its own distinctive approach, within a UK-wide policy framework. The Scottish government (2008a) pledged to tackle problem drug use through policies on the economy, poverty, and support for families and children; a new approach to drugs education targeted at parents and grandparents; and improvements in drug treatment services, particularly for prisoners. Wales combined alcohol and drugs within its substance misuse strategy (NAfW, 2000b; Welsh Assembly Government, 2008b). This strategy identified four main areas for action: prevention, targeting efforts on children and young people and involving parents and carers more in prevention activity; supporting substance misusers, with more investment in outreach services and expansion of harm-reduction services and more effective commissioning of services; supporting families, to reduce the risk to children and adults as a result of substance abuse; and protecting communities by, for example, law enforcement. The strategy for Northern Ireland also combined efforts to tackle alcohol and drug harm (DHSSPS, 2006c). It set out a range of priorities including improvements in drug and alcohol education, efforts to reduce antisocial behaviour related to alcohol and drugs, and the development of a regional commissioning framework for services.

Further Developments

Further developments in drug policy were heralded by the Cameron government. Amid media concern about the availability and dangers of 'legal high' party drugs, the Conservative–Liberal programme stated that it would introduce a system of temporary bans while health issues were being considered by independent experts. It was made clear that a substance would not be permanently banned without full advice from the ACMD. In 2010, the Brown government had introduced a ban on the legal high, mephedrone. The Cameron government followed this with a ban on naphyrone. Both are now class B drugs. The coalition government also announced a consultation on drug policies, promising a new strategy by the end of 2010. Its programme pledged to tackle drug smuggling. It also stated that it would ensure that sentencing for drug use helped offenders to come off drugs, while exploring the possibilities for secure treatment-based accommodation for drug offenders. In a further move, the Cameron government announced its intention to abolish the NTA, transferring its functions to the newly proposed public health service.

The Impact of Policy

It is difficult to measure the impact of drug policies, not least because targets and measures have constantly changed. Nonetheless, some success is evident. In England, the drug harm index rose between 1998 and 2001, then fell between 2002 and 2005, to 17 per cent below its 1998 level (Goodwin, 2007). With regard to specific harms, the initial targets to reduce levels of reoffending by drug users could not be accurately measured. The Labour government claimed a 20 per cent fall in acquisitive crime related to drugs (HM Government, 2008c). It is difficult to say whether drug-related crime rates have declined because many crimes such as fraud, violence and vice are excluded from these figures. Moreover, other factors (the economy, regeneration, policing, criminal justice reforms) may have had more effect on these figures than the drug strategy. Disappointingly, the drug interventions programme had mixed results. Although crime committed by those on the programme fell by 26 per cent overall, over a quarter of those participating showed a sharp increase in their volume of offending (NAO, 2010a). Meanwhile, drug-related deaths rose 10 per cent between 1998 and 2005 (which, as already noted, is likely to be an underestimate of their actual level).

With regard to lifetime use, the proportion of 16–24 year olds in England and Wales reporting using any drug decreased from 54 per cent to 45 per cent between 1998 and 2006/7 (NHS Information Centre, 2008b). Those reporting use in the past year declined from 32 per cent to 24 per cent, while past-month use fell from 21 per cent to 14 per cent. This was reflected in the use of specific drugs. Those reporting cannabis use in the past year fell from 28 per cent to 21 per cent, amphetamines from 10 per cent to less than 4 per cent, and LSD from 3.2 per cent to less than one per cent. Reported class A drug use fell only slightly (from 8.6 per cent to 8 per cent) as did reported use of ecstasy (5.1 per cent to 4.8 per cent). However, the percentage of young adults admitting to cocaine use in the past year doubled (3.2 per cent to 6.1 per cent between 1998 and 2006/7), leading some to call for tougher enforcement (Home Affairs Committee, 2010). Heroin use increased sharply between 1998 and 2000 (0.3 per cent to 0.8 per cent) before falling (to 0.2 per cent by 2007). Among school-children in England, rates of self-reported drug use in the past month decreased between 2001 and 2007 from 12 per cent to 10 per cent. Reported drug use in the previous year fell from 20 per cent to 17 per cent (NHS Information Centre, 2008b). Class A drug use among schoolchildren fell slightly (4.3 per cent to 4.0 per cent in reported past year use) while cocaine use increased. Cannabis use in the previous year fell from 13 per cent to 9 per cent between 2001 and 2007.

There are huge difficulties in measuring the impact of policy on the supply of drugs. However, street prices are regarded as a good indicator. It appears that between 2000 and 2005, the price of heroin fell by almost a fifth, cocaine prices by a third, and ecstasy and cannabis prices by two-thirds between 1994 and 2005 (Owen, 2006). This suggests that supply is not being significantly disrupted by enforcement authorities. The UK enforcement agency, SOCA, claimed that recent efforts to block supplies led to rising wholesale prices of cocaine (*Guardian*, 2009), but this is not likely to be sustainable as suppliers redouble their efforts to meet demand. Moreover, in the short term, high wholesale prices may have serious adverse effects on health as drug dealers increasingly dilute their products with contaminants.

The target to double the number of people in drug treatment was achieved in 2004/5, two years ahead of schedule. However, this is a crude measure. There is double counting due to people dropping out and later re-entering treatment (although the Labour government's target to increase the proportion of drug users sustaining or completing treatment year on year was achieved for the period 2002–6). Also the measure does not indicate the quality or appropriateness of treatment.

Criticism of Government Policies

Government policies have been criticized by several external policy reviews (RSA Commission, 2007; Police Foundation, 2000; Reuter and Stevens, 2007; Home Affairs Select Committee, 2002, 2010; Science and Technology Committee, 2006) and by its own policy advisors (Prime Minister's Strategy Unit, 2003a; ACMD, 2006a). The main criticisms are that current policies do not fully address the problem of drug abuse, place too great an emphasis on crime reduction and prohibition rather than harm reduction, are not sufficiently evidence-based, and do not take into account the harms associated with legal addictions such as alcohol and tobacco. Further problems include implementation, poor coordination between agencies, and shortcomings in the accessibility and quality of services. Some critics also point out that the current approach is expensive and wasteful and that regulation rather than prohibition of drugs is a more cost-effective policy (Transform Drug Policy Foundation, 2009). Others assess the underlying reasons why policies suffer from such shortcomings, acknowledging that the media have exerted much influence over the agenda and that politicians fear being seen as soft on drugs (Critchley, 2008; Monaghan, 2008b).

There has been particular criticism of drugs law and enforcement. Government has faced pressure to overhaul the system of drugs classification. The existing system has been criticized for failing to reflect the relative harm associated with different drugs (The Police Foundation, 2000; Science and Technology Committee, 2006; Reuter and Stevens, 2007; RSA Commission, 2007; Nutt et al., 2007; UK Drug Policy Commission, 2009; Levitt et al., 2006). Some drugs, it is argued, such as cannabis, LSD and ecstasy, do not warrant being placed in higher categories. Meanwhile, alcohol and tobacco, which cause much harm (see Chapter 15) are not covered by drug legislation. Initially, the Blair government responded to these concerns by tinkering with the system. Cannabis was reclassified as a class C drug in 2004. However, evidence about the effects of more potent varieties of the drug (Di Forti et al., 2009), led to its being reinstated as a class B drug in 2008. This decision went against the advice of the Advisory Committee on the Misuse of Drugs and occurred in the context of falling levels of cannabis use among young people (ACMD, 2006b). Subsequently, ACMD's (2009) advice to reclassify ecstasy as a class B (from class A) drug was also rejected. Later, in 2009, the Home Secretary sacked the chair of the ACMD, Professor Nutt, following his public comments that cannabis should not have been elevated to class B and that alcohol and tobacco were relatively more harmful than cannabis, ecstasy and LSD.

A similarly confused approach is evident in law enforcement. Many critics believe that excessive resources are allocated to low-level drug offences, such as the possession of class B and C drugs, particularly cannabis (Newcombe, 2007). In 2001/2, the police in Lambeth relaxed law enforcement on cannabis possession for personal use. This experiment was successful in enabling the police to target suppliers, particularly of class A drugs. Nationally, following the downgrade of cannabis to class C, penalties for possession were reduced. The maximum penalties for possession were restored following the reversal of this policy. The reclassification of cannabis was accompanied by a new 'escalation' penalty system for adults to punish repeat offending. First-time offenders receive a warning, with subsequent offences punishable by penalty notices, caution and then prosecution. A similar escalator system already in place for under-18s – reprimand, final warning and charge – has been retained. Meanwhile, the therapeutic uses of cannabis have been explored (see Exhibit 14.2).

Exhibit 14.2

Cannabis Therapy

Cannabis has been used for therapeutic purposes. Its use in pain relief and to alleviate symptoms of some neurological diseases, in particular MS, was employed as an argument for decriminalization. In addition, there were calls to explore the efficacy of cannabis-based medicines as a step towards licensing them as prescription drugs (see BMA, 1997; House of Lords, 1998b, 2001b). Initially, GPs were permitted to prescribe a cannabis-based mouth spray (Sativex). UK drug regulators allowed the drug to be imported from Canada, where it was licensed in 2005. In 2010, Sativex was finally licensed by the UK authorities, opening the way for it to be more widely prescribed. However, NICE has not yet ruled on the drug's cost-effectiveness. This means that local NHS bodies remain reluctant to fund the treatment and that most patients will have to pay privately for the drug, thereby restricting its availability.

Drug education has attracted criticism. Successive governments have placed faith in educational campaigns and programmes, resulting in increased activity. By 2004, four-fifths of primary schools had a drug education policy (compared with two-fifths in 1997). Among secondary schools, 90 per cent also had such policies (compared with less than 75 per cent in 1997) (Ofsted, 2005b). Ofsted found that planning and provision of drugs education had improved. However, it concluded that the quality of policies and provision varied widely and that the lack of specialist subject teachers was a particular problem (see also Advisory Group on Drug and Alcohol Education, 2008).

Governments have funded mass media campaigns, such as those on heroin in the 1980s and 90s and more recently the multimedia Frank campaign. After three years, the Frank campaign had achieved recognition among a majority of young people (68 per cent were aware when prompted, 39 per cent unprompted), and its website had over 3.5 million hits in the six months to March 2006 (Home Office et al., 2006). However, the number of referrals from Frank to local treatment services (10,893) and the number of interactive calls with young people (9,909) fell considerably short of their targets (18,000 and 15,000 respectively).

There is little to suggest that drug education and campaigns alone are effective in reducing drug use (McInnes and Barrett, 2007; ACMD, 2006a; Reuter and Stevens, 2007). However, the evidence base is poor, with many programmes being inadequately evaluated. The available evidence suggests that some programmes increase awareness of drug issues and increase the life skills of children and young people. They may reduce harm by delaying the onset of drug use or the escalation of drug use. But there appears to be no long-term benefit from such programmes in preventing drug use. Some may be counterproductive, particularly programmes that use shock and scare tactics.

Lack of proven effectiveness has not stopped governments from backing educational initiatives. Although expensive, educational programmes have obvious political benefits, reassuring parents and the public that something is being done. Similar reasons may explain the growing interest of politicians in zero tolerance school policies, the use of drug testing and sniffer dogs. Yet these are problematic in terms of criminalization, possible injustice, social exclusion and infringement of human rights, while having no significant impact on drug use (McKeganey, 2005; Reuter and Stevens, 2007; ACMD, 2006a).

A further area of criticism relates to treatment. Although there is much support for recent policies to encourage treatment, there is disquiet that policy is dominated by criminal justice priorities (McSweeney, 2007; Reuter and Stevens, 2007). Community sentencing with requirements for testing and treatment has had limited success (NAO, 2004c, 2010; Hough et al., 2003). Arrest referral schemes can improve access to treatment and reduce reoffending, but do not reach all who need help (including the most vulnerable) (Crowther-Dowey, 2007). Increased powers to test offenders and require drugs assessment have been criticized as ineffective and wasteful (RSA Commission, 2007).

The availability of treatment remains a problem, particularly in some parts of the country and for those who have not committed offences (RSA Commission, 2007). The NTA was created to oversee and improve drug treatment programmes. Capacity has increased since, reflected in increases in numbers treated, although the quality of services is variable (Reuter and Stevens, 2007). Drop out rates continue to be high, however (NAO, 2010a), reflecting a need for better support and follow-on services, as well as more flexible and responsive services. In this context, NICE (see for example NICE 2007a, b and c) has issued guidance on the effectiveness of treatment in this field, including guidance on community-based interventions to reduce substance abuse among vulnerable and disadvantaged young people; treatment guidelines for people receiving opioid detoxification; and psychosocial interventions for drug misusers. Some critics of policy, however, believe that too many resources have been allocated to treatment and that more should be done to prevent addiction and enforce drug laws more effectively (Gyngell, 2009).

Others have proposed more radical measures to treat drug addicts and reduce harm associated with illegal drugs, particularly heroin. One idea is to make drugs more available to addicts on prescription. Methadone (a heroin substitute) has been used for a number of years in an attempt to wean addicts off heroin (Farrell et al., 1994). Although successful to some extent in reducing heroin use, harm and crime (Webster, 2007; Bennett and Holloway, 2005), methadone has adverse consequences, including overdoses, accidental poisonings (including children), and deaths (Newcombe, 1996; Dalrymple, 2003). Heroin (and cocaine) can also be prescribed to addicts, although this is exceptional, requiring a Home Office licence. The Home Affairs Committee (2002) supported moves to expand heroin prescribing, providing that this was done in a carefully controlled way. Another idea is to provide 'drug consumption rooms' (DCRs) for heroin (or cocaine) addicts, where drugs may be taken in a safe and hygienic environment (Reuter and Stevens, 2007; Independent Working Group on Drug Consumption Rooms, 2006). This gives access to basic facilities, support and advice, which may further prevent harm. DCRs have been credited with decreasing drug-related illness and death, reducing public nuisance arising from injecting in public, and lowering risks to the public from discarded needles. In some schemes, drugs are also provided. Here, there may be reduced incentives for addicts to engage in crime to fund their habit, and a reduction in demand for illegal drugs supplied by criminals. DCRs have been used in Norway, Germany, Holland and Switzerland, among others. However, they are controversial and have been labelled by their critics as 'shooting galleries' or 'drug dens', encouraging drug taking. Such schemes are also likely to face opposition from local residents. However, if these areas are already frequented by addicts and dealers, the local community may actually suffer fewer problems from the introduction of DCRs.

Another area of criticism is the lack of aftercare and community-based facilities for drug users. The Home Affairs Committee (2002) found that GPs were not adequately trained to deal with addiction. It also noted that there was little interest in addictions within general practice and that many drug users lacked access to primary care facilities. Others have found that GPs are unwilling to provide treatment for drug addicts (RSA Commission, 2007). Yet primary care has an essential role in providing initial help for people with addictions and in managing patients in community settings.

Other Countries' Approaches

Some countries take a hard line approach, dominated by an authoritarian criminal justice perspective. This involves severe legal penalties for drug trafficking, dealing and possession. Huge resources are allocated to law enforcement and to disrupt the supply chain. Little distinction is made between soft and hard drugs, the former seen as a gateway to the latter. Education and information policies emphasize abstinence from drugs and use shock tactics to deter potential users. Care and treatment policies tend to be linked to the criminal justice system. Although drug addicts are often helped, the emphasis is on criminal rehabilitation rather than harm reduction.

The above describes the approach pursued by the USA, at least until recently (see Wisotsky, 1986; Epstein, 1977). During the 1970s, the federal government under President Nixon declared a 'War on Drugs'. This policy was reiterated in the 1980s under President Reagan, supplemented with prohibitionist educational campaigns promoting a 'Just Say No' message. Moves towards a treatment and health-oriented approach in the late 1980s, and efforts by some states to decriminalize cannabis possession, were reversed in 1989 with the appointment of a drugs czar who explicitly favoured supply-side control policies. More recently, the pendulum has swung back towards a more compassionate approach (such as drug courts and extended treatment facilities), although the emphasis remains on treatment sanctioned by the criminal justice system. However, there is considerable variation between states. Some take a more liberal approach than others, with a number (including Oregon, Massachusetts and California) pursuing policies to decriminalize soft drugs or reduce penalties for possession.

The shortcomings of the prohibitionist approach are well documented (see Mishan, 1990). It criminalizes those who experiment with drugs, perhaps increasing the likelihood that they will become more marginalized and try harder drugs. It makes the drugs trade extremely profitable as shortages raise prices. It gives greater incentives for dealers to adulterate drugs – creating further health problems. Prohibition creates a greater role for organized crime, which has wider social consequences in terms of gang warfare and links with other 'rackets' such as vice and people trafficking. The war on drugs is expensive and absorbs resources that could be used to treat addicts and prevent drug abuse. It is relatively ineffective: drug abuse rates in the US, for example, are relatively high compared with other countries (UNODC, 2008).

Some countries have pursued a more liberal policy aimed at minimizing harm. The Netherlands is the classic example (see Spruit, 1998). In the mid-1970s, the Dutch government policy distinguished sharply between hard and soft drugs. While legal penalties remained, suppliers and users of cannabis were not prosecuted, providing they obeyed certain guidelines. Hence coffee shops were allowed to sell cannabis, providing they did not supply hard drugs, refused to sell to those under 18 years of age, kept limited stocks, sold only small quantities, and did not cause a public nuisance. Meanwhile, drugs such as heroin faced a stricter regime in terms of penalties and law enforcement, although even here the main emphasis was upon harm reduction. For example, drug addicts who were repeatedly arrested were offered treatment options as an alternative to long prison sentences.

Dutch policy became more restrictive during the second half of the 1990s when measures were introduced to limit the number of coffee houses and to reduce the amount of cannabis that could be sold to each customer. This resulted from both internal and external pressures. After initially declining, cannabis use increased in Holland from the mid-1980s. However, this was in line with many other countries and did not appear to result from decriminalization. Indeed, comparative studies found that decriminalization of cannabis does not increase prevalence (MacCoun and Reuter, 2001; Reinarman et al., 2004). Within Holland, there was concern about nuisance caused by coffee houses and by drug tourism. It was claimed that the liberality of the Dutch drug laws attracted drug users from other countries. The Dutch government was also under pressure from other countries, particularly EU member states, concerned about the implications for the abolition of border controls. They argued that if the Dutch did not impose further restrictions, they would be unable to prevent drugs being imported into their own countries. At the time of writing, the Dutch government is considering proposals to further restrict the supply of cannabis by coffee houses to tourists.

Domestic drug policies do not operate in a vacuum but are influenced by other countries' experiences. Hence some of the language of the 'War on Drugs' in the USA was imported into the UK, which for a brief period appointed its own drug czar. But other, more liberal US approaches, such as drug courts for example, have also been adopted. At the same time, the Dutch case and other countries' experiences with decriminalization led to pressures in the UK to relax the regulation of cannabis, although, as noted, this was later reversed.

International Policies

The global market for illicit drugs has been estimated at $400 billion per annum, making it one of largest industries in the world (UNDCP, 1998). Around 185 million people worldwide use illicit drugs (WHO, 2009c). Drug control is a matter for several global institutions, which set the context for EU and national policies. The UN has been the main source of global initiatives in this field. The UN Commission on Narcotic Drugs (CND) was established in 1946 as the central policymaking body of the UN on drug issues. It develops proposals to combat drug abuse and implements UN conventions and protocols, such as the Single Convention on Narcotic Drugs (1961 – amended by the 1972 protocol on drugs), the Convention on Psychotropic Substances (1971), and the Convention Against the Illicit Traffic in Narcotic Drugs and Psychotropic Substances (1988). An International Narcotics Control Board (INCB), a quasi-judicial body, promotes compliance with international agreements and identifies weaknesses in current arrangements.

Dissatisfaction with the existing drug control system led to the UN Drug Control Programme (UNDCP) in 1990. A global action programme was launched in the same year with the aim of reducing drug use and harm. The UN designated the 1990s as the Decade Against Drug Abuse. UN initiatives have been developed in conjunction with WHO (the Global Initiative on Primary Prevention of Substance Abuse, for example, is a joint WHO/UNDCP initiative). In addition, WHO has an advisory role in relation to the UNDCP and runs its own programme to promote health by preventing and reducing the adverse consequences of substance use. The common themes of both UN and WHO initiatives in this field are to promote global cooperation on drug issues, to promote partnerships at all levels and to mobilize communities against the consequences of drug abuse. However, a review of the UNDCP found evidence of poor coordination between UN agencies, a need for greater cooperation between the UNDCP and INCB, confusion about the role of CND, and inadequate funding for the drug control programme (UN Commission for Narcotic Drugs, 1999). Efforts were already underway to address this. The UNDP merged with the Centre for International Crime Prevention to form the UN Office on Drugs and Crime in 1997. A new political declaration on drugs was adopted by the UN General Assembly in 1998. This called for greater efforts to reduce drug demand and supply through international cooperation, treatment and rehabilitation, education and information, elimination of illicit crops, action on synthetic stimulants (such as ecstasy), and to tackle criminal and terrorist networks involved in illicit drug production and supply.

The EU has adopted anti-drug policies. In 1990, the first European action plan on drugs was devised, followed by initiatives to combat drug money laundering. In 1993, the European Monitoring Centre for Drugs and Drug Addiction (EMCDDA) was established to provide evidence and information for decision makers. The EU has since promoted research on illicit drugs to improve the evidence base. The Maastricht Treaty of 1992 explicitly referred to the problem of drug addiction. It was followed by a further drug action plan in 1994, covering the next five years. This aimed to encourage cooperation between organizations in member states, to encourage research and dissemination of information about drugs, and to improve health education and training in this field. EU states also agreed to approximate their laws on drug control laws and cooperate more closely to combat drug trafficking. A commitment to joint action was reiterated by the Amsterdam Treaty of 1997, which specifically mentioned the need to complement member states' action to reduce drug-related damage.

A further five-year action plan on drugs was subsequently launched (Commission of the European Communities, 1999). It aimed to substantially reduce levels of drug use, particularly among those under 18; reduce drug-related health damage and deaths; increase the number of successfully treated addicts; reduce the availability of illicit drugs; reduce the number of drug related crimes; and reduce money laundering and illegal trafficking of precursors (chemicals used in the manufacture of illicit drugs). Despite these aspirations, the plan did not achieve its objectives on drug prevalence or availability (Commission of the European Communities, 2004b). Some improvements in drug-related health harms and treatment were achieved, however. Other measures included additional funding for drug prevention projects, joint action on synthetic drugs, minimum provisions on drug-related criminal acts and penalties for drug trafficking and joint efforts to counter trafficking and money laundering.

A strategy for 2005–12 was subsequently introduced (Council of European Union, 2004), which provided a framework for two consecutive action plans (for 2005–8 and 2009–12). These set out a range of objectives with targets to improve coordination, reduce demand and reduce supply. A new coordinating mechanism was introduced (the European Council High level Working Group on Drugs). Specific priorities were identified to reduce demand, including improving access and effectiveness of programmes to prevent drug use, early intervention measures especially for young people, targeted and diverse treatment programmes and services to prevent drug-related diseases. With regard to supply, the key priorities were to strengthen EU law enforcement, prevent import and export of illicit drugs, intensify cooperation on enforcement between member states, and bolster law enforcement efforts in drug producing countries.

The EU continues to promote cooperation between member states on drug issues. It works with other international bodies on drug strategy and policy, such as the UNDCP, and regional institutions such as ASEAN (the Association of South East Asian Nations) and the Pompidou group (the Cooperation Group to Combat Drug Abuse and Illicit Trafficking in Drugs – which operates under the auspices of the Council of Europe and includes both EU and non-EU European countries). Improving international cooperation on drugs has been a key theme of EU strategies. For example, the most recent strategy was committed to 'coordinated, effective and more visible action by the Union in international organizations and fora enhancing and promoting a balanced approach to the drugs problem' (Council of the European Union, 2004, p. 17). It also pledged to assist non-EU countries, including producer and transit countries, to be more effective in reducing drug supply and demand.

Conclusion

The problems associated with drugs are intractable. As Gossop (1996) has observed, every society has its own particular drugs, and campaigns to rid society of drugs entirely are futile. He argued that we must learn to live with drugs, seeking to reduce their harms, rather than simply prohibiting them. Successive governments have attempted to deal with the illicit drug misuse by controlling supply and encouraging abstinence. These policies have been strongly driven by criminal justice perspectives and priorities, co-existing with a medical model of treatment for addicts. The main emphasis of policy has been upon prohibition and punishment of offenders, although harm reduction and prevention of illness have been influential, particularly in recent years. Although drugs policy has had some success, as indicated by reductions in some drug use, increase in treatment 'throughput' and a decline in some indicators of harm, the impact on public health and wellbeing in a broader sense is less clear. UK drug use is relatively high compared with mid-twentieth-century standards and in comparison with similar countries today.

What more could be done? A further shift away from prohibition towards regulation has been advocated. This may well be more cost-effective, freeing up resources for initiatives to prevent and treat drug addiction. But this is opposed by those who want stricter enforcement (Gyngell, 2009). Substantial decriminalization of drug use is a leap in the dark. No one really knows what might happen and the ramifications of an increase in drug problems are such that no politician is ever likely to take the risk. The best that can be hoped for is a more effective balance of policies that reflects risks of harm and where availability is controlled alongside high-quality health promotion and treatment services. The contents of this policy package must be based on evidence and experimentation, rather than knee-jerk reaction. It must include policies, however unpalatable to the media and sections of public opinion, that can reduce harm, such as DCRs and a risk-based drug classification system. Finally, it must incorporate the whole range of addictions, legal and illegal, substance-based and non-substance-based (such as gambling, for example) and seek to address the circumstances and reasons why people indulge in such activities.

Alcohol and Tobacco 15

It is often agreed that the consequences of legal substances such as alcohol and tobacco receive less attention than illicit drugs. Governments have often been accused of not giving sufficient priority to these 'legal addictions'. In recent decades, however, the impact of alcohol and tobacco has been taken more seriously. This chapter explores the extent of alcohol- and tobacco-related problems and the responses of policymakers.

Tobacco

The appeal of tobacco has varied since it was introduced to Britain during the sixteenth century. Its popularity increased sharply in the early twentieth century, reaching a peak in the 1950s, when around three-quarters of the male population and 40 per cent of women smoked. Although smoking declined in the second half of the century – to less than a third of the adult population by the late 1990s – it remained popular among some groups. By 2007, 21 per cent of adults in England aged 16 and over smoked (NHS Information Centre, 2009b). Among children aged 11–15 years, 6 per cent claim to smoke at least once a week, with girls more likely than boys to smoke regularly. Smoking is slightly more common among men (22 per cent) than women (19 per cent), and is higher in routine and manual groups (26 per cent) than in professional and managerial groups (15 per cent). It is more popular among some ethnic groups (Black Caribbean people, Irish people, Pakistani and Bangladeshi men) than in others. There are regional variations, smoking prevalence being significantly higher than average in northern England and in Scotland than elsewhere in Britain.

The Health Risks of Smoking

In 2007, over 100,000 deaths in the UK – a fifth of the total – were related to smoking (Allender et al., 2009). About half of regular smokers will die from the habit, and lifelong smokers die on average ten years younger than non-smokers (Doll et al., 2004). Smoking is associated with many diseases (NHS Information Centre, 2009b) including cancers (lung, mouth, pharynx, oesophagus, trachea, bronchus, larynx, stomach, pancreas, cervix, kidney and leukaemia), respiratory diseases (including chronic obstructive pulmonary disease, bronchitis and emphysema) and cardiovascular diseases (such as stroke and heart disease). Smoking may also be linked to breast and bowel cancers (Reynolds et al., 2004; Botteri et al., 2008). Smokers are at greater risk from a range of other medical conditions including stomach and duodenal ulcers, psoriasis, Crohn's disease, cataracts, blindness and impaired vision, and hip fracture. Smoking is also linked to male impotence, impairment of male and female fertility, low birthweight, miscarriages, stillbirths and cot deaths (BMA, 2004b). Smoking is a major cause of morbidity, responsible for over 440,000 hospital admissions each year in England among adults aged 35 and over, accounting for 5 per cent of all hospital admissions for this age group (NHS Information Centre, 2009b). The cost of smoking to the NHS has been estimated at £5.2 billion per annum (Allender et al., 2009). The total lifetime health costs saved by smoking cessation have been estimated at €24,800 for a 35-year-old man and €34,100 for a 35-year-old woman (Rasmussen et al., 2005).

The health consequences of smoking have been evident for almost as long as the habit has been practised. In the seventeenth century, initial enthusiasm among the medical profession for tobacco as a panacea gave way to concern about its adverse effects (Harrison, 1986). Medical opinion hardened further following King James I's 'Counterblaste to Tobacco' in 1604 (King James I, 1616), which vilified smoking as 'loathsome to the eye, hateful to the nose, harmful to the brain, dangerous to the lungs'. This early anti-smoking campaign was accompanied by higher taxes on tobacco and the introduction of licensing (see Harrison, 1986). Such measures were, however, less draconian than those in some other countries. For example, in seventeenth-century Russia, smokers were mutilated and purveyors of tobacco flogged to death (Skrabanek, 1994; Corti, 1931). Despite restrictions, smoking flourished and governments became highly dependent on the tobacco trade. Tobacco raised vital tax revenues and generated other economic benefits such as export revenues, jobs and profits. Although its harmful effects were known, the trade was rarely challenged. Indeed, when new epidemiological evidence about smoking became available in the second half of the twentieth century, it took decades to persuade policymakers to address the problem seriously (see Pollock, 1999; Berridge, 2007).

During the 1950s, the British government privately acknowledged new evidence linking tobacco smoking to lung cancer and other diseases (Doll and Hill, 1950, 1956). In 1953, an official committee suggested that there was a causal association between smoking and cancer of the lung (Pollock, 1999), although its advice to ministers was toned down. Concerns about implications of anti-smoking policies for employment, exports and tax revenues led to a cautious approach. Ministers emphasized uncertainties surrounding the link between smoking and lung cancer and called for more research. By 1956, following pressure from Parliament, the government publicly acknowledged a causal connection between smoking and lung cancer. However, tensions within government were evident when the Chancellor of the Exchequer let it slip that 'we at the Treasury do not want too many people to stop smoking' (*Hansard*, 1957). Following a Medical Research Council report in 1957, calls for a substantial health education campaign and a ban on tobacco advertising were rejected. Pressures continued during the early 1960s, following a landmark report from the Royal College of Physicians (RCP) (1962), which summarized the compelling evidence on smoking and ill health. Subsequently, a small health education campaign was launched and, following a change of government, a ban on TV advertising of cigarettes was imposed in 1965. Efforts by backbench MPs to extend this ban to all forms of tobacco advertising were blocked by the government and MPs sympathetic to the tobacco industry.

A second RCP (1971) report on smoking was published, and a pressure group, Action on Smoking and Health (ASH), formed. While the RCP operated chiefly through elite medico-political networks, ASH was a high-profile, media-oriented campaigning organization (Popham, 1981). Despite overwhelming evidence linking smoking and ill health, the UK government would not adopt policies – such as higher taxation, comprehensive advertising bans, and bans on smoking in public places – advocated by the anti-smoking lobby (Taylor, 1984). Throughout the 1970s, attempts by backbench MPs to legislate were frustrated by tobacco industry lobbying. The industry had allies within Whitehall too. The Treasury, Trade, Industry and Employment departments all opposed further restrictions on smoking. Instead of legislation, voluntary agreements were introduced on tobacco advertising and sponsorship, health warnings and tar levels. These were periodically renegotiated, usually in response to some new revelation about the health risks of tobacco (Royal College of Physicians, 1977, 1983). The agreements were heavily criticized by anti-smoking campaigners, who saw them as an opportunity for the tobacco industry to buy time in order to diversify into other non-tobacco product areas (including, ironically, life insurance), produce 'low-tar' tobacco products and market their products more aggressively to Third World countries. Consequently, smoking rates in developing countries increased. Today about half the 5.4 million deaths from tobacco occur in the developing world and it is expected that by 2030 over 80 per cent of tobacco-related deaths will be in these countries (WHO, 2008d).

Smoking Policy in the 1980s and 90s

During the 1980s, the anti-smoking campaign was reinforced by the BMA (1986), which launched a high-profile attack on government and the tobacco industry. Even so, the prospects of a comprehensive ban on tobacco advertising receded in the context of the Thatcher government's anti-interventionist, pro-business approach. Nonetheless, the Thatcher government did raise tobacco taxes and increased resources for anti-smoking education programmes. It was also forced to adopt stronger health warnings on tobacco products, as a result of a European directive in 1989. Subsequently, the Major government adopted explicit targets for reducing smoking in its *Health of the Nation* strategy (Cm 1986, 1992). It aimed to cut the death rate from lung cancer by at least 30 per cent in men under 75, and 15 per cent in women under 75 by the year 2010 (using 1990 as a baseline); to reduce the prevalence of cigarette smoking in men and women aged 16 or over to no more than 20 per cent by the year 2000; to reduce the consumption of cigarettes by 40 per cent by the year 2000; to ensure that at least a third of women smokers stopped smoking at the start of their pregnancy; and to reduce smoking prevalence among 11–15 year olds by a third.

These targets proved difficult to achieve and, in the case of smoking among teenage girls, the trend actually moved in the opposite direction. The Major government committed funds to an anti-smoking advertising campaign and pledged to increase tobacco taxes by 3 per cent above the rate of inflation each year. However, anti-smoking campaigners believed that stronger policies were necessary, particularly with regard to the promotion of tobacco products. The UK policy on tobacco promotion was weak compared with the approach taken by some countries. In Norway, a comprehensive advertising ban was imposed in 1975. Others, such as France, Canada, Australia and New Zealand, followed suit. Research into the effects of tobacco advertising bans (DoH, 1992) demonstrated their effectiveness in reducing smoking. However, throughout the 1990s supporters of such a ban were frustrated by the government's reluctance to confront the tobacco lobby. Instead, another set of voluntary agreements was negotiated, including a reduction in shopfront advertising, stronger health warnings on advertisements and a ban on advertisements in teenage magazines.

The White Paper on Smoking

The Blair government adopted a more robust policy than its predecessor (Cairney, 2007a; Amos, 2007). The level of priority was indicated in a white paper, *Smoking Kills* (Cm 4177, 1998). The main targets of this strategy were to reduce smoking among schoolchildren from 13 per cent to 9 per cent or less by 2010; to cut adult smoking from 28 per cent to 24 per cent; and to reduce the percentage of women smoking during pregnancy from 23 per cent to 15 per cent by the year 2010. New commitments included plans to raise tobacco tax above inflation; better law enforcement on tobacco sales to children; additional funds for services helping people to stop smoking; wider access to nicotine replacement therapies; a new health education campaign on smoking; a ban on tobacco advertising; and efforts to reduce exposure to environmental tobacco smoke. These policies were extended by further commitments in the NHS Plan (Cm 4818, 2000) and the *Choosing Health* white paper (Cm 6374, 2004), discussed below. The government aimed to reduce the higher smoking prevalence among routine and manual groups to 26 per cent or less by 2010. In 2007, a more stringent overall target was set to reduce adult smoking prevalence to 21 per cent or less by 2010. In order to drive forward implementation, these targets were incorporated in NHS planning and priority statements.

Price and Taxation

Increasing the price of tobacco through taxation is regarded as one of the most effective instruments for reducing tobacco use (WHO, 2008d). It has been estimated that in industrialized and higher income countries such as the UK a 10 per cent price rise is associated with a 4 per cent fall in consumption (Jha and Chaloupka, 1999). Following *Smoking Kills*, tobacco taxation increased substantially. Between 1996 and 2008, rates of duty increased by almost 70 per cent. As a result, tobacco prices increased at more than twice the average rate of inflation and became less affordable in real terms (NHS Information Centre, 2009b). Indeed, tobacco was 14.5 per cent less affordable in 2008 than in 1980.

Although tax is an effective instrument, some argue that it does not take into account the circumstances of people on low incomes. As Graham (1993) and Dorsett and Marsh (1998) have shown, poorer people find it more difficult to stop smoking. Raising the price of cigarettes may increase hardship as they spend more of their small income on tobacco to maintain consumption levels (Marsh and McKay, 1994). However, other researchers have shown that poorer socioeconomic groups and young people are actually more responsive to increases in price (Ogilvie et al., 2005; Townsend et al., 1994; Joossens and Raw, 2006). The impact of higher prices and taxes is reduced by the relaxation of border controls, which has encouraged legitimate cross-border purchasing as well as illegal smuggling of tobacco. The illegal trade in tobacco is big business (Joosens and Raw, 2000). Around a fifth of tobacco consumed in the UK is smuggled (Health Committee, 2009). It is the poorest that are most likely to use illicit tobacco. According to West et al. (2008), the availability of cheap tobacco through smuggling may be responsible for as many as 6500 deaths annually in the UK. The government has tried to reduce the illegal trade in tobacco and stepped up enforcement (HM Treasury, 2006b). In 2008, responsibility for controlling smuggling passed to the new UK Border Agency. However, more could be done, including signing up to legally binding EU agreements with tobacco companies (involving fines on companies for failure to control smuggling) to strengthen control over production and distribution, thereby reducing the opportunities for illicit trading (Health Committee, 2009). It should be noted that in the past, UK tobacco companies have been complicit in illicit trading, although no charges have ever been brought against them (Lee and Collin, 2006).

Restrictions on Availability

Additional restrictions have been imposed on sales of tobacco products. In 2007, the legal minimum age for purchasing tobacco in England, Scotland and Wales was raised to 18 years. In some countries, the minimum age has been raised even higher. In most Canadian provinces, where the legal age for purchasing tobacco is 19, smoking rates among 18-year-olds are lower than the national average. Evidence suggests that, although raising the legal age can reduce access to tobacco, enforcement is crucial to the success of such measures (Sundh and Hagquist, 2006; Ahmad and Billimek, 2007; Tutt et al., 2009). Without high compliance from retailers, it is difficult to reduce access (Stead and Lancaster, 2005). In 2006, almost two-thirds of underage smokers in England said that they obtained their cigarettes from shops. Only 52 per cent were refused on at least one occasion (although this was an improvement on 1990, when 37 per cent were refused purchases). This perhaps reflects improved enforcement, in particular the introduction of test purchasing of retailers and a new protocol to promote consistency in law enforcement by local authorities. Even so, retailers continue to break the law, with one in five retailers in England failing test purchases (LACORS, 2008a). From 2009, new on the spot fines were introduced for retailers caught selling tobacco to under-18s and those persistently doing this will face tobacco banning orders, which prohibit their selling tobacco.

Health campaigners called for new restrictions to prevent access to vending machines by children and young people (BMA, 2007b). A voluntary code was agreed between government and cigarette machine operators concerning the siting and supervision of such machines. However, this was ineffective in preventing access by children and young people (DoH, 2008e). Consequently a statutory ban on tobacco vending machines was introduced in the UK, to be implemented in October 2011. Also included in this legislation were powers to ban the display of tobacco products at point of sale, to be phased in between 2011 and 2013. This has also been recommended by anti-smoking groups (see BMA, 2007b).

Some have called for a licensing system for tobacco retailers. A system of tobacco licensing was abandoned some years ago as it proved uneconomic. Such a system might be useful in ensuring higher standards of retailing with regard to sales to minors. However, as the experience of alcohol licensing has shown (see below), licensing systems are ineffective without adequate enforcement. Arguments for a new licensing system have not so far been accepted by the UK government, although the Scottish government is introducing a new registration scheme for retailers.

Advertising and Promotion

Advertising and promotion bans can prevent the onset of smoking and help people to stop (WHO, 2008d; Jha and Chaloupka, 1999). They may also help to prevent the normalization of smoking and bolster health warnings. In the light of evidence that comprehensive tobacco bans reduce consumption (Saffer and Chaloupka, 2000), anti-smoking campaigners pressed for further restrictions on advertising and promotion. In 1997, the Blair government pledged to ban tobacco advertising, reflecting a commitment in the Labour party manifesto. Meanwhile, an EU directive in the following year sought to phase out tobacco advertising and sponsorship by 2006. The Blair government was criticized for supporting moves to give certain international events, such as Formula One motor racing, more time to comply with the provisions of the directive. It was later revealed that funds had been donated to the Labour party by Bernie Ecclestone, a businessman and the vice president of Formula One's governing body. Ecclestone and the Labour party denied this was an attempt to influence the UK government's position on tobacco advertising and promotion. The donation was later returned. Subsequently, the tobacco industry successfully appealed to the European Court of Justice against the EU directive. Although fresh legislation was brought forward, this was more limited than the original directive. To fulfil its manifesto commitment, the Blair government banned press and billboard advertising of tobacco products following the passage of the Tobacco Advertising and Promotion Act 2002. It also acquired new legal powers to regulate internet advertising, point of sale advertising and brand-sharing (where non-tobacco products are marketed using tobacco branding and logos). Sponsorship by tobacco companies in the UK was also banned by this legislation.

Health Warnings and Education

In the 1970s, health warnings were included on tobacco packaging and later on advertisements. Larger, more explicit and specific warnings about the dangers of smoking were introduced in the 1990s, required by EU directives. More recently, a new range of health warnings on tobacco packaging was introduced, again prompted by the EU. In 2003, larger and more prominent warning messages were introduced. From 2009, cigarette packets must now include pictorial images of smoking-related harm, an approach used previously in other countries including Australia, Canada and Brazil. There is evidence that stronger warnings discourage smoking (Givel, 2007; Willemson, 2005).

Health education has been expanded. In England, for example, the Department of Health budget for advertising expenditure on tobacco control increased from £6 million to £25 million between 1999/2000 and 2004/5 (*Hansard*, 2006). Health education media campaigns have become more sophisticated. Rather than simply informing the public of the dangers of smoking, these campaigns now aim to persuade people to give up their habit. Sometimes this involves using 'shock' images, including a campaign in 2004 that showed fat oozing out of a cigarette to illustrate the effects of smoking on the cardiovascular system. Another, in 2007, depicted smokers being pierced through the mouth by giant fishhooks to illustrate their addiction to cigarettes. (This campaign was later adjudged to have broken the advertising standards rules by causing distress to children!) Alongside negative messages, anti-tobacco advertisements are now more often linked to positive help with addiction, such as smoking cessation services, discussed below. There has also been a greater effort to understand the context and motivations of the target audience and to tailor messages to particular social groups (parents, pregnant women, routine and manual workers).

The evidence on the effectiveness of health education on smoking is mixed. This is partly because there are many different ways of delivering health education and various target audiences, some of whom are more resistant to messages than others. There is evidence that mass media campaigns can influence smoking behaviour in young people, although much depends on the intensity and duration of the messages and on the design of the programme (Sowden and Arblaster, 1998). The use of 'tailored messages' and of media appropriate to the target population is recommended. Although mass media campaigns get most attention, health education is also provided as part of broader health promotion activities in a variety of settings. For example, health promotion about smoking occurs in schools (see Chapter 9). It appears that these achieve only limited success, with social reinforcement programmes being more effective than knowledge-based interventions (NHS Centre for Reviews and Dissemination, 1999). Community-based approaches using different intervention components (mass media, school-based health promotion and community action) have been shown to be effective in reducing smoking among young people (Sowden et al., 2003). Moreover, it is acknowledged that health promotion about smoking aimed at young people must be based on a better understanding of their culture and identity (Denscombe, 2001a, 2001b). Health promotion can also happen in workplaces (see Chapter 10 and NICE, 2007d) and in the wider community. Smoking-related health promotion is also undertaken by NHS organizations and professionals, discussed further, in the context of NHS smoking cessation services, below.

NHS Advice and Smoking Cessation Services

Nicotine is a highly addictive substance (Royal College of Physicians, 2002). People often need help to overcome their addiction. This can take a number of forms, including advice from a primary health care professional, such as a GP, pharmacist, dentist, nurse, health visitor or midwife. Although brief advice is regarded as effective (NICE, 2006d; Silagy et al., 2004; Rice and Stead, 2004), opportunities through contact with patients are not fully exploited (BMA, 2007b). Efforts to encourage such activities included bringing smoking cessation within the quality and outcomes framework for GPs, (although it has been argued that more weight should be given to incentives to help patients stop smoking rather than simply recording smoking status). Other initiatives have encouraged professionals to target advice on specific groups, such as pregnant women or schoolchildren.

Alongside conventional channels of professional advice, there is a new set of specialist services, specifically aimed at helping people stop smoking. These services developed out of smoking cessation services established by health action zones (HAZs, see Chapter 7) and other partnerships established in the 1990s. They now constitute a nationwide service. Specific services include group and individual support for self-help and pharmacological therapies (such as nicotine replacement therapies, now available on prescription and in some cases over the counter). In 2008/9, almost 700,000 people in England used NHS Stop Smoking Services, half of whom stopped smoking for at least four weeks (NHS Information Centre, 2009b). Smoking cessation services are regarded as highly cost-effective in terms of lives saved and future health costs (Godfrey et al., 2005), although the longer term effectiveness of these interventions is likely to be less, as many smokers resume their habit (Wanless, 2004; Milne, 2005). Indeed, some are critical of smoking cessation services for using resources that could be more effectively spent on preventing smoking through health promotion and regulation. Some have noted that most smokers quit alone, without the assistance of support services (Chapman, 2009).

There is scope for improvement. Disadvantaged areas have been targeted by NHS smoking cessation services (Chesterman et al., 2005) and PCTs' performance in deprived areas has been adjudged as better than those in more affluent areas (Healthcare Commission, 2007b). Even so, smoking cessation services have less success in reducing smoking rates among routine and manual workers and other vulnerable groups such as pregnant women, compared with other social groups (NICE, 2008e; BMA, 2007b). Moreover, these services have not so far targeted underage smokers; surprising given the additional benefits of stopping smoking at a younger age (Denscombe, 2007; Bokoh et al., 2007). NICE (2008e) published comprehensive guidance on comprehensive smoking cessation services. It recommended that smoking cessation services target minority ethnic and socioeconomically disadvantaged groups in the population. It pointed out that some groups, notably pregnant women in routine and manual groups and those under 20 years of age, may need additional support to give up smoking. The Healthcare Commission (2007b) also identified room for improvement, particularly with regard to collecting data on local tobacco use, service usage and effectiveness, improving local partnership working, and continuing to place high priority on smoking cessation and tobacco control.

Increasingly, there is an emphasis on comprehensive, multi-agency approaches to tobacco control. This covers a range of activities such as smoking cessation services, smokefree environments, underage sales and providing health promotion about smoking. To improve partnerships, central government encouraged the formation of tobacco control alliances between different local agencies (such as local government, the NHS and the voluntary sector). Some of these originated from the healthy alliances established by the Major government in the 1990s, others from the HAZs established by the Blair government. In 2000, funds were allocated by the NHS Cancer Plan to promote tobacco control alliances. These have since been encouraged by strategic health authorities and government regional offices, which established regional tobacco control offices to coordinate and support local alliances.

European and International Action

The UK has one of the strongest anti-tobacco policies among comparable countries (Joossens and Raw, 2006). However, domestic policy has developed in the context of efforts at the European and international level to reduce smoking. In the 1980s and 90s, when UK policy was relatively weak, the European Community began to take an interest in preventing tobacco-related illness as part of its programme on cancer prevention. It promoted stronger health warnings on tobacco products, set a maximum tar level for cigarettes, and sought restrictions on advertising and sponsorship. After 2000, the EU introduced stronger health warnings, reduced tar, nicotine and carbon monoxide content, and banned misleading descriptions such as low tar, mild and light cigarettes (European Parliament and Council of the European Union, 2001, 2003). In 2007, the European Commission introduced a green paper on smokefree environments to encourage a comprehensive ban on smoking in public places (European Commission, Health and Consumer Directorate-General, 2007). It also proposed raising the taxation on cigarettes across Europe. Even so, the EU has often faced both ways on the tobacco issue, reflected in the granting of subsidies to tobacco producers.

On a global level, WHO has introduced strategies and action plans on tobacco (see WHO, 1996, 1997b; WHO Regional Office for Europe, 1993d).

Until recently this posed little threat to the tobacco trade. WHO relied mainly on persuading member states to adopt stronger policies. But tobacco control now has a much higher priority. In the late 1990s, the World Bank shifted its policy away from supporting the tobacco trade towards tobacco control (although other international trade bodies, such as the IMF, continued to promote the tobacco trade – Gilmore et al., 2009). WHO launched its Tobacco Free Initiative, to promote more effective global controls, including the development of an international framework for tobacco control. This has now come to fruition with the formulation of the Framework Convention on Tobacco Control (FCTC) (WHO, 2003). The FCTC is wide-ranging and covers issues such as a price and tax measures, tobacco advertising and sponsorship, regulation of content of tobacco products, packaging and labelling, health education, passive smoking and smoking cessation as well as reducing the availability of tobacco products (including sales to minors and illicit trade in tobacco). The UK ratified the treaty in 2004 and 168 countries have now signed up. However, the extent to which this new global initiative will succeed against continued opposition from the powerful tobacco industry and its allies remains to be seen.

Tobacco Industry

The tobacco industry has fought doggedly against anti-smoking policies. It had much success in the early years, persuading governments that anti-smoking policies were unpopular, undermined personal freedom, reduced tax revenues, and damaged employment (Taylor, 1984). The tobacco industry was supported by others, such as the advertising industry. It also received support from sport and art organizations dependent on tobacco sponsorship. The tobacco industry remains a powerful political player. It continues to seek to dilute policies at national and international levels. The industry's methods have been revealed by internal documents, some leaked, others disclosed through the legal process (Glantz et al., 1996). For example, the industry mounted a sustained campaign against the European Community's tobacco advertising legislation in the 1990s, exerting influence at the highest level, especially in the UK and German governments, the main opponents of the directive (Neuman et al., 2002). The industry mobilized strongly against the World Bank's shift in policy against the tobacco trade and the introduction of the FCTC (Mamudu et al., 2008; Assunta and Chapman, 2006). Tobacco companies paid lobbyists to try to block and reverse these policies in both international and domestic policy arenas.

Since the 1990s, the industry has been subject to litigation from individuals with smoking-related illnesses and from states seeking to recoup medical expenses (Orey, 1999). Most cases have centred on allegations that tobacco companies knowingly sold a product injurious to health and conspired to conceal the facts. Cases have also been brought against employers for illnesses caused or exacerbated by passive smoking. For anti-smoking campaigners, litigation has brought two main benefits. It has had financial implications as the industry has been forced to settle compensation claims. Meanwhile, passive smoking judgments have encouraged the development of no-smoking environments, which have implications for the industry's sales and profitability (see Exhibit 15.1).

Tobacco companies have responded by diversifying into different product lines (providing scope for cross-branding) and expanding markets in countries where regulation is weak. They have tried to improve their image by openly admitting that tobacco is addictive and harmful to health. They have also adopted corporate social responsibility policies, much to the disgust of anti-smoking campaigners who point to the industry's appalling track record (Chapman, 2007). The ethical inconsistency between the tobacco industry's CSR aspirations and the differential standards of consumer protection it pursues in different countries has been noted (Nuffield Council on Bioethics, 2007).

Exhibit 15.1

Passive Smoking and Smoking Bans

The emergence of evidence about the dangers of breathing in external tobacco smoke (ETS) provided a powerful argument for banning smoking in public places (Nuffield Council on Bioethics, 2007; Chapman, 2007). Studies in the 1990s found that passive smoking was linked to a range of diseases including lung cancer, heart disease, respiratory disease, sudden infant death syndrome and ear infections (US Department of Health and Human Services, 1986; US Environmental Protection Agency, 1992; UK Scientific Committee on Tobacco and Health, 1998; Boffeta et al., 1998; Law et al., 1997; He et al., 1999). Reviews of the evidence (International Agency for the Research on Cancer, 2002b; UK Scientific Committee on Tobacco and Health, 2004; Royal College of Physicians, 2005b) found that the risk of lung cancer and heart disease in non-smokers exposed to ETS increased by around a quarter. Further research suggested the increased risks of heart disease were even higher, at 50–60 per cent (Whincup et al., 2004). Meanwhile, it was estimated that in the UK passive smoking in the workplace was responsible for over 600 deaths per annum. A further 10,700 deaths were due to passive smoking at home (Jamrozik, 2005). However, it is difficult to isolate the effect of passive smoking as people encounter tobacco smoke in a wide range of settings over a long period of time. Moreover, the presence of other carcinogens in the environment, such as radon, complicates matters further (Nilsson, 1999). Evidence linking passive smoking to increased risk of ill health has been challenged (Booker and North, 2007; Enstrom and Kabat, 2003).

Initially, governments responded to this evidence cautiously. The Major government produced a voluntary code of practice on smoking in public places and guidance on how to address passive smoking in the workplace. Initially the Blair government appeared willing to consider banning smoking in all public places, including pubs and restaurants. However, after discussions with businesses, it adopted an approach not dissimilar to its predecessor. A charter was introduced to encourage establishments to introduce their own measures to improve indoor air quality, including, for example, the use of more efficient ventilation systems. The government sought to persuade employers to voluntarily impose smoking bans at work through a code of practice.

This voluntary approach was superseded by legislation. Bans on smoking in public places across the UK were introduced, beginning with Scotland in 2006 (England, Wales and Northern Ireland followed suit in 2007). This occurred partly because of new evidence about the impact of passive smoking, mentioned above. A crucial factor was the experience of countries that had already banned smoking in public places (the Irish Republic, US states such as Montana, California and New York, Thailand, and some Canadian and Australian states) (see, for example, Allwright et al., 2005; Juster et al., 2007; Sargent et al., 2004). Evidence from these jurisdictions indicated that a smoking ban could reduce smoking and ill health. Early evidence from the UK bans confirms this. In Scotland, exposure to ETS among non-smokers from non-smoking households fell almost 50 per cent, and there was a smaller but statistically non-significant fall in exposure of non-smokers from smoking households of 16 per cent (Haw and Gruer, 2007). Children were also less exposed to tobacco smoke (Akhtar et al., 2007) following the ban. In addition, the number of admissions for acute coronary syndrome fell by 17 per cent in the 10 months following the ban compared with a 4 per cent decline in England in the same period and a 3 per cent annual average decrease in Scotland in the previous decade (Pell et al., 2008). Following the English ban, there was a small but significant reduction (2.4 per cent) in hospital admissions for heart attack (Sims, et al., 2010). The UK data forms part of a growing evidence base that suggests that smoking bans reduce deaths from cardiovascular disease due to passive smoking (Institute of Medicine, 2009).

The anti-smoking lobby (comprising medical organizations, health research charities, anti-smoking pressure groups and public health groups) campaigned vociferously for smoking bans. Scotland, using its devolved powers, was able to bring in legislation first, showing that a ban was politically feasible. Notably, this legislation was intro-duced in a much more favourable political context. Scotland faced a higher level of smoking-related illness, there was strong leadership from politicians, a cross-party consensus, and a weaker pro-smoking lobby (Donnelly and Whittle, 2008; Cairney, 2007b). The momentum of the Scottish decision led other parts of the UK to introduce their own proposals. In England, a hasty compromise was reached to satisfy the tobacco industry and the licensed trade, by excluding pubs and bars that did not serve food and private membership clubs from their initial proposals. This went against the strong advice of the Chief Medical Officer (who considered resigning over the issue) and the Health and Safety Commission. Following a highly critical report from the Health Committee (2005b), which recommended a comprehensive ban including licensed premises, and a groundswell of support for this option among MPs, the government was forced to retreat. One of the key arguments against a partial ban was that it would have less effect on smoking in poorer and less healthy areas (where most pubs, bars and clubs would be exempt from the ban because they didn't serve food)

(Health Committee, 2005b; Woodall et al., 2005; Tocque et al., 2005). Another crucial factor was the hospitality industry, which became increasingly concerned about the inconsistencies of a partial ban and the risk of legal action from staff exposed to ETS. In the end, very few exemptions to the ban were granted (including prisons, mental hospitals, private hotel rooms, residential care homes and hospices). There was concern that the ban would be flouted, but this was not confirmed by enforcement agencies, which found high levels of compliance. Indeed, four out of five people in Britain supported it (NHS Information Centre, 2009b).

Further Developments

UK tobacco policy has developed considerably in recent years, with a favourable international context, coherent policy direction and additional resources from central government. There has also been increased local activity, extended service provision and improved partnership working. Smoking rates have declined, but continued implementation is needed to maintain this momentum. More needs to be done to reduce smoking among young people, pregnant women, routine and manual workers, and minority ethnic groups as well as vulnerable groups such as prisoners and homeless people (BMA, 2007b). In 2010, the Brown government set out further proposals to reduce smoking (HM Government, 2010b). It aimed to reduce the smoking rate among 11–15 year olds to one per cent or less, and the rate among 16–17 year olds to 8 per cent by 2020. Another aim was to reduce adult smoking rates to 10 per cent or less by 2020, while halving smoking rates for pregnant women, routine and manual groups and people in disadvantaged areas. A further target was to increase by 2020 the proportion of homes where parents smoke but which are entirely smokefree indoors. In order to achieve these aims, the Brown government stated that it would make tobacco less affordable through duties and by preventing illicit trade in cigarettes, and ensure that advertising of tobacco accessories is not being used to encourage tobacco use. It pledged to implement the bans in tobacco vending machines and point of sale displays. The government also said it would review current restrictions on retail of tobacco to children and young people. It stated that it would encourage research into links between tobacco packaging and smoking, which could lead to tobacco products being sold in plain packaging. Further marketing campaigns to help people to quit were promised alongside a radical approach to stopping smoking, with more routes to support people who cannot give up abruptly, including extending the availability of nicotine delivery products. In addition, the government promised to promote smokefree communities, focusing on the most disadvantaged communities, and to review whether further action was needed to extend smokefree legislation to other areas.

Despite its achievements, the anti-smoking lobby is constantly vigilant about the tobacco industry and its political influence. Although many legislative changes have been introduced on the 'policy wish list' of the anti-smoking lobby (Chapman, 2007), further policy options include the establishment of a nicotine regulatory authority for the UK with jurisdiction over tobacco products and nicotine delivery products to ensure coherent regulation of this addiction (Royal College of Physicians, 2002), or alternatively, a tobacco regulatory authority (Health Committee, 2000) to regulate the introduction of lower-risk tobacco products. Other ideas include coordinated increases in tobacco taxes, ring-fencing of tobacco taxation for anti-smoking policies and a positive licensing scheme for tobacco (BMA, 2007b), as well as greater efforts to tackle illicit trade and illegal sales (Health Committee, 2009). Other legislative restrictions might include restrictions on smoking in cars, in the home or outdoor environments (Royal College of Physicians, 2010).

At the time of writing, however, there is concern that the advances made in smoking policy over the previous decade may be coming to a halt. The Cameron government imposed a freeze on mass media health campaigns, including smoking, reduced the size of the smoking policy team in the DoH and the regions, and decided not to review or extend the smoking ban. In addition, it hesitated over the implementation of bans on tobacco displays and vending machines, enacted by the previous government (Aveyard et al., 2010).

Alcohol

Alcohol is a popular and legally available drug. Unlike tobacco, alcohol consumed in moderation and in a socially responsible manner can confer net benefits for individual health and social wellbeing (Edwards, 2003; Academy of Medical Sciences, 2004). Alcohol is consumed by the vast majority (around 90 per cent) of the UK adult population. However, alcohol can have adverse consequences, including:

- *Health and illness*. The number of deaths directly linked to alcohol in England doubled between 1991 and 2005, reaching over 6500 in 2006 (NHS Information Centre, 2009c). As many as 22,000 deaths per year, however, could be attributable to alcohol (Prime Minister's Strategy Unit, 2003b), and the overall figure could be even higher (Health Committee, 2010). Specifically, there have been significant increases in death rates from particular diseases, such as chronic liver disease (a 466 per cent increase in adults aged 25–64 between 1970 and 2000 – Academy of Medical Sciences, 2004). In 2007/8, there were over 860,000 hospital admissions related to alcohol in England, two-thirds more than in 2002/3

(NHS Information Centre, 2009c). Around 7 per cent of the adult population are believed to be dependent on alcohol (Academy of Medical Sciences, 2004). The consequences of drinking in pregnancy are also of concern with the identification of foetal alcohol spectrum disorders, associated with learning and physical disabilities and behavioural problems (BMA, 2008).

- *Crime and public order.* Over half the victims of violent crime believed their attackers were under the influence of alcohol (NHS Information Centre, 2008c). A third of domestic violence incidents may be alcohol-related (Prime Minister's Strategy Unit 2003b). Alcohol is a factor in 30 per cent of sexual offences and a third of burglaries (POST, 2005). Drunkenness convictions, however, have declined (from over 100,000 annually in the 1980s), partly due to the introduction of fixed penalty fines for some drunkenness offences in 2004 and also to changes in policing practices.

- *The welfare of children and young people.* Although the percentage of school-children reporting never having drunk alcohol has risen in recent years, from 39 per cent to 46 per cent between 2001 and 2007, one in five 11–15 year olds report drinking alcohol in the previous week (NHS Information Centre, 2009c). In 2007, the average consumption of those who did drink was 12.7 units per week (see Exhibit 4.1). A quarter of 11–15 year olds stated that they believed that it was 'okay' for someone of their age to get drunk. Campaigns to tackle underage drinking have found that almost 40 per cent of premises targeted served alcohol to minors (Home Office, 2007). Alcohol also impacts on family life, with an estimated 780,000 to 1.3 million children affected by parental alcohol problems (Prime Minister's Strategy Unit, 2003b).

- *Productivity.* Alcohol is linked to absenteeism and reduced work performance. Approximately 17 million working days are lost through alcohol-related absence every year (Prime Minister's Strategy Unit 2003b).

- *Sexual health.* Alcohol has been associated with sexual health problems such as teenage pregnancy and sexually transmitted infections (see Independent Advisory Group on Sexual Health and HIV, 2007).

- *Accidents.* Drink-driving causes over 500 deaths and around 15,000 injuries every year in Great Britain. Although the number of drink-driving deaths has fallen since the 1960s, there was an increase between 2000 and 2005. Alcohol is also implicated in other accidents such as fires, falls and drownings (Institute for Alcohol Studies, 2009).

Alcohol problems are linked to overall levels of consumption (Academy of Medical Sciences, 2004; Babor et al., 2003). The annual level of consumption per capita in 2009 was over two and a half times that of 1950, at 9.5

litres of pure alcohol. Official figures, which exclude smuggled goods and alcohol brought in legitimately by travellers, underestimate consumption. The true level may be 20 per cent higher (Academy of Medical Sciences, 2004). The culture of drinking is also a factor in alcohol-related problems. Binge drinking is a feature of northern European drinking cultures, especially among younger people (POST, 2005). Although definitions vary, binge drinking essentially refers to excessive drinking in a short period of time (a common definition is double the daily maximum recommended levels – 8 units for men and 6 for women – on any one day). Current estimates indicate that a quarter of men and 16 per cent of women binge drink according to this definition (NHS Information Centre, 2009c), and that 41 per cent of men and 34 per cent of women exceed the maximum daily recommended levels (4 units of alcohol for men, 3 for women). In addition, around a third of men and a fifth of women report drinking above weekly maximum recommended levels (21 units for men, 14 for women). Also 9 per cent of men and 6 per cent of women consume at over 50 and 35 units a week respectively (NHS Information Centre, 2009c). UK alcohol consumption and problems have increased relative to other industrialized countries. Although UK consumption levels are close to the EU average of 13 litres of pure alcohol per person per annum (after adding in estimates of unrecorded consumption – see above) (Anderson and Baumberg, 2006), chronic liver disease is falling in most European countries, while rising in the UK (Academy of Medical Sciences, 2004).

Alcohol and Policies

The health and social problems associated with alcohol are centuries old (Barr, 1995), while legislation restricting alcohol dates back to the fifteenth century (Plant and Plant, 2006). A complex array of regulation, including laws, taxes and enforcement practices, has since developed. This has been punctuated by periods of crisis where alcohol has been regarded as a major threat to society, the most prominent of these being the Gin Epidemic of the eighteenth century, the Victorian and Edwardian temperance campaign against the 'evils of drink', and the restriction of alcohol during the First World War (see Abel, 2001; Greenaway, 2003). Closer to modern times, alcohol has once again become a prominent public policy issue (Baggott, 1990; Plant and Plant, 2006). Rising alcohol consumption and problems in the 1960s and 70s led to concerns among key professional groups – in health, social work, police and criminal justice. These professionals, along with voluntary organizations in the alcohol field, became the vanguard of the new anti-alcohol lobby, filling the gap left by the decline in the temperance movement. The 'discovery' of alcohol problems by the media helped propel the issue onto the political agenda. Government was drawn into the fray, with ministers from both parties taking a special interest, notably Sir Keith Joseph (who facilitated an extension of services for people with alcohol problems) and Barbara Castle (who introduced the breathalyser to combat drink-driving).

Although central government began to address alcohol problems during the 1970s and 80s, bureaucratic, interest group, electoral and ideological factors inhibited its response. Central government bureaucracies, organized on departmental lines, were in conflict over how to respond. Departments sponsoring trade and commercial interests (Ministry of Agriculture, Fisheries and Food and the Department of Trade) took a different view from those dealing with alcohol problems (such as the Home Office and Department of Health and Social Security). Despite a commitment to devise an alcohol strategy, departments could not agree on the way forward. The task of developing a joined-up approach fell to a cross-government think tank, the Central Policy Review Staff (CPRS). It called for a comprehensive government strategy on alcohol aimed at preventing further increases in alcohol consumption and in the longer term reducing it. It also urged alcohol taxes to at least maintain the real price of alcohol; to maintain existing licensing laws and enforce them; to implement further restrictions on drink-driving; and ensure that advertising and the media should reinforce moderate drinking habits. The UK government refused to publish the CPRS report, but it was later leaked, spurring further media coverage of the issue (CPRS, 1982).

The UK government was unwilling to adopt the CPRS recommendations, largely because it would offend the drinks industry. The industry was a major contributor to the economy, a key source of tax revenues, a substantial exporter, and a significant source of employment. Indeed, the drinks industry had important allies in the form of trade unions, which opposed measures that might adversely affect employment. The economic leverage of the industry was combined with strong political connections (especially with the Conservative party) and had direct links with Parliament (through MPs' consultancies, directorships and shareholdings). It also engaged extensively with government departments on a range of issues affecting its business.

The industry was able to block policies, such as the use of taxation and legislation to restrict price and availability. It was successful in persuading government to approach alcohol misuse as an individual rather than a social issue, focusing on symptoms of alcohol-related illness and disorder rather than on preventing problems through population-wide policies to control overall alcohol consumption. Another factor was that politicians of all parties feared a public backlash if they intervened too strongly in regulating alcohol consumption. They were worried about accusations of introducing a nanny state. Although politicians of all parties weighed these considerations carefully, such fears were particularly strong among neoliberal Conservatives who dominated the policy process in the 1980s.

Thatcherism and Alcohol

The Thatcher government did publish a policy document on alcohol, entitled *Drinking Sensibly* (DHSS, 1981b). It was a pale shadow of the CPRS report and provided a stark illustration of industry influence and political weakness. *Drinking Sensibly* did not support the use of taxation as an explicit instrument of policy, refused to control overall consumption, and emphasized the importance of the alcohol industry to the economy. Minor concessions to the alcohol misuse lobby included a modification of alcohol advertising practices and a programme of health education. The document stated that the government had no plans to relax the licensing laws, although backbenchers were encouraged to introduce legislation on this topic throughout the 1980s (Baggott, 1990).

During the late 1980s, problems associated with alcohol misuse were increasingly highlighted by professional groups including doctors, police and criminal justice organizations. The media also gave increasing coverage to alcohol problems, notably public disorder, highlighting the impact of so called 'lager louts'. The government responded by relaxing licensing hours in 1988. However, at the same time it created a ministerial committee on alcohol abuse to devise an overall strategy and to coordinate action across government. The committee endorsed proposals to discourage underage drinking and alcohol-related disorder, review alcohol advertising codes of practice, promote health education and information about alcohol, and combat drinking and driving.

Alcohol and the Major Government

Under the Major government, alcohol became part of a broader public health strategy. Targets to reduce excessive drinking by 30 per cent in men and women (but not to reduce overall levels of consumption as recommended by the WHO Regional Office for Europe, 1985) were included as 'risk factors' in the *Health of the Nation* strategy (Cm 1986, 1992). Nonetheless, even these targets were not met (women's alcohol consumption actually increased). To make matters worse, the government relaxed the sensible drinking recommendations that formed the basis of these targets, a move heavily criticized by alcohol agencies, doctors and WHO.

During the mid-1990s, there was increasing anxiety about alcopops – heavily marketed and attractively packaged fruit-flavoured alcoholic drinks – which some believed were deliberately aimed at children and young people. This was strenuously denied by the drinks industry. However, these drinks appealed to young people and were associated with excessive drinking and drunkenness (McKeganey et al., 1996; Hughes et al., 1997). Following pressure from professional groups, voluntary organizations and the Labour opposition, the Major government increased excise duty on these products. In an effort to avert a government ban on alcopops, the drinks producers' social responsibility organization, the Portman Group, drew up a voluntary code of practice on the naming, packaging and merchandizing of alcoholic drinks.

Alcohol and the Blair and Brown Governments

Although the Labour government initially promised an alcohol strategy (Cm 3852, 1998), this was not forthcoming. Instead, following advice from the Better Regulation Task Force and lobbying from the drinks industry, the leisure and tourism industries and some local authorities, the government decided to reform the licensing laws. The Licensing Act 2003 established a new system of licensing in England and Wales that brought together previous regimes for alcohol, public entertainment and late-night refreshment. Although the new Act contained new measures to regulate premises, persons selling alcohol, and alcohol availability (including new powers for police to close premises), it allowed premises to apply for longer opening hours, up to 24 hours a day.

The legislation was opposed by a coalition of groups concerned that increased availability of alcohol would produce more problems. Supporters argued that the measures would actually reduce alcohol problems by bringing about a more relaxed continental drinking culture. There was, however, little public controversy at this stage. It was only when the government began to implement the changes, amid increased media coverage of alcohol problems (and, in particular, binge drinking), that opposition to the changes began to mount (Plant and Plant, 2006). Police chiefs and local authorities (which had previously expressed support for the changes) publicly criticized the reforms. Meanwhile, criticism intensified from doctors, health professional organizations and voluntary organizations.

The Blair government responded by resurrecting its earlier commitment to an alcohol strategy. The Prime Minister's Strategy Unit was given the task of reviewing the evidence on the extent of the problem and the policy options. Its interim report estimated the overall costs of alcohol misuse at around £20 billion per annum and catalogued the range of problems related to alcohol (Prime Minister's Strategy Unit, 2003b). However, it was criticized by campaigners against alcohol misuse for overemphasizing the benefits of alcohol consumption, and for downplaying the link between the price and availability of alcohol, overall consumption and the level of problems. Subsequently the Prime Minister's Strategy Unit (2004) produced a final report, which the government adopted as its alcohol strategy for England (other parts of the UK developed their own approaches – see below). The strategy placed emphasis on providing information about alcohol to individuals, promoting changes in drinking cultures and improving services for people with drink problems, reducing crime and disorder, and working with industry to reduce alcohol problems. The strategy did not adopt measures to regulate the availability of alcohol, such as price controls, higher taxes or reducing licensed outlets or drinking hours, despite evidence that such measures could be effective in reducing alcohol consumption and harm (Babor et al., 2003; Edwards et al., 1994).

The alcohol strategy proposals included 'improved and better targeted education and communication' about alcohol (Prime Minister's Strategy Unit, 2004). A new social marketing campaign was promised, to make the sensible drinking message easier to understand and apply and to target campaigns at those most at risk. The 'Know Your Limits' campaign was launched in 2006, aimed primarily at 18–24 year olds. It used TV advertisements and other promotional materials and established a new website. In 2008, this was followed up by two TV advertising campaigns at a total cost of £10 million. The first aimed to inform people about the unit levels of alcohol drinks, the second to discourage binge drinking among young people.

The Blair government pledged improvements in services for people with alcohol problems. It promised new pilot programmes to establish the efficacy of early identification and treatment services; an audit of alcohol treatment and aftercare as a basis for improving services; and improvements in commissioning and monitoring standards in this field. Commitments were made to improve services for vulnerable groups by commissioning integrated care pathways for people with drug problems, homeless people, young people and those with mental illness. However, alcohol early intervention and treatment services are under-resourced and have a low priority within the NHS (NAO, 2008b).

The Labour government's strategy gave a substantial role to the Portman Group. This body coordinated drink industry activities on alcohol education and harm prevention and operated a self-regulatory scheme on marketing alcoholic drinks (Baggott, 2006). The Portman Group has been heavily criticized by campaigners against alcohol misuse for being a lobbyist for the industry, although it vigorously denies this (Coussins, 2004). Some alcohol researchers are concerned that the Portman Group has sought to influence research agendas and thereby the evidence base (Edwards et al., 2004). They were deeply critical of a decision in 2004 to appoint the then chief executive of the Portman Group to the governing body of the Alcohol Education and Research Council, which disburses funds for research and educational projects (Mayor, 2004).

The emphasis on working with the drinks industry led to the development of various self-regulatory and voluntary schemes. National social responsibility standards were drawn up, covering issues such as sensible drinking, underage drinking, and alcohol marketing. Concerns that the national standards and other industry codes would not reduce bad practices were later found to be justified (Baggott, 2006). A review of standards found that commercial imperatives dominated, there was little enforcement or monitoring of standards, and no evidence that they improved practice or reduced alcohol-related harm (KPMG, 2008).

The government drew up an agreement with the industry on labelling. Some producers and retailers had already placed sensible drinking messages on containers, advertising and at point of sale. In 2007, the industry agreed to place information on containers, including alcohol unit guidelines, sensible drinking messages and health warnings about drinking in pregnancy. When this was audited (CCFRAG, 2008), only a minority of samples contained the agreed formats on drinking guidelines. Shortcomings were also found in unit labelling, responsibility messages and warnings about drinking in pregnancy.

The third area of cooperation with the industry was the Drinkaware Trust. After prolonged negotiations between the government and the industry, a fund for alcohol misuse projects was established. It was based on the Portman Group's existing trust, which funded educational and community projects. The governing body of the new trust included industry and non-industry stakeholders, as well as two lay people with no professional interest in alcohol, and an independent chair. The Drinkaware Trust is funded by the industry, supplemented by other sources, including the National Lottery. It has three objectives: to increase awareness of safe and responsible drinking, and the impact of alcohol misuse on society and individuals; to improve attitudes towards safe and responsible drinking and the unacceptability of binge drinking; and to effect positive changes in behaviour related to alcohol consumption. In seeking to meet these objectives, the trust is required to act in the public interest and undertake evidence-based programmes.

Policy Shifts

Amid continued concern about alcohol problems, in particular underage drinking, binge drinking and the impact of cheap alcohol, pressure grew for a more robust approach to alcohol problems (ACMD, 2006a; Home Affairs Committee, 2005, 2008; Nuffield Council on Bioethics, 2007; BMA, 2008; Academy of Medical Colleges, 2004). Groups campaigning against alcohol misuse began to coordinate their activities more effectively, marked by the creation of Alcohol Health Alliance UK, a coalition of organizations led by the Royal College of Physicians.

The government began to strengthen its policy in 2005, proposing a range of measures to deal with problems of alcohol-related disorder and crime (DCMS, Home Office and Office of the Deputy Prime Minister, 2005). This included new alcohol disorder zones (ADZs), where police and local authorities could impose levies on local drinks outlets to fund measures to reduce alcohol problems. The scheme was heavily criticized for being counterproductive and bureaucratic, not least by those expected to use the powers. To date, this legislation has not been used. It was enacted in 2006, along with other measures such as new police powers to close outlets persistently selling to underage drinkers, to disperse drinkers where disorder was likely, and to review licensed premises associated with crime and disorder. In addition, new banning orders for troublemakers were introduced as well as further on the spot fines for alcohol offences.

The replacement of Tony Blair as Prime Minister by Gordon Brown was accompanied by a new strategy (HM Government, 2007e). This involved renewed efforts to prioritize alcohol policy and coordinate it across government departments. Although there were continuities, including a desire to work with the industry, further public information campaigns and improvements in law enforcement, there were signs of a tougher approach (Anderson, 2007). Alcohol was included within a new cross-government PSA delivery agreement that contained specific performance measures (HM Government, 2007f). A study of the link between price, drinks promotions and harm was announced. This found that price and promotions were significant factors in alcohol misuse and that measures to raise prices could reduce alcohol consumption and harm (Booth et al., 2008a, 2008b). Government support for this approach was reflected in an above-inflation rise in alcohol taxation in subsequent budgets. The government also agreed to introduce new licensing regulations, with new penalties for minors possessing alcohol, changes in criteria for withdrawing licences from those who persistently sold alcohol to children, new probationary periods for licensees and increased sanctions for breaching licensing conditions. This followed evidence that the Licensing Act 2003 had not significantly changed the drinking culture or reduced alcohol-related problems (DCMS, 2008a; DCMS, 2008b; Hough et al., 2008; LACORS, 2008; Roberts and Eldridge, 2007; Durnford et al., 2008). To be fair, the much-feared 24-hour drinking spree had not materialized, with less than one in twenty outlets granted all day opening. However, there was much variation locally, with licensing powers not being fully used to reduce alcohol problems (NAO, 2008a).

The Brown government was under pressure to increase regulation of the drinks industry. It now estimated the costs of alcohol misuse at a higher level than previously – at £25 billion per annum (NAO 2008b). Concern about underage drinking continued. Although enforcement campaigns indicated that fewer outlets were serving children, some outlets were continuing to break the law. Price discounting and loss leading were still evident, despite the adverse effects of cheap alcohol. Indeed, in 2009, the CMO caused a stir by calling for a minimum unit price for alcohol. At this stage, his idea was rejected by the government. Attempts were made, however, to address the weaknesses of self-regulation. Following the KPMG (2008) report on industry standards, the Brown government announced a national mandatory code of practice. The necessary legal powers were contained in the Police Act of 2009. The first part of the code, which contained a ban on irresponsible promotions and serving practices and a requirement that free tap water would be available, came into force in April 2010. The second part – relating to age verification policies and the availability of smaller alcohol measures – was due to be implemented later that year. In addition, powers were introduced to enable amendments to the Licensing Act and to increase the ability of local licensing authorities to take action against problem outlets.

Nonetheless, alcohol problems continued to attract concern. The House of Commons Health Committee, reporting on the issue in 2010, recommended minimum pricing, tightening of rules on advertising and sponsorship, and a mandatory labelling scheme. It also called for better law enforcement, particularly in relation to serving people who are drunk, and improvements in health services for people with alcohol problems. The Health Committee was also critical of the government for responding too much to the industry's concerns rather that those expressed by health experts. This echoed the sentiments of a report from the BMA (2009) that examined the effects of alcohol marketing on young people. This report was critical of policies influenced and implemented by the drinks industry. It called for a much tougher approach including a comprehensive ban on all alcohol marketing communications, minimum prices, taxation to rise above inflation and be linked to the strength of different alcoholic drinks, a reduction in licensing hours, and a compulsory levy on the drinks industry to fund an independent public health body to oversee alcohol-related research, health promotion and policy advice.

The Cameron government came to office committed to further action on alcohol problems. The Conservative–Liberal coalition programme contained several proposals including review of alcohol taxation and pricing and a ban on the sale of alcohol at below cost price. It also promised a review of alcohol licensing to give councils and police stronger powers to refuse and remove licences from premises causing problems. It also proposed greater powers for police and councils to permanently close premises selling to underage drinkers, increasing the maximum fine for selling to underage drinkers (to £20,000), and allowing councils to charge for late-night licences to cover the cost of policing. On the other hand, the Cameron government's first budget reversed a 10 per cent above-inflation increase in cider duty imposed by Labour earlier in the year, to the annoyance of some alcohol misuse campaigners.

Alcohol Policies in Other parts of the UK

In the past there have been differences in alcohol policy across the countries of the UK. Until fairly recently, for example, Wales had a more restrictive approach, with some districts not permitting the sale of alcohol on Sundays. In contrast, Scotland relaxed its licensing laws in the 1970s, allowing pubs and bars to open longer. Since devolution, opportunities to develop a distinctive approach have increased. Scotland has now adopted a more restrictive approach. Its licensing reforms followed a review of alcohol misuse and, as a result, gave more weight to the prevention of alcohol problems than was the case in England. In Scotland, public health is clearly identified as one of the key objectives of licensing: not the case in England and Wales. Scotland also introduced new powers to control underage drinking and cut-price alcohol. The Scottish government's alcohol plan (Scottish Executive, 2002c) set targets to reduce drinking over sensible levels and created stronger local networks to address alcohol misuse. In 2009, the Scottish Nationalist government introduced a revised strategy (Scottish Government, 2009c) that proposed a range of measures, including raising the purchase age of alcohol to 21, preventing the sale of cheap alcohol (through minimum pricing), and increasing resources for prevention and treatment of alcohol problems.

Wales has also taken a distinctive approach. Wales has integrated its alcohol, drugs and substance misuse strategies for some time (Welsh Office, 1996; NAfW, 2000b; Welsh Assembly Government, 2008b). It introduced integrated drug and alcohol action teams (DAATs) at local level in the 1990s. The revised strategy for Wales focuses on prevention, supporting misusers, supporting families and tackling the availability of illicit drugs and inappropriate availability of alcohol and other substances. The Welsh substance misuse strategy will be underpinned by a specific alcohol action plan. The Welsh approach, by including legal and illegal substances, has created the scope for a more comprehensive and holistic approach to addictions.

Northern Ireland devised its alcohol strategy in 2000 (DHSSPS, 2000). It has since moved towards a more integrated approach. Northern Ireland has a regional coordinator for alcohol and drugs and four regional drug and alcohol control teams. The latest strategy (DHSSPS, 2006c) covers both alcohol and drugs. It should be noted that Scotland and England have also been moving in a similar direction. Scotland introduced alcohol and drug action teams covering 22 geographical areas (these are now known as alcohol and drug partnerships). In England the remit of most drug action teams now includes alcohol. DATs also work closely with local crime and disorder reduction partnerships (CDRPs), which are now required to have an alcohol strategy.

International/EU Responses to Alcohol

Alcohol policy has appeared on global and European Union agendas. WHO has passed a series of resolutions about alcohol since the late 1970s. It has brought together and disseminated evidence about the scale of alcohol problems, highlighting for example that over 76 million people worldwide have an alcohol disorder and that 3.2 per cent of deaths globally are due to alcohol (WHO, 2004b). WHO commissioned studies into the causes of alcohol problems and the effectiveness of policy interventions (WHO, 2004b, 2007; Babor et al., 2003). In recent years it has moved from providing the evidence base to a more proactive approach (WHO, 2008c). In 2008, WHO embarked on the development of a global strategy on alcohol. This strategy, approved by the World Health Assembly in 2010, identified five objectives: raising global awareness of alcohol problems and increasing government commitment to act to address harmful use; strengthening the knowledge base on harms and interventions; increasing technical support to member states to prevent alcohol misuse and manage alcohol-use disorders; strengthening partnerships and better coordination among stakeholders and increasing the mobilization of resources; improving systems of monitoring and surveillance, with more effective dissemination and use of information for advocacy, policy development and evaluation (WHO, 2010). The strategy also set out important guiding principles, including that public policies and interventions to prevent and reduce alcohol harms should be guided and formulated by public health interests, based on clear goals and evidence, and that public health should be given proper deference in relation to competing interests in this field. It also identified a range of policy options and interventions for member states, including policies on health services, community action, drink-driving, regulation of alcohol availability, restrictions on marketing of alcohol products, pricing policies, and measures to reduce the public health impact of illicit alcohol. Furthermore, the strategy included a commitment to global action on alcohol misuse through greater cooperation between WHO and other UN and international agencies to provide leadership, strengthen advocacy, formulate policy options, strengthen partnerships and promote networking.

An international approach is necessary for a number of reasons. First, it enables all the evidence about policy interventions to be brought together and shared between governments. Second, because the alcohol industry is global there is a need to ensure that problems are tackled in a coordinated way. Weaknesses in regulation in particular regions or countries can be easily exploited by the industry. Third, as many trade decisions are made at an international level, it is important that these decisions fully reflect the public health consequences.

The WHO Regional Office for Europe has also been active in promoting action on alcohol. The European *Health for All* strategy set a target of cutting alcohol consumption by 25 per cent by the year 2000 (WHO Regional Office for Europe, 1985). An expert committee was established to provide a scientific basis for an action plan on alcohol (Edwards et al., 1994). The committee's report was at the centre of major controversy when it was revealed that the drinks industry had offered academics money to criticize it (*Independent on Sunday*, 1994). The first European alcohol action plan (EAAP) covered the period up to 2000 (WHO Regional Office for Europe, 1993c) and aimed to encourage member states to adopt an alcohol policy. This was relatively unsuccessful, with about half the countries failing to comply. An attempt had been made to create a stronger momentum on alcohol policy with the agreement of European Alcohol Charter (1995), which set out ethical principles and goals for the development of alcohol policies, such as the right to be protected from the harmful consequences of alcohol, the right to impartial information about alcohol and for those with problems the right to treatment and care. A revised EAAP was subsequently introduced (WHO Regional Office for Europe, 2000c). This set out policy recommendations in more detail, including, for example, advocating the use of tax to reduce harm, the protection of children from exposure to alcohol marketing, reduction of the alcohol limit for drivers, and restrictions on the availability of alcohol. In 2001, a Declaration on Young People and Alcohol was agreed by European health ministers. This had several objectives, including reducing alcohol consumption in this age group, minimizing pressures to drink (including advertising and sponsorship), and controlling availability.

The European Union has also developed an alcohol strategy (see Anderson and Baumberg, 2006). From the 1980s, concerns about alcohol misuse led to some action, including funding for health promotion and research. Subsequently, EU directives in specific areas such as broadcast advertising and road safety provided a basis for alcohol policy development. On the other hand, some EU decisions, notably on tax harmonization and with regard to subsidies for the wine industry through CAP, undermined alcohol policies by making alcohol more available at cheaper prices. The need for a strategic approach was recognized and the European Commission given the task of drawing this up. The Commission funded a review of alcohol policy in Europe (Anderson and Baumberg, 2006) which estimated the cost of alcohol misuse in the EU at €125 billion per annum with a further €270 billion in intangible costs, including loss of life and human suffering. The report argued that alcohol misuse damaged EU competitiveness and social cohesion, and was a major cause of inequalities. The EU strategy was finalized in 2006 (Commission of the European Communities, 2006). Its key themes were to protect children and the unborn, reduce deaths from traffic accidents, reduce harm among adults, increase awareness of alcohol problems and create a better evidence base. The strategy did state that the health impact of alcohol would be taken into account in future EU decisions. But, largely due to intense lobbying from the drinks industry, it failed to deal with the health consequences of wine subsidies, and did not back policies to raise taxes, place health warnings on products, or restrict marketing of alcohol products at the

European level (McKee, 2006). Instead, it opted for softer policies such as monitoring drinking habits, collecting data on harm, supporting collaboration and promoting research.

Conclusion

Public health policy must bring together all aspects of drugs use. Alcohol and tobacco are major public health issues, but for too long they have been given lower priority than illicit drugs (Goldstein and Kalant, 1993). Comprehensive policies and integrated strategies are required, in spite of the political obstacles. There are signs of an increased willingness to look at the problems of alcohol and tobacco in the broader context of drug abuse. Education programmes increasingly address legal as well as illegal drugs. National strategies also address both types of substance. But in terms of priorities, alcohol, tobacco and drugs are treated differently. It seems sensible that drug policies should incorporate a balanced assessment of the risks and benefits of the different types of drugs used. These policies should also be realistic and should prioritize harm minimization. Furthermore, they must be based on a clearer understanding of why individuals and societies use and misuse drugs and therefore should be linked with broader policies aimed at improving individual and social welfare.

Socioeconomic Factors and Health   16

Health is not simply a matter of individual choice but is shaped by one's social and economic context (Raphael, 2006). As this chapter will show, socio-economic conditions influence health in a number of ways: by depriving some people of essential material resources; through social structures and processes that give fewer opportunities to enjoy good health to some compared with others; and by exposing some people to higher risks of disease, illness and injury. The first part of this chapter clarifies some key concepts. This is followed by an analysis of various aspects of deprivation and inequality and their relationship with ill health.

Concepts of Poverty and Inequality

When examining the role of socioeconomic factors, it is important to clarify a number of key concepts: poverty, deprivation, social exclusion, inequality and inequity.

Poverty is a contested concept (Alcock, 2006). Different definitions exist, based on value judgements about the nature of poverty and what should be done to alleviate it. A distinction is often made between *absolute* and *relative* poverty. Absolute poverty is defined as having a level of resources below that needed to sustain human life. It is defined in terms of basic needs, such as food, clothing and shelter. In wealthier societies, however, it is argued that the poverty line should be higher than subsistence level because people need more resources to participate as citizens. Hence, people may have their basic needs met but live in relative poverty. The notion of relative poverty is defined in relation to an average level of resources for that society. In the UK and other industrialized countries, the poverty threshold is defined as a percentage (60 per cent in the UK) of the national median income.

Deprivation is often used synonymously with poverty, although it is also applied to specific non-income disadvantages, such as difficulties in access to housing, to good quality education, employment opportunities, transport, communication and health services. It is also used to describe local areas or regions where there is a high level of poverty or where people face particular disadvantages. In recent times, the term *social exclusion* has been coined to describe the processes whereby people are unable to participate as consumers and citizens in society (Hills et al., 2002; Levitas, 1998). This focuses on removing the barriers faced by people in participating in key social and economic activities, rather than simply increasing their income.

The terms inequality and inequity are often used interchangeably. However, they have different meanings. Inequalities are empirical constructions – they are neither good nor bad. An inequity is a normative concept, based on judgements about fairness and justice. The fact that someone earns twice as much as someone else is a statistical inequality. If we think this unjustifiable, it then becomes an inequity. This distinction can be further illustrated by exploring the concept of health inequalities.

Health Inequalities

Not all health inequalities are inequitable (Graham, 2007). For example, inequality in health status related to ageing is not normally regarded as inequitable. In contrast, differences in health status between rich and poor are often judged as inequitable. However, much depends on explanations for inequality. If older people's health is worse because of relatively poor access to services, this would be regarded by many as inequitable. Furthermore, as we shall see, some argue that inequalities between rich and poor are not inequitable where these are due to different preferences for health behaviours. Hence, as Graham (2007) observes, empirical research on the causes of health inequalities is important. It can have an impact on how we judge them as inequities.

Judgement about inequity is rooted in normative theories of justice (see Pereira, 1993; Graham, 2007; Le Grand, 1987). This is not the place for reviewing these complex arguments and debates. However, as Graham (2007) notes, there are essentially two main ethical approaches that provide justification for addressing health inequities. The first, associated with the philosopher John Rawls' (1999) theory of justice, argues that there should be some minimum set of 'primary goods' that all must have and that inequalities are only justified if the least well-off person benefits from these arrangements. Many view health as an essential element and apply Rawls' theory to argue that the health of the most disadvantaged must be maximized. The second, Sen's (1985) 'basic capabilities' approach, argues that health is a fundamental condition of human life and vital constituent of human capability. Therefore the aim should be to equalize opportunities for good health (see also Whitehead, 1992).

Both ethical approaches justify action to reduce health inequalities. Health inequalities are also regarded by many as a key public health priority. This is associated with the 'stewardship model' of public health (Nuffield Council on Bioethics, 2007) where the state has responsibility for the individual and the collective needs of its people. According to this, the state must provide conditions that allow people to thrive and be healthy including reducing health inequalities.

The Concept of Health Inequalities in the UK

In the UK, health inequality has become a proxy term for health inequity (Graham, 2004). Health inequalities are referred to in policy documents and by campaigners as a problem to be addressed rather as a neutral statistic. This imprecision is complicated further by the use of different meanings of health inequality. According to Graham (2004), the meaning of health inequalities has shifted between: health disadvantage (some social groups being worse off than others); as a health 'gap' between higher and lower social groups; and as a gradient where health is related to position in the social hierarchy. These different conceptualizations of health inequalities are important as they imply different foci and frameworks for policy. Addressing health disadvantage is a less ambitious strategy than narrowing health gaps or reducing gradients. These issues will be picked up later in the next chapter in the context of policy developments.

Dimensions of Health Inequality in the UK

Social Class

Differences in mortality and morbidity between social classes are well documented (Townsend et al., 1992; Whitehead and Drever, 1997; Shaw et al., 1999). Previous evidence, using the Registrar General's classification of social class, found that men in social class V (unskilled manual workers) had an almost threefold-higher death rate compared with professional and managerial staff. Using a new classification of social class (see Exhibit 16.1) for 2001–3 in England and Wales, gave similar results. The standardized mortality rate for males aged 25–64 was 2.8 times higher for routine workers compared with those in higher managerial occupations (White et al., 2007). The mortality rate is higher for routine and manual occupations than for those in the highest social class for almost all diseases (exceptions being leukaemia, and breast and skin cancer). Routine workers have 2.8 times the standardized mortality rate from circulatory diseases of higher managerial and professional occupations, 1.8 times the death rate from cancer, 4.9 times the death rate from respiratory disease, 3.5 times the death rate from digestive diseases and 3.3 times the death rate from accidents (White et al., 2008). Deaths rates for women also exhibit a social class gradient. The standardized mortality rate for women aged 25–69 in this period was 1.9 times higher for those in routine occupations than those in higher managerial and professional groups (Langford and Johnson, 2009). Variations in death rates feed through into life expectancy statistics. For 2001–3, men in professional occupations (social class I of the Registrar General's social class classification) had a life expectancy at birth of 80 (compared with 72.7 years for people in social class V (unskilled manual) while among women the difference was seven years exactly (ONS, 2007).

There are significant differences in maternal, infant and child mortality between social classes (BMA, 1999). Maternal mortality is associated with social disadvantage (Spencer and Law, 2007). In 2003, the infant mortality rate in the routine and manual class was almost a fifth higher than the average (Dorling et al., 2007a). Children in social class V are five times more likely to suffer accidental death compared with those in social class I (Towner, 2005). Children of unemployed parents are 13 times more likely to die of external causes and injuries than those born into the top social class (Edwards et al., 2006).

Inequality in mortality rates is mirrored in differences in self-reported ill health. Men and women in routine and manual occupations have significantly higher rates of self-reported ill health than those in higher managerial and professional occupations (Walker et al., 2001; Babb, 2004). Moreover, social inequalities in self-reported ill health increase from middle to early old age (Chandola et al., 2007). People in lower social classes are more likely to suffer from mental illnesses than those further up the hierarchy (Meltzer et al., 2004; Murali and Oyebode, 2004). Mental health is both a cause and a consequence of social, economic and environmental inequalities (Friedli, 2009; Rogers and Pilgrim, 2003). It may also play a role as a pathway between such inequalities and health, discussed further below in the context of income distribution and health.

Exhibit 16.1

Social Class Categories

The Registrar General's social class classification placed people into one of six occupational groups:

I   professional
II   managerial, technical, intermediate
IIIN skilled non-manual

IIIM　skilled manual

IV　　partly skilled manual

V　　unskilled manual

In 2001, this was superseded by a new classification, the National Statistics Socioeconomic Classification (NS-SEC), of which there are three different versions using nine, five and three classes respectively. The nine-class model is shown below:

1.1　Large employers and higher managerial occupations

1.2　Higher professional occupations

2　Lower managerial, administrative and professional occupations

3　Intermediate occupations

4　Small employers and self-employed people

5　Lower supervisory and technical occupations

6　Semi-routine occupations

7　Routine occupations

8　Never worked, long-term unemployed

Source: ONS (2008a)

Differences in health status are often depicted as a gap between 'higher' and 'lower classes', or alternatively between routine or unskilled manual workers and the rest of the population. It is more accurate to see them as a gradient where the risks of death, disease and illness are progressively and inversely related to location in the occupational hierarchy. This was confirmed by a major study of the health of civil servants – the Whitehall programme (Marmot et al., 1978, 1991; Fernie, 2004). This found that the more senior you are in the hierarchy, the longer you are likely to live. Lower grade civil servants had four times the risk of dying between ages 40 and 64 compared with top grades (Marmot, 2004). In particular, workers with imbalance between demands, control and rewards at work were likely to face higher risks of heart and circulatory diseases, mental health problems and poor health (Stansfield et al., 1999; Kuper et al., 2002). Marmot (2004) argued that the findings from the Whitehall studies can be extended to other aspects of life. He points out that the health impact of hierarchy and 'status syndrome' has been observed in many other settings. Oscar winners, for example, have longer life expectancy than their fellow actors.

The relationship between health and position in the employment hierarchy is hardly surprising given the importance of paid employment as a marker of social status and a source of income in contemporary society. Health is also linked to unemployment (Waddell and Burton, 2006). In one study, even after adjustment for other variables such as social class, health status and lifestyle, risks of mortality for middle-aged men doubled for those who became unemployed compared with those still in employment (Morris et al., 1994). Unemployment also adversely affects the health of young people, trapping them in a downward spiral of worsening health and reduced opportunities (Lakey, 2001). Studies have also revealed that job insecurity has a deleterious effect on health (Ferrie et al., 2001, 2005).

Is the Social Class Health Gap Widening?

An examination of UK trends reveals that inequalities linked to social class have widened over time. Between the periods 1972–6 and 1997–2001, life expectancy at birth for men in non-manual classes grew faster than for those in manual classes. Consequently, the life expectancy gap grew from 2.1 years to 3.8 years (ONS, 2007). There was a slight narrowing of this gap between the periods 1997–2001 and 2002–5 (to 3.3 years). For women, the pattern is more complicated. The life expectancy gap between females in non-manual and manual classes (2.5 years in the 1972–6 period) narrowed in the 1970s and early 1980s (reaching 1.9 years in 1982–6). It then widened dramatically between 1987 and 1991 (to 2.9 years) and has stayed at a similar level since.

When one compares changes in life expectancy between the highest and lowest social class, the gap is even wider. For example, the gap in life expectancy at birth between men in social classes I and V increased from 5.4 years to 7.3 years from 1972–6 to 2002–5. In women, the life expectancy difference grew from 4.8 years to 7 years.

Another indicator of the health gap is infant mortality rates. The infant mortality rate for social class I fell during the 1990s but increased in social class V (there was also a slight rise in social class IIIN in the late 1990s). Between 2000 and 2003, the gap between the infant mortality rate of routine and manual workers and the rest of the population actually widened (Dorling et al., 2007a). It has since narrowed, but is still wider than in the period 1997–99 (DoH, 2009f).

Explaining Inequalities

There are several different explanations for health inequalities, each of which carries different implications for policy (Townsend et al., 1992; Bartley, 2004; Asthana and Halliday, 2006). One explanation (known as the artefactual explanation) is that health inequalities are exaggerated by the use of poor quality data, in particular resulting from the use of occupation as a proxy for social class (Illsley, 1986). There are a number ways in which this might happen. For example, it is possible that changes in occupation in later life or unemployment may lead to misclassification of individuals. Another possibility is that health inequalities based on occupation could reflect changes in occupational structure (that is, the growth of non-manual jobs and the decline of manual work) rather than differential risks of illness between social classes. Statistical artefacts do not, however, explain the magnitude of health equalities and may even underestimate their magnitude (Goldblatt, 1989; Fox et al., 1990; Davey Smith et al., 1994).

Another explanation is that social class health differences arise from a process of social selection (Stern, 1983; Illsley, 1986). According to this, health inequalities are produced by healthy people moving up the social structure and less healthy people being downwardly mobile. It is based on an assumption that healthy people are better able to secure and retain higher status occupations. Hence health inequalities are a cause rather than a consequence of social class inequalities. There is evidence that health status can influence job selection, particularly in manual occupations where physical fitness is important (Goldblatt et al., 1990). Nonetheless, studies have confirmed that social selection is not a main cause of health inequalities (Donkin et al., 2002; Chandola et al., 2003; Power et al., 1996).

The third explanation attributes health inequalities to cultural and behavioural factors. Variations in health status are associated with differences in lifestyle between social classes. For example, smoking and obesity are both higher in routine and manual social classes. This perspective has often been labelled the 'victim-blaming' approach as it ignores the wider socioeconomic context that shapes individual lifestyle choices (Backett and Davison, 1995; Graham, 1993). This is discussed further below.

The fourth explanation is that material and structural factors are the main cause of health inequalities. This posits that social, economic and political factors can determine health outcomes. There are many different approaches, however, and these have developed beyond the basic proposition that social class is associated with health inequality (Townsend et al., 1992). Income has been identified as a major factor in health inequalities (Benzeval et al., 2001). It appears to have a stronger impact on health than education (which is strongly linked to social class – Marmot, 2004). However, indicators of access to specific resources (such as car ownership and housing tenure) are important markers of health status (Macintyre et al., 2001). There has also been much interest in income inequalities as a potential explanation for health inequalities at the population level.

The Relative Income Thesis

The *relative income thesis* states that countries with greater income inequality have worse levels of health (Wilkinson, 1996; Wilkinson and Pickett, 2006,

2007, 2009; Lynch and Kaplan, 1997; Kahn et al., 2000). Although changes in overall material standards have little impact on health, income differentials are associated with differences in mortality and life expectancy. Mortality tends to be lower in societies where income differentials are smaller, even after controlling for average income levels, absolute poverty levels and other socioeconomic factors (see also Kennedy et al., 1996; Wolfson et al., 1999; Ben-Shlomo et al., 1996; Stanistreet et al., 1999; Ram, 2005; Dahl et al., 2006; Kondo et al., 2008; Babones, 2008; Kim et al., 2008; Dorling et al., 2007).

Although the precise causal link between income distribution and health is unclear, a number of potential causes have been suggested (Bartley, 2004). Material inequalities are thought to affect stress-related illness through the perception of social injustice and lower resilience (Abbott, 2007; Friedli, 2009; Crepaz and Crepaz, 2004; Wilkinson, 1996; Wilkinson and Pickett, 2009). Others, however, cast doubt on a direct relationship between stress and vulnerability to disease (Kunst et al., 1998). Another possibility is that inequality could affect social cohesion through its impact on 'social capital', the networks, norms and trust within communities, the broader civic importance of which has been identified by a number of authors, including Putnam (2000), Coleman (1988), and Bordieu (1986). It has been argued that culture, social networks and institutions can affect health (Hall and Lamont, 2009). Wilkinson (1997) cites research that identifies social trust (as indicated by membership of voluntary groups and levels of trust in the community) as a factor linking income distribution and health (Kawachi et al., 1997; Kawachi and Kennedy, 1997). Others studies have also found a relationship between social capital measures and health (Kaplan et al., 1996; Li, 2007; Veenstra et al., 2005). Importantly, some have identified a link between social capital and mental health (McCulloch, 2001; Freidli, 2009), although social capital is a complex concept and may be both an asset and a liability with respect to health (see Almedom, 2005). Others, while accepting that social networks might well play a role in promoting health, have similarly expressed concern about a lack of clarity surrounding the term and have questioned its impact on health (see Muntaner et al., 2001; Cattell, 2001).

Critics have attacked the relative income thesis on several grounds. It has been argued that the link between income inequality and overall health standards is tenuous and that health inequalities are more closely related to specific factors, such as absolute poverty and unemployment. Furthermore, it has been claimed that the relationship between income inequality and general levels of heath is largely a statistical artefact, and that relationships between variables at an aggregate level are wrongly interpreted as applying at the individual level (Robinson, 1950; Gravelle et al., 1998, 2002 – see also Ellison, 2002). Others argue that the relative income hypothesis is based on flawed measures of income distribution (Judge, 1995). Further research into compara tive health inequalities has challenged the evidence base of the relative income thesis. Several studies, covering a number of countries, did not find a link between income inequality and health (Lynch et al., 2004; Mellor and Milyo, 2001; Sturm and Gresenz, 2002; Osler et al., 2002; Shibuya et al., 2002; Backlund et al., 2007). Some identified individual risk factors (including low levels of income), rather than income inequalities, as key factors behind health inequalities.

The overall picture is that, although some (but not all) studies have found an association between income inequality and poor health in the USA (which is characterized by a highly unequal income distribution), there is less evidence of an association outside the USA. Nonetheless, Wilkinson and Pickett (2006) conclude that the majority of properly designed studies support a link between income inequality and health. The issue remains disputed. The field is bedevilled by complex methodological debates about the quality of data, confounding variables (for example educational attainments and racial composition), time lags, analysis and interpretation (Subramanian and Kawachi, 2004). Indeed, some studies that found no supporting evidence have been reanalysed or reinterpreted as giving support to the relative income hypothesis (Subramanian et al., 2003; Subramanian and Kawachi, 2007). Defenders of the thesis adduce various reasons why some studies have not found a relationship (Wilkinson and Pickett, 2006; Lobmayer and Wilkinson, 2000). These include the failure of studies measuring inequality in small areas to reflect the scale of social class differences in society (but see Hou and Myles, 2005), the inclusion by some studies of control variables that are likely to mediate between class and health rather than confound the relationship; and the temporary loss of the relationship between income inequality and health in international studies in the mid-1980s – attributed to a number of factors including a shift in the age distribution of relative poverty from elderly people to younger people (who have lower death rates, creating a longer time lag between inequality and mortality).

Dynamics of Disadvantage

Others have investigated structures, patterns and processes through which people are disadvantaged and how this might affect health inequalities. Scambler and Scambler (2007) identify six types of asset flows that affect health and longevity.

- Biological or body assets can be affected by class relations prior to birth, as evidenced by the greater likelihood of low-birthweight babies in low-income families.

- Psychological assets provide a capacity to cope with adverse events,

- Social assets refer to social capital, networks and support.

- Cultural assets include learning and education.

- Spatial assets relate to the characteristics of particular geographical areas.

- Material assets include income and other material resources.

It is hypothesized that the distribution of these resources is related to health inequalities. This distribution is in turn related to broader political and social trends, such as increased political and social inequality arising from economic trends and public policies in recent decades (Coburn, 2004).

The particular impact of socioeconomic environments on health attitudes, belief and behaviours on health inequalities has been highlighted. According to Singh-Manoux and Marmot (2005), these contexts shape health behaviours, psychological vulnerability, participation in social networks and future time perspective (placing high value on future goals) – all of which have implications for health attitudes and choices. This may explain why people from different socioeconomic contexts indulge more in health-damaging lifestyles than others. It may also highlight the processes through which health inequalities are produced and sustained across the lifespan and between generations.

There is much interest in lifecourse approaches to health and health inequalities (Asthana and Halliday, 2006; Bartley, 2004; Davey Smith and Lynch, 1997; Siegrist and Marmot, 2006; Kuh et al., 2003). Socioeconomic factors in pregnancy, infancy and childhood have an effect on the future health of adults (see Chapter 9). For many observers, it is these that contribute most to variations in illness. Even so, at the other end of the age range health inequalities persist and, according to some accounts, widen in later life (Marmot and Shipley, 1996; Huisman et al., 2003; Chandola et al., 2007). Although there may be critical periods when health inequalities are influenced by social circumstances, it is possible that a range of socioeconomic factors over the lifetime affect health and the risk of premature death (Davey Smith et al., 1997). From this perspective, early life experiences (and indeed pre-life experiences and family background) may place individuals on trajectories that produce greater health risks or expose them to cumulative health risks at later stages in their life.

Health and Place

Where you live is a powerful indicator of your health status. Across the UK, life expectancy varies widely. Regionally in England, there is a north–south divide, with health being poorer in the north than the south (Seigler et al., 2008). England has better levels of health than Wales, Northern Ireland and Scotland (Babb, 2004; Doran et al., 2004). However, this masks differences between local areas (ONS, 2009a). For example, life expectancy for men in

Glasgow is almost 14 years less than in Kensington and Chelsea, London. A slightly smaller gap (11.7 years) exists for women. Health inequalities between different areas are widening. Inequalities in premature mortality continued to rise steadily in the first decade of the twenty-first century, reaching an extent not seen since the 1920s and 30s (Thomas et al., 2010). Moreover, as we shall see in the next chapter, the relative mortality gap between the most deprived areas and the rest of England has widened since the late 1990s, despite explicit policy commitments to reduce it (DoH, 2009f). Statistics on health behaviour also reveal inequalities between local areas. Across PCTs there is a two and a half fold variation in smoking rates, a fourfold variation in fruit and vegetable consumption, a twofold difference in obesity levels, and five-fold variation in binge drinking (Appleby, 2005).

However, location is not necessarily a cause of health or ill health. Indeed, it is difficult to unravel the impact of place, deprivation and other factors. This is because the least healthy areas contain a high proportion of socioeco-nomically deprived people (Drever and Whitehead, 1995; Sloggett and Joshi, 1994). The picture is complicated further because 'place' is a complex aggre-gation of factors such as housing (see Exhibit 16.2), neighbourhood context, and wider environmental factors. Indeed, there are many theoretical links between place and health (Curtis, 2004; Blackman, 2006; Macintyre et al., 2002; Cummins et al., 2007). The concept of therapeutic landscapes has been used to make sense of the various factors relating to a particular place, such as cultural attachment, identity and physical salubrity, all of which may have a bearing on psychological wellbeing and health. These factors can apply to different dimensions of place such as home, neighbourhood and natural spaces. Other factors mediating between place and health include material conditions and facilities, physical environmental hazards and social capital.

Place seems to have an impact over and above individual socioeconomic circumstances (Macintyre et al., 1993; Blackman, 2006; Curtis, 2004; Shouls et al., 1996). This contextual effect is generally found to be smaller than that associated with characteristics of individuals living in a particular area (Kawachi and Berkman, 2003). However, individual characteristics and place-specific characteristics may be mutually reinforcing and it is possible that the complexity of their relationship with health may not be detected by conven-tional statistical analysis (Cummins et al., 2007).

The literature on health and place is growing rapidly. Some studies suggest that residential conditions in early life may explain health in later life (Curtis et al., 2004). People living in areas that have high levels of greenery are three times more likely than those living elsewhere to be physically active and 40 per cent less likely to be obese. Those living in areas with high levels of litter and graffiti are about 50 per cent less likely than others to be more physically active and have a 50 per cent greater likelihood of being obese (Ellaway et al., 2005). The level of resources available to people in different areas has also been explored, with findings that poorer neighbourhoods are not necessarily deprived of resources (such as public services and outdoor play areas) as is often assumed (Macintyre et al., 2008). There also appears to be a link between areas that have high levels of socioeconomic deprivation and environmental pollution (see Briggs et al., 2008), suggesting a further pathway of inequity although the associations found so far are weak, subtle and complex.

Exhibit 16.2

Housing and Health

Historically, the link between inadequate housing and poor health is well established. The overcrowded slums of the Victorian era were breeding grounds for disease (Chadwick, 1842). In the years that followed, a range of policies were developed to address the housing question. This included slum clearance, the provision of affordable housing, town planning, regulation of landlords, building regulations and controls over the setting of rent levels (Lund, 2006).

Today, four key aspects of housing have implications for public health (BMA, 2003; Dunn, 2000; Hunt, 1997; Marsh et al., 1999; Marsh, 2007; Bonnefoy, 2007; Pevalin et al., 2008).

- *Physical risks from inadequate housing.* These include damp, mould, extremes of temperature, hazardous materials such as asbestos and lead, infestation, and accidents. These are linked to specific conditions (for example, cold is linked to increased risks of respiratory infection and cardiovascular conditions; damp and mould to respiratory problems, eczema, asthma, and allergies – BMA, 2003). Also included in this category are the physical risks associated with overcrowding, such as increased risks of infection, for example respiratory conditions, meningitis, TB, and helicobactor pylori, a risk factor for stomach cancer (ODPM, 2004b).

- *Risks to mental health and wellbeing.* Living in poor or inadequate housing is stressful. Poor housing quality and living in multi-dwelling housing is associated with adverse psychological health (Evans et al., 2003). Overcrowding is also linked to mental health problems (ODPM, 2004b).

- *Neighbourhood effects.* There are additional physical and mental health risks associated with living in particular neighbourhoods, including crime and antisocial behaviour (BMA, 2003). These are often difficult to separate from the physical characteristics associated with a particular dwelling (Blackman, 2006). For example, poor insulation can exacerbate problems associated with neighbour noise.

- *Homelessness.* The absence of permanent accommodation is linked to higher risks of mental and physical illness. Single homeless people have an average life expectancy of 42 (Griffiths, 2002) and much higher rates of respiratory disease, musculoskeletal disorders, skin disorders and infestations (Royal College of Physicians, 1994; Wilkinson, 1999). They have higher rates of mental illness and alcohol and drug dependence (Griffiths, 2002). People living in temporary accommodation also face a higher risk of mental and physical health problems (Marsh et al., 1999; Royal College of Physicians, 1994) and children are particularly at risk (Vostanis and Cumella, 1999).

Although there is much evidence linking poor housing and ill health, it is difficult to prove that the former causes the latter (Marsh, 2007). Poor health increases the likelihood of living in poor or inadequate housing. Some health conditions, such as mental illness, are linked to increased risks of being homeless. It is possible that illness and housing problems are caused by a third factor (for example, marital breakdown can be a cause of mental illness and homelessness). In addition, many housing characteristics interact with each other and it is difficult to quantify the specific effects of, for example, damp, overcrowded housing in a noisy neighbourhood. It is also difficult to disentangle housing factors from other risk factors, such as low income, unhealthy lifestyles, social class and ethnicity, and assess their relative importance. The 'triangular relationship' between housing, health and deprivation in particular requires further scrutiny (Goodchild, 1998; Brimblecombe et al., 1999). To make matters even more complex, housing can affect the health of some groups more than others, with children, chronically ill people, elderly people and gypsies and travellers being more vulnerable (Barnes et al., 2008; BMA, 2003; Parry et al., 2004; Shelter, 2006). Given the difficulties of evaluating the impact of housing on health, it has been suggested that a better approach would be to conceptualize housing and health in a holistic way (Thomson et al., 2001). Indeed, it is argued that insufficient attention has been given to the cultural importance of housing and the link between the concept of 'home' and wellbeing (Dunn, 2000; Evans et al., 2003). A house is more than a collection of physical characteristics. It is an important place where people's identities are shaped, from which they derive social status, and where they can create a positive sense of themselves (Bratt, 2002). It has an important role as a foundation of family life, a secure and stable place, and as a basis for important social support activities that underpin wellbeing. By recognizing the cultural significance of housing, it may be seen to have a far greater impact on health than is apparent from assessments based on health risks associated with specific housing characteristics.

There is a paucity of evidence about which interventions are effective in reducing health problems associated with housing (Marsh, 2007). Reviews of the literature have found only weak evidence that interventions work (NICE, 2005; Saegert et al., 2003; Thomson et al., 2001). However, it does appear that specific initiatives may be effective in improving health and wellbeing, including home insulation (Howden-Chapman et al., 2007), upgrading (such as central heating, ventilation, rewiring, insulation and reroofing – Barton et al., 2007) and rehousing for those with medical needs (Blackman et al., 2003). There is also evidence from reviews that accidental injuries among children and young people in the home can be prevented by home visits and advice on home hazards combined with media campaigns and by the provision of free or discounted home safety equipment (NICE, 2005). It has also been found that home hazard modification reduces falls among elderly people.

Despite their close association in the early development of the welfare state, housing and health policy developed separately. Hence important housing policies, such as the building of high-rise social housing in the 1960s and 70s, and, in the decades that followed, the sale of council houses, the reduction in social housing, and the deregulation of the private rented sector, did not benefit from any assessment of health consequences (Stewart, 2005). By 1996, a sixth of households lived in poor housing conditions (DETR, 2000d).

More recently, however, there has been an attempt to bring health and housing policies more closely together (Stewart, 2005). The Acheson report (Independent Inquiry into Inequalities in Health, 1998), echoing the suppressed Black report of the late 1970s, identified housing as a key determinant of health inequalities. It recommended: policies to improve availability of social housing for less well people, within a framework of environmental improvement, planning and design that takes into account social networks and access to goods and services; policies that improve housing provision and access to health care for homeless people; and policies to improve the quality of housing, including measures to improve heating and insulation and reduce fuel poverty. The Acheson report also recommended that government should aim to reduce the fear of crime and violence and create safe environments.

Health aspects of housing have been referred to in policy documents, including the cross-government strategy on health inequalities (DH, 2003a) and the Sustainable Communities Plan (ODPM, 2003b; Cm 6424, 2005; Cm 6467, 2005).

Homelessness – Targets were set for reducing different types of homelessness, such as rough sleepers and families in bed and breakfast accommodation. In 2007, a PSA target was set to halve the numbers of households in temporary accommodation to 50,500 by 2010. Specific guidance was issued on health and homelessness in England (ODPM/DOH, 2004). In Scotland, NHS boards are required to produce health and homelessness plans which they and local authorities must incorporate in their wider plans. The number of new homeless households in England in 2008 was 75,000, and has fallen dramatically since 2003 when over 200,000 households were officially recognized as newly homeless. This figure excludes people deemed intentionally homeless and those who are 'concealed' in other households of relatives and friends (www.poverty.org.uk, 2009).

Substandard homes – The government in England set a number of targets including that by 2010 all social housing (and 70 per cent of private housing occupied by vulnerable individuals) should meet a new decent homes standard. The devolved governments have their own targets, which differ in emphasis and detail (for example different target dates and different coverage of tenures). The decent homes standard is based on statutory minimum standards, state of repair, access to modern facilities and thermal comfort. Although many houses have been improved (1.3 million according to the government's estimates – DCLG, 2007c) and the proportion of non-decent homes has fallen since the mid-1990s (www. poverty.org.uk, 2009), the percentage of homes that do not meet the decent homes standard has remained high, at around a third of all dwellings and 29 per cent of social housing (ODPM, 2003c; DCLG, 2009b). In 2006, a health and safety rating system was introduced for the regulation of housing standards. This was based on an assessment of risks to health and safety and linked to enforcement based on the severity of these risks.

Overcrowding – Around 3 per cent of households are deemed overcrowded housing, the same as a decade ago (DCLG, 2009b). An action plan (DCLG, 2007b) was introduced, funding pathfinder schemes to address overcrowding in local areas with the worst problems. The government also promised to update the statutory overcrowding standards.

Fuel poverty – This is defined as where households are spending more than a tenth of their income on gas and electricity. In 2000, the government stated that it would seek to abolish fuel poverty by 2016 (and by 2010 for vulnerable groups). Several initiatives have been introduced, including grants for insulating homes and improving energy efficiency and cold weather payments to vulnerable groups. In 2006, 11 per cent of households were in fuel poverty, a lower proportion than in the 1990s when over a fifth of households were in this position (www.poverty.org.uk). However, rising energy prices have exacerbated the situation and by 2008 over 4 million households in England were in fuel poverty (treble the number in 2004) (Fuel Poverty Advisory Group, 2008). Fuel poverty policies have been heavily criticized for failing to reach those in need (Energy and Climate Change Committee, 2010). Government targets to end fuel poverty are unlikely to be met.

Housing stock and affordability – The shortage of good quality, affordable housing remains (Barker, 2004). The government has sought to address this by offering help to particular groups wishing to buy homes, such as 'key workers' in high-price housing areas. It has also encouraged the building of new homes for ownership. However, the number of new homes built in the social housing sector fell between the mid-1990s and 2003/4. Although it has risen since, the number of social housing dwellings built annually is less than in the last years of the Major government (www.poverty.org.uk, 2009). The Labour government (DCLG, 2007c) planned to build 240,000 additional new homes a year by 2016, with at least a quarter of these being 'affordable homes', although initially the number of new homes has fallen short of this target. Furthermore, housing has been linked to regeneration policy to promote across the board improvements in housing, neighbourhoods and the wider socioeconomic context of particular areas (see Exhibit 17.1; Mullins et al., 2006).

Despite some welcome changes, much more could be done to improve the contribution of housing policy to public health (Chartered Institute of Environmental Health, 2007; BMA, 2003). Many households still live in homes that do not meet their needs, some of which is below acceptable standards. Homelessness remains a problem. Efforts to address overcrowding are overdue and have yet to meet the scale of the problem.

Other Health Inequalities

Ethnicity

Some ethnic groups living in the UK have higher mortality rates and poorer health than the rest of the population (Bartley, 2004; POST, 2007; Sproston and Mindell, 2006; Bradby and Chandola, 2007). For example, after adjusting for age, people from Pakistani and Bangladeshi communities and Black Caribbean women are more likely to report poor health than the general population. Indian, East African and Black African people report a similar level of health to the White British population, while Chinese people have the best health of all ethnic groups (ONS, 2004).

This overall picture masks important variations, however. Some ethnic groups are at higher risk of specific illnesses. For example, cardiovascular disorders are higher than average among people from the Indian subcontinent. There is also a disproportionately high incidence of diabetes in these communities, and also in Black Caribbean women. Although some cancers (such as liver cancer, for example) are more common in black and minority ethnic groups, overall cancer rates are lower than in the general population. People originating from the Indian subcontinent have a much higher than average rate of tuberculosis infection. In addition, a small number of diseases are wholly or mainly confined to ethnic populations, including rickets (predominantly affecting people of Asian origin) and sickle-cell anaemia and thalassaemia (affecting people originating from Africa, Asia, the Middle East and the Mediterranean). There are also variations in mental health. Pakistani people and Bangladeshi men have higher than average levels of psychiatric morbidity (Sproston and Mindell, 2006). People from the Black Caribbean community are more likely to be diagnosed with a serious mental illness than the general population (Cochrane and Bal, 1989; Cope, 1989) but this may be due to differences in interpretation of symptoms and diagnosis (Sharpley et al., 2001; Nazroo, 1998; Rogers and Pilgrim, 2003).

There are several explanations for variations in ethnic health and illness, each carrying different policy implications (Nazroo, 1998; Bradby and Chandola, 2007). Some variation may be due to biases from inadequate research methods. The methods used to categorize people can produce misleading conclusions. In mortality studies, ethnic status is based on country of birth, which is a very crude indicator of ethnicity.

Ethnic differences may be due to cultural factors. These include variations in healthy lifestyles between different ethnic groups (Nazroo, 1998; Sproston and Mindell, 2006). For example, Indian, Pakistani and Bangladeshi men report lower levels of physical exercise than the general population, while Black Caribbean, Irish, Pakistani and Bangladeshi men report higher rates of smoking. Obesity rates vary between different ethnic groups, being higher than average among Black African and Pakistani women, Black Caribbean men and women, and Irish men. Most ethnic groups, with the exception of Irish people and Black Caribbean men, undertake lower than average levels of physical activity.

Material explanations relate excess mortality and ill health among ethnic groups to socioeconomic disadvantage. Notably Black Caribbean, Pakistani and Bangladeshi people are significantly overrepresented in manual households and in lower income groups (Nazroo, 1998). Two-thirds of Pakistani and Bangladeshi people are in the bottom income quintile, as are 28 per cent of Black Caribbeans and 35 per cent of Black non-Caribbeans (Babb, 2004).

Social class, material living conditions and local deprivation may explain much of the differences in health between minority ethnic groups and the general population (Chandola, 2001). However, other forms of disadvantage might affect ethnic health including overt and implicit racism. Institutional race discrimination and insensitivity in service provision may further affect mortality rates if people from ethnic backgrounds receive inadequate or inappropriate health care or face difficulties accessing services (see Exhibit 16.3).

It is possible that genetic factors may play some part in ethnic health inequalities (Collins, 2004). Further light may be shed on such risk factors through ongoing research into the health implications of the mapping of the human genome. However, one must be careful not to adopt a deterministic approach that automatically attributes inequalities in health to genetic factors within a cultural group (Bradby and Chandola, 2007; Pearce et al., 2004). As Bartley (2004) commented, ethnicity is not genetically determined, so the link between genes, ethnicity and disease is tenuous. At present it would appear that material, cultural and service factors are more important influences on the health of ethnic groups.

Gender

There are important differences in health status between men and women (Doyal, 1995; Bartley, 2004; Annandale and Hunt, 2000). Women live longer than men, and death rates are lower for women compared with men in every age group. Women report slightly higher rates of long-standing illness and limiting long-standing illness than men (ONS, 2010). Men and women differ in their susceptibility to different kinds of illness. For example, disorders and diseases of the reproductive system are more commonly found in women, and women report higher levels of psychiatric morbidity (Singleton et al., 2001; Rogers and Pilgrim, 2003). However, men are more at risk from injury and accidental death compared with women.

Aside from obvious anatomical differences between the sexes, a range of factors explain variations in health status. Socioeconomic factors have a differential impact on male and female health: the class gradient for mortality and life expectancy is steeper for men than women. Women are not invulnerable to the health effects of socioeconomic disadvantage. Indeed, a strong socioeconomic gradient exists for psychosocial health: disadvantaged women and, in particular, single mothers, have poor levels of psychosocial health (Macran et al., 1996; Graham, 1993).

The changing role of women in society is also extremely relevant to gender differences in health. Increased female participation in the labour market – often including casual, part-time and relatively low-paid jobs – has ambiguous health implications. Although paid work brings in extra income, which may improve the quality of life, it can bring added stress, particularly when coupled with family responsibilities (Doyal, 1995). Much seems to depend on the aspect of health under consideration and the kind of work undertaken. The association between paid work and better health is less apparent for physical than mental health, and applies less to women in full-time work and those in professional and managerial posts (Bartley et al., 1992). Interestingly, no relationship was found between employment status and domestic conditions, suggesting that paid work and improved income may outweigh the negative effects of combining domestic workload with employment. In general, employed women have better mental health than those not employed and other positive effects on physical health can be demonstrated. Even so, in some circumstances participation in the work-place may bring additional risks and hazards, including stress, offsetting the benefits of paid work (Doyal, 1995).

Women's role in society has changed in other ways relevant to their health. Many women have greater financial independence and more freedom of choice than a generation ago. They now participate more in further and higher education, in the professions and in other institutions that were almost exclusively male less than half a century ago. Women's lifestyles have changed and this too has implications for health. Women are becoming more similar to men in aspects of health behaviour. Alcohol consumption is increasing in young women, paralleled by an increase in drink-related problems (Plant and Plant, 2006). Although smoking has declined among both men and women, the difference between male and female smoking rates is very small (NHS Information Centre, 2009b).

When examining health variations associated with gender, however, cultural and ethnic dimensions are important. Many of the changes in female working patterns and lifestyles have not occurred uniformly across ethnic groups. Therefore one must take into account the interaction between ethnic background and gender, as well as social class, when evaluating the impact of social change on health of women.

Men's health is seen as an increasingly important topic. Men are more at risk from certain diseases and conditions than women. This has raised questions about 'male disadvantage' in health (Cameron and Bernades, 1998; Hayes and Prior, 2003). The conventional wisdom that, irrespective of morbidity, women are heavier users of health services than men has also come under attack (Hunt et al., 1999; Hayes and Prior, 2003). Moreover, 'masculinity' and in particular men's risk-taking behaviour has also been identified as a key factor in their health and wellbeing (Sabo and Gordon, 1993). Rather than seeing gender issues in health as being concerned with the neglect of women's health needs, some have argued that the distinctive needs of both sexes must be taken into account in medical research, service delivery and also in wider social policies (Doyal, 2001; Hayes and Prior, 2003; Exhibit 16.3).

In addition to variations between men and women's health, there are also inequalities in health between people of different sexual orientation. For example, lesbian, gay, bisexual and transgender people have higher levels of suicide, alcohol and substance dependence, smoking, deliberate self-harm and mental disorders (Care Services Improvement Partnership, 2007; King et al., 2003). The specific needs of these groups went largely unrecognized until recently (Fish, 2006) and there is growing evidence that these needs are still not being met (see Exhibit 16.3).

Exhibit 16.3

Inequalities in Access to Health Services

To some extent health inequalities can be attributed to problems faced by social groups in accessing and using health services. Although the NHS provides a service that is comprehensive and mostly free at point of delivery, it does not necessarily provide an equitable service. Indeed, some argue that there is an inverse care law, whereby the availability of health care for a particular group or community varies inversely with the level of need (Tudor Hart, 1971, 2006).

Although this has been hotly debated (see Powell, 1990), there is evidence that some social groups may not have their health needs met as well as others:

- Areas with high health needs have fewer doctors (Appleby and Deeming, 2001).

- People on low incomes and in areas of high deprivation with high health needs do not have the highest rates of treatment, including cardiac and cancer services (Dixon et al., 2003; Hippisley Cox et al., 1997; Chaturvedi and Ben Schlomo, 1995; Morris et al., 2005; Graham et al., 2002). These variations are mainly found in secondary rather than in primary care settings. Survival rates for most common cancers are lower for people living in poorer neighbourhoods than for those in affluent areas (Rachet et al., 2008). However, some studies have not found a link between social position and access to treatment (see, for example, Britton et al., 2004).

- Ethnic minorities are more likely to consult their GP than the rest of the population but less likely to receive secondary care (Morris et al., 2005). Some ethnic groups with high levels of illness have lower levels of service utilization, for example Pakistani women and GP services, South Asian people and CHD treatment services, and South Asian women and cervical cancer screening services (Morris et al., 2005; Smaje and Le Grand, 1997; Chaturvedi et al., 1997; Feder et al., 2002; Aspinall and Jacobson, 2004). Minority ethnic groups also report lower than average levels of satisfaction with health services (Aspinall and Jacobson, 2004; Bradby and Chandola, 2007).

- Women have experienced poorer access than men to CHD treatments and hip replacements (Raine, 2000; Raine et al., 2003; Shaw et al. 2004) but better access to liver transplant and cataract operations (Raine, 2000).

- There is evidence that older people do not get access to the care they need and that the quality of services they receive is lower (Reid et al., 2002; Roberts et al., 2002; Shaw et al., 2004). Disabled people and people with learning disabilities experience problems of access and poor quality care, despite their greater health needs (Disability Rights Commission, 2006; Healthcare Commission, 2007d; Mencap, 2007). People with different sexual orientations have faced difficulties in having their health needs recognized and in accessing services (Fish, 2006). There are specific inequalities in access relating to distance from GP and specialist services, particularly but not exclusively in rural areas (see Haynes et al., 1999).

Conclusion

This chapter has shown that health inequalities represent a major public health challenge. Socioeconomic differences in health status are not a statistical artefact but arise from a range of factors relating to income, material deprivation and other structural factors. There is much evidence that social inequality has an impact on levels of health. Although more needs to be known about the precise causal mechanisms that link deprivation and social inequalities to ill health, enough is known to justify intervention. Other inequalities relating to ethnicity, gender, sexuality, age and disability must also be addressed. In the next chapter, the policy response to these issues is examined.

Inequities and Inequalities Policy

17

Having explored the main dimensions of health inequality in some depth, this chapter is devoted to an analysis of the policy context. It begins with an examination of the approach of the Conservative governments of the 1980s and 90s, before moving on to consider the Blair, Brown and Cameron governments' initiatives in this field. The chapter also considers the European and international response to health inequalities.

The Conservative Governments of Thatcher and Major

The Thatcher and Major governments' main priorities were to curb inflation and reduce public expenditure and taxation while improving incentives to private enterprise and increase its role in the provision of public services. Other important postwar policy objectives, such as full employment and income redistribution, were disregarded. Policies were introduced that reduced the burden of taxation for those on high incomes, cut entitlements to welfare benefits for the poor and abandoned low wage regulation. The power of trade unions was curbed. Important public services were privatized, leading to windfall gains for some, but reduced entitlements for others. These policies were compounded by broader social and economic changes, such as the decline in long-term, full-time employment and the growth of low-paid, casual work, the rise of dual-income families, increased levels of divorce, and the growth of single parenting.

Unsurprisingly, these policies widened income inequalities (Goodman et al., 1997). Income inequality grew rapidly from the late 1970s up to the early 1990s reaching a level not seen since 1945 (Joseph Rowntree Foundation, 1995). Between 1979 and 1992, the top tenth of the income distribution enjoyed more than a 60 per cent increase in income (after housing costs were taken into account) while the income of the bottom 10 per cent fell by 17 per cent. These inequalities persisted throughout the 1990s. By 1995, the richest fifth of the population received 40 per cent of total household disposable income (up from 36 per cent in 1979) while the share of the poorest fifth fell from 9.4 per cent to 7.9 per cent. Deprivation levels also increased. By 1996, one quarter of all households were living on below half the average income (after deduction of housing costs), compared with 9 per cent in 1979 (Department of Social Security, 1998). The welfare state continued to redistribute towards the poor, however (Hills, 1997). The average income of the top fifth households in 1995/6 was 16 times that of the bottom fifth before taxes and benefits in kind were taken into account, but only three and a half times greater afterwards (ONS, 1998, p. 101). Other measures of inequality – based on expenditure rather than income – indicated a less dramatic increase in inequality (see Goodman et al., 1997).

The growth in inequality was blamed for undermining economic performance and creating social divisions (Commission for Social Justice, 1994; Hutton, 1996). It was also linked to widening health inequalities, discussed in the previous chapter. The Thatcher government denied that health inequalities were caused by material factors and attributed them to statistical artefact, social mobility or, more often than not, individual behaviour. This was reflected in its rejection of the Black report of 1980, which argued for policies to improve the material conditions for the poor (DHSS, 1980; Townsend et al., 1992; Berridge and Blume, 2003). Throughout the 1980s the Thatcher government denied that health inequalities were widening as a result of its policies. But when the Health Education Council commissioned a study to update the Black report, it found health inequalities were growing in line with social and economic inequalities (Whitehead, 1987; Townsend et al., 1992). In particular, the report noted the growing threats to health posed by homelessness, unemployment and child poverty and criticized the government's failure to tackle these problems.

The Major Government

The Major government accepted the need for a national health strategy but refused to incorporate equity as a key objective. Subsequently, its *Health of the Nation* strategy was criticized for not targeting health inequalities. The Major government acknowledged 'variations' in health status (chosen in preference to the more politically charged term, 'inequalities') between different socioeconomic groups and attributed these to 'a complex interplay of genetic, biological, social, environmental, cultural and behavioural factors' (Cm 1986, 1992, p. 122). However, it became increasingly difficult to ignore the impact of inequalities on health (see Benzeval et al., 1995). Indeed, the government's overall health targets were being undermined by variations in health status between socioeconomic groups. Consequently, following pressure to examine the issue further, particularly from professionals encountering adverse socio-economic conditions in everyday practice (see BMA, 1995, 1999; Health Visitors' Association, 1996), the Department of Health established a review of 'health variations'. The review was narrowly confined to recommendations about what the DoH and the NHS could do about the problem. Unsurprisingly, it produced a rather cautious report, urging local service commissioners to identify and reduce health variations and calling for more research evidence (DoH, 1995).

The failure to acknowledge that health inequalities were related to socioeconomic factors was political. The disadvantaged tended not to vote for the Conservative party. Davey Smith and Dorling (1996, 1997) showed a strong negative association between voting Conservative and mortality rates (and correspondingly, a strong positive association between voting Labour and mortality rates) at the general elections in the 1980s and 90s. Although Conservative governments realized there were no votes in tackling socioeconomic inequalities, they did address some aspects of health inequality. They aimed to improve women's health by expanding screening services for breast and cervical cancer (see Chapter 8). Practitioners were encouraged to develop services more closely geared to women's needs in areas such as maternity services and general practice. Some measures were specifically geared to the health of ethnic minorities, such as the Stop Rickets Campaign and the Asian Mother and Baby Campaign, although such initiatives were regarded as piecemeal (Smaje, 1995; Johnson, 1993). In the early 1990s, policy focused more on the health needs of ethnic groups and there was an increase in the amount of research in this field. Although these initiatives were welcomed, they did not equate to a comprehensive and coordinated strategy to improve the health of ethnic minorities (Ahmad, 1993; Smaje, 1995).

The Blair and Brown Governments

When the Blair government entered office most observers believed that equity in health would have a much higher priority. In opposition, the Labour party had frequently criticized the Conservatives' refusal to acknowledge the relationship between health inequity and material inequalities. Furthermore, Labour was traditionally closer to bodies such as trade unions and welfare organizations, which had campaigned vigorously for action in this area.

Shortly after taking office, an independent inquiry into inequalities was appointed under the chairmanship of Sir Donald Acheson, a former Chief Medical Officer. The Acheson inquiry made 39 recommendations. These included: incorporating inequalities within health impact assessment (see Exhibit 11.2), giving a high priority for policies aimed at improving health and reducing inequalities among women of childbearing age, expectant mothers and young children, and endorsing policies to reduce income inequalities and improve living standards for those receiving social security benefits (Independent Inquiry into Inequalities in Health, 1998). The inquiry made a range of specific recommendations such as additional resources for schools in deprived areas, nutrition policies for schools, policies to increase work opportunities, and to improve the availability and quality of housing and public transport, policies to reduce poverty, and to tackle ethnic and gender inequalities in health. Its report also recommended establishing mechanisms to monitor inequalities in health and to evaluate the effectiveness of measures to reduce them.

These recommendations were welcomed by those campaigning for action on health inequalities for being comprehensive and for addressing key socio-economic factors affecting health and health inequalities. Some, however, were critical that the recommendations were not ranked in any order of priority (Dorling et al., 2007a). Moreover, Acheson did not identify targets to reduce inequalities, to the disappointment of some campaigners, although this issue was to resurface later. The inquiry was criticized for not costing its recommendations. The government's terms of reference having constrained the inquiry by insisting that the review be carried out within the broad framework of its financial strategy (Dorling et al., 2007a).

The Blair government responded positively to the Acheson report by reiterating a commitment to improving the health of the worst-off in society and narrowing the health gap (Cm 4386, 1999; DoH, 1999d). It proposed a cross-government approach reflecting the key policy areas identified by Acheson (Exworthy et al., 2003). This involved a range of measures, many already underway, aimed at tackling social and economic causes of ill health and health inequalities. These included broader policies to reduce poverty and social exclusion, regenerate deprived areas, and to improve housing and the education and welfare of children. Two key programmes were launched, which reflected Acheson's approach. Sure Start (see Chapter 9), aimed to provide support to disadvantaged families with young children in an effort to improve health and emotional development in the early years. Health action zones (HAZs) (see Exhibit 7.2) sought to improve health in local areas with high health needs through multi-agency partnerships. Both these problems held potential to reduce health inequalities between different social groups.

Most of Acheson's specific recommendations were accepted by the government. Some, however, were not immediately pursued (including the key recommendation that all policies be evaluated for their impact on health inequalities and should favour the less well off). Nonetheless, the Acheson report should be evaluated not only in terms of its direct influence on the government's agenda, but also for creating a 'window of opportunity' that campaigners were able to exploit, subsequently persuading government to prioritize particular measures (Dowler and Spencer, 2007). During the formulation of the NHS Plan, another opportunity arose. One of the committees established as part of this exercise, which had been given the task of recommending ways of improving public health, endorsed national health inequality targets. The government agreed and in 2001 set out two targets for the NHS in England to be achieved by 2010:

- To reduce by at least 10 per cent the gap in infant mortality (deaths in children under one year of age) between manual groups and the population as a whole.

- To reduce by at least 10 per cent the gap between the fifth of areas with the lowest life expectancy at birth and the population as a whole.

These targets were incorporated within the government's PSA targets, and subsequently modified (Dorling et al., 2007a). The infant mortality target was altered to reduce the gap between 'routine and manual' groups and the rest of the population. The life expectancy target was amended to reduce the gap between areas with the worst health and deprivation indicators (the so-called spearhead areas – see below) and the population as a whole. Additional targets were set in 2004, aimed at reducing the inequalities gap between the fifth of areas with the worst health and deprivation indicators and the rest of the population by at least 40 per cent for cardiovascular disease and 6 per cent for cancer, as well as a new target to reduce smoking among routine and manual groups to 26 per cent or less by 2010.

Although the identification of targets to reduce health inequalities was broadly welcomed (see Health Committee, 2001, 2009), critics pointed out that they were not sufficiently challenging. In particular, the health gap was defined rather narrowly by the government as the difference between the worst off and the average, not between the worst and best (Low, 2004; Dorling et al., 2007a). Aiming to reduce the gap between those with the best and worst health would have been a more accurate reflection of the actual scale of health inequalities, and a much more challenging task.

In order to achieve the new targets, the government realized it had to strengthen policy on health inequalities, particularly in coordinating activity across departments and agencies. A cross-cutting review was initiated, leading to a renewed programme of action (HM Treasury/DoH, 2002; DoH, 2003a). This set out over 80 commitments across four areas: supporting families, mothers and children; engaging communities and individuals; preventing illness and providing effective treatment and care; and addressing the underlying determinants of health and the long-term causes of health inequalities. The programme also identified a number of specific commitments including: an expansion of Sure Start, childcare and children's centres; improvements in children's mental health services; and an expansion in school-based health initiatives. Targets were set in a number of health-related areas such as housing, diet, exercise, drug abuse, smoking and poverty.

Within the NHS, health inequality was identified as a priority for the 2003–6 planning cycle (DoH, 2002e). The 2006/7 planning framework selected health inequalities as one of the top six NHS priorities (DoH, 2006a). PCTs were required to undertake health equity audits to review inequities in the causes of ill health and in access to services, to ensure action was agreed and incorporated into local plans and evaluate the impact of these actions on inequity. In 2004, 'spearhead areas' – those with the worst health and deprivation indicators – were identified. These were expected to take forward the government's agenda as set out in *Choosing Health*, being among the first to adopt new initiatives to encourage healthier lifestyles. These areas received additional funding and support (including support from a national support team). New funding streams included the Communities for Health programme, established in 2005 to provide funds for pilot projects in deprived areas. In addition, the funding system for PCTs was changed in an effort to increase resources for areas with higher health needs due to poverty and deprivation. The government also sought to increase access to primary care for deprived populations by experimenting with new service models (such as nurse-led practices and walk-in centres) and by reducing waiting times for emergency, outpatient and elective care for all NHS patients.

Despite these efforts the outcome was disappointing. As shown in the previous chapter, health inequalities remained problematic. The Labour government claimed some success, however. Almost all departmental commitments set out in the cross-cutting programme for action were achieved and most of the government's indicators relating to its action plan had moved in a positive direction (DoH, 2008f). Another source of comfort for the government was that a greater proportion of spearhead PCT areas than non-spearhead areas achieved key public health targets with regard to long-term conditions, suicide prevention, mortality, older people, drug misuse, smoking, cancer and mental health (Healthcare Commission and Audit Commission, 2008). However, for two other targets (GP measurement of BMI and sexual health), the situation was reversed. Notably, a greater proportion of spearhead PCTs achieved health inequality reduction targets compared with non-spearhead areas. However, it was subsequently found that less than a fifth of spearhead areas were on track to meet their 2010 life expectancy gap targets for both men and women (DoH, 2009f). Moreover, in terms of outcomes, there was little progress. Although the infant mortality rate among the routine and manual groups had improved since the baseline period set for the target (1997–9), it had not improved at the same rate as the rest of the population, so the gap widened. The relative gap increased by 3 per cent between the baseline period and 2006–8, although there were some fluctuations in between these periods (DoH, 2009f). For both men and women, the relative gap in life expectancy between the poorest areas and England as a whole was wider in 2006–8 than at the baseline (1995–7, in this case). For men, the inequalities gap had grown by 7 per cent, for women 14 per cent (DoH, 2009f). Moreover, since the late 1990s, the gap in cancer death rates had not narrowed, while inequalities in smoking and cardiovascular disease actually widened.

There are several reasons why the government's policy failed to meet its objectives (Health Committee, 2009; Healthcare Commission and Audit Commission, 2008; Audit Commission, 2010b; Asthana and Halliday, 2006; Dowler and Spencer, 2007; Exworthy et al., 2003; Shaw et al., 2005; Marks, 2006). First, some initiatives were not given sufficient time or resources to have a sustained impact. HAZs, for example, were downgraded and discontinued (Exhibit 7.2). Second, shifts in policy in this field did not help. For example, the initial emphasis on structural and material conditions underpinning inequalities gave way to the *Choosing Health* agenda, which placed more emphasis on individual lifestyles. Third, government programmes lacked clear objectives and were not properly evaluated. This made it difficult to assess what worked in reducing inequalities and why. Fourth, despite giving health inequality priority status and bringing it within performance frameworks, in reality it remained a lower priority than others such as waiting times and other acute sector targets. Fifth, although resources to PCTs were reallocated on the basis of population need arising from deprivation, the move towards full needs-based allocations was slow. Wealthier and healthier populations are still more generously funded relative to their needs compared with poorer localities. Sixth, although relationships between local NHS bodies, local government and other agencies improved in this field, much more was required to promote effective joint working, such as sharing information, pooling budgets and engaging in joint action. Finally, the government's health inequalities policy was undermined by its failure to adequately address wider social and economic inequalities. This is explored in more detail in the following section.

Social and Economic Policies

The Blair governments introduced a range of policies to reduce poverty and social exclusion. These included: action on child poverty (see Exhibit 9.1), housing (see Exhibit 16.2), teenage pregnancy (Exhibit 9.2.) and regeneration (Exhibit 17.1) A programme of welfare reform was set in motion, which included 'New Deals' for young people, long-term unemployed, for communities, older workers, lone parents and disabled people (Cm 3805, 1998). A minimum wage was also introduced. Taxes were raised and expenditure on public services such as education and health increased (representing an important 'benefit in kind' – see Jones et al., 2009). Tax credits were introduced for working families, pensioners and disabled people. Although the Labour government's taxation policies had only a small redistributive effect, the net effect of its budgets (including tax credits and benefits) has been progressive, redistributing in particular towards pensioners and low-income families (Jones et al., 2009).

These policies had some impact in reducing child and pensioner poverty and narrowing economic divisions between deprived and other areas (Hills et al., 2009). The percentage of people living in poverty fell from 25 per cent of the population in 1996/7 to just over a fifth in 2004/5, but has since risen to 22 per cent (Palmer et al., 2008; Brewer et al., 2008). However, child poverty levels, although declining, remained high (see Exhibit 9.1). Wealth and income was still unequally distributed (Babb, 2005). The top fifth of UK households in the income distribution received over 40 per cent of disposable income in 2006/7, while the share of the bottom fifth was below 10 per cent. The top fifth of households have four times the disposable income of the bottom fifth after redistribution through tax and benefits (ONS 2009b; Jones et al., 2008). Wealth also continues to be unequally distributed: around a quarter of wealth is held by the top one per cent of the population in the UK (Paxton and Dixon, 2004). Although the gap between the very rich and very poor widened between 1996/7 and 2001/2, it has since fallen and remains about the same as in 1996/7 (Brewer et al., 2008). There is evidence that rich and poor are increasingly polarized and now live further apart (Dorling et al., 2007a). A further report, from the National Equality Panel (2010) found that inequalities in earnings and incomes in Britain were high compared with 30 years ago and in comparison with other countries. Although in recent years the gap had narrowed slightly, the large growth in inequality in the 1980s had not been reversed. The report found some narrowing of the widest gaps between social groups, such as male and female earnings. But it noted that deep-seated and systematic differences remained. The panel's report commented that gaps within social groups were significant and had grown. It also found that many inequalities accumulated across the life cycle, especially in socioeconomic groups, and through generations, making it difficult to achieve equality of opportunity.

Hills et al. (2009) found that initially the Labour government was strongly committed to policy initiatives aimed at reducing inequality but that subsequently (from around 2002/3) momentum was lost. Palmer et al. (2008) found that out of 56 statistical indicators of poverty and social exclusion, 30 improved while 7 deteriorated between 1997 and 2002/3. But between 2003 and the latest available data, 14 improved while 15 deteriorated.

Social Mobility

Another aspect of poverty and social exclusion is restricted social mobility. Social mobility reflects the degree of equal opportunity in society. It relates to the ability of people from low-income and working-class backgrounds to move to higher income and social groups if they choose. Several studies have concluded that social mobility in the UK has not improved in recent decades (Goldthorpe and Mills, 2008; Prime Minister's Strategy Unit, 2008b) while others have found a decline (Paxton and Dixon, 2004; Blanden and Gibbons, 2006; Blanden and Machin, 2008). One of the crucial factors in social mobility is education, which is strongly influenced by income and wealth. Wealthy parents are able to secure education for their children at the best schools and universities that enable them to secure the better-paid jobs of the future. This is done either by paying for private education or by access to the best performing state schools, which tend to be selective. This system reinforces existing biases and inequalities in society (Adonis and Pollard, 1997; Paxton and Dixon, 2004).

Some have called for a radical approach to social inequality and social mobility to address the structural bias in British society (see, for example, Diamond, 2005). This would involve greater redistribution through tax and benefit systems, direct public funding to services for the poor, a widening of asset ownership, increased spending on education and policies to redistribute opportunities towards disadvantaged people. Others have focused on the plight of disadvantaged children and have called for a range of policies to reduce child poverty, improve support in the early years, reduce social class differences in education, improve employment and training opportunities for poorer groups, reduce health inequalities and improve communities where poor people live (Independent Commission on Social Mobility, 2009). With regard to health outcomes, it has been argued that a policy of redistribution of income and wealth would have a major impact on health inequalities (Mitchell et al., 2000; Shaw et al., 2005).

Brown's Britain

Following the replacement of Blair by Brown, the Labour government reviewed its approach to social mobility. Following the Prime Minister's Strategy Unit (2008b) report, a white paper was subsequently issued (HM Government, 2009c), setting out priorities in investing in early years; schools; young adults; training; supporting families and communities. There was little new here. It was merely an extension of initiatives from the previous decade. Most proposals focused on addressing specific barriers to mobility, such as improving training opportunities and providing support for families with children. The white paper was silent on tackling the structural causes of injustice and inequality and redistributing wealth, income and opportunities. However, a new duty on the public services to tackle socioeconomic disadvantage and narrow the gaps between rich and poor was proposed. Legislation incorporating a duty on certain public authorities to consider socioeconomic disadvantage when taking strategic decisions was introduced into Parliament in 2009, alongside duties to promote equal opportunities for ethnic groups, men and women, people of different religions or beliefs, disabled people, people of different ages and lesbian, gay, bisexual and transgender (LGBT) people.

Further Steps on Health Inequalities

To be effective, policies to reduce health inequality must tackle all dimensions of the problem (Dahlgren and Whitehead, 1992). This includes action to tackle: general socioeconomic cultural and environmental conditions; living and working conditions; social and community influences; and individual lifestyle factors. In particular, there needs to be a much stronger link between social justice policies and inequality policies combined with a greater effort to address macro-environmental factors. This is the case not just in the UK but elsewhere (Crombie et al., 2005).

Although the Labour governments of Blair and Brown adopted a powerful rhetoric of social justice and concern for the disadvantaged, and introduced a raft of measures on social exclusion, equal opportunities and anti-discrimination, and extended rights, as well as specific measures on health inequalities, they continued the overarching socioeconomic policies of their Conservative predecessors. This involved an emphasis on markets, privatization and protecting the interests of the wealthy (Sampson, 2004). These policies made it impossible to tackle the fundamental socioeconomic inequalities that underpin health inequalities, and it is hardly surprising that the health gap persisted (Graham, 2007; Asthana and Halliday, 2006; Dowler and Spencer, 2007).

Turning from this bigger picture, the Health Committee (2009) made many recommendations on how health inequalities might be more effectively addressed in England. These included: better evaluation of initiatives (including piloting, randomization or use of quasi-experimental methods where this was not possible, collection of baseline data and monitoring of costs and outcomes); a closer match between PCTs' financial allocations and the needs of their populations; and better information about how effectively PCTs allocate budgets to reduce health inequalities. More specifically, the committee recommended a comprehensive traffic light system of labelling for food (see Chapter 13), the implementation of quantitative indicators for the Healthy Schools programme (see Chapter 9), changes to the planning system to encourage walking and cycling (Chapter 13), and further action on smuggled tobacco (see Chapter 15).

Meanwhile, the Labour government appeared to be increasingly concerned about its failure to achieve reductions in health inequalities and realized that more needed to be done (DoH, 2008f). The DoH placed faith in stronger partnerships between local agencies and on the development of assessment tools to identify, and incentives to promote, an appropriate response to health inequalities. Better performance management and a stronger evidence base were also part of its renewed strategy. The DoH also announced that it would commission a review of progress on inequalities covering the period since the Acheson report and contributing to the development of future strategy. The department also said that it would lead work across government on inequalities and would seek to ensure that health inequalities be included in policy impact assessments (as recommended by Acheson a decade earlier).

The review was chaired by Professor Marmot (who also chaired the WHO inquiry into social determinants of health – see Exhibit 17.2). Its report (Strategic Review of Health Inequalities in England, 2010) concluded that reducing health inequality was a matter of fairness and social justice, and that action should focus on reducing the social gradient in health. It also stated that health inequalities resulted from social inequalities and therefore action was needed across all social determinants. The review argued that actions must be universal but with a scale and intensity proportionate to the level of disadvantage. Focusing solely on the most disadvantaged would not reduce health inequalities. A further observation was that society and the economy would benefit from a narrowing of health inequalities. The report was critical of economic growth as the key indicator of success, arguing that fair distribution of health, wellbeing and sustainability were also important goals. The review identified six objectives: give every child the best start in life; enable children, young people, and adults to maximize their capabilities and have control over their lives; create fair employment and good work for all; ensure a healthy standard of living for all; create and develop healthy and sustainable places and communities; and strengthen the role and impact of ill health prevention. It called on various parties – central government, the NHS, the voluntary and private sectors and community groups – to help attain these objectives. Furthermore, it noted that national policies would not work without effective local delivery systems focused on health equity across all policies and that effective local delivery required participation and empowerment of individuals and communities.

The strategic review was inherited by the Cameron government, which acknowledged its findings and the six policy objectives it identified. Before becoming Prime Minister, Cameron had acknowledged the problem of health inequalities and pledged to allocate additional NHS public health resources to disadvantaged areas with high health needs (Conservative Party, 2010a).

He also acknowledged the role of poverty in health inequalities and that social inequalities could be damaging to society (Cameron, 2009). He endorsed the previous government's commitment to ending child poverty and pledged to create a fairer society by removing barriers to social mobility. Even so, the suspicion that the Cameron government would not place high priority on reducing health inequalities remained. First, there was no major commitment forthcoming on reducing underlying socioeconomic inequalities between the wealthy and the poor. The focus was instead on improving the position of the most disadvantaged. Second, the solutions proposed to reduce poverty and improve opportunities for the poor relied heavily on voluntary action. Cameron's vision of a 'Big Society' emphasised the contribution of private and charitable activities, a strengthening of individual responsibility, and a reduced role for the state within a decentralized system of governance (Cameron, 2009, 2010b). Yet many would argue that 'Big Government' is needed to protect the poor and uphold their rights as citizens. Third, the Cameron government has imposed tax increases and proposed large cuts in public expenditure. At the time of writing, these policies, and the underlying economic instability affecting the UK and other countries, have huge implications for poverty and social inequality. Future health inequalities are affected by current economic conditions (Van den Berg et al., 2009). Some fear that if the current economic conditions continue, the health gap will widen further (Thomas et al., 2010), and even may lessen the chances of sustained government action on inequalities in future (Graham, 2009).

Exhibit 17.1

Regeneration and Social Exclusion

Regeneration policy can be traced back to efforts to address the economic and social problems associated with the long-term decline of heavy industry concentrated in particular areas. It also has roots in postwar reconstruction, town planning, and slum clearance programmes. During the twentieth century, these various strands grew into a complex web of initiatives, funds and agencies. Although substantial resources were involved in these programmes, they were piecemeal, fragmented and poorly coordinated. Initiatives were often ad hoc and short term. They failed to address the complex and multiple aspects of the problem and, in particular, the needs of people living in deprived areas. Furthermore policies were 'top-down', and although local authorities were actively involved in regeneration, there was a failure to engage with the grassroots, the very people whose lives were blighted by living in run-down areas.

During the 1990s, the Conservative government attempted to rationalize regeneration programmes. Urban development corporations were set up to encourage the redevelopment of derelict urban land left by industry. The Single Regeneration Budget (SRB) was introduced in 1994, amalgamating various schemes. However, criticism remained of the lack of strategic purpose, poor accountability, lack of involvement of stake-holders and a lack of genuine assessment of the relative needs of the regions and localities (see Regional Policy Commission, 1996). There was also a concern that too much emphasis was placed on the physical aspects of regeneration (new buildings, infrastructure) and not enough on the needs of communities.

The New Labour government sought to bring regeneration under the aegis of its poli-cies to combat social exclusion and address the multiple causes of deprivation. A Social Exclusion Unit was established, which set out plans for a comprehensive effort to improve the welfare of communities (Cm 4045, 1998). It recommended a national strategy for neighbourhood renewal aimed at reducing the gap between deprived neighbourhoods and the rest of England, and in the worst neighbourhoods to improve health, and education, while reducing crime and longer term worklessness. This was carried forward by 18 Policy Action Teams, which brought together officials, experts and stakeholders to explore specific aspects of social exclusion, such as housing, employment, skills, antisocial behaviour, sport and the arts.

This strategy developed alongside various regeneration and support programmes, introduced by New Labour, aimed at reducing social exclusion. The New Deal for Communities was introduced as a long-term plan to invest in neighbourhoods with multiple problems arising from deprivation. The Blair government initially retained the SRB but initiated a number of changes with a view to relating allocation of resources more closely to needs, promoting greater involvement by communities and stake-holders, and providing a more strategic overview at regional level, through new regional development agencies (RDAs). This was replaced by a new funding regime in 2002, bringing together all the current RDA funding schemes.

A further aim of the Blair government was to improve the link between regeneration and other area-based programmes located in deprived areas. These included Sure Start (see Chapter 9), which sought greater integration of services for children at risk of social exclusion in order to improve their emotional, physical, intellectual, and social development. Also, health action zones (see Chapter 7), as well as education and employment action zones, located in areas of high need, were expected to dovetail with the broader regeneration programmes. Regeneration continued to be linked to traditional policies such as housing renewal (see Exhibit 16.2) and economic develop-ment. But it also became more closely associated with new policy agendas such as sustainable development and community safety initiatives (see Chapter 11).

In 2000, the Blair government launched its *National Strategy for Neighbourhood Renewal* (Social Exclusion Unit, 2000, 2001). This was based on the Policy Action Team reports. Following a period of consultation, an action plan was introduced. This aimed to reduce worklessness and crime as well as improve health, skills, housing, and the physical environment in the most deprived neighbourhoods. The plan was seen as an improvement on previous attempts to address the problems of deprived areas in several respects. It was long term. It sought to address a range of problems in a coor-dinated and coherent way. It aimed to work with communities, emphasizing the impor-tance of social capital, cohesion and community development. It was not simply aimed at promoting economic development and improved physical infrastructure (although these were important objectives). There were also encouraging signs that policies might be better coordinated than in the past. The Neighbourhood Renewal Unit was estab-lished to coordinate policy at central government level (now part of the Department of

Communities and Local Government). At local level, local strategic partnerships were established to coordinate the efforts of local agencies (now rolled out to all local authority areas, not just those targeted by the Neighbourhood Renewal strategy). Funding was provided for those areas involved in the programme. In addition, targets were set for improving outcomes in areas including employment, education, health, crime, housing and (from 2004) the quality of the environment. Notably, these were aimed at reducing inequalities and set minimum standards for poor areas and disadvantaged groups (known as 'floor targets').

It is difficult to assess the impact of the regeneration and social exclusion initiatives, particularly as it is a long-term plan. Although there has been some specific improvement in indicators for crime, employment, education and housing, it is impossible to generalize (Blackman, 2006). Even though health has been increasingly recognized as an important part of the regeneration agenda, it is one of many competing considerations. It is also relatively easy to overlook, particularly when health priorities conflict with economic priorities. To put it another way, economic regeneration must incorporate a philosophy of health promotion and this has been rather slow to develop (although national guidance has been issued on health and regeneration – DoH and Neighbourhood Renewal Unit, 2002). Moreover, the regeneration strategy says little about geographical areas that are arguably 'overdeveloped' or individuals whose wealth and income are extremely high. Yet these factors contribute much to social exclusion and inequity. Indeed, it can be argued that social exclusion policies which tend to concentrate on the poor and deprived areas and the people living in them tend towards victim-blaming (Scott-Samuel, 1998). A broader agenda, and one which the New Labour government occasionally acknowledged, was to focus on improving health and wellbeing in all areas, not just those that are deprived (Cm 4911, 2000; Cm 4909, 2000). Relevant to this was the report of the Urban Task Force (Rogers, 1999) which identified not only specific measures to address particularly deprived areas but broader approaches to improving the urban environment as a whole. The needs of rural areas also need to be addressed. Often there is considerable social exclusion in areas outside deprived urban neighbourhoods (Commission for Rural Communities, 2005; Cm 4909, 2000).

The future of regeneration policy is uncertain. The Cameron government proposed abolishing RDAs and other regional bodies (see Chapter 7). Furthermore, given the likely scale of impending public sector budget cuts, it is probable that regeneration programmes will be substantially reduced.

Other Inequalities

As the Health Committee (2009) noted, policy has focused mainly on socio-economic health inequalities. But, as shown in the previous chapter, other health inequalities such as those relating to ethnicity, gender, disability and age are important. With regard to these groups, the New Labour government and the NHS adopted a three-tier approach: efforts to improve access to services; specific prevention initiatives; and broader social and economic policies.

Ethnic Groups

Perhaps the most important measure affecting ethnic health inequalities has been legislative change (in particular the Race Relations Amendment Act 2000) to outlaw discrimination in public services and promote equality between ethnic groups. However, compliance varies in practice, and the NHS has often been slow to develop proactive policies in this field (Healthcare Commission, 2007c). Policy initiatives include the Delivering Racial Equality initiative in mental health services, which involves PCTs providing race equality training, appointing race equality leads and community development workers (POST, 2007). National guidance on mental health services for ethnic communities was also issued. A number of initiatives are aimed at spreading good practice in race equality and mainstreaming this into health and social care, including 'Race for Health', a DoH-funded programme that works with PCTs and NHS trusts to improve services. Ethnic groups have also benefited from local initiatives to improve access to care and to promote health, especially in cities with diverse and multicultural communities, such as Leicester, Birmingham and some London boroughs. Some ethnic groups may benefit from wider programmes to reduce social exclusion and poverty. However, this is not guaranteed as many ethnic minority people live outside areas benefiting from these programmes. Moreover, even those that do may face additional language and cultural barriers that prevent them from benefiting fully.

Gender and Sexuality

Policies have focused on expanding services that target gender-specific conditions (such as cervical and breast cancer screening for women and testicular and prostate cancer in men). Services have attempted to address men's and women's health issues in a broader sense (for example well woman/well man clinics). There have been attempts to tailor services to specific gender needs, as in the case of maternity services (although the choices available to women have often fallen short of expectations – see Health Committee, 2003c). Women have benefited to some extent from the government's gender equality agenda and from specific measures to increase female participation in the workforce. The Equal Pay Act, introduced in 1970, was strengthened in 2003. In 2006, a new Equality Act created a duty on public authorities to create equal opportunities between men and women and to prohibit sexual discrimination in the workplace. In recent years, specific health initiatives have focused on inequalities from a male perspective and have sought to target these through improved policies and services (for example mental health problems in young men and suicide prevention). Some health services have also attempted to tailor their services to the needs of LGBT communities (Fish, 2006).

Age and Disability

Government has sought to rid the NHS of ageism and of discrimination against people with long-term conditions and disabilities, although evidence of such practices persists (see Exhibit 16.3). For older people, an effort was made to focus on prevention and public health as part of the older people's national service framework. Among other things, this sought to promote healthy and active lifestyles and prevent falls among elderly people. Some PCTs along with local authorities and the voluntary sector have been innovative in creating local projects to promote older people's health, for example by encouraging exercise and also smoking cessation (DoH, 2007c). However, services remain underdeveloped and more needs to be done to shift resources towards health promotion. Other policies, such as the Expert Patients' Programme, have sought to maintain health and improve the quality of life of older people (as well as people of other ages) with long-term conditions. Breast cancer screening has been extended to women aged 70, and older people have benefited from flu vaccination programmes. More broadly, pensioners benefited from the Labour governments' broader social and economic policies, notably from specific policies such as free prescriptions, bus travel and swimming, as well as winter fuel payments and grants for home insulation, all of which have health implications. Disabled people have potentially benefited from a wider definition of disability and increased scope of discrimination provisions in the Disability Discrimination Act 2005, but again, much depends on the implementation in practice. The 2009 equality legislation, mentioned earlier, strengthens the position of older people and disabled people facing discrimination. Age discrimination in employment and training was made unlawful in 2006. The new legislation seeks to extend this to services, including health and social care services.

International Developments

Health inequalities are not confined to the UK (Mackenbach, 2005; Commission on Social Determinants of Health, 2008). Many countries seek to reduce health inequalities (Crombie et al., 2005; Judge et al., 2005; Mackenbach and Stronks, 2002). Such policies have been encouraged by WHO, which has long emphasized the importance of promoting equity in health. This was a key theme of the Declaration of Alma Ata (WHO/UNICEF, 1978). This message was reiterated subsequently by WHO conferences and policy statements in the 1980s and 90s, such as the Ottawa Charter on Health Promotion (WHO, 1986), the Adelaide Recommendations (WHO, 1988), and the Jakarta Declaration (WHO, 1997a) (see Chapter 5). Reducing inequalities was also an important aspect of WHO programmes such as Healthy Cities (see Exhibit 7.1).

Equity was a key feature of the *Health for All* strategy (WHO, 1981). In 1985 specific targets were set for the WHO European region that included a reduction of at least 25 per cent in the differences in health status between groups and countries by improving the health of disadvantaged groups (WHO Regional Office for Europe, 1985). The emphasis on equity in health was maintained when *Health for All* was revised (see WHO, 1998a). The European regional targets were updated, the equity target now stating that, 'By the Year 2020 the health gap between socioeconomic groups within countries should be reduced by one fourth in all member states, by substantially improving the health of disadvantaged groups' (WHO Regional Office for Europe, 1999c).

Amid criticism that it was not doing enough to reduce inequalities within countries (see, for example, Braveman et al., 2001), WHO has strengthened efforts to promote action on health inequalities. It established a Commission on Social Determinants of Health in 2005 to conduct an analysis of health inequalities and possible policies and interventions. Its report (Commission on Social Determinants of Health, 2008) called for a closing of the health gap within a generation, setting out a number of targets. These included: reducing by 10 years between 2000 and 2040 the life expectancy at birth (LEB) gap between the one third of countries with highest and the one third with the lowest LEB levels by levelling up the latter; halving in the same period the LEB gap between social groups within countries by levelling up the lower socioeconomic groups; reducing mortality rates in all countries and in all social groups within countries in this period, halving adult mortality rates, reducing the under-5 mortality rate by 90 per cent and the maternal mortality rate by 95 per cent.

The Commission made three overarching recommendations. First, improve daily living conditions, the circumstances in which people are born, grow, live, work and age. In particular, the Commission identified the improvement of conditions for girls and women and of the circumstances in which children are born, an emphasis on early child development and education for girls and boys, improvement of living and working conditions, a social protection policy for all, and the creation of conditions for a flourishing older life. Second, the Commission recommended that the inequitable distribution of power, money and resources must be tackled. This would require a strong public sector, committed, capable and adequately funded. It would also need strengthened governance, legitimacy, space and support for civil society, an accountable private sector and collective action. Third, the Commission recommended that health inequity be measured within countries and globally. It also urged that the impact of policies and actions on equity be evaluated. In order to create the necessary capacity, the Commission recommended investment in training of policymakers and practitioners and greater public understanding of social determinants of health, as well as more research into social determinants. More specifically, the Commission made a number of recommendations aimed at international agencies, governments and others such as NGOs and donors (see Exhibit 17.2).

Exhibit 17.2

Commission on Social Determinants of Health

Key Recommendations:

- Universal coverage of comprehensive package of quality early development programmes and services regardless of ability to pay.
- Quality education that pays attention to children's physical, social/emotional, language/cognitive development starting in pre-primary school.
- Quality compulsory primary and secondary education, regardless of ability to pay.
- The establishment of participatory mechanisms to enable people to engage in building healthier and safer cities.
- Greater availability of affordable housing.
- Promotion of physical activity through investment in active transport.
- Encourage health eating through retail planning of access to food.
- Reduce violence through environmental design, including controls on alcohol outlets.
- The implementation of programmes to promote equity between rural and urban areas.
- Consider the health equity impact of strategies concerned with adaptation and mitigation of climate change.
- Fair, full employment and strengthened representation of workers in policy and programmes in this field.
- Economic and social policies that provide secure work and a living wage.
- Stronger enforcement of work standards and employment.
- Reduced insecurity and fairer pay for informal, temporary and part-time workers.
- Occupational health and safety be extended to all workers and beyond material work-related hazards to include stress and behavioural factors.
- Establish universal social protection systems at a level that is sufficient for healthy living.
- Health care should be universal, focused on primary care and available regardless of ability to pay.
- Improving health equity should be a measure of government performance.
- Health equity should be a cross-government responsibility chaired at the highest political level possible.
- The monitoring of social determinants must be institutionalized and health equity impact assessment used for all policies, including finance.

- The health sector should adopt a social determinants of health approach, with leadership from the minister of health.

- National capacity for progressive taxation should be strengthened.

- New national and global mechanisms such as special health taxes and global tax options should be developed.

- Donor countries should increase aid to 0.7 per cent of GDP (under existing commitments), expand debt relief and coordinate aid through a social determinants of health framework.

- Measures should be implemented to avoid future unsustainable debt in international borrowing.

- Governments should establish a cross-government mechanism to allocate a budget for action on social determinants of health.

- Public resources be equitably allocated and monitored between regions and social groups.

- Health equity impact assessments be incorporated in international economic agreements.

- Public health should have stronger representation in international and domestic economic policy negotiations.

- Strengthen public sector leadership in the provision of health goods and services and control of health-damaging products.

- Address gender biases in structures of society and organizations.

- Increase investment in sexual and reproductive health services.

- Empower all groups in society through fair representation in decision-making.

- Make health equity a global development goal and adopt a social determinants framework to strengthen multilateral action on development.

- WHO to institutionalize social determinants approach across all sectors.

- Ensure routine monitoring systems for health equity and social determinants of health are in place locally, nationally and internationally.

- Invest in generating and sharing new evidence on social determinants of health and effectiveness of measures to reduce health inequities.

- Provide training on social determinants of health to policy actors, stakeholders, and practitioners and invest in raising public awareness.

- Build capacity for health equity impact assessment.

Source: Adapted from Commission on Social Determinants of Health (2008). *Closing the Gap in a Generation: Health Equity Through Action on the Social Determinants of Health.* Final Report. Geneva: World Health Organization. Reproduced with permission.

At the European level, action on health inequalities has been stimulated by European level WHO commitments and targets mentioned above. Another stimulus has been the concern to address issues of poverty and social exclusion at the European level, which addresses the social determinants of health. The EU (and previously the European Community) built on articles in the original Treaty of Rome which advocated close cooperation on social policy (Nugent, 2006; Hantrais, 2007). Subsequent treaties and European Court judgments strengthened the ability of the EU to introduce a range of policies on poverty, social exclusion, equal opportunities and anti-discrimination, social cohesion, employment and economic development. These included projects to improve the welfare of elderly and disabled people, the promotion of equal opportunities and extended rights for workers and citizens. In 2000, the EU identified poverty and social inclusion as a priority and established a process for reviewing the action plans of member states in this field (Official Journal of the European Communities, 2000).

More specifically the EU has identified health inequalities as an important issue and has funded projects in this field. This includes DETERMINE, an EU Consortium for action on socioeconomic determinants of health, consisting of government agencies, health bodies, networks and other organizations. EU health strategy has as one of its aims the reduction of health inequalities (see Chapter 5). The focus was strengthened in 2005, when the British presidency of the EU chose to highlight health inequalities (Arie, 2005). During this period, the European Commission established a new expert group to produce reports on health inequality in Europe. At the time of writing, action on health inequalities is being considered as a possible cross-cutting area for the EU new health strategy. The European Commission has proposed using EU funding for public health projects to reduce health inequalities.

Exhibit 17.3

The UK Devolved Governments' Strategies on Health Inequalities

Wales has placed great emphasis on equity, both with regard to health inequalities and unequal access to health care. This was acknowledged in *Better Health, Better Wales* (NAfW, 1998). Subsequently, the Welsh Assembly commissioned a report on health inequalities, which recommended a dual approach involving a range of actions within and outside the NHS. Specific recommendations included renewed efforts to tackle poverty and inequality, a health inequalities fund, better evaluation of the impact of NHS spending on equity, and a new formula to allocate health resources on the basis of need (Townsend, 2001). A health inequalities fund was established in 2001 to stimulate action by targeting resources at disadvantaged populations. The initial focus was on coronary heart disease, and a number of projects have been funded in areas such as workplace health, lifestyle advice and risk assessment. Welsh health strategies have continued the commitment to reduce health inequalities (Welsh Assembly Government, 2005a). A revised health inequalities strategy has been promised for 2010.

The Scottish government has also shown a strong commitment to tackling health inequalities as part of a wider programme of social justice. In 1999, a social justice strategy was introduced (Scottish Executive, 1999b, 1999c). This was followed by a new cross-departmental poverty and social exclusion strategy, *Closing the Opportunity Gap* (Scottish Executive, 2002d, 2004). As part of this, targets were set to reduce health inequalities between people in deprived and affluent areas by improving health in deprived areas by 15 per cent. Subsequently, the Scottish government responded positively to recommendations that health inequalities be included in health impact assessment (HIA). Such a move was also backed by a ministerial task force appointed to review strategy on health inequalities (Scottish Government, 2008b). The ministerial review's report (*Equally Well*) set out a range of recommendations including action in four main areas: children's early years, mental illness and wellbeing; the 'big killers', such as cancer and heart disease; and drug and alcohol problems. The underlying philosophy was to improve the range of circumstances and environments to improve people's lives and their health; to address intergenerational factors that perpetuate inequalities; to engage individuals, families and communities in their own health; to deliver public services that are targeted to those most in need and geared to prevention. Specific recommendations included further development of support services for families with young children, action to improve the physical environment and transport to promote healthy weight, and more help for people with depression and anxiety living in deprived areas. The task force report was followed by an implementation plan, which identified a number of local test sites to take forward specific recommendations from the task force (Scottish Government, 2008c). In addition, a new poverty and social inclusion framework was introduced in 2008 (Scottish Government, 2008d). This gave a commitment to increase the proportion of income received by the poorest 30 per cent of households by 2017, decrease the proportion of people living in poverty and increase healthy life expectancy at birth in the most deprived areas.

Northern Ireland has pursued a broad strategy on social justice and equality since the early 1990s. The policy of 'targeting social need' introduced by the Conservative government aimed to tackle socioeconomic differences between Protestant and Catholic communities. It was reinforced with a new initiative (known as New Targeting Social Need) by the Blair government. This began to focus more effectively on the underlying causes of inequalities and social exclusion and was developed further by the devolved adminstration (Office of First Minister and Deputy First Minister, 2004, 2007b). More specifically, Northern Ireland's cross-departmental strategy, *Investing for Health*, sought to address those factors that shape health inequalities (DHSSPS, 2002a). Northern Ireland has a target to halve the gap in life expectancy between deprived areas and the average by 2010, and to reduce the gap in long-standing illness between the highest and most deprived socioeconomic groups by 20 per cent.

Conclusion

The governments of Blair and Brown acknowledged the existence of health inequalities. This represented an important shift in policy compared with the Conservative governments of the 1980s and 90s, which attempted to ignore or downplay the problem. Since 1997 there has been a large amount of policy activity in this field. This included broader social and economic policies and specific health inequality initiatives.

However, the continuation of the previous Conservative government's neoliberal approach in economic and fiscal policy was a major barrier to progress. And there was a failure to strongly link the social justice, regeneration and health agendas. Furthermore, despite attempts to target and prioritize health inequalities, progress was difficult in the face of continuing and widening socioeconomic inequalities that marked British society. It is unlikely that the 'health gap' will be narrowed as long as these trends continue. Indeed, in the present economic and political climate of economic instability and public expenditure cuts, and with a government that is, arguably, less likely to pursue strategies of equality than Labour, inequalities are likely to widen further.

Conclusion

18

Chapter 1 outlined three broad approaches as a framework for analysing public health policy: ideological perspectives, theories of risk, and models of the policy process. Having explored public health issues in detail in the intervening chapters, it is now possible to draw some conclusions within the context of this framework.

Ideological Perspectives

Different ideological perspectives have been influential in different historical periods. In the Victorian and Edwardian periods, liberal ideas were powerful. Health considerations were subjugated to market forces, profit-making and private commercial interests. Nonetheless, other ideologies did exert influence. Paternalism and utilitarianism had much impact on the response to public health problems of the Victorian era, as Chapter 2 illustrated. During the twentieth century, as socialism became more influential, policies reflected collectivist welfare principles, culminating in the creation of the postwar welfare state. Somewhat paradoxically, the NHS, one of the flagships of the welfare state, did not give priority to public health or preventive medicine, although it did contribute to improved levels of health by improving access to health care.

Turning to more modern times, public health rose up the agenda with the focus initially on the collectivist, socialist and egalitarian principles of 'Health for All'. However, neoliberal ideas became more entrenched among the political elite from the late 1970s onwards. These began to shape the state's response to public health, with a greater emphasis on individual responsibilities, personal choices and on the role of business interests as a partner, rather than an enemy, of public health. A key impetus behind such approaches was that investment in public health and health promotion could reduce the costs of the welfare state. It was, however, shown that prevention did not necessarily reduce costs. Nonetheless, these ideas were influential not only in

Conservative party circles but among the Labour party leadership, increasingly attracted to a Third Way approach combining elements of collectivism and neoliberalism. Consequently, the emphasis on individual responsibility intensified, as reflected in Tony Blair's comments in 2006:

> Our public health problems are not, strictly speaking, public health questions at all, they are questions of individual lifestyle. (www.politics.co.uk, 26/7/06)

The Third Way also encouraged efforts to bring commercial organizations into partnership with the state to promote health. Voluntary agreements were drawn up with a number of industries whose products were linked to ill health, such as the food and drink industries. As the Nuffield Council on Bioethics (2007) argued, commercial organizations should help to minimize health harms. For example, food and drink firms have an ethical duty to assist individuals to make healthy choices. The Nuffield Council on Bioethics further maintained that the state has a responsibility to undertake regulation when the market fails to uphold its responsibility and where the health of the population is at risk. Although the Blair and Brown governments did strengthen regulation of commercial interests where self-regulation did not succeed, as in the case of the tobacco industry, they were extremely tolerant of inadequate self-regulation in other areas, such as alcohol and nutrition.

Other ideologies have also been influential. Green perspectives shaped the public health agenda. The growth of Green values, coupled with the persistence of collectivist ideas in society, acted as a brake on neoliberalism and the liberal elements of the Third Way. Issues such as pollution, global warming and sustainability have promoted an extension in the state's role. Many of these interventions have important benefits for public health. Public health policies have also been influenced by feminist ideas. Reforms to improve child and maternal health in the early decades of the twentieth century were influenced by a growing awareness of women's rights and needs. Services have continued to develop to meet specific health needs of women, such as screening for breast and cervical cancer. However, as Chapter 8 showed, the benefits of some interventions have been challenged. Public health policies have tended to address specific diseases of women, rather than to address the public health consequences of women's social and economic roles. They have also ignored the role of environmental factors in the onset of diseases that affect women disproportionately.

Public health interventions are often disliked by neoliberals, who have reacted by restating the importance of individual liberties and the dangers of the nanny state. The dangers of the overpowerful and interfering state have a powerful resonance that is not confined to right-wing liberals. Moreover, opposition to public health intervention on libertarian grounds is not new. Campaigns against fluoridation and for smokers' rights have their antecedents in the Victorian anti-vaccination campaigns and the opponents of the Contagious Diseases Acts. Fears about health fascism are not groundless, as illustrated by the more extreme reactions to public health problems in history. People fear and dislike compulsion. The danger is that such fears may be used by powerful interests to prevent policies that may contribute to the public good. It is important therefore that the least intrusive means are used to achieve public health objectives (Nuffield Council on Bioethics, 2007). These may include better information about health risks, a context that allows real choice and incentives (such as taxes and subsidies) to encourage healthier outcomes (Durante, 2007). A more participatory approach, which involves people in the assessment of health risks and seeks to operate with a more sympathetic approach to their social context, may also help to build greater trust between the individual and the state on these matters and avoid 'victim-blaming'. This is discussed further below. Of course, there will be situations where a draconian approach is needed, such as a mass outbreak of a highly infectious fatal disease for example. But such infringements of liberty must be kept to a minimum and commensurate with the risks of harm. It is also crucial that interventions are based on good evidence, discussed further below.

Risk

As noted in the introductory chapter, there is much controversy about the nature of risk in modern societies. According to some, modern societies are host to an array of high consequence risks. For others, risk is exaggerated through processes of social construction. What light has this book shed on this debate?

It has been shown that ill health is associated with risks arising from a range of factors including accidents, pollution, climate change, harmful agents in food, diet, drug and alcohol consumption and smoking. Furthermore people's risk in many of these areas varies according to their socioeconomic status. Whether they face greater risks now than in the past is difficult to substantiate. In many respects, there have been improvements in public health and the risks associated with some activities have declined, such as accidents in the workplace for example. Even so, there is evidence of increased risks in some areas in recent decades (for example drugs, alcohol, environmental risks) although even these kinds of problems are not unprecedented.

Two things are evident. First, contemporary health risks appear to be more complex than was previously the case. Concerns about specific pollutants have been overtaken to some extent by systemic risks, such as those associated with climate change. Problems are interlocking, such as the environmental effects of the food system for example. Risks are often manifested globally, not just in one country. Although infectious diseases have often in the past spread from country to country, the risks are perhaps greater now with the advent of globalization and the increased travel and interaction it brings. The risk of transferring diseases between countries is also now applicable to chronic illness. The burgeoning global consumer culture appears to have enhanced the spread of lifestyle-related diseases associated with smoking, alcohol and obesity, for example.

Second, there is heightened sensitivity about health risks. This is partly because there is more information about such risks. However, more is not necessarily better as this information is often of poor quality. The research evidence base is often weak and findings sometimes contradictory. There is a significant gap between researchers, policymakers and practitioners (Hunter, 2009). Moreover, findings are often manipulated by vested interests or misinterpreted (sometimes deliberately) by the media (Goldacre, 2008). This can lead to risk amplification in some areas while understating other risks. For example, the risk of illegal drugs has tended to be exaggerated by the media while those associated with legal addictions (at least until recently) have been underplayed.

The precautionary principle, a key element in responding to future risks, is a way of dealing with uncertainty. But it is criticized by some for exaggerating risks in the absence of clear evidence. The culture of fear (Furedi, 1997) that this creates engenders irrational behaviour and ill-founded policies. As a result, entrepreneurialism and creativity are stifled. Social control and regulation increase and individual liberty is eroded (Booker and North, 2007). This can be a real danger. Policymakers are in a difficult position, however. Faced with scientific evidence of the possibility of a large-scale public health problem, they are damned if they act and the problem is less than anticipated (as with new variant CJD) and damned if they do nothing and the problem deteriorates. Where a major systemic threat to health, such as climate change, is predicted policymakers must act on incomplete evidence, as to do nothing could foreclose options further down the line. It is easy to criticize with the benefit of hindsight.

The emphasis on health risks has increased the power of some groups, notably those who highlight, study and manage risks, such as health pressure groups, scientific experts and risk managers. This has had a disempowering effect on people who are often sceptical about prescriptions and processes emerging from the 'risk business'. There is a pressing need to involve and engage people in their health in order to balance lay and expert perspectives. This may entail giving people accurate, intelligible, evidence-based information about risks. It also might involve greater public engagement in health, allowing them to put forward their ideas based on personal experience about how their health and that of the wider community can be improved (Labonte, 1998). Communicating risks must not be a one-way street (Irwin and Wynne, 1996). In this context some have highlighted the importance of lay epidemiology and community development, which place greater emphasis on lay perspectives. By being sensitive to the concerns of people who might be at higher risk of health problems, it may be possible to identify contextual and subjective factors that affect health and wellbeing but that are not easily detectable by conventional scientific methods. As already noted, this may help to avoid the victim-blaming often associated with public health policies. By seeking to understand social and cultural processes associated with lifestyles involving greater risk of illness, policy-makers and professionals can reach a fuller understanding of risk attitudes and behaviours that undermine public health policies and interventions. These may include risk compensation, where people take greater risks in a safer environment, and the deliberate choice of unhealthy lifestyles as a protest against perceived state control and surveillance. At the same time, greater lay involvement in public health issues may enable people to take more informed decisions about their own individual health risks while providing a basis for community action to improve health.

Policy Processes

What conclusions can be drawn about the policy processes in public health? One of the most obvious points is that these involve many different layers of government. National policies are shaped by international and European policies, agreements, institutions and processes. Some of these have a primary focus on health, such as global strategies on alcohol, tobacco and diet. Others, though having important health implications, are located in other policy arenas such as trade, environment, and agriculture. Examples include WTO processes, the Common Agricultural Policy and agreements on pollution and climate change. While global and European institutions and processes are not new influences on public health policies, it appears that they are becoming more important in many areas including food and drink, illegal drugs, alcohol, tobacco and the environment.

National policies in turn are moderated by devolved and subnational government structures. In the UK, devolved powers have enabled Wales, Scotland and Northern Ireland to adopt distinctive policies, placing emphasis on different priorities or using different policy instruments. Although constraints have been imposed by the need to respect UK-wide policies and international and European frameworks, there are many examples of devolved governments using their powers to develop innovative public health policies and processes. In some cases, these experiences have created political pressures to undertake reforms in other parts of the UK (as in the case of Scotland's smoking ban in public places, for example).

The regional and local levels of government also became increasingly important. Regional bodies acquired influence over policies affecting public health (such as economic development, planning, transport). However, recent proposals by the Cameron government, aimed at removing regional government in all areas of England outside London, will transfer these powers to local bodies and consortia. Local authorities and partnership bodies have scope to address public health priorities in their individual and joint plans. While such priorities may have been neglected in the past, there are signs that local bodies are beginning to take their responsibilities in this area more seriously.

A problem that faces governing institutions at all levels is the multi-sectoral nature of public health. A wide range of policy sectors affect health – such as trade, environment, agriculture, transport. Yet there is poor coordination of these various arenas. For example, WTO processes and the Common Agriculture Policy have been criticized for failing to place sufficient emphasis on health. The same arguments apply at national and subnational level. There has been poor coordination of public health between government departments. At regional and local level, more could be done to prioritize public health and improve partnerships between the various agencies involved. There have been some improvements at all these levels in recent years, including commitments to healthy public policies, more explicit coordinating and partnership working arrangements and the championing of health impact assessment as a means of incorporating health consequences into decision-making. However, the reality of multi-sector public health often falls short of the rhetoric.

This problem must be addressed. As this book has shown, public health issues are often interrelated in complex ways Health inequalities are associated with a range of specific public health problems (smoking, obesity and accidents, for example). There are important links between the problems of food production, obesity and climate change. Transport is linked to a range of public health issues (accidents, obesity, pollution). Planning systems have a wide range of implications for health, including pollution, physical activity and access to food products. Governments at all levels must be much more intelligent in tackling these interrelated problems. A holistic approach to public health, marshalling the resources of all governmental agencies is necessary (Durante, 2007).

Public health has been accorded much higher priority at all levels of government than in the recent past. As noted, concerns about future costs of illness and health services have provided impetus and projected public health issues onto the agenda. Public health has benefited from the high priority accorded to environmental issues, such as pollution and climate change, which have significant health implications. Another reason for the increasing attention given to public health by government is effective campaigning by pressure groups and coalitions. Action on smoking, alcohol and obesity, for example, has arisen partly because of well-organized lobbies that include health professionals.

Those campaigning for improvements in public health have been successful in getting issues on the agenda by advocating policies in various arenas. The media have taken up issues and helped create wider public concern on issues such as alcohol abuse and obesity, for example. Parliament has also been a useful arena in which to advocate policy recommendations and amplify them, through the reports of select committees, for example. But Parliament and the media can also be significant barriers to action. Commercial lobbies have influence over both. In addition, sections of the media have been highly critical of the nanny state and what they see as undue interference in individual lifestyles.

The public health lobby is stronger and better organized than in the recent past. This is partly because of the greater role played by experts in policy advocacy. The BMA and some Royal Colleges, for example, now play a leading role in campaigns to strengthen policies, such as in the fields of alcohol and tobacco. New alliances have been formed and there is much more coherence in campaigns to change policy. What is perhaps lacking is a common agenda for public health. Even here, though, there have been efforts to promote this. The public health manifesto launched by the Faculty of Public Health and the Royal Society for Public Health (2010) is a step in the direction of a more unified approach.

The manifesto contained 12 key recommendations, which applied across the contemporary field of public health:

- a minimum price of 50p per unit of alcohol by 2011

- no junk food advertising on pre-watershed TV by 2011

- 20 mph limit in built up areas by 2011

- a dedicated school nurse for every secondary school by 2012

- 25 per cent increase in cycle lanes and cycles racks by 2015

- compulsory and standard front-of-pack labelling on all pre-packaged food by 2011

- a commitment to expand and upgrade school sports facilities and playing fields by 2012

- introduce presumed consent for organ donation by 2011

- stop the use of transfats by 2011

- ban smoking in cars with children by 2011

- free school meals for all children under 16 by 2014

- chlamydia tests for all new university and college students by 2013

Another problem for the public health lobby is that it lacks a mass membership. It mainly comprises expert groups and small lobbying organizations. On Green issues, in contrast, there are large membership organizations that give additional legitimacy to lobbying efforts. Although one can identify a coherent public health lobby, one cannot at present identify a public health movement. Much more remains to be done to engage with the public and gain their active support for public health objectives and policies.

The higher priority given to public health by government has been reflected in the setting of public health targets. Many public health advocates see such targets as a good thing, underlining an official commitment to health improvement. However, targets can be counterproductive, particularly if there are too many, or if government constantly changes the target for political expedience (Healthcare Commission/Audit Commission, 2008). Targets may also skew priorities by shifting efforts away from areas where targets have not been set or where performance is difficult to measure. Moreover, despite the political attention being given to public health in the past two decades, it has somewhat paradoxically been marginalized despite being firmly on the political agenda. For example, although the subject of no fewer than three white papers between 1992 and 2004, public health has continued to lack weight compared with other issues, such as health service reform for example. Despite the rhetorical commitment, the public health function remains under-resourced and lacks coherence and capacity. Where there have been advances, as in smoking policy for example, this has been underpinned by a strong and coherent lobby, which has persisted over time.

Although governments at all levels could do more to improve public health, it should not be exclusively a government responsibility. As already noted, it is important that individuals and communities, and the organizations that represent them, are engaged. The voluntary sector and charities have a key part to play in improving health. Recent governments have also identified a role for commercial organizations, including the food and drinks industries. This is controversial, as already noted, because private industry has often been perceived as the enemy of public health in the past. One thinks of the water companies' campaign against the Victorian sanitary reforms, the asbestos industry's efforts to evade responsibility for fatal lung diseases and the tobacco industry's attempts to deny the impact of smoking on health.

However, not all industries are bad for health. In some cases, such as the food industry, voluntary cooperation might bring benefits, as the expertise of the corporate sector can be used to improve health (by marketing healthier foods, for example). Indeed, companies may have an incentive to develop healthier products; increasing profit margins and gaining market share over rivals. However, there are dangers in working with private interests. Governments can be manipulated by large corporations, which are highly skilled in the arts of lobbying. Commercial interests may use voluntary approaches as a means of diluting or delaying policies that might damage profits but be better for health. This is an accusation that has been levelled at the alcoholic drinks industry, for example (Health Committee, 2010).

Commercial organizations are extremely active in policy networks that affect health. They are regarded as insider groups that have good access to ministers and civil servants across a range of departments. They are particularly influential in trade, agriculture, transport and environment policy arenas where they may be regarded as 'core insiders'. Even in health policy, they are effective lobbyists, notwithstanding the involvement in these policy networks of countervailing insider groups such as the medical profession and other professional groups.

Another key element is the role of evidence in policymaking. The Blair government often emphasized its commitment to evidence-based policy. However, much depends on the availability of evidence and the extent to which the policy processes draws upon it. Public health policies have suffered on both counts (Hunter, 2009). The evidence base is relatively weak (Health Committee, 2009; Healthcare Commission/Audit Commission, 2008). All too often it has been difficult to establish links conclusively between certain activities and health. Sometimes this is because there are so many factors involved that causation is difficult to prove. In other cases it is because little or no research has been undertaken. There has also been insufficient evaluation of public health interventions, which undermines their legitimacy and prevents lessons from being learned for future policy development. There is an element of policy transfer where initiatives are taken up as a result of experience elsewhere – examples include the smoking ban, food safety agencies and congestion charges. Policy transfer can also be encouraged by international and European policy frameworks that advocate particular interventions. It is important to note that evidence does not operate in a political vacuum. It feeds into ideas about how to solve problems. But much depends on how these ideas are taken up by policy advocates and the nature of the political context. Policy windows open up when the various problem, policy and political streams converge. Evidence can be a catalyst in this process – the case of smoking bans in enclosed public places is one example. But it doesn't guarantee action, particularly when the political stream – public opinion, party leaderships and the media – is not conducive to action.

Finally, the role of party politics must be considered. Although there has been a high degree of continuity in public health policies since the 1990s, the governing party has set the context for policy development. The Blair and Brown governments developed policies in particular areas neglected by their Conservative predecessors – for example in relation to poverty and health inequalities. They strengthened policies in some areas, notably food policy, smoking and, more recently, alcohol. However, as this book has shown, both public health policy and achievement fell short of the promises of New Labour in opposition.

At the 2010 general election, the Labour government was replaced by a Conservative–Liberal Democrat coalition government with David Cameron (the leader of the Conservatives) as Prime Minister. This was the first coalition government for over 60 years. The majority partner in the coalition, the Conservatives, had earlier developed a range of policy proposals on public health and had indicated that public health would be an early priority should they gain office (Conservative Party, 2010a, 2010b). The Liberal Democrats also made several commitments in this area (Liberal Democrats, 2010).

The Cameron government brought together these various commitments into a programme (HM Government, 2010c). This contained 25 policy commitments on public health issues (not including those on climate change and sustainable development, which also have public health implications). Subsequently, these were developed further and new ones added (Lansley, 2010a; Cm 7881, 2010). At the time of writing the key policy commitments are:

- a white paper on public health due to be published in 2010

- the focus of the Department of Health to be on public health (although an earlier Conservative proposal to rename the department as the Department for Public Health was not followed up in the Conservative manifesto nor the coalition programme agreement)

- a new Cabinet subcommittee on public health, chaired by the Secretary of State for Health

- a new, ring-fenced public health budget

- a new national public health service

- clear outcomes and measures to judge progress on public health

- an enhanced role for directors of public health to improve the health of their communities

- a strengthened role for local government in improving public health

- an expansion in the numbers of health visitors and minimum service guarantees for health visiting services

- a greater role for employers in promoting health of workers

- a 'responsibility deal' with business to ensure that industry contributes to better health in its marketing and product development combined with less direct regulation (see Public Health Commission, 2009)

- 'Change4Life' to become less of a central government campaign and more a social movement, with a bigger financial input from business, the voluntary sector and local government

- more information and   stronger incentives to enable people to make healthy choices

- action on health inequalities, including a 'health premium' targeting public health resources to areas with the poorest health. The new government backed the six policy objectives of the Marmot review established by the Brown government (see Chapter 17)

- measures to reduce binge drinking and underage drinking, including bans on the sale of alcohol below cost, increased penalties for serving alcohol to under-18s, and greater powers to close licensed premises. In addition, reviews of alcohol licensing legislation and price/taxation of alcohol were proposed

In addition, other policy commitments have implications for public health, notably the proposed abolition of strategic health authorities and other regional government bodies, the abolition of PCTs and their replacement by consortia of GPs. These organizational changes will almost certainly weaken public health, at least in the short term, through a loss of strategic focus, a weaker emphasis on population health, a reduction in capacity and expertise and disruption of partnerships at both regional and local levels. Other policies also have ramifications, such as the review of government 'arms length' agencies that proposed the abolition of some national public health bodies and cast a dark shadow of doubt over others. The new government's budget cuts also have implications for public health, including a freeze on national health promotion campaigns and cutbacks in regeneration programmes, housing funds and welfare benefits. At the time of writing, further public expenditure cuts are being explored.

Many of the new government's policies represent a continuation of the Labour government's policies. Some policies, such as retrenchment in public expenditure, are likely to have been pursued to some extent by Labour had they been returned to office. Even so, there are some potentially radical departures, notably the creation of a distinct public health service and the abolition of some regional bodies that probably would not have happened had Labour remained in power.

All governments, irrespective of their political composition, must face political realities. The Cameron coalition government will be no different. Its policies and commitments on public health reform will be tested by vested interests, by existing health bureaucracies and by media and public pressure. It also faces the added pressure of severe economic instability. These circumstances, coupled with the complex dynamics of coalition politics, make it extremely difficult to chart the future course of public health policy with any accuracy.

Bibliography

Abbasi, K., Roberts, I. and Mohan, D. (2002) 'War on the Roads', *British Medical Journal*, 324: 1107–8.

Abbott, S. (2007) 'The Psychosocial Effects on Health of Socioeconomic Inequalities', *Critical Public Health*, 17(2): 151–8.

Abbott, S. and Kiloran, A. (2005) *Mapping Public Health Networks* (London: Health Development Agency).

Abbott, S., Chapman, J., Shaw, S. et al. (2005) 'Flattening the National Health Service Hierarchy: The Case of Public Health', *Policy Studies*, 26(2): 133–48.

Abbott, S., Florin, D., Fulop, N. and Gillam, S. (2001) *Primary Care Groups and Trusts: Improving Health* (London: King's Fund).

Abel-Smith, B. (1964) *The Hospitals 1800–1948* (London: Heinemann).

Abel, B. (2001) 'The Gin Epidemic: Much Ado About What?', *Alcohol and Alcoholism*, 36(5): 401–5.

Abramson, J. and Wright, J. (2007) 'Are Lipid-lowering Guidelines Evidence-based?', *The Lancet*, (369)9557: 168–9.

Academy of Medical Sciences) (2004) *Calling Time: The Nation's Drinking as a Major Health Issue* (London: AMS).

ACMD (Advisory Committee on the Misuse of Drugs) (2000) *Reducing Drug Related Deaths* (London: TSO).

ACMD (2006a) *Pathways to Problems – Hazardous Use of Tobacco, Alcohol and Other Drugs by Young People in the UK and its Implications for Policy* (London: TSO).

ACMD (2006b) *Further Consideration of the Classification of Cannabis Under the Misuse of Drugs Act 1971* (London: Home Office).

ACMD (2009) *MDMA ('Ecstasy'): A Review of its Harms and Classification Under the Misuse of Drugs Act 1971* (London: Home Office).

ACRE (Advisory Committee on Releases to the Environment) (2004) *Advice on the Implications of the Farm Scale Evaluations of Genetically Modified Herbicide Tolerant Crops* (London: DEFRA).

ACRE (2005) *Advice on the Implications of the Farm Scale Evaluations of Genetically Modified Herbicide Tolerant Winter Oilseed Rape* (London: DEFRA).

Adams, C., Baeza, J. and Calnan, M. (2001) 'The New Health Promotion Arrangements in General Medical Practice in England: Results From a National Evaluation', *Health Education Journal*, 60(1): 45–58.

Adams, I. (1993) *Political Ideology Today* (Manchester: Manchester University Press).

Adams, J. (1995) *Risk* (London: UCL Press).

Adler, M. (1997) 'Sexual Health – A Health of the Nation Failure', *British Medical Journal*, 314: 1743.

Adonis, A. and Pollard, S. (1997) *A Class Act* (London: Hamish Hamilton).

Advisory Committee on the Microbiological Safety of Food (1999) *Report on Microbial Antibiotic Resistance in Relation to Food Safety* (London: TSO).

Advisory Group on Drug and Alcohol Education (2008) *Drug Education: An Entitlement for All – A Report to Government by the Advisory Group on Drug and Alcohol Education* (London: DCSF).

Aggleton, P. (1990) *Health* (London: Routledge).

Agriculture and Environmental Biotechnology Commission (2002) *Animals and Biotechnology* (London: Department of Trade and Industry).

Agriculture Committee (1989) *Salmonella in Eggs, 1st Report 1988/9*, HC 108 (London: HMSO).

Agriculture Committee (1990) *BSE, 5th Report 1989/90*, HC 449 (London: HMSO).

Ahmad, S. and Billimek, J. (2007) 'Limiting Youth Access to Tobacco: Comparing the Long-Term Health Impacts of Increasing Cigarette Excise Taxes and Raising the Legal Smoking Age to 21 in the United States', *Health Policy*, 80: 378–91.

Ahmad, W. (ed.) (1993) *Race and Health in Contemporary Britain* (Buckingham: Open University Press).

Akhtar, P., Currie, D., Currie, C. and Haw, S. (2007) 'Changes in Child Exposure to Environmental Tobacco-Smoke (CHETS) Study After Implementation of Smoke-Free Legislation in Scotland: National Cross-Sectional Survey', *British Medical Journal*, 335: 545–9.

Alcock, P. (2006) *Understanding Poverty* (3rd edn) (London: Palgrave Macmillan).

Alcock, P. and Scott, D. (2002) 'Partnerships and the Voluntary Sector: Can Compacts Work?' in Glendinning, C., Powell, M. and Rummery, K. (eds) *Partnerships, New Labour and Governance* (Bristol: Policy Press), pp. 113–30.

Alcohol Concern (2004) *Addressing Alcohol Through the New GP Contract: A Briefing for Primary Care Organisations* (London: Alcohol Concern).

Alexander, F.E., Anderson, T.J., Brown, H.K. et al. (1999) '14 Years of Follow Up from the Edinburgh Randomised Trial of Breast Cancer Screening', *The Lancet*, 353: 1903–8.

Alexander, M. (2003) *Calling the Shots: Childhood Vaccinations – One Family's Journey* (London: Jessica Kingsley).

Alford, R. (1975) *Health Care Politics* (Chicago: University of Chicago Press).

Allender, S., Balakrishnan, R., Scarborough, P. et al. (2009) 'The Burden of Smoking Related Ill Health in the UK', *Tobacco Control*, 0: 1–7 (doi: 10.1136/tc.2008.026294).

Allgood, P., Warwick, J., Warren, R. et al. (2008) 'A Case Control Study of the Impact of the East Anglian Breast Screening Programme on Breast Cancer Mortality', *British Journal of Cancer*, 98: 206–9.

Alloway, B. and Ayres, D. (1997) *Principles of Environmental Pollution* (2nd edn) (London: Chapman and Hall).

Allsop, J. (1990) 'Does Socialism Necessarily Mean the Public Provision of Health Care?' in Carrier, J. and Kendall, I. *Socialism and the NHS: Fabian Essays in Health Care* (Aldershot: Avebury), pp. 31–41.

Allwright, S., Paul, G., Greiner, B. et al. (2005) 'Legislation for Smoke-Free Workplaces and Health of Bar Workers in Ireland: Before and After Study', *British Medical Journal*, 331: 1117.

Alm, J., Swartz, J., Lilja, G. et al. (1999) 'Atopy in Children of Families with an Anthroposophic Lifestyle', *The Lancet*, 353(9163): 1485–8.

Almedom, A. (2005) 'Social Capital and Mental Health: An Interdisciplinary Review of Primary Evidence', *Social Science & Medicine*, 61: 943–64.

Amos, A. (2007) 'From Self-Regulation to Legislation: The Social Impact of Public Health Action on Smoking' in Scriven, A. and Garman, S. *Public Health: Social Context and Action* (Maidenhead: Open University Press), pp. 193–206.

Amos, M. (2002) 'Community Development' in Adams, L., Amos, M. and Munro, J. *Promoting Health: Politics and Practice* (London: Sage), pp. 63–71.

Anderson, D. (1985) 'Interfering, Unrealistic Know-alls?. The Image and Reality of Health Educators', *Health Education Journal*, 44(1): 43.

Anderson, P. (2007) 'A Safe, Sensible and Social AHRSE: New Labour and Alcohol Policy,' *Addiction*, 102(10): 1515–27.

Anderson, P. and Baumberg, B. (2006) *Alcohol in Europe: A Public Health Perspective. A Report for the European Commission* (London: Institute of Alcohol Studies).

Anderson, W., Florin, D., Gillam, S. and Mountford, L. (2002) *Every Voice Counts: Primary Care Organisations and Public Involvement* (London: King's Fund).

Andersson, I., Aspergen, K., Janzon, L. et al. (1988) 'Mammographic Screening and Mortality from Breast Cancer: The Malmo Mammographic Screening Programme,' *British Medical Journal*, 297: 943–50.

Annandale, E. (1998) *The Sociology of Health and Medicine. A Critical Introduction* (Cambridge: Polity).

Annandale, E. and Hunt, K. (2000) *Gender Inequalities in Health* (Buckingham: Open University Press).

Antonovsky, A. (1979) *Health, Stress and Coping* (San Francisco: Jossey-Bass).

Antonovsky, A. (1996) 'The Salutogenic Model as a Theory to Guide Health Promotion', *Health Promotion International*, 11(1): 11–18.

Appleby, J. (2005) 'Public Health', *Health Service Journal*, 20 October, 21.

Appleby, J. and Deeming, C. (2001) 'Inverse Care Law', *Health Service Journal*, 21 June, 37.

Appleyard, B. (2000) *Brave New World – Genetics and the Human Experience* (London: Harper Collins).

Arason, V., Kristinnson, K., Sigurdsson, J.A. et al. (1996) 'Do Antimicrobials Increase the Carriage Rate of Penicillin Resistant Pneumococci in Children? Cross Sectional Prevalence Study', *British Medical Journal*, 313: 387–91.

Arie, S. (2005) 'UK Pushes EU to Tackle Health Gap Between Rich and Poor', *British Medical Journal*, 332(7522): 923.

Armingeon, K. and Beyeler, M. (2004) *The OECD and European Welfare States* (Cheltenham: Edward Elgar).

Armstrong, D. (1993) 'Public Health Spaces and the Fabrication of Identity', *Sociology*, 27(3): 393–410.

Arnold, P., Topping, A. and Honey, S. (2004) 'Exploring the Contribution of District Nurses to Public Health', *British Journal of Community Nursing*, 9(5): 216–22.

Arnold, S.F., Klotz, D.M., Collins, B.M. et al. (1996) 'Synergestic Activation of Estrogen Reception with Combinations of Environmental Chemicals', *Science*, 272: 1489–92.

Arnstein, S. (1969) 'A Ladder of Citizen Participation', *AIP Journal*, July, 216–24.

Aronson, A., Miller, A., Woolcottt, C. et al. (2000) 'Breast Adipose Tissue Concentrations of

Polychlorinated Biphenyls and Other Orga-nochlorines and Breast Cancer Risk', *Cancer Epidiomological Biomarkers Prevention*, 9(1): 55–63.

Ashcroft, R. (2007) 'Should Genetic Information be Disclosed to Insurers? No', *British Medical Journal*, 334(7605): 1197.

Ashton, J. (1990) 'Public Health and Primary Care: Towards a Common Agenda', *Public Health*, 104(6): 387–98.

Ashton, J. (1992) 'The Origin of Healthy Cities', in Ashton, J. (ed.) *Healthy Cities* (Milton Keynes: Open University), pp. 1–12.

Ashton, J. (2000) 'Public Health Service Needs to be Independent', *British Medical Journal*, 321: 1473.

Ashton, J. and Seymour, H. (1988) *The New Public Health* (Milton Keynes: Open University Press).

Ashworth, M., Medina, J. and Morgan, M. (2008) 'Effect of Socio-Economic Deprivation on Blood Pressure Monitoring and Control in England: A Survey of Data From the Quality and Outcomes Framework', *British Medical Journal*, 337: 2030.

Aspinall, P. and Jacobson, B. (2004) *Ethnic Disparities in Health and Health Care: A Focussed Review of the Evidence and Selected Examples of Good Practice* (London: London Health Observatory).

Association of Directors of Public Health (2005) *'Memorandum' in Health Committee (2005) Health – Minutes of Evidence HC 358i, Session 2004/5* (London: TSO).

Association of Directors of Public Health, British Heart Foundation, Campaign for Better Transport, et al. (2008) *Take Action on Active Travel* (London: ADPH).

Assunta, M. and Chapman, S. (2006) 'Health Treaty Dilution: A Case Study of Japan's Influence on the Language of the WHO Framework Convention on Tobacco Control', *Journal Epidemiology Community Health*, 60: 751–6.

Asthana, S. and Halliday, J. (2006) *What Works in Tackling Health Inequalities? Pathways, Policies and Practice Through the Lifecourse* (Bristol: Policy Press).

Aswani, K. (2007) 'Primary Care as the Gateway to Public Health' in Griffiths, S. and Hunter, D.J. *New Perspectives in Public Health* (2nd edn) (Oxford: Radcliffe), pp. 230–9.

Atkins Transport Planning in Association with PricewaterhouseCoopers and Warwick Business School (2006) *Long-Term Process and Impact Evaluation of the Local Transport Plan Policy Monitoring and Reporting of LTP Outcomes* (Epsom: Atkins Transport Planning).

Atrens, D. (1994) 'The Questionable Wisdom of a Low Fat Diet and Cholesterol Reduction', *Social Science & Medicine*, 39(3): 433–7.

Audit Commission (1990) *Environmental Heath Survey of Food Premises*, Information Paper 2 (London: HMSO).

Audit Commission (1996) *What the Doctor Ordered: A Study of GP Fundholders in England and Wales* (London: HMSO).

Audit Commission (1998) *Effective Partnership Working* (London: Audit Commission).

Audit Commission (2003) *Survey of Practice Nurses* (London: Audit Commission).

Audit Commission (2004a) *Transforming Health and Social Care in Wales* (London: Audit Commission).

Audit Commission (2004b) *Transforming Primary Care* (London: Audit Commission).

Audit Commission (2005) *Governing Partnerships: Bridging the Accountability Gap* (London: Audit Commission).

Audit Commission (2006) *Early Lessons in Implementing Practice Based Commissioning* (London: Audit Commission).

Audit Commission (2007) *Improving Health and Well-being* (London: Audit Commission).

Audit Commission (2008) *Are We There Yet? Improving Governance and Resource Management in Childrens' Trusts* (London: Audit Commission).

Audit Commission (2009) *Working Better Together? Managing Local Strategic Partnerships* (London: Audit Commission).

Audit Commission (2010a) *Giving Children a Healthy Start* (London: Audit Commission).

Audit Commission (2010b) *Healthy Balance* (London: Audit Commission).

Audit Commission and Healthcare Commission (2007) *Better Safe than Sorry: Preventing Unintentional Injury to Children* (London: Audit Commission).

Audit Scotland (2006) *Tackling Waiting Times in the NHS in Scotland* (Edinburgh: Audit Scotland).

Aveyard, P., Amos, A., Bauld, L. et al. (2010) 'Is the UK's Coalition Government Serious about Public Health?' *The Lancet*, 376(9741): 589.

Axelrad, J., Howard, C. and McLean, W. (2002) 'Interactions Between Pesticides and Components of Pesticide Formulations in an in Vitro Neurotoxicity Test', *Toxicology*, 173(3): 259–68.

Azjen, I. and Fishbein, M. (1980) *Understanding Attitudes and Predicting Behaviour* (England Cliffs, NJ: Prentice Hall).

Babb, P. (2004) *Focus on Social Inequalities* (London: ONS).

Babb, P. (2005) *A Summary of Focus on Social Inequalities* (London: Office for National Statistics).

Babones, S. (2008) 'Income Inequality and Population Health: Correlation and Casualty', *Social Science & Medicine*, 66: 1614–26.

Babor, T., Caetano, R., Casswell, S. et al. (2003) *Alcohol: No Ordinary Commodity. Research and Public Policy* (Oxford: Oxford University Press).

Bachrach, P. and Baratz, M. (1962) 'Two Faces of Power', *American Political Science Review*, 56(4): 1947–52.

Backett, K.C. and Davison, C. (1995) 'Lifecourse and Lifestyle – The Social and Cultural Location of Health Behaviours', *Social Science & Medicine*, 40(5): 629–30.

Backlund, E., Rowe, G., Lynch, J. et al. (2007) 'Income Inequality and Mortality: A Multilevel Prospective Study'. *International Journal of Epidemiology*, 36(3): 590–6.

Baer, P. and Mastrandrea, M. (2006) *High Stakes: Designing Emissions Pathways to Reduce the Risk of Dangerous Climate Change* (London: Institute for Public Policy Research).

Baeza, J. and Calnan, M. (1998) 'Beating the Bands', *Health Service Journal*, 24 September, 26–7.

Baggott, R. (1990) *Alcohol, Politics and Social Policy* (Aldershot: Avebury).

Baggott, R. (1995) *Pressure Groups Today* (Manchester: Manchester University Press).

Baggott, R. (1998) 'The BSE Crisis: Public Health and the Risk Society', in Gray, P. and t'Hart, P. (eds) *Public Policy Disasters in Western Europe* (London: Routledge), pp. 61–78.

Baggott, R. (2004) *Health and Healthcare in Britain* (3rd edn) (Basingstoke: Palgrave Macmillan).

Baggott, R. (2005) 'A Funny Thing Happened on the Way to the Forum? Reforming Patient and Public Involvement in the NHS in England', *Public Administration*, 83(3): 533–51.

Baggott, R. (2006) *Alcohol Strategy and the Drinks Industry: A Partnership for Prevention?* (York: York Publishing Services).

Baggott, R. (2007) *Understanding Health Policy* (Bristol: Policy Press).

Baggott, R., Allsop, J. and Jones, K. (2005) *Speaking for Patients and Carers* (Basingstoke: Palgrave Macmillan).

Baird, G., Pickles, A., Simonoff, E. et al. (2008) 'Measles, Vaccine, and Antibody Response in Autism Spectrum Disorders', *Archives of Disease in Childhood,* 93: 832–7.

Bakan, S. (2005) *The Corporation: The Pathological Pursuit of Profit and Power* (London: Constable).

Baker, D. and Middleton, E. (2003) 'Cervical Screening and Health Inequality in England in the 1990s', *Journal of Epidemiology and Community Health*, 57: 417–23.

Baksh, F., Butcher, J., Wrelton, E. and Morgan, P. (2007) *Young People, Smoking and Health* (London: National Children's Bureau).

Baldwin, E. (1997) 'Reclaiming Our Future: International Efforts to Eliminate the Threat of Persistent Organic Pollutants', *Hastings International and Comparative Law Review*, 20: 855–99.

Ball, D. (2006) *Understanding Environmental Health Policy* (Maidenhead: Open University Press).

Ball, J. and Pike, G. (2005) *Results from a Census Survey of RCN School Nurses* (London: RCN).

Balloch, S. and Taylor, M. (2001) *Partnership Working: Policy and Practice* (Bristol: Policy Press).

Banks, E., Reeves, G., Beral, V. et al. (2004) 'Influence of Personal Characteristics of Individual Women on Sensitivity and Specificity of Mammography in the Million Women Study: Cohort Study', *British Medical Journal*, 329(7464): 477.

Banks, P. (2002) *Partnerships Under Pressure* (London: King's Fund).

Bara, J. and Budge, I. (2001) 'Party Policy and Ideology: Still New Labour', *Parliamentary Affairs*, 54(4): 590–606.

Barker, A. and Peters, B.G. (1993a) 'Science, Policy and Government' in Barker, A. and Peters, B.G. *The Politics of Expert Advice* (Edinburgh: Edinburgh University Press), pp. 1–6.

Barker, A. and Peters, B.G. (1993b) *The Politics of Expert Advice* (Edinburgh: Edinburgh University Press).

Barker, D. (1994) *Mothers, Babies and Health in Later Life* (2nd edn) (London: British Medical Journal Publishing Group).

Barker, D. and Osmond, C. (1987) 'Inequalities in Health in Britain: Specific Explanations in Three Lancashire Towns', *British Medical Journal*, 294: 749–52.

Barker, K. (2004) *Review of Housing Supply – Delivering Stability: Securing our Future Housing Needs – Final Report – Recommendations* (Norwich: HMSO).

Barker, K. (2006) *Barker Review of Land Use Planning – Final Report Recommendations* (London: HM Treasury).

Barling, D. and Lang, T. (2003) 'A Reluctant Food Policy? The First Five Years of Food Policy Under Labour', *The Political Quarterly*, 74(1): 8–18.

Barnard, M., Becker, E., Creegan, C. et al. (2009) *Evaluation of the National Healthy Schools Programme Interim Report* (London: National Centre for Social Research).

Barnes, J., Ball, M., Meadows, P. and Belsky, J. (2009) *Nurse Family Partnerships: Second Year Pilot Sites Implementation in England: The Infancy Period* (London: Institute for the Study of Children, Families and Social Issues).

Barnes, M., Bauld, L., Benzeval, M. et al. (2005) *Health Action Zones: Partnerships for Health Equity* (London: Routledge).

Barnes, M., Butt, S. and Tomaszewski, W. (2008) *What Happens to Children in Persistently Bad Housing?* (London: Shelter).

Barnes, M., Harrison, S., Mort, M. and Shardlow, P. (1999) *Unequal Partners: User Groups and Community Care* (Bristol: Policy Press).

Barr, A. (1995) *Drink – An Informal Social History* (London: Bantam Press).

Barrett, S. (2004) 'Implementation Studies: Time for a Revival?', *Public Administration*, 82(2): 249–62.

Bartholomew, M. (2002) 'James Lind's Treatise of the Scurvy (1753)', *Postgraduate Medical Journal*, 78: 695–6.

Bartley, M. (2004) *Health Inequality an Introduction to Theories, Concepts and Methods* (Cambridge: Polity Press).

Bartley, M., Popay, J. and Plewis, I. (1992) 'Domestic Conditions, Paid Employment and Women's Experience of Ill Health', *Sociology of Health and Illness*, 14(3): 313–45.

Barton, A., Basham, M., Foy, C. and Torbay Healthy Housing Group et al. (2007) 'The Watcombe Housing Study: The Short Term Effect of Improving Housing Conditions on the Health of Residents', *Journal of Epidemiology Community Health,* 61(9): 771–7.

Bartrip, P. (1996) *Themselves Writ Large: The BMA 1832–1966* (London: British Medical Journal Publishing Group).

Baskin, D.G., Seeley, R.J., Kuijper, J.L. et al. (1998) 'Increased Expression of mRNA for the Long Form of the Leptin Receptor in the Hypothalmus is Associated with Leptin Hypersensitivity and Fasting', *Diabetes*, 47(4): 538–43.

Bassil, K., Vakil, C., Sanborn, M. et al. (2007) 'Cancer Health Effects of Pesticides: Systematic Review', *Canadian Family Physician*, 53(10): 1704–11.

Bateman, B., Warner, J., Hutchinson, E. et al. (2004) 'The Effects of a Double Blind, Placebo Controlled, Artificial Food Colourings and Benzoate Preservative Challenge on Hyperactivity in a General Population Sample of Preschool Children', *Archives of Disease in Childhood*, 89: 506–11.

Batniji, R. and Woods, N. (2009) *Averting a Crisis for Global Health: 3 Actions for the G20* (Oxford: Global Economic Governance Programme).

Batt, S. (1994) *Patient No More: The Politics of Breast Cancer* (London: Scarlett Press).

Batterham, R., Cohen, M., Ellis, S. et al. (2003) 'Inhibition of Food Intake in Obese Subjects by Peptide YY3-36', *New England Journal of Medicine*, 349(10): 941–8.

Battisti, D. and Naylor, R. (2009) 'Historical Warnings of Food Insecurity with Unprecedented Seasonal Heat' *Science,* 9 January 323(591): 240–4.

Bauld, L. and Judge, K. (eds) (2002) *Learning from Health Action Zones* (Chichester: Aeneas Press).

Bauld, L. and Judge, K. (2005) *Health Improvement Planning In Scotland: An Analysis of Joint Health Improvement Plans and Regeneration Outcome Agreements* (Edinburgh: NHS Health Scotland).

Bauld, L. and McKenzie, M. (2007) 'Health Action Zones: Multi-agency Partnerships to Improve Health' in Scriven, A. and Garman, S. (eds) *Public Health: Social Context and Action* (Basingstoke: Palgrave Macmillan), pp. 131–43.

Baum, F. (2002) *The New Public Health* (2nd edn) (Oxford: Oxford University Press).

Baum, M. (1999) 'Money May Be Better Spent on Symptomatic Women,' *British Medical Journal*, 318: 398.

Bauman, Z. (2007) *Liquid Times Living in an Age of Uncertainty* (Cambridge: Polity Press).

Baumgartner, F. and Jones, B. (1993) *Agendas and Instability in American Politics* (Chicago: University of Chicago Press).

Bayer, R. (1993) 'The Great Drug Policy Debate: What Means This Thing Called Decriminalisation' in Bayer, R. and Oppenheimer, G. (eds) *Confronting Drugs Policy: Illicit Drugs in a Free Society*, (Cambridge: Cambridge University Press), pp. 1–23.

BBC (2002) 'Tainted Food Clampdown Call', 6 February 2002, (http://news.bbc.co.uk/1/hi/health/1805059.stm accessed 13.8.10).

BBC (2006) 'Cameron Wants 'Independent' NHS', *BBC News Online*, (news.bbc.co.uk/l/hi/uk_politics/6032473.stm accessed 11.12.06).

BBC (2010a) 'Meat of cloned cow offspring in UK food chain, FSA says', *BBC News Online* (ww.bbc.co.uk/news/uk-10859866 accessed 13.8.10).

BBC (2010b) 'Minister Rejects Jamie Oliver Approach on Health' (http://news.bbc.co.uk/1/hi/10459744.stm accessed 14.8.10).

Beaglehole, R. and Bonita, R. (2004) *Public Health at the Crossroads: Achievements and Prospects* (2nd edn) (Cambridge: Cambridge University Press).

Beattie, A. (2002) 'Education for Systems Change: A Key Resource for Radical Action on Health' in Adams, L., Amos, M. and Munro, J. *Promoting Health: Politics and Practice* (London: Sage), pp. 157–65.

Beauchamp, D. (1988) *The Health of the Republic. Epidemics, Medicine and Moralism as Challenges to Democracy* (Philadelphia: Temple University Press).

Beaver, M. (1997) 'Misuse of Epidemiology', *Public Health*, 111: 63–6.

Beck, U. (1992) *The Risk Society* (London: Sage).

Becker, M. (1974) 'The Health Belief Model and Personal Health Behaviour', *Health Education Monographs*, 2(4): 324–508.

Bedford, H. (2007) 'Immunisation: Ethics, Effectiveness, Organisation' in Cowley, S. (ed.) *Community Public Health in Policy & Practice: A Sourcebook* (London: Bailliere Tindall), pp. 337–56.

Beecham Review (2006) *Beyond Boundaries: Citizen-Centred Local Services for Wales. Review of Local Service Delivery. Report to the Welsh Assembly Government* (Cardiff: Welsh Assembly Government).

Bell, D. and Gray, T. (2002) 'The Ambiguous role of the Environment Agency in England and Wales', *Environmental Politics*, 11(3): 76–98.

Belot, M. and James, J. (2009) *Healthy School Meals and Educational Outcomes* (Essex: Institute for Social and Economic Research).

Belsky, J., Melhuish, E., Barnes, J. et al. (2006) 'Effects of Sure Start Local Programmes on Children and Families: Early Findings from a Quasi-Experimental, Cross Sectional Study', *British Medical Journal*, 332: 1476.

Ben-Shlomo, Y., White, I.R. and Marmot, M. (1996) 'Does the Variation in the Socioeconomic Characteristics of an Area Affect Mortality?', *British Medical Journal*, 312: 1013–14.

Benetou, V., Trichopoulou, B., Orfanos, P. et al. (2008) 'Conformity to Traditional Mediterranean Diet and Cancer Incidence: The Greek EPIC Cohort', *British Journal of Cancer*, 99(1): 191–5.

Bennett, J. and Dilorenzo, F. (1999) *The Food and Drink Police: America's Nannies, Busybodies and Petty Tyrants* (New York: Transaction).

Bennett, T. and Holloway, K. (2005) *Understanding Drugs, Alcohol and Crime* (Maidenhead: Open University Press).

Bentham, G. and Langford, I. (1994) *GEC-1994–15: Climate Change and the Incidence of Food Poisoning in England and Wales* (Centre for Social and Economic Research on the Global Environment (CSERGE), University of East Anglia).

Benzeval, M., Judge, D. and Whitehead, M. (1995) 'Unfinished Business' in Benzeval, M., Judge, D. and Whitehead, M. (eds) *Tackling Inequalities in Health: An Agenda for Action* (London: King's Fund), pp. 122–40.

Benzeval, M., Judge, K. and Shouls, S. (2001) 'Understanding the Relationship Between Income and Health: How Much Can be Gleaned from Cross-sectional Data?' *Social Policy and Administration*, 35: 376–96.

Beral, V. and Million Women Study Collaborators (2003) 'Breast Cancer and Hormone-Replacement Therapy in the Million Women Study', *The Lancet*, 362(9382): 419–27.

Beresford, S., Johnson, K., Ritenbaugh, C. et al. (2006) 'Low-Fat Dietary Pattern and Risk of Colorectal Cancer', *Journal of American Medical Association*, 295: 643–54.

Berger, P. (ed.) (1991) *Health, Lifestyle and Environment: Counteracting the Panic* (London: Social Affairs Unit).

Bergstrom, A., Pisani, P., Tenet, V. et al. (2001) 'Overweight as an Avoidable Cause of Cancer in Europe', *International Journal of Cancer*, 193: 421-30.

Berkeley, D. and Springett, J. (2006) 'From Rhetoric to Reality: Barriers Faced by Health for All Initiative', *Social Science & Medicine*, 63: 179–88.

Berki, R. (1975) *Socialism* (London: Dent).

Berlin, I. (1969) *Four Essays on Liberty* (Oxford: Oxford University Press).

Berlinguer, G. (1999) 'Globalisation and Global Health', *International Journal of Health Services*, 29(3): 579–95.

Berman, S. (1998) 'Path Dependency and Political Action: Re-examining Responses to the Depression', *Comparative Politics*, 20(4): 379–400.

Berridge, V. (1989) 'History and Addiction Control: The Case of Alcohol' in Robinson, D., Maynard, A. and Chester, R. *Controlling Legal Addictions* (Basingstoke: Macmillan – now Palgrave Macmillan).

Berridge, V. (1996) *AIDS in the UK: The Making of Policy 1981–1994* (Oxford: Oxford University Press).

Berridge, V. (1998) 'AIDS and British Drug Policy A Post War Situation' in Bloor, M. and Wood, F. *Addiction and Problem Drug Use: Issues in Behaviour, Policy and Practice* (London: Jessica Kingsley), pp. 85–108.

Berridge, V. (2005) *Temperance* (York: Joseph Rowntree Foundation).

Berridge, V. (2007) *Marketing Health: Smoking and the Discourse of Public Health in Britain, 1945–2000* (Oxford: Oxford University Press).

Berridge, V. and Blume, S. (2003) *Poor Health: Social Inequality Before and After the Black Report* (London: Cass).

Berridge, V. and Edwards, G. (1981) *Opium and the People* (London: Allen Lane).

Berridge, V., Christie, D. and Tansey, E. (2006) *Public Health in the 1980s and 1990s: Decline and Rise (Volume 26)* (London: Wellcome Trust).

Berrington de Gonzales, A. and Reeves, G. (2005) 'Mammographic Screening Before Age 50 Years in the UK: Comparison of Radiation Risks with the Mortality Benefits', *British Journal of Cancer*, 93(5): 590–6.

Berrington de Gonzalez, A., Sweetland, S. and Spencer, E. (2003) 'A Meta-Analysis of Obesity and the Risk of Pancreatic Cancer', *British Journal of Cancer*, 89: 519–23.

Bhatti, N., Law, M.R., Morris, J.K. et al. (1995) 'Increasing Incidences of Tuberculosis in England and Wales: A Study of Likely Causes', *British Medical Journal*, 310: 967–9.

Biddle, L., Brock, A., Brookes, S. and Gunnell, D. (2008) 'Suicide Rates in Young Men in England and Wales in the 21st Century: Time Trend Study' *British Medical Journal* doi: 10.1136/bmj.39475.603935.25 (accessed 16.7.10).

Billingham, K. and Perkins, E. (1997) 'A Public Health Approach to Nursing in the Community', *Nursing Standard*, 11(35): 43–6.

Bingham, S., Luben, R., Welch, A. et al. (2007) 'Epidemiologic Assessment of Sugars Consumption Using Biomarkers: Comparisons of Obese and Nonobese Individuals in the European Prospective Investigation of Cancer Norfolk', *Cancer Epidemiology Biomarkers & Prevention*, 16: 1651–4.

Bingham, S.A., Day, N.E., Luben, R. et al. (2003) 'Dietary Fibre in Food and Protection Against Colorectal Cancer in the European Prospective Investigation into Cancer and Nutrition (EPIC): An Observational Study', *The Lancet*, 361(9368): 1496–501.

Bird, J. and Lockwood, M. (2009) *The Prospects for Personal Carbon Trading* (London: IPPR).

Black, C. (2008) *Working for a Healthier Tomorrow: Dame Carol Black's Review of the Health of Britain's Working Age Population* (London: TSO).

Black, R., Allen, L., Bhutta, Z. and for the Maternal and Child Undernutrition Study Group et al. (2008) 'Maternal and Child Undernutrition: Global and Regional Exposures and Health Consequences', *The Lancet*, 371(9608): 243–60.

Blackman, S. (2007) 'See Emily Play: Youth Culture, Recreational Drug Use and Normalisation' in Simpson, M., Shildrick, T. and Macdonald, R. *Drugs in Britain – Supply, Consumption and Control* (Basingstoke: Palgrave Macmillan).

Blackman, T. (2006) *Placing Health: Neighbourhood Renewal, Health Improvement and Complexity* (Bristol: Policy Press).

Blackman, T., Anderson, J. and Pye, P. (2003) 'Change in Adult Health Following Medical Priority Rehousing: A Longitudinal Study', *Journal of Public Health Medicine*, 25(1): 22–8.

Blackwell, D. (2007) 'Health Benefits of Physical Activity across the Lifespan' in Merchant, J., Griffin. B.A. and Charnock, A. *Sport and Physical Activity – The Role of Health Promotion* (Basingstoke: Palgrave Macmillan).

Blair, S., Shaten, J., Brownell, K. et al. (1993) 'Body Weight Change, All Cause Mortality in the Multiple Risk Factor Intervention Trial', *Annals of Internal Medicine*, 119(2): 49–57.

Blanchflower, D. and Oswald, A. (2008) 'Is Well Being U-shaped Over the Life Cycle?', *Social Science & Medicine*, 66(6): 1733–49.

Blanden, J. and Gibbons, S. (2006) *The Persistence of Poverty Across Generations* (York: Joseph Rowntree Foundation).

Blanden, J. and Machin, S. (2008) 'Up and Down the Generational Income Ladder in Britain: Past Changes and Future Prospects', *National Institute Economic Review*, 205(1): 101–16.

Blanks, R., Moss, S.M., McGahan, C.E. et al. (2000) 'Effect of NHS Breast Screening Programme on Mortality from Breast Cancer in England and Wales 1990–8: A Comparison of Observed with Predicted Mortality', *British Medical Journal*, 321(7262): 665–9.

Blaxter, M. (2004) *Health* (Cambridge: Polity).

Blenkinsop, S., Bradshaw, S., Cade, J. et al. (2007) *Further Evaluation of the School Fruit and Vegetable Scheme* (London: Department of Health).

Blenkinsop, S., Eggers, M., Schagen, I. et al. (2004) *Evaluation of the Impact of the National Healthy School Standard. Final Report* (London: National Foundation for Educational Research, Thomas Coram Research Unit, Institute of Education, University of London).

Blouin, C., Chopra, M. and Hoeven, R. (2009) 'Trade and Social Determinants of Health', *The Lancet*, 373: 502–7.

Blume, S. (2006) 'Anti-Vaccination Movements and Their Interpretations', *Social Science & Medicine*, 62: 628–42.

BMA (British Medical Association) (1986) *Smoking Out the Barons: The Campaign Against the Tobacco Industry*, Report of the BMA Public Affairs Division (Chichester: J. Wiley).

BMA (1995) *Inequalities in Health*, Board of Science and Education Occasional Paper (London: British Medical Association).

BMA (1997) *The Misuse of Drugs* (Amsterdam: Harwood).

BMA (1998) *Health and Environmental Impact Assessment – An Integrated Approach* (London: Earthscan).

BMA (1999) *Growing Up in Britain* (London: British Medical Association).

BMA (2001) *Preventing Injuries* (London: British Medical Association).

BMA (2003) *Housing & Health: Building for the Future* (London: British Medical Association).

BMA (2004a) BMA Response to the Consultation 'Choosing Health', July 2004 (http://www.bma.org.uk/ap.nsf/Content/choosehlth accessed 11 7 07).

BMA (2004b) *Smoking and Reproductive Life* (London: British Medical Association).

BMA (2005a) *Population Screening and Genetic Testing* (London: British Medical Association).

BMA (2005b) *Preventing Childhood Obesity* (London: British Medical Association).

BMA (2007a) *A Rational Way Forward for the NHS in England* (London: British Medical Association).

BMA (2007b) *Breaking the Cycle of Children's Exposure to Tobacco Smoke* (London: British Medical Association).

BMA (2008) *Alcohol Misuse: Tackling the UK Epidemic* (London: British Medical Association).

BMA (2009) *Under the Influence: The Damaging Effect of Alcohol Marketing on Young People* (London: British Medical Association).

Bochel, C. (2006) 'New Labour Participation and the Policy Process', *Public Policy and Administration*, 21(4): 10–22.

Body, R. (1991) *Our Food: Our Land* (London: Random Century).

Boffeta, P., Agudo, P., Ahrens, W. et al. (1998) 'Multicentre Case Control Study of Exposure to Environmental Tobacco Smoke and Lung Cancer in Europe', *Journal of the National Cancer Institute*, 90: 1440–50.

Boffeta, P., Couto, E., Wichmann, J. et al. (2010) 'Fruit and Vegetable Consumption and Overall Cancer Risk in the European Prospective Investigation into Cancer and Nutrition', *Journal of National Cancer Institute* (doi: 10.1093/jnci/djq072 accessed 13.5.10).

Bonell, C., Fletcher, A. and McCambridge, J. (2007) 'Improving School Ethos May Reduce Substance Misuse and Teenage Pregnancy', *British Medical Journal*, 334(7594): 614–16.

Bonnefoy, X. (2007) 'Inadequate Housing and Health: An Overview', *International Journal of Environment and Pollution*, 30(3/4): 411–29.

Booker, C. (2009a) *The Real Global Warming Disaster* (London: Continuum).

Booker, C. (2009b) 'Climate Change: Is this the Worst Scientific Scandal of Our Generation?' Telegraph.co.uk 28 November 2009 (accessed 19.11.09).

Booker, C. and North, R. (1994) *The Mad Officials* (London: Constable).

Booker, C. and North, R. (2005) *The Great Deception: Can the European Union Survive?* (London: Continuum).

Booker, C. and North, R. (2007) *Scared to Death: From BSE to Global Warming: Why Scares Are Costing Us the Earth* (London: Continum).

Booth, A., Meier, P., Stockwell, P. et al. (2008a) *Independent Review of the Effects of Alcohol Pricing and Promotion Part A* (Sheffield: University of Sheffield).

Booth, A., Meier, P., Stockwell, P. et al. (2008b) *Independent Review of the Effects of Alcohol Pricing and Promotion Part B* (Sheffield: University of Sheffield).

Booth, C. (1902) *Life and Labour of the People in London* (London: Macmillan).

Bordieu, P. (1986) 'The Forms of Capital' in Richardson, J. *Handbook of Theory and Research for the Sociology of Education* (New York: Greenwood), pp. 241–58.

Boseley, S. (2004) 'United States Accused of Sabotaging Obesity Strategy', *International Journal of Health Services*, 34(3): 553–4.

Boseley, S. (2006) 'Safe Sex Advertising Campaign Offers the Bare Facts', *The Guardian*, 11 November (http://guardian.co.uk/uk/2006/nov/11/health.politics accessed 21.4.08).

Bosma, H., Marmot, M., Hemingway, H. et al. (1997) 'Low Job Control and Risk of Coronary Heart Disease in Whitehall II', *British Medical Journal*, 314: 558–65.

Botteri, E., Iodice, S., Bagnardi, V. et al. (2008) 'Smoking and Colorectal Cancer', *Journal of the American Medical Association*, 300(23): 2765–78.

Bowcott, O. and Campbell, D. (2009) 'Thirteen Children in Hospital after Contracting E.Coli at Godstone Farm' (Guardian.co.uk accessed 15/9/09).

Bowyer, C., Monkhouse, C., Skinner, I. and Willis, R. (2005) *Business Action on Climate Change: Where Next After Emissions Trading?* (London: Green Alliance).

Boyce, T., Robertson, R. and Dixon, A. (2008) *Commissioning and Behaviour Change: Kicking Bad Habits Final Report* (London: King's Fund).

Boyd Orr, J. (1936) *Food, Health and Income* (London: Macmillan).

Boydell, L. and Rugkåsa, J. (2007) 'Benefits of Working in Partnership: A Model', *Critical Public Health*, 17: 217–28.

Bradby, H. and Chandola, T. (2007) 'Ethnicity and Racism in the Politics of Health' in Garman, S. and Scriven, A. *Public Health: Social Context and Action* (Maidenhead: Open University Press), pp. 76–85.

Bradshaw, J. (ed.) (2002) *The Well-being of Children in the UK* (London: Save the Children: University of York).

Bradshaw, J. and Mayhew, E. (eds) 2005 *The Well-being of Children in the UK* (2nd edn) (London: Save the Children).

Bratt, R.G. (2002) 'Housing and Family Well-being', *Housing Studies*, 17(1): 13–26.

Braveman, P., Starfield, B. and Geiger, H.J. (2001) 'World Health Report 2000: How it Removes Equity from the Agenda for Public Health Monitoring and Policy', *British Medical Journal*, 323: 678–81.

Breen, J. (2002) 'Protecting Pedestrians Politicians Must Put Public Interests Before That of the Car Industry', *British Medical Journal*, 324: 1109–10.

Brett, J. and Austoker, J. (2001) 'Women who are Recalled for Further Investigation for Breast Screening: Psychological Consequences Three Years after Recall and Factors Affecting Re-attendance', *Journal of Public Health Medicine*, 23(4): 292–300.

Brewer, M., Goodman, A., Muriel, A. and Sibieta, L. (2008) *Poverty and Inequality in the UK: 2007* (London: Institute for Fiscal Studies).

Briggs, A. (1959) *The Age of Improvement* (London: Longman).

Briggs, D., Abellan, J.J. and Fecht, D. (2008) 'Environmental Inequity in England: Small Area Associations between Socio-Economic Status and Environmental Pollution', *Social Science & Medicine*, 67: 1612–29.

Brimblecombe, N., Dorling, D. and Shaw, M. (1999) 'Where the Poor Die in a Rich City: The Case of Oxford', *Health and Place*, 5: 287–300.

Brinton, L.A., Reeves, W., Brenes, M.M. et al. (1989) 'The Male Factor in the Etiology of Cervical Cancer among Sexually Monogamous Women', *International Journal of Cancer*, August, 44(2): 199–203.

Britton, A., Shipley, M., Marmot, M. and Hemingway, H. (2004) 'Does Access to Cardiac Investigation and Treatment Contribute to Social and Ethnic Differences in Coronary Heart Disease? Whitehall II Prospective Cohort Study', *British Medical Journal*, 329(7461): 318.

Broadbent, J. (1998) 'Practice Nurses and the Effects of the New GP Contract in the British NHS: The Advent of a Professional Project', *Social Science & Medicine*, 47(4): 497–506.

Brown, B. and Liddle, B. (2005) 'Service Domains – The New Communities: A Case Study of Peterlee Sure Start UK', *Local Government Studies*, 31(4): 449–73.

Brown, G. (2008) Prime Minister's Speech on the National Health Service, 7 January (www.pm.gov.uk accessed 7.3.08).

Brown, N., Manzolillo, P., Zhang, J. et al. (1998) 'Prenatal TCDD Predisposition to Mammary Cancer in Rats', *Carcinogenesis*, 19(9): 1623–9.

Brown, P. and Zavestoski, S. (eds) (2004) *Sociology of Health and Illness*, Volume 26(6), Special Issue: Social Movements in Health (Oxford: Blackwell).

Bruce, M. (1968) *The Coming of the Welfare State* (4th edn) (London: Batsford).

Brugts, P., Yetgin, T., Hoeks, S. et al. (2009) 'The Benefits of Statins in People Without Established Cardiovascular Disease but with Cardiovascular Risk Factors Meta Analysis of Randomised Controlled Trials', *British Medical Journal*, 338 (b2376 doi: 10.1136/bmj.2376).

Bruyinckx, E., Mortelmans, D., Van Goethen, M. and Van Hove, E. (1999) 'Risk Factors of Pain in Mammographic Screening', *Social Science & Medicine*, 49: 933–41.

Bryson, C. (2004) *The Fluoride Deception* (New York: Seven Stories Press).

Bunker, J. (2001) 'The Role of Medical Care in Contributing to Health Improvements Within Societies', *International Journal of Epidemiology*, 30: 1260–3.

Bunker, J., Frazier, H. and Mostelle, F. (1994) 'Improving Health: Measuring Effects of Medical Care', *Milbank Quarterly*, 72(2): 225–58.

Bunton, R. and Macdonald, G. (2002) 'Health Promotion Disciplinary Developments' in Bunton, R. and Macdonald, G. (eds) *Health Promotion Disciplines, Diversity and Developments* (2nd edn) (London: Routledge), pp. 9–27.

Burke, S., Gray, I., Paterson, K. and Meyrick, J. (2002) *Environmental Health 2012: A Key Partner in Delivering the Public Health Agenda* (London: Health Development Agency).

Burkitt, D. (1973) 'Some Disease Characteristics of Modern Western Civilisations', *British Medical Journal*, 1: 274–8.

Burley, V. (1997) 'Sugar Consumption and Cancers of the Digestive Tract', *European Journal of Cancer Prevention*, 6(5): 422–34.

Burley, V. (1998) 'Sugar Consumption and Cancer in Sites Other than the Digestive Tract', *European Journal of Cancer Prevention*, 7(4): 253–77.

Burton, P., Croft, J., Hastings, A. et al. (2004) *What Work in Community Involvement in Area Based Initiatives Home Office On line Report 53/04* (London: Home Office).

Business and Enterprise Committee (2008) *1st Report 2008/9 Energy Policy: Future Challenges,* HC 32 (London: TSO).

Butt, Y. (2007) 'The Role of Public Health Nursing' in Griffiths, S. and Hunter, D. *New Perspectives in Public Health* (2nd edn) (Oxford: Radcliffe), pp. 240–3.

Bynum, W. (1994) *Science and the Practice of Medicine in the Nineteenth Century* (Cambridge: Cambridge University Press).

Byrne, D. (2004) *Partnerships for Health in Europe* (Non-paper) (Brussels: European Commission).

Byrne, P. (1997) *Social Movements in Britain* (London: Routledge).

C 281 (1871) *Report of the Royal Commission on the Sanitary Laws*, House of Commons Sessional Papers, Volume 35, 1.

Cabinet Office (2007) *Capability Review of the Department of Health* (London: Cabinet Office).

Cairney, P. (2007a) 'A 'Multiple Lenses' Approach to Policy Change: The Case of Tobacco Policy in the UK', *British Politics*, 2: 45–68.

Cairney, P. (2007b) 'Using Devolution to Set the Agenda? Venue Shift and the Smoking Ban in

Scotland, *British Journal of Politics and International Relations*, 9: 73–89.

Cairns, J. (1995) 'The Costs of Prevention', *British Medical Journal*, 311: 1520.

Calle, E., Frumkin, H., Henley, J. et al. (2002) 'Organochlorines and Breast Cancer Risk', *A Cancer Journal for Clinicians*, 52(5): 301.

Calle, E., Rodriguez, C., Walker-Thurmond, K. and Thun, M. (2003) 'Overweight, Obesity, and Mortality from Cancer in a Prospectively Studied Cohort of U.S. Adults', *New England Journal of Medicine*, 348(17): 1625–38.

Calman, K. and Smith, D. (2001) 'Works in Theory but not in Practice? The Role of the Precautionary Principle in Public Health Policy', *Public Administration*, 79(1): 185–204.

Cameron, C. and Bernardes, J. (1998) 'Gender Disadvantage and Health: Men's Health for a Change', *Sociology of Health and Illness*, 20: 673–93.

Cameron, D. (2009) 'The Big Society', www.conservatives.com/News/Speeches/2009 (accessed 24.8.10).

Cameron, D. (2010a) 'I'll Cut the Deficit, not the NHS' www.conservatives.com/news/speeches/2010 (accessed 31.8.10).

Cameron, D. (2010b) 'Supporting Parents', www.conservatives.com/News/Speeches/2010 (accessed 24.8.10).

Cameron, S. and Christie, G. (2007) 'Exploring Health Visitors' Perceptions of the Public Health Nursing Role', *Primary Care Research and Development*, 8: 80–90.

Campbell, F. (2000) *Building Healthy Communities: The Role of Local Government in Health Improvement* (London: Democratic Health Network).

Campbell, F. (2002) *Health and the New Political Structures in Local Government* (London: Local Government Information Unit).

Campbell, S., Steiner, A., Robison, J. et al. (2005) 'Do Personal Medical Contracts Improve Quality of Care? A Multimethod Evaluation', *Journal of Health Services Research and Policy*, 10(1): 31–9.

Campos, P., Saguy, A., Ernsberger, P. et al. (2006) 'The Epidemiology of Overweight and Obesity: Public Health Crisis or Moral Panic', *International Journal of Epidemiology*, 35: 55–60.

Canadian Institutes of Health Research (2003) *The Future of Public Health in Canada: Developing a Public Health System for the 21st Century* (Ottowa: CIHR).

Cannon, G. (1987) *The Politics of Food* (London: Century Hutchinson).

Care Services Improvement Partnership (2007) *Mental Disorders, Suicide, and Deliberate Harm in Lesbian, Gay and Bisexual People: A Systematic Review* (London: National Institute for Mental Health in England).

Carnegie Research Institute (2007) *The National Evaluation of LEAP: Final Report on the National Evaluation of the Local Exercise Action Pilots* (London: Department of Health).

Carter, N. (2007) *The Politics of the Environment: Idea, Activism, Policy* (2nd edn) (Cambridge: Cambridge University Press).

CASH (Consensus Action on Salt and Health) (2007) *Salt in ReadyMeals 45% Lower Than Four Years Ago* (London: CASH) (www.actiononsalt.org.uk accessed 23.11.07).

Cashmore, E. (2006) *Celebrity Culture* (London: Routledge).

Castel, R. (1991) 'From Dangerousness to Risk' in Burchell, G., Gordon, G. and Miller, P. (eds) *The Foucault Effect: Studies in Governmentality* (Hemel Hempstead: Harvester Wheatsheaf), pp. 281–98.

Castelli, D., Hillman, C., Buck, S. and Erwin, H. (2007) 'Physical Fitness and Academic Achievement in Third and Fifth Grade Students', *Journal of Sport and Exercise Psychology*, 29: 2329–52.

Cattell, V. (2001) 'Poor People, Poor Places and Poor Health: The Mediating Role of Social Networks and Social Capital', *Social Science & Medicine*, 52: 1501–46.

CCFRAG (Campden and Chorleywood Food Research Association Group) (2008) *Monitoring Implementation of Alcohol Labelling Regime* (Chipping Campden: CCFRAG).

Cd 1507 (1903) Report of the Royal Commission on Physical Training (Scotland) (London: HMSO).

Cd 2175 (1904) Report of the Inter-departmental Committee on Physical Deterioration (London: HMSO).

Cd 4499 (1909) *Royal Commission on the Poor Laws and Relief of Distress*, Majority and Minority Report (London, HMSO).

Central Policy Review Staff (CPRS) (1982) *Alcohol Policies in the UK* (Stockholm: Sociologiska Institutionen).

Centre for Agricultural Strategy (1979) *National Food Policy in the UK* (Reading: CAS).

Centre for Public Scrutiny (2005) *Tackling the Democratic Deficit in Health: An Introduction to the Power of Local Authority Health Scrutiny* (London: Centre for Public Scrutiny).

Chadda, D. (1996) 'The Narked Civil Servants', *Health Service Journal*, 21 March, 11.

Chadwick, E. (1842) *Report on the Sanitary Condition of the Labouring Population of Great Britain* (London: Poor Law Commission).

Chamberlain, J. (1984) 'Which Prescriptive Screening Programmes are Worthwhile?', *Journal of Epidemiology and Community Health*, 38: 270–7.

Chandola, T. (2001) 'Ethnic and Class Differences in Health in Relation to British South Asians: Using the New National Statistics Socio-economic Classification', *Social Science & Medicine*, 252(8): 1285–96.

Chandola, T., Bartley, M., Sacker, A. et al. (2003) 'Health Selection in the Whitehall II Study, UK', *Social Science & Medicine*, 56: 2059–72.

Chandola, T., Britton, A., Brunner, E. et al. (2008) 'Work Stress and Coronary Heart Disease: What are the Mechanisms?', *European Heart Journal* (doi: 10.1093/eurheart/ehm584).

Chandola, T., Ferrie, J., Sacker, A. and Marmot, M. (2007) 'Social Inequalities in Self reported Health in Early Old Age: Follow-Up of Prospective Cohort Study', *British Medical Journal*, 334: 990.

Chapman, J., Shaw, S., Carter, Y. et al. (2003) *Capacity and Development Needs of Primary Care Trusts and Strategic Heath Authority Specialists in Public Health* (London: City University).

Chapman, J., Shaw, S., Congdon, P. et al. (2005) 'Specialist Public Health Capacity in England: Working in the New Primary Care Organisations', *Public Health*, 119: 22–31.

Chapman, S. (2007) *Public Health Advocacy and Tobacco Control – Making Smoking History* (Oxford: Blackwell).

Chapman, S. (2009) 'The Inverse Impact Law of Smoking Cessation', *The Lancet*, 373.

Chapple, A., Halliwell, S., Sibbald, B. et al. (2000) 'A Walk-in? Now You're Talkin', *Health Service Journal*, 4 May, 28–9.

Charles, C. and De Maio, S. (1993) 'Lay Participation in Health Care Decision Making: a Conceptual Framework', *Journal of Health Politics, Policy and Law*, 18(4): 881–904.

Charlton, B. (2001) 'Public Health and Personal Freedom' in Marinker, M. (ed.) *Personal Freedom or Public Health?* (London: King's Fund), pp. 55–69.

Charny, M. (1994) 'The Costs of Screening' in Le Fanu, J. *Preventionitis* (London: Social Affairs Unit), pp. 106–17.

Chartered Institute of Environmental Health and the Royal Society for the Promotion of Health (2004) *Choosing Health?* (http://www.cieh.org/library/Knowledge/CIEH_Consultation_responses/2004-06-choosingHealth-Final.pdf accessed 23.8.10).

Chartered Institute of Environmental Health (2007) *Commission on Housing Renewal and Public Health: Final Report* (London: CIEH).

Chatham House (2008a) *UK Food Supply: Storm Clouds on the Horizon* (London: Chatham House).

Chatham House (2008b) *Thinking about the Future of food: The Chatham House Food Supply Scenarios* (London: Chatham House).

Chaturverdi, N. and Ben-Shlomo, Y. (1995) 'From the Surgery to Surgeon: Does Deprivation Influence Consultation and Operation Rates?', *British Journal of General Practice*, 45: 127–31.

Chaturvedi, N., Rai, H. and Ben-Shlomo, Y. (1997) 'Lay Diagnosis and Health Care Seeking Behaviour for Chest Pain Among South Asians and Europeans', *The Lancet*, 35: 1578–83.

Chave, S. (1974) 'The Medical Officer of Health 1847–74', *Proceedings of the Royal Society of Medicine*, 67: 1243–7.

Chesterman, J., Judge, K. and Bauld, L. (2005) 'How Effective are the English Smoking Treatment Services in Reaching Disadvantaged Smokers?', *Addiction*, 100: 36–45.

CHI (Commisssion for Health Improvement) (2003) *Getting Better? A Report on the NHS* (London: CHI).

CHI (2004) *What CHI found in Primary Care Trusts* (London: CHI).

Chief Medical Officer (2006) *On the State of the Public Health Annual Report of the Chief Medical Officer 2005* (London: HMSO).

Chief Medical Officer (2007) *On the State of the Public Health Annual Report of the Chief Medical Officer 2006* (London: HMSO).

Children's Society, The (2009) *The Good Childhood Inquiry* (London: The Children's Society).

Chlebowski, R.T., Kuller, L.H., Prentice, R.L. et al. (2009) 'Breast Cancer after Use of Estrogen plus Progestin in Postmenopausal Women', *New England Journal of Medicine*, 360: 573–87.

Chui, L.F. (2003) *Inequalities of Access to Cancer Screening: A Literature Review* (Sheffield: NHS Cancer Screening Programmes).

Clapp, R., Howe, G. and Jacobs, M. (2006) 'Environmental and Occupational Causes of Cancers Revisited', *Journal of Public Health Policy*, 27: 61–76.

Clarke, A. (1995) 'Population Screening for Genetic Susceptibility to Disease', *British Medical Journal*, 311: 35–8.

Clarke, J. and Glendinning, C. (2002) 'Partnership and the Remaking of Welfare Governance' in Glendinning, C., Powell, M. and Rummery, K. (eds) *Partnerships, New Labour and Governance* (Bristol: Policy Press).

Clarke, J. and Newman, J. (1997) *The Managerial State* (London: Sage).

Clarke, K. (2006) 'Childhood, Parenting and Early Intervention: A Critical Examination of the Sure Start National Programme', *Critical Social Policy*, 26(4): 699–721.

Clarke, M. and Stewart, J. (1994) 'The Local Authority and the New Community Governance', *Regional Studies*, 28: 201–19.

Cm 249 (1987) *Promoting Better Health* (London: HMSO).

Cm 289 (1988) *Public Health in England* (London: HMSO).

Cm 555 (1989) *Working for Patients* (London: HMSO).

Cm 1523 (1991) *The Health of the Nation: A Consultative Document for Health in England* (London: HMSO).

Cm 1986 (1992) *The Health of the Nation: A Strategy for Health in England* (London: TSO).

Cm 2426 (1994) *Sustainable Development: The UK Strategy* (London: HMSO).

Cm 2674 (1994) *18th Report of the Royal Commission on Environmental Pollution: Transport and the Environment* (London: HMSO).

Cm 2846 (1995) *Tackling Drugs Together: A Strategy for England* (London: HMSO).

Cm 3234 (1996) *Transport: The Way Forward* (London: HMSO).

Cm 3805 (1998) *New Ambitions for Our Country: A New Contract for Welfare* (London: TSO).

Cm 3807 (1997) *The New NHS; Modern, Dependable* (London: TSO).

Cm 3830 (1998) *The Food Standards Agency: A Force for Change* (London: TSO).

Cm 3852 (1998) *Our Healthier Nation* (London: HMSO).

Cm 3854 (1998) *Working Together for a Healthier Scotland: A Consultation Document* (London: TSO).

Cm 3945 (1998) *Tackling Drugs to Build a Better Britain* (London: TSO).

Cm 3950 (1998) *A New Deal for Transport* (London: TSO).

Cm 3992 (1998) *Better Health, Better Wales Consultation Document* (London: TSO).

Cm 4014 (1998) *Modernising Local Government – In Touch with the People,* (London: TSO).

Cm 4045 (1998) *Bringing Britain Together: A National Strategy for Neighbourhood Renewal* (London: TSO).

Cm 4177 (1998) *Smoking Kills* (London: TSO).

Cm 4269 (1999) *Towards A Healthier Scotland, Scottish White Paper* (London: TSO).

Cm 4345 (1999) *A Better Quality of Life: A Strategy for Sustainable Development for the UK* (London: TSO).

Cm 4386 (1999) *Saving Lives; Our Healthier Nation* (London: TSO).

Cm 4445 (1999) *Opportunity for All: Tackling Poverty and Social Exclusion* (London: TSO).

Cm 4548 (2000) *The Air Quality Strategy for England, Scotland, Wales and Northern Ireland – Working together for clean air* (London: TSO).

Cm 4693 (2000) *A Waste Strategy for England and Wales* (London: TSO).

Cm 4749 (2000) *22nd Report of the Royal Commission on Environmental Pollution: Energy: the Changing Climate* (London. HMSO).

Cm 4818 (2000) *The NHS Plan: A Plan for Investment – A Plan for Reform* (London: TSO).

Cm 4909 (2000) *Our Countryside the Future: A Fair Deal for Rural England* (London: TSO).

Cm 4911(2000) *Our Towns and Cities. The Future: Developing an Urban Renaissance* (London: TSO).

Cm 4913 (2000) *Climate Change: The UK Programme* (London: TSO).

Cm 5730 (2003) *The Victoria Climbié Inquiry: Report of an Inquiry by Lord Laming* (London: TSO).

Cm 5827 (2003) *Chemicals in Products: Safeguarding the Environment and Human Health. 24th Report of the Royal Commission on Environmental Pollution* (London: TSO).

Cm 5860 (2003) *Every Child Matters: Green Paper* (London: TSO).

Cm 6079 (2003) *Building on the Best: Choice, Responsiveness and Equity in the NHS* (London: TSO).

Cm 6234 (2004) *The Future of Transport* (London: TSO).

Cm 6374 (2004) *Choosing Health: Making Healthy Choices Easier* (London: TSO).

Cm 6424 (2005) *Sustainable Communities: Homes for All* (London: TSO).

Cm 6467 (2005) *Securing the Future: Delivering the UK Sustainable Development Strategy* (London: TSO).

Cm 6737 (2006) *Our Health, Our Care, Our Say: A New Direction for Community Services* (London: TSO).

Cm 6764 (2006) *Climate Change the UK Programme* (London: TSO).

Cm 6939 (2006) *Strong and Prosperous Communities: The Local Government White Paper* (London: TSO).

Cm 7009 (2007) *26th Report of the Royal Commission on Environmental Pollution; The Urban Environment* (London: TSO).

Cm 7047 (1977) *Prevention and Health* (London: HMSO).

Cm 7124 (2007) *Meeting the Energy Challenge: A White Paper on Energy* (London: TSO).

Cm 7169 (2007) *The Air Quality Strategy for England, Scotland, Wales and Northern Ireland* (London: TSO).

Cm 7296 (2008) *Meeting the Energy Challenge a White Paper on Nuclear power* (London: TSO).

Cm 7432 (2008) *High Quality Care for All* (London: TSO).

Cm 7775 (2009) *NHS 2010–2015: From Good to Great. Preventative, People-Centered, Productive* (London: TSO).

Cm 7881 (2010) *Equity and Excellence: Liberating the NHS* (London: TSO).

Cmd 693 (1920) *Interim Report on the Future Provision of Medical and Allied Services* (London: HMSO).

Cmnd 3569 (1968) *Report of the Royal Commission on Medical Education* (London: HMSO).

Cmnd 3703 (1968) *Committee on Local Authority and Allied Personal Services* (London: HMSO).

Cmnd 6684 (1976) *Fit for the Future: Report of the Committee on Child Health Services* (London: HMSO).

Cmnd 7047 (1977) *Prevention and Health* (London: HMSO).

Cmnd 7615 (1979) *Report of the Royal Commission on the National Health Service* (London: HMSO).

Cmnd 9716 (1986) *Report of the Committee of Inquiry into an Outbreak of Food Poisoning at Stanley Royal Hospital Wakefield* (London: HMSO).

Cmnd 9771 (1986) *Primary Health Care: An Agenda for Discussion* (London: HMSO).

Cmnd 9772 (1986) *First Report of the Committee of Inquiry into the Outbreak of Legionnaire's Disease in Stafford, April 1985* (London: HMSO).

Coaffee, J. (2005) 'Shock of the New: Complexity and Emerging Rationales for Partnership Working' *Public Policy and Administration*, 20(3): 23–41.

Coburn, D. (2004) 'Beyond the Income Inequality Hypothesis: Class, Neo-Liberalism, and Health Inequalities', *Social Science & Medicine*, 58: 41–56.

Cochrane, R. and Bal, S. (1989) 'Mental Hospital Admission Rates of Immigrants to England: A Comparison of 1971 and 1981', *Social Psychiatry and Psychiatric Epidemiology*, 24: 2–11.

Coggon, D., Reading, I., Croft, P. et al. (2001) 'Knee Osteoarthritis and Obesity', *International Journal of Obesity*, 25(5): 622–7.

Coghlan, A. (2007) 'Dying for Some Quiet: The Truth about Noise Pollution', *New Scientist*, 22 August, 2618.

Coker, R., McKee, M. and Atun, R. (2008) *Health Systems and the Challenge of Communicable Diseases: Experiences form Europe and Latin America* (Maidenhead: Open University Press).

Coleman, A. and Glendinning, C. (2004) 'Local Authority Scrutiny of Health: Making the Views of the Community Count?', *Health Expectations*, 7: 29–39.

Coleman, J. (1988) 'Social Capital in the Creation of Human Capital', *American Journal of Sociology*, 94: 95–120.

Colhoun, H., McKeigue, P. and Davey Smith, G. (2003) 'Problems of Reporting Genetic Associations with Complex Outcomes', *The Lancet*, 361(9360): 865–72.

Collaborative Group on Hormonal Factors in Breast Cancer (1996) 'Breast Cancer and Hormonal Contraceptives: Collaborative Reanalysis of Individual Data on 53,297 Women with Breast Cancer and 100,239 Women Without Breast Cancer from 54 Epidemiological Studies', *The Lancet*, 347(9017): 1713–27.

Collin, J. and Lee, K. (2007) 'Globalisation and Public Health Policy', in Scriven, A. and Garman, S. (eds) *Public Health, Social Context and Action* (Maidenhead: Open University Press).

Collingridge, D. and Reeve, C. (1986) *Science Speaks to Power: The Role of Experts in Policy Making* (London: Pinter).

Collins, F.S. (2004) 'What We Do and Don't Know About "Race", "Ethnicity", Genetics and Health at the Dawn of the Genome Era', *Nature Genetics Supplement*, 36(11): s13–5.

COMA (Committee on Medical Aspects of Food) (1974) *Diet and Coronary Heart Disease* (London: DHSS).

COMA (1984) *Diet and Cardiovascular Disease* (London: HMSO).

COMA (1994) *Nutritional Aspects of Cardiovascular Disease* (London: HMSO).

COMA (1997) *Nutritional Aspects of the Development of Cancer* (London: HMSO).

COMARE (Committee on Medical Aspects of Radiation in the Environment) (2005) *10th Report: The Incidence of Childhood Cancer around Nuclear Installations in Great Britain* (Oxon: COMARE).

COMARE (2008) *12th Report: The Impact of Personally Initiated X-ray Computed Tomography Scanning for the Health Assessment of Asymptomatic Individuals* (London: Department of Health).

COMEAP (Committee on the Medical Effects of Air Pollutants) (1998) *The Quantification of the Effects of Air Pollution on Health in the UK* (London: HMSO).

COMEAP (2006) *Cardiovascular Disease and Air Pollution: A Report by the Committee on the Medical Effects of Air Pollution and Appendices* (London: Department of Health).

COMEAP (2007) *Long-term Exposure to Air Pollution: Effect on Mortality* (London: Department of Health).

Commission for Integrated Transport (2002) *Initial Assessment Report on the 10 year Transport Plan* (London: CIT).

Commission for Integrated Transport (2007) *Transport and Climate Change* (London: CIT).

Commission for Rural Communities (2005) *Rural Disadvantage Priorities for Action* (London: CRC).

Commission for Social Justice (1994) *Social Justice: Strategies for Social Renewal* (London: Verso).

Commission of the European Communities (1999) *Communication From the Commission to the Council, the European Parliament, the Economic and Social Committee and the Committee of the Regions on a European Union Action Plan to combat drugs (2000–4)* COM 1999 239 final 26.5.99. (Brussels: European Commission).

Commission of the European Communities (2000) *White Paper on Food Safety, 12 January 2000 COM (1999) 719 Final* (Brussels: Commission of the European Communities).

Commission of the European Communities (2001) *Communication from the Commission. A Sustainable Europe for a Better World: A European Strategy for Sustainable Development Com (2001) 264 Final* (Brussels: European Commission).

Commission of the European Communities (2003) *Communication from the Commission to the Council, The European Parliament, The European Economic and Social Committee: A European Environment and Health Strategy COM (2003) 338 Final* (Brussels: Commission of the European Communities).

Commission of the European Communities (2004a) *Communication from the Commission to the Council, The European Parliament, The European Economic and Social Committee: The European Environment and Health Action Plan 2004–2010 COM (2004) 416 Final* (Brussels: Commission of the European Communities).

Commission of the European Communities (2004b) *Communication From the Commission to the Council and the European Parliament – On the Results of the Final Evaluation of the EU Drugs Strategy and Action Plan on Drugs (2000–2004)* (Brussels: European Commission) 22.10.2004 COM (2004)707 Final.

Commission of the European Communities (2005) *Green Paper: Promoting Healthy Diets and Physical Activity: A European Dimension for the Prevention of Overweight, Obesity and Chronic Diseases COM (2005) 637 Final* (Brussels: Commission of the European Communities).

Commission of the European Communities (2006) *Communication from the Commission to the Council, The European Parliament, The European Economic and Social Committee and the Committee of the Regions. An EU Strategy to Support Member States in Reducing Alcohol Related Harm* (Brussels: Commission of the European Communities).

Commission of the European Communities (2007a) *White Paper on A Strategy for Europe on Nutrition, Overweight and Obesity Related Health Issues COM (2007) 279 Final* (Brussels: Commission of the European Communities).

Commission of the European Communities (2007b) *White Paper on Sport* (Brussels: Commission of the European Communities) (http://ec.europa.eu/sport/white-paper/index_en.htm accessed 15.5.10).

Commission of the European Communities (2007c) *White Paper. Together for Health: A Strategic Approach for the EU 2008–2013 COM (2007) 630 Final* (Brussels: European Commission).

Commission of the European Communities (2009) *Report from the Commission on Food Irradiation for the Year 2007 Official Journal of the EU* 9.10.09 C242/2.

Commission on Social Determinants of Health (2008) *Closing the Gap in a Generation: Health Equity Through Action on the Social Determinants of Health* (Geneva: World Health Organisation).

Committee on Climate Change (2008) *Building a Low Carbon Economy: The UK's Contribution to Tackling Climate Change* (London: TSO).

Committee on Food Marketing and the Diets of Children and Youth (2006) *Food Marketing to Children and Youth: Threat or Opportunity?* (Washington: National Academies Press).

Committee on the Carcinogenity of Chemicals in Food, Consumer Products and the Environment (2000) *COC Statement on Breast Cancer Risk and Exposure to Organochlorine Insecticides:* Consideration of the Epidemiology Data on Dieldrin, DDT and Certain Hexachlorocyclohexane Isomers (London: Department of Health).

Committee on the Carcinogenity of Chemicals in Food, Consumer Products and the Environment (2004) *Breast Cancer Risk and Exposure to Organochlorine Insecticide: Consideration of the Epidiomology Data on Dieldrin, DDT and Certain Hexachlorocyclohexane Isomers Statement COC/04/S3* (London: Department of Health).

Committee on Toxicity (2002) *Risk Assessment of Mixtures of Pesticides and Similar Substances* (London: Committee on Toxicity).

Connelly, J. (1999) 'Public Health Policy: Between Victim Blaming and the Nanny State – Will the Third Way Work?' *Policy Studies*, 20(1): 51–67.

Connelly, J., McAveary, M. and Griffiths, S. (2005) 'National Survey of Working Life in Public Health after Shifting the Balance of Power: Results of First Survey', *Public Health*, 119: 1133–7.

Conservative Party (2010a) *A Healthier Nation. Policy Green Paper no. 12* (London: Conservative Party).

Conservative Party (2010b) *Invitation to Join the Government of Britain* (London: Conservative Party).

Cook, D. (2002) 'Consultation for a Change? Engaging Users and Communities in the Policy Process', *Social Policy and Administration*, 36(5): 516–31.

Cooper, C., Snow, S., McAlindon, T.E. et al. (2001) 'Risk Factors for the Incidence and Progression of Radiographic Knee Osteoarthritis', *Arthritis Rheumatism*, 43(5): 995–1000.

Cooper, L., Coote, A., Davies, A. and Jackson, C. (1995) *Voices Off Tackling the Democratic Deficit in Health* (London: IPPR).

Coote, A. (2002) *Claiming the Health Dividend* (London: King's Fund).

Coote, A. (2004) *Prevention Rather Than Cure: Making the Case for Choosing Health* (London: King's Fund).

Cope, R. (1989) 'The Compulsory Detention of Afro Caribbeans Under the Mental Health Act', *New Community*, 15(3): 343–56.

Corcoran, N. (ed.) (2007) *Communicating Health: Strategies for Health Promotion* (London: Sage).

Cornish, Y., Russell-Hodgson, C., Fani-Kayode, S. et al. (1997) *Review of Health of the Nation in North Thames* (London: South East Institute of Public Health).

Corrigan, P. (2007) 'New Social Democratic Politics of Health in England Today' in Griffiths, S. and Hunter, D. *New Perspectives in Public Health* (2nd edn) (Oxford: Radcliffe), pp. 79–86.

Corti, Count Egon Caesar (1931) *A History of Smoking* (London: Harrap).

Cosford, P., Mahony, M., Angell, E. et al. (2006) 'Public Health Professionals' Perceptions Toward Provision of Health Protection in England: A Survey of Expectations of Primary Care Trusts and Health Protection Units in the Delivery of Health Protection', *BMC Public Health*, 6: 297.

Costongs, C. and Springett, J. (1997) 'Joint Working and the Production of a City Health Plan: The Liverpool Experience', *Health Promotion International*, 12(1): 9–19.

Cottam, R. (2005) 'Is Public Health Coercive Health?', *The Lancet*, 366(5): 1593–4.

Coulter, A. (2003) 'Engaging Patients and Citizens' in Leatherman, K. and Sutherland, K. *The Quest for Quality in the NHS: A Mid Term Evaluation of the Ten Year Quality Agenda* (London: TSO), pp. 183–201.

Coulter, A. (2007) 'Patient Engagement: Why is it Important?' in Andersson, E., Tritter, J. and Wilson, R. (eds) *Healthy Democracy: The Future of Involvement in Health and Social Care* (London: Involve), pp. 27–36.

Council of Europe (1996) *European Social Charter* (http://conventions.coe.int/treaty/en/treaties/html/163.htm accessed 23.8.10).

Council of the European Communities (1980) Council Directive 80/778/EEC of 15 July 1980 Relating to the Quality of Water Intended for Human Consumption.

Council of the European Communities (1998) Council Directive 98/83/EC of 3 November 1998 on the Quality of Water Intended for Human Consumption.

Council of the European Union (2004) *EU Drugs Strategy (2005–2012)*, Brussels, 22 November 2004.

Council of the European Union (2005) *EU Drugs Action Plan (2005–2008)*, Brussels, 19 May 2005.

Council of the European Union (2006) *Renewed Sustainable Development Strategy 10917/06* (Brussels).

Coussins, J. (2004) 'The Portman Group Does Not Represent Alcohol Industry', *British Medical Journal*, 329(14): 404.

Cowley, S., Caan, W., Dowling, S. and Weir, H. (2007) 'What do Health Visitors do? A National Survey of Activities and Service Organisation', *Public Health*, 121: 869–79.

Coxall, W. (2001) *Pressure Groups in British Politics* (London: Longman).

Coyle, E. (2007) 'Public Health in Wales' in Griffiths, S. and Hunter, D. (eds) *New Perspectives in Public Health* (London: Routledge), pp. 37–44.

Crabbe, T. (2006) Knowing *the Score: Positive Futures Case Study Research Report* (London: Crime Concern).

Craig, C. (2003) 'Reterritorialising Health: Inclusive Partnerships, Joined up Governance and Common Accountability Platforms in Third Way New Zealand', *Policy and Politics*, 31(3): 335–52.

Craig, C., Taylor, M. and Parkes, T. (2004) 'Protest or Partnership? The Voluntary and Community Sectors in the Policy Process', *Social Policy and Administration*, 38(3): 221–39.

Craig, G. and Taylor, M. (2002) 'Dangerous Liaisons: Local Government and the Voluntary and Community Sectors' in Glendinning, C., Powell, M. and Rummery, K. (eds) *Partnerships, New Labour and Governance* (Bristol: Policy Press), pp. 131–48.

Craig, G., Adamson, S., Ali, N. et al. (2007) *Sure Start and Black and Minority Ethnic Populations* (London: Department for Education and Skills (DfES)).

Crawford, R. (1980) 'Healthism and the Medicalisation of Everyday Life', *International Journal of Health Services*, 10(3): 365–88.

Crawshaw, P., Bunton, R. and Gillen, K. (2003) 'Health Action Zones and the Problem of

Community', *Health and Social Care in the Community*, 11(1): 36–44.

Crayford, T. (2007) *Choosing Health Survey Headlines: Press Release 18 October* (Cambridge: Association of Directors of Public Health).

Creighton, C. (1965) *A History of Epidemics*, Vol. 2, London: Frank Cass.

Crepaz, M. and Crepaz, N. (2004) 'Is Equality Good Medicine? Determinants of Life Expectancy in Industrialised Democracies', *Journal of Public Policy*, 24(3): 275–98.

Crick, B. (1987) *Socialism* (Milton Keynes: Open University Press).

Critchley, J. (2008) 'All the Experts Admit That We Should Legalise Drugs', *The Independent* 14 August (www.independent.co.uk accessed 17.5.10).

Crombie, I., Irvine, L., Elliott, L. and Wallace, H. (2005) *Policies to Reduce Inequalities in 13 Developed Countries* (Copenhagen: WHO Regional Office for Europe).

Crossley, N. (2004) 'Fat is a Sociological Issue: Obesity Rates in Late Modern "Body Conscious" Societies', *Social Theory and Health*, 2: 222–53.

Crossman, R. (1972) *Inside View: Three Lectures on Prime Ministerial Government* (London: Jonathan Cape).

Crown, J. (1999) 'The Practice of Public Health Medicine: Past, Present and Future' in Jenkins, S. and Hunter, D. *Perspectives on Public Health* (Oxford: Radcliffe), pp. 214–71.

Crowther-Dowey, C. (2007) 'The Police and Drugs', in Simpson, M., Shildrick, T. and Macdonald, R. *Drugs in Britain – Supply, Consumption and Control* (Basingstoke: Palgrave Macmillan).

Cuckle, H. and Wald, N. (1984) 'Principles of Screening Antenatal and Neonatal Screening' in Wald, N.J. (ed.) *Antenatals and Neonatal Screening* (Oxford: Oxford University Press).

Cummins, S. and Macintyre, S. (2002) '"Food Deserts" – Evidence and Assumption in Health Policy Making', *British Medical Journal*, 325: 436–8.

Cummins, S., Curtis, S., Diez-Roux, A.V. and Macintyre, S. (2007) 'Understanding and Representing "Place" in Health Research: A Relational Approach', *Social Science & Medicine*, 65: 1825–38.

Cunningham-Burley, S. and Amos, A. (2002) 'The New Genetics and Health Promotion' in Bunton R. and MacDonald, G. (eds) *Health Promotion: Disciplines and Diversity* (London: Routledge), pp. 284–301.

Currie, E. (1989) *Lifelines* (London: Pan).

Curtice, C. (1992) 'Strategies and Values: Research and the WHO Healthy Cities Project in Europe' in Davies, J. and Kelly, M. *Healthy*

Cities (Buckingham: Open University Press), pp. 34–54.

Curtis, S. (2004) *Health and Inequality: Geographical Perspectives* (London: Sage).

Curtis, S., Southall, H., Congdon, P. and Dodgeon, B. (2004) 'Area Effects on Health Variation Over the Life-Course: Analysis of the Longitudinal Study Sample in England Using New data on Area of Residence in Childhood', *Social Science & Medicine*, 58: 57–74.

Dahl, E., Elstad, J.I., Hofoss, D. and Martin-Mollard, M. (2006) 'For Whom is Income Inequality Most Harmful? A Multi-Level Analysis of Income Inequality and Mortality in Norway', *Social Science & Medicine*, 63: 2562–74.

Dahlgren, G. and Whitehead, M. (1992) *Policies and Strategies to Promote Social Equity in Health* (Copenhagen: WHO).

Dales, L., Hammer, S. and Smith, N. (2001) 'Time Trends in Autism and in Measles, Mumps, Rubella Immunisation Coverage in California', *Journal of American Medical Association*, 285(9): 1183–5.

Dalrymple, T. (2003) 'We Must Kick Our Methadone Habit', 30 May *Times Online* (www.timesonline.co.uk accessed 17.5.10).

Dalziel, Y. (2008) 'Community Development as a Public Health Function', in Cowley, S. (ed.) *Community Public Health in Policy and Practice* (London: Balliere Tindall Elsevier), pp. 108–28.

Damro, C. and Mendez, P. (2003) 'Emissions Trading at Kyoto: From EU Resistance to Union Innovation' *Environmental Politics*, 12(2): summer, 71–94.

Dangour, A., Dodhia, S., Hayter, A. et al. (2009) *Comparison of Composition of Organically and Conventionally Produced Foodstuffs: A Systematic Review of the Available Literature* (London: London School of Hygiene and Tropical Medicine).

Darbre, P. (2006) 'Environmental Oestrogens, Cosmetics and Breast Cancer', *Best Practice Research Clinical Endocrinology and Metabolism*, 20(1): 121–43.

Darbre, P. (2009) 'Underarm Perspirants, Deodorants and Breast Cancer' *Breast Cancer Research*, 11 Supp. 3: S5 doi:10.1186/bcr2424 (accessed 16.7.10).

Darlow, A., Percy-Smith, J. and Wells, P. (2007) 'Community Strategies: Are They Delivering Joined up Governance?', *Local Government Studies*, 33(1): 117–29.

Davey Smith, G. (ed.) (2003) *Health Inequalities: Lifecourse Approaches* (Bristol: Policy Press).

Davey Smith, G. (2004) 'Lifestyle, Health and Health Promotion in Nazi Germany', *British Medical Journal*, 329 1424–5

Davey Smith, G. and Dorling, D. (1996) 'I'm Alright John: Voting Pattern and Mortality in England and Wales 1981–92', *British Medical Journal*, 313: 1573–7.

Davey Smith, G. and Dorling, D. (1997) 'Associations between Voting Patterns and Mortality Remain', *British Medical Journal*, 315: 430–1.

Davey Smith, G. and Lynch, J. (1997) 'Life Course Approaches to Socioeconomic Differentials in Health' in Kuh, D. and Schlomo, Y. *A Life Course Approach Chronic Disease Epidemiology* (Oxford: Oxford University Press), pp. 77–115.

Davey Smith, G., Blane, D. and Bartley, M. (1994) 'Explanations for Socio-economic Differentials in Mortality', *European Journal of Public Health*, 4: 131–44.

Davey Smith, G., Hart, C., Blane, D. et al. (1997) 'Lifetime Socioeconomic Position and Mortality: Prospective Observational Study', *British Medical Journal*, 314: 547–52.

Davey Smith, G., Ebrahim, S., Lewis, S. et al. (2005) 'Genetic Epidemiology and Public Health: Hope, Hype, and Future Prospects', *The Lancet*, 366(9495): 1484–98.

David, P. (1985) 'Clio and the Economics of Qerty', *America Economic Review*, 75(2): 332–7.

Davies, A. (1997) *Reporting the Public Health* (London: Institute of Public Policy Research).

Davies, C. (1995) *Gender and the Professional Predicament in Nursing* (Buckingham: Open University Press).

Davies, J. and Foley, P. (2007) 'Partnerships and Alliances for Health' in Lloyd, C., Handsley, S., Douglas, J. et al. (eds) *Policy and Practice in Promoting Public Health* (Maidenhead: Open University Press/Sage), pp. 127–54.

Davies, J. and Kelly, M. (1992) *Healthy Cities* (Buckingham: Open University Press).

Davis, L., Dowler, E., Hunter, D. et al. (2007) *Food and Wellbeing: A Review of the Nutrition Strategy for Wales 2003–6* (Coventry: University of Warwick).

Davison, C., MacIntyre, S. and Davey Smith, G. (1994) 'The Potential Impact of Predictive Genetic Testing for Susceptibility to Common Chronic Diseases: A Review and Proposed Research Agenda', *Sociology of Health and Illness*, 16(3): 340–71.

Dawson, S., Morris, Z., Erickson, W. et al. (2007) *Engaging with Care: A Vision for the Health and Social Care Workforce of England* (London: Nuffield Trust).

Day, P. and Klein, R. (1989) 'Interpreting the Unexpected: The Case of AIDS Policy Making in Britain', *Journal of Public Policy*, 9(3): 337–53.

Daykin, N., Evans, D., Petsoulas, C. and Sayer, A. (2007) 'Evaluating the Impact of Patient and Public Involvement Initiatives on UK Health Services: A Systematic Review', *Evidence and Policy*, 3(1): 47–65.

DCLG (Department of Communities and Local Government) (2007a) *Planning Policy Statement: Planning and Climate Change Supplement to Planning Policy Statement 1* (London: DCLG).

DCLG (2007b) *Tackling Overcrowding in England* (London: DCLG).

DCLG (2007c) *Homes for the Future: More Affordable, More Sustainable* (London: TSO).

DCLG (2009a) *Statutory Homelessness: 1st Quarter 2009, England* (London: National Statistics).

DCLG (2009b) *Housing Surveys Bulletin* (London: DCLG).

DCMS (Department for Culture, Media and Sport) (2008a) *Written Ministerial Statement by Andy Burnham on the Evaluation of the Impact of the Licensing Act 2003* (London: DCMS).

DCMS (2008b) *Evaluation of the Licensing Act 2003* (London: DCMS).

DCMS, Home Office, and ODPM (Office of Deputy Prime Minister) (2005) *Drinking Responsibly: The Government's Proposals* (London: DCMS, Home Office and ODPM).

DCSF (Department for Children Schools and Families) (2007) *The Children's Plan: Building Brighter Futures* (London: TSO).

DCSF (2008a) *Children and Young People's Workforce Strategy* (London: DCMS).

DCSF (2008b) *The Play Strategy* (London: DCSF).

DCSF (2008c) *Staying Safe: Action Plan* (London: DCSF).

DCSF (2009) *The Impact of the Commercial World on Childrens' Wellbeing: Report of An independent Assessment* (London: DCMS).

DCSF and DCMS (2008) *Physical Education and Sports Strategy for Young People* (London: DCSF/DCMS).

DCSF and DoH (Department of Health) (2009) *Healthy Lives, Brighter Futures: The Strategy for Children's and Young People's Health* (London: DoH).

de Leeuw, E. and Skovgaard, T. (2005) 'Utility-Driven Evidence for Healthy Cities: Problems with Evidence Generation and Application', *Social Science & Medicine*, 61: 1331–41.

DeBell, D. (2007) *Public Health Practice and the School-Age Population* (London: Hodder Arnold).

Decision of the European Parliament and of the Council (2001) *Adopting a Programme of Community Action in the field of Public Health* (2001–6), amended proposal, 2000/0119 (COD).

Decision of the European Parliament and of the Council (2006) *Establishing a Second Programme of Community Action in the Field* of Health (2007–13), amended proposal, 2004/0042 A (COD).

DEFRA (Department for Environment, Food and Rural Affairs) (2002) *The Strategy for Sustainable Farming and Food: Facing The Future* (London: DEFRA).

DEFRA (2006a) *Food Industry Sustainability Strategy* (London: DEFRA).

DEFRA (2006b) *UK Pesticides Strategy: A Strategy for the Sustainable use of Plant Protection Products* (London: DEFRA).

DEFRA (2007) *Waste Strategy for England 2007* (London: DEFRA).

DEFRA (2008a) *UK Emissions of Air Pollutants: 2006 Results* (London: DEFRA).

DEFRA) (2008b) *Family Food: A Report in the 2007 Food and Expenditure Survey* (London: DEFRA).

DEFRA (2009) UK Climate Projections (http://ukclimateprojections.defra.gov.uk accessed 13.8.09).

DEFRA, Welsh Assembly Government, Scottish Executive and Department of the Environment Northern Ireland (2007) *National Implementation Plan for the Stockholm Convention on Persistent Organic Pollutants UK of Great Britain and Northern Ireland* (London: DEFRA).

Dembe, A., Erickson, J., Delbos, R. and Banks, S. (2005) 'The Impact of Overtime and Long Work Hours on Occupational Injuries and Illnesses: New Evidence from the United State', *Occupational and Environmental Medicine*, 62: 588–97.

Denman, S. (1999) 'Health Promoting Schools in England – A Way Forward in Development', *Journal of Public Health Medicine*, 21(2): 215–20.

Denscombe, M. (2001a) 'Peer Group Pressure, Young People and Smoking: New Developments and Policy Implications', *Drugs, Education, Prevention and Policy*, 8(1): 7–32.

Denscombe, M. (2001b) 'Smoking Cessation Among Young People: The Need for Qualitative Research on Young People's Experiences of Giving up Tobacco Smoking', *Health Education Journal*, 60(3): 221–31.

Denscombe, M. (2007) 'UK Health Policy and "Underage" Smokers: The Case for Smoking Cessation Services', *Health Policy*, 80: 69–76.

Department of Education for Northern Ireland (DENI) (2008) *New Nutritional Standards for School Lunches and Other Food in Schools* (Belfast: DENI).

Department of Health, Education and Welfare (1979) *Healthy People: The Surgeon General's Report on Health Promotion and Disease Prevention* (Washington: Public Health Service).

Department of Social Security (1990) *Households Below Average Income 1979–1996/7* (London: TSO).

Depression Alliance/Sane (2007) *New Survey Reveals GP Contract Compromises People with Depression* (London: Sane/Depression Alliance).

Derrett, C. and Burke, L. (2006) 'The Future of Primary Care Nurses and Health Visitors', *British Medical Journal*, 333: 1185–6.

DeStefano, F., Bhasin, T.K., Thompson, W.W. et al. (2004) 'Age at First Measles-Mumps-Rubella Vaccination in Children with Autism and School-Matched Control Subjects: A Population Based Study in Metropolitan Atlanta', *Paediatrics*, 113(2): 259–66.

DETR (Department for the Environment, Transport and Regions), DFEE, DoH (1999) *School Travel* (London: DETR).

DETR (2000a) *Tomorrow's Roads Safer For Everyone* (London: DETR).

DETR (2000b) *Transport 2010: The 10 Year Plan* (London: DETR).

DETR (2000c) *Transport 2010: Meeting the Local Transport Challenge* (London: DETR).

DETR (2000d) *The English House Conditions Survey* (London: TSO).

Devine, A., Criddle, R.A., Dick, I.M. et al. (1995) 'Longitudinal Study of the Effect of Sodium and Calcium Intakes on Regional Bone Density in Postmenopausal Women', *American Journal of Clinical Nutrition*, 62: 740–5.

Devlin, R. and Henry, J. (2008) 'Clinical Review: Major Consequences of Illicit Drug Consumption', *Critical Care* 12(1): 202 (Epub Jan8 accessed 17.5.10).

Dewailly, E., Dodin, S., Verrault, R. et al. (1994) 'High Organochlorine Body Burden in Women with Estrogen Receptor-Positive Breast Cancer', *Journal of the National Cancer Institute*, 86(3): 232–4.

DFEE (Department for Education and Employment) (1999) *National Healthy School Standard Guidance* (London: DFEE).

DfES (Department for Education and Skills) (2004a) *Every Child Matters: Next Steps* (London: DfES)

DfES (2004b) *Every Child Matters: Change for Children* (London: DfES)

DfES (2004c) *Drugs: Guidance for Schools* (London: DfES).

DfES (2005) Statutory Guidance on inter-agency cooperation to improve the wellbeing of children: Children's Trusts (London: DfES)

DfES and DCMS (Department for Culture Media and Sport) (2003) *Learning Through PE and Sport. A Guide to the Physical Education School Sport and Club Link Strategy* (London: TSO).

DfT (Department for Transport) (2005) *Travelling to School Initiative: Report on the Findings of the Initial Evaluation* (London: DfT).

DfT (2007) *Child Road Safety Strategy* (London: DfT).

DHSS (Department of Health and Social Security) (1972) *Report of the Working Party on Medical Administrators* (London: HMSO).

DHSS (1976a) Prevention and Health: Everybody's Business (London: DHSS).

DHSS (1976b) *Priorities for Health and Personal Social Services in England: A Consultative Document* (London: HMSO).

DHSS (1977) *The Way Forward* (London: DHSS).

DHSS (Department of Health and Social Security) (1980) *Inequalities in Health: Report of A Research Working Party* (The Black Report) (London: DHSS).

DHSS (1981a) Care in Action (London: DHSS).

DHSS (1981b) *Drinking Sensibly* (London: DHSS).

DHSS (1983) *NHS Management Inquiry* (London: DoH).

DHSS (1986) *Neighbourhood Nursing: A Focus for Care. Report of the Community Nursing Review* (The Cumberlege Report) London: HMSO).

DHSSNI (Department of Health and Social Security for Northern Ireland) (1996) *Health and Well-being towards the new Millennium* (Belfast: DHSSNI).

DHSSNI (1997) *Well in 2000* (Belfast: DHSSNI).

DHSSPS (Department of Health, Social Security and Public Safety, Northern Ireland) (2000) *Strategy for Reducing Alcohol-related Harm* (Belfast: DHSSPS).

DHSSPS (2002a) *Investing for Health* (Belfast: DHSSPS).

DHSSPS (2002b) *Teenage Pregnancy and Parenthood: Strategy and Action Plan 2002–2007* (Belfast: DHSSPS).

DHSSPS (2003) *Strengthening the Nursing Contribution to Public Health* (Belfast: DHSSPS).

DHSSPS (2004a) *The Review of the Public Health Function in Northern Ireland* (Belfast: DHSSPS).

DHSSPS (2004b) *Investing for Health Update* (Belfast: DHSSPS).

DHSSPS (2004c) *A Healthier Future: A twenty-year vision for health and wellbeing in Northern Ireland* (Belfast: DHSSPNI).

DHSSPS (2005) *Realising the Vision. Nursing for Public Health* (Belfast: DHSSPS).

DHSSPS (2006a) *Our Children and Young People – Our Shared Responsibility.* Inspection of Child Protection Services in Northern Ireland. An Overview Report (Belfast: DHSSPS).

DHSSPS (2006b) *Fit Futures* (Belfast: DHSSPS).

DHSSPS (2006c) *New Strategic Direction for Alcohol and Drugs 2006–11* (Belfast: DHSSPS).

Diamond, P. (2005) *Equality Now The Future of Revisionism* (London: Fabian Society).

DiCenso, A., Guyatt, G., Willan, A. and Griffith, L. (2002) 'Interventions to Reduce Unintended Pregnancies Among Adolescents: Systematic Review of Randomised Controlled Trials', *British Medical Journal*, (324): 1426.

Di Forti, M., Morgan, C., Dazzan, P. et al. (2009) 'High Potency Cannabis and the Risk of Psychosis', *The British Journal of Psychiatry*, 195: 488–91.

Dingle, A. (1980) *The Campaign for Prohibition in Victorian England* (London: Croom Helm).

Disability Rights Commission (2006) *Equal Treatment: Closing the Gap* (London: DRC).

Dixon, A., Le Grand, J., Henderson, J. et al. (2003) *Is the NHS Equitable? A Review of the Evidence* (London: London School of Economics).

Dixon, H., Scully, M., Wakefield, M. et al. (2007) 'The Effects of Television Advertisements for Junk Food Versus Nutritious Food on Children's Food Attitudes and Preferences', *Social Science & Medicine*, 65(7): 1311–23.

Dixon, M. (2006) 'Screening for Breast Cancer', *British Medical Journal*, 332(7540): 499–500.

Dobbs, L. and Moore, C. (2002) 'Engaging Communities in Area-based Regeneration: The Role of Participatory Evaluation', *Policy Studies*, 23(3/4): 157–71.

Dobson, A. (1990) *Green Political Thought: An Introduction* (London: Unwin Hyman).

Docherty, I. and Shaw, J. (2008) Traffic Jam: Ten Years of Sustainable Transport in the UK (Bristol: Policy Press).

DoE (Department of the Environment) (1996) *National Air Quality Strategy* (London: HMSO).

DoH (Department of Health) (1992) *Effect of Tobacco Advertisements on Tobacco Consumption: A Discussion Document Reviewing the Evidence* (London: DoH).

DoH (Department of Health) (1993) *Working Together for Better Health* (London: DoH).

DoH (1995) *Variations in Health: What can the Department of Health and the NHS do?* (London: DoH).

DoH (1996) *Task Force to Review Services for Drug Misusers* (London: DoH).

DoH (1997) *Breast Cancer Services in Exeter and Quality Assurance for Breast Screening: Report to the Secretary of State* (London: DoH).

DoH (1998) *The Health of the Nation: A Policy Assessed* (London: TSO).

DoH (1999a) *Making a Difference* (London: DoH).

DoH (1999b) *National Service Framework for Mental Health: Modern Standards and Service Models* (London: TSO).

DoH (1999c) *Patient and Public Involvement in the New NHS* (London: DoH).

DoH (1999d) *Reducing Health Inequalities: An Action Report* (London: DoH).

DoH (2001a) *Report of the Chief Medical Officer's Project to Strengthen the Public Health Function* (London: DoH).

DoH (2001b) *Vision to Reality* (London: DoH).

DoH (2001c) *Shifting the Balance of Power within the NHS: Securing Delivery* (London: DoH).

DoH (2001d) *Making it Happen: A Guide to Delivering Mental Health Promotion* (London: DoH).

DoH (2001e) *Better Prevention, Better Services, Better Sexual Health: The National Strategy for Sexual Health and HIV* (London: TSO).

DoH (2002a) *Getting Ahead of the Curve: A Strategy for Combating Infectious Diseases (including other aspects of health protection)* (London: DoH).

DoH (2002b) *National Suicide Prevention Strategy for England* (London: TSO).

DoH (2002c) *The National Strategy for Sexual Health and HIV Implementation Action Plan* (London: DoH).

DoH (2002d) *Preventing Accidental Injury: Priorities for Action* (London: DoH).

DoH (2002e) *Planning and Priorities Framework 2003–06* (London: DoH).

DoH (2003a) *Tackling Health Inequalities: Programme for Action* (London: DoH).

DoH (2003b) *Winning Ways: Working Together the Reduce Healthcare Associated Infection in England – Report from the Chief Medical Officer* (London: DoH).

DoH (2003c) *Our Inheritance, Our Future: Realising the Potential of Genetics in the NHS* (London: DoH).

DoH (2003d) *Annual Report of the Chief Medical Officer 2002* (London: TSO).

DoH (2004a) *Towards Cleaner Hospitals and Lower Rates of Infection* (London: DoH).

DoH (2004b) *The Chief Nursing Officer's Review of the Nursing, Midwifery and Health Visiting Contribution to Vulnerable Children and Young People* (London: DoH)

DoH (2004c) *Making Partnership Work for Patients, Carers and Service Users: A Strategic Agreement between the Department of Health, the NHS and the Voluntary and Community Sector* (London: DoH).

DoH (2004d) *Action Plan on Hospital Hygiene* (London: DoH).

DoH (2004e) *A Least Five a Week: Evidence in the Impact of Physical Activity and its Relationship to Health – A Report from the Chief Medical Officer* (London: DoH).

DoH (2004f) *Celebrating Our Culture* (London: DoH).

DoH (2004g) *Better Heath in Old Age* (London: DoH).

DoH (2005a) *Delivering Choosing Health: Making Healthier Choices Easier* (London: DoH).

DoH (2005b) *Choosing Health through Pharmacy: A Programme for Pharmaceutical Public Health* (London, DoH).

DoH (2005c) *Choosing Activity: A Physical Activity Action Plan* (London: DoH).

DoH (2005d) *Choosing A Better Diet: A Food and Health Action Plan* (London: DoH).

DoH (2006a) *Health Reform in England: Update and Commissioning Framework* (London: DoH).

DoH (2006b) *Essence of Care: Benchmarks for Promoting Health* (London: DoH).

DoH (2006c) *Strengthening Regional Partnerships for Health and Wellbeing* (London: DoH).

DoH (2007a) *Commissioning Framework for Health and Wellbeing* (London: DoH).

DoH (2007b) *Health is Global: Proposals for a UK Wide Government Strategy* (London: DoH).

DoH (2007c) *Communities for Health: Learning From the Pilots* (London: DoH).

DoH (2008a) *The NHS in England: The Operating Framework for 2008/10* (London: DoH).

DoH (2008b) *A High Quality Workforce: NHS Next Stage Review* (London: DoH).

DoH (2008c) *Ambitions for Health: A Strategic Framework for Maximising the Potential of Social Marketing and Health-Related Behaviour* (London: DoH).

DoH (2008d) *Changes in Food and Drink Advertising and Promotion to Children: A Report Outlining the Changes in the Nature and Balance of Food and Drink Advertising and Promotion to Children, From January 2003 to December 2007* (London: DoH).

DoH (2008e) *Consultation on the Future of Tobacco Control* (London: DoH).

DoH (2008f) *Tackling Health Inequalities: 2007 Status Report on the Programme for Action* (London: DoH).

DoH (2009a) *The NHS Operating Framework for England for 2010/11* (London: DoH).

DoH (2009b) *NHS Health and Well-being, Final Report* (London: DoH).

DoH (2009c) *Moving Forward: Progress and Priorities – Working Together for High Quality Sexual Health* (London: DoH).

DoH (2009d) *Securing Better Health for Children and Young People through World Class Commissioning* (London: DoH).

DoH (2009e) *Let's Get Moving: Commissioning Guidance: A New Physical Activity Pathway for the NHS* (London: DoH).

DoH (2009f) *Tackling Health Inequalities: 2006-08 Policy and Data Update for the 2010 National Target* (London: DoH).

DoH/CPHVA (2003) *Liberating the Public Health Talents of Community Practitioners and Health Visitors* (London: DoH).

DoH and DCSF (2008) *Child Health Promotion Programme: Pregnancy and the First Five Years of Life* (London: DoH/ DCSF).

DoH and DCSF (2009) *Healthy Lives: Brighter Futures: The Strategy for Children and Young People's Health* (London: DoH)

DoH and DfES (Department for Education and Skills) (2004) *National Service Framework for*

Children, Young People and Maternity Services (London: DoH/DfES).

DoH and DfES (2005) *National Healthy School Status: A Guide for Schools* (London: DoH/DfES).

DoH and Health Protection Agency (HPA) (2008) *The Health Effects of Climate Change in the UK* (London: DoH).

DoH and Neighbourhood Renewal Unit (2002) *Health and Neighbourhood Renewal* (London: DoH).

DoH and NHSE (National Health Service Executive) (1999) *Resistance to Antibiotics and other Antimicrobial Agents* (London: NHSE).

DoH/NHSE (2000) *The Management and Control of Hospital Infection* (London: TSO).

DoH and National Treatment Agency for Substance Misuse (2007) *Reducing Drug-Related Harm: An Action Plan* (London: DoH).

DoH, NTF (Nutrition Task Force) and PATF (Physical Activity Task Force) (1995) *Obesity: Reversing the Increasing Problem of Obesity in England* (London: DoH).

DoH and NTF (1996) *Low Income Project Team Low Income, Food Nutrition and Health: Strategies for Improvement* (London: DoH).

DoH and SMAC (Standing Medical Advisory Committee) (1998) *The Path of Least Resistance* (London: DoH).

DoH and UK Advisory Committee on the Microbiological Safety of Food (1999) *Microbial Antibiotic Resistance in Relation to Food Safety* (London: TSO).

Dolan, P., Peasgood, T., Dixon, A. et al. (2006) 'Research on the Relationship Between Well-Being and Sustainable Development', (London: Defra).

Dolk, H., Vrijhend, M., Armstrong, B. et al. (1998) 'Risk of Congenital Anomalies Near Hazardous Waste Landfill Sites in Europe', *The Lancet*, 352: 423–7.

Doll, R. and Hill, A. (1950) 'Smoking and Carcinoma of the Lung', *British Medical Journal*, 2: 739–48.

Doll, R. and Hill, A. (1956) 'Lung Cancer and Other Causes of Death in Relation to Smoking', *British Medical Journal*, 2: 1071–81.

Doll, R., Peto, R., Boreham, J. and Sutherland, I. (2004) 'Mortality in Relation to Smoking: 50 Years' Observations on Male British Doctors', *British Medical Journal*, 328(7455): 1519 (doi: 10.1136/bmj.38142.554479 accessed 17.5.10).

Donaldson, L. and May, R. (1999) *Health Implications of Genetically Modified Foods* (London: DoH).

Donkin, A., Goldblatt, P. and Lynch, K. (2002) 'Inequalities in Life Expectancy by Social Class 1972–1999', *Health Statistics Quarterly*, 15: autumn, 5–15.

Donnelly, P. (2007) 'Public Health in Scotland: The Dividend of Devolution' in Griffiths, S. and Hunter, D. (eds) *New Perspectives in Public Health* (London: Routledge), pp. 22–8.

Donnelly, P. and Whittle, P. (2008) 'After the Smoke has Cleared – Reflections on Scotland's Tobacco Control Legislation', *Public Health*, 122: 762–6.

Donovan, R. and Henley, N. (2003) *Social Marketing: Principles and Practice* (East Hawthorn, VIC: IP Communications).

Dooris, M. (2006) 'The Challenge of Developing Corporate Citizenship for Sustainable Public Health', *Critical Public Health*, 16(4): 331–43.

Doran, T., Drever, F. and Whitehead, M. (2004) 'Is There a North–South Divide in Social Class Inequalities in Health in Great Britain? Cross Sectional Study Using Data from the 2001 Census', *British Medical Journal*, 328: 1043–5.

Doran, T., Fullwood, C., Kontopantelis, E. and Reeves, D. (2008) 'Effect of Financial Incentives on Inequalities in the Delivery of Primary Clinical Care in England: Analysis of Clinical Activity Indicators for the Quality and Outcomes Framework', *The Lancet*, 372(9460): 728–36.

Dorgan, J.F., Brock, J.W., Rothman, N. et al. (1999) 'Serum Organochlorine Pesticides and PCBs and Breast Cancer Risk: Results From a Prospective Analysis', *Cancer Causes and Control*, 10: 1–11.

Dorling, D., Mitchell, R. and Pearce, J. (2007b) 'The Global Impact of Income Inequality on Health by Age: An Observational Study', *British Medical Journal* (doi: 10.1136/bmj.39349.507315.DE).

Dorling, D., Shaw, M. and Davey Smith, G. (2007a) 'Inequalities in Mortality Rates Under New Labour' in Dowler, E. and Spencer, N. *Challenging Health Inequalities – From Acheson to 'Choosing Health'* (Bristol: Policy Press), pp. 31–46.

Dorn, N., Baker, O. and Seddon, T. (1994) *Paying for Heroin: Estimating the Financial Costs of Acquisitive Crime by Dependent Heroin Users in England and Wales* (London: Institution of Drug Dependence).

Dorsett, R. and Marsh, A. (1998) *Poverty, Smoking and Lone Parenthood* (London: Policy Studies Institute).

Dos Santos Silva, I., Mangtani, P., McCormack, V. et al. (2004) 'Phyto-oestrogen Intake and Breast Cancer Risk in South Asian Women in England: Findings From a Population-Based Case-Control Study', *Cancer Causes Control*, 15(8): 805–18.

Douglas, M. and Wildavsky, A. (1982) *Risk and Culture* (Los Angeles: University of California).

Dowler, E. and Spencer, N. (2007) *Challenging Health Inequalities – From Acheson to 'Choosing Health'* (Bristol: Policy Press).

Dowling, B. (1997) 'Effect of Fundholding on Waiting Times: A Database Study', *British Medical Journal*, 315: 290–2.

Downie, R., Tannahill, L. and Tannahill, A. (1996) *Health Promotion Models and Values* (Oxford: Oxford University Press).

Downs, A. (1972) 'Up and Down with Ecology: The Issue-Attention Cycle', *The Public Interest*, 28(1): 38–50.

Doyal, L. (1979) *The Political Economy of Health* (London: Pluto).

Doyal, L. (1995) *What Makes Women Sick? Gender and the Political Economy of Health* (London: Macmillan – now Palgrave Macmillan).

Doyal, L. (2001) 'Sex, Gender and Health: Time for a New Approach', *British Medical Journal*, 323: 1061–3.

Doyal, L. (ed.) (1998) *Women and Health Services: An Agenda for Change* (Buckingham: Open University Press).

Doyle, T. and McEachern, D. (2001) *Environment and Politics* (London: Routledge).

Dr Foster (2008) *Weighing Up the Burden of Obesity: A Review by Dr Foster Research* (London: Dr Foster).

Drakeford, M. (2006) 'Health Policy in Wales: Making a Difference in Conditions of Difficulty', *Critical Social Policy*, 26(3): 543–61.

Draper, G., Vincent, T., Kroll, M. and Swanson, J. (2005) 'Childhood Cancer in Relation to Distance from High Voltage Power Lines in England and Wales: A Case Control Study', *British Medical Journal*, 330: 1290.

Draper, P. (ed.) (1991) *Health Through Public Policy: The Greening of Public Health* (London: Greenprint).

Drever, F. and Whitehead, M. (1995) 'Mortality in Regions and Local Authority Districts in the 1990s: Exploring the Relationship with Deprivation,' *Population Trends*, 82: 19–27.

Drinking Water Inspectorate (DWI) (2007) *Drinking Water in England and Wales 2006* (London: DWI).

Drinking Water Inspectorate (DWI) (2008) *Drinking Water in England and Wales 2007* (London: DWI).

Driver, S. and Martell, L. (2002) *Blair's Britain* (Cambridge: Polity Press).

Druce, M., Small, C. and Bloom, S. (2004) 'Mini-review: Gut Peptides Regulating Satiety', *Endocrinology*, 145(6): 2660–5.

Duffy, S.W., Agbaje, O., Tabar, L. et al. (2005) 'Overdiagnosis and Overtreatment of Breast Cancer: Estimates From Two Trials Of Mammographic Screening for Breast Cancer' *Breast Cancer Research*, 7: 258–65.

Dugdill, L. and Springett, J. (1994) 'Evaluation of Workplace Health Promotion: A Review', *Health Education Journal*, 53: 337–47.

Duhl, L.J. (1986) 'The Healthy City: Its Function and its Future', *Health Promotion*, 1: 55–60.

Dummer, T., Dickinson, H. and Parker, L. (2003) 'Adverse Pregnancy Outcomes Around Incinerators and Crematoriums in Cumbria, North West England 1956–93', *Journal of Epidemiology and Community Health*, 57(6): 456–61.

Duncan, B. (2002) 'Health Policy in the European Union: How it's Made and How to Influence it', *British Medical Journal*, 324: 1027–30.

Dunn, J.R. (2000) 'Housing and Health Inequalities: Review and Prospects for Research', *Housing Studies*, 15(3): 341–66.

Dunsire, A. (1978) *Implementation in a Bureaucracy* (Oxford: Martin Robertson).

Durante, L. (2007) *Improving our Health: A Holistic Approach* (London: IPPR).

Durham, M. (1991) *Sex and Politics: The Family and Morality in the Thatcher Years* (Basingstoke: Macmillan – now Palgrave Macmillan).

Durnford, A., Perkins, T. and Perry, J. (2008) 'An Evaluation of Alcohol Attendances to an Inner City Emergency Department Before and After the Introduction of the UK Licensing Act 2003', *BMC Public Health*, 8: 379.

Dworkin, R. (1972) 'Paternalism', *Monist*, 56(1): 64–84.

Dworkin, R. (2005) 'Paternalism' in *Stanford Encyclopedia of Philosophy* (http://plato.stanford.edu/entries/paternalism/).

EAC (Environmental Audit Committee) (2003a) *5th Report 2002–03: Waste – an Audit* (London: TSO).

EAC (2003b) *2nd Report 2002–03: Johannesburg and Back: the World Summit on Sustainable Development,* HC 169 (London: TSO)

EAC (2004a) *13th Report 2004–05 The Sustainable Development Strategy: Illusion or Reality?,* HC 624 (London: TSO).

EAC (2004b) *2nd Report 2003–04: GM Foods Evaluating the Farm Scale Trials,* HC 90 (London: TSO).

EAC (2005) *8th Report 2004–05: Progress on the Use of Pesticides: the Voluntary Initiative,* HC 258 (London: TSO).

EAC (2006a) *9th Report 2005–06: Reducing Carbon Emissions from Transport,* HC 981 (London: TSO).

EAC (2006b) *6th Report 2005–06 Keeping the Lights on: Nuclear, Renewables and Climate Change,* HC 584 (London: TSO).

EAC (2007a) *7th Report 2006–07: Beyond Stern. From the Climate Change Programme Review to the Draft Climate Change Bill* HC 460 (London: TSO)

EAC (2007b) *9th Report 2007–08: The Structure of Government and the Challenge of Climate Change*, HC 740 (London: TSO).

EAC (2008a) *9th Report 2007–08: Carbon Capture and Storage,* HC 654 (London: TSO).

EAC (2008b) *10th Report 2007–08: Vehicle Excise Duty as an Environmental Tax,* HC 907 (London: TSO).

EAC (2008c) *4th Report 2007–08: Are Biofuels Sustainable?,* HC 528 (London: TSO).

EAC (2008d) *2nd Report 2007–08 Reducing Carbon Emissions from UK Business: The Role of the Climate Change Levy and Agreements,* HC 354 (London: TSO).

EAC (2008e) *8th Report 2007–08: Climate Change and Local Regional and Devolved Government* HC 225 (London: TSO).

EAC (2008f) *6th Report 2007–08: Reaching an International Agreement on Climate Change,* HC 355 (London: TSO).

EAC (2010a) *5th Report 2009–10: Air Quality,* HC 229 (London: TSO).

EAC (2010b) *4th Report 2009–10: The Role of Carbon Markets in Preventing Dangerous Climate Change,* HC 290 (London: TSO).

EAC (2010c) *3rd Report 2009–10: Carbon Budgets,* HC 228 (London: TSO).

Earle, S. (2007a) 'Promoting Health in a Global Context' in Lloyd, C., Handsley, S., Douglas, J. et al. (2007) *Policy and Practice in Promoting Public Health* (London: Sage/Open University), pp. 1–32.

Earle, S. (2007b) 'Focusing on the Health of Children and Young People' in Earle, S., Lloyd, C., Sidell, M. and Spurr, S. *Theory and Research in Promoting Public Health* (London: Sage Publications), pp. 164–93.

EarlyBird (2010) Key Findings from EarlyBird (www.earlybirddiabetes.org/findings.php accessed 12.2.10).

East Midlands Public Health, Government Office for the East Midlands and NHS East Midlands (2009) *The East Midlands Public Health Strategy: Next Steps for Investment in Health* (Nottingham: Government Office for the East Midlands).

East Midlands Regional Assembly (2003) *Investment for Health: A Public Health Strategy for the East Midlands* (Melton Mowbray: EMRA).

Easterlin, R. (1974) 'Does Economic Growth Improve the Human Lot? Some Empirical Evidence' (http://graphics8.nytimes.com/images/2008/04/16/business/Easterlin1974.pdf accessed 21.5.10).

Eaton, C.B. (2004) 'Obesity as a Risk Factor for Osteoarthritis: Mechanical Versus Metabolic', *Medicine and Health Rhode Island*, 87(7): 201 4.

Eddington, R. (2006) *The Eddington Transport Study* (London: HM Treasury).

Edelman, M. (1977) *Political Language: Words that Succeed and Policies that Fail* (New York: Institute for the Study of Poverty).

Education and Skills Committee (2005) *Every Child Matters, Ninth Report, Session 2004–5,* HC 40-1 (London: TSO).

Edwards, A., Barnes, M., Plewis, I. and Morris, K. (2006) *Working to Prevent the Social Exclusion of Children and Young People: Final Lessons from the National Evaluation of the Children's Fund* (University of Birmingham, School of Education).

Edwards, G. (2003) *Alcohol: The World's Favourite Drug* (New York: St Martins).

Edwards, G., Anderson, P., Babor, T.F. et al. (1994) *Alcohol Policy and the Public Good* (Oxford: Oxford University Press).

Edwards, G., West R., Babor, T.F. et al. (2004) 'An Invitation to the Alcohol Industry Lobby to Help Decide Public Funding of Alcohol Research and Professional Training: A Decision that Should Be Reversed', *Addiction*, 99(10): 1235–6.

Edwards, L. (2001) 'Walk in Centres Checked Out', *Which?*, January, 7–9.

Edwards, N. (2006) 'Scrutiny and the Bounty', *Health Service Journal*, 1 June, 18–19.

Edwards, P., Roberts, I., Green, J. and Lutchman, S. (2006) 'Deaths from Injury in Children and Employment Status in Family: Analysis of Trends in Class Specific Deaths Rates', *British Medical Journal*, 333: 119 (doi: 10.1136/bmj.38875.757488.4F accessed 19.5.10).

EFRAC (Environment Food and Rural Affairs Committee) (2002) *9th Report 2001–02: The Future of Agriculture in a Changing World,* HC 550 (London: TSO).

EFRAC (2005a) *4th Report 2004–05: Waste Policy and the Landfill Directive,* HC 102 (London: TSO).

EFRAC (2005b) *9th Report 2004–05: Climate Change – Looking Forward,* HC 130 (London: TSO).

EFRAC (2006) *7th Report 2005–06: The Environmental Agency,* HC 780 (London: TSO).

EFRAC (2007) *4th Report 2006–07: The UK Government's Vision for the Common Agricultural Policy,* HC 546 (London: TSO).

EFRAC (2008) *5th Report 2007–08: Energy Efficiency and Fuel Poverty,* HC 1099 (London: TSO).

EFRAC (2009) *4th Report 2008–09: Securing Food Supplies up to 2050: The Challenges Faced by the UK,* HC 213 (London: TSO).

Egger, G. and Swinburn, B. (1997) 'An Ecological Approach to the Obesity Pandemic', *British Medical Journal*, 315: 477–80.

Egred, M. and Davis, G. (2005) 'Cocaine and the Heart', *Postgraduate Medical Journal*, 81(959): 568–71.

Eldridge, J. (1999) 'Risk Society and the Media: Now You See it, Now You Don't' in Philo, G. (ed.) *Message Received* (London: Longman), pp. 106–27.

Elinder, L., Joossens, L., Raw, M. et al. (2003) *Public Health Aspects of the Common Agricultural Policy: Developments and Recommendations for Change in Four Sectors: Fruit and Vegetables, Dairy, Wine and Tobacco* (Swedish National Institute of Public Health).

Ellaway, A. Macintyre, S. and Bonnefoy, X. (2005) 'Graffiti, Greenery and Obesity in Adults: Secondary Analysis of European Cross Sectional Survey' *British Medical Journal,* 331: 611-12.

Elliott, L. (2004) *The Global Politics of the Environment* (London: Palgrave Macmillan).

Elliott, P., Eaton, N., Shaddick, G. and Carter, R. (2000) 'Cancer Incidence Near Municipal Solid Waste Incinerators in Great Britain 2 Histopathological and Case Note Review of Primary Liver Cancer Cases', *British Journal of Cancer,* 82(5): 1103–6.

Elliott, P., Shaddick, G., Kleinschmidt, I. et al. (1996a) 'Cancer Incidence Near Municipal Solid Waste Incinerators in Great Britain', *British Journal of Cancer,* 73(5): 702–10.

Elliott, P., Stamler, J., Nichols, R. et al. (1996b) 'Intersalt Revisted: Further Analyses of 24 Hour Sodium Excretion and Blood Pressure Within and Across Populations', *British Medical Journal,* 312: 1249–53.

Elliott, P., Briggs, D., Morris, S. et al. (2001) 'Risk of Adverse Birth Outcomes in Populations Living Near Landfill Sites', *British Medical Journal,* 323: 18 August, 363–8.

Elliott, P., Shaddick, G., Wakefield, J. et al. (2007) 'Long-term Associations of Outdoor Air Pollution with Mortality in Great Britain', *Thorax,* 62: 1088–94.

Ellison, G. (2002) 'Letting the Gini Out of the Bottle? Challenges Facing the Relative Income Hypothesis', *Social Science & Medicine,* 54: 561–76.

EMCDDA (European Monitoring Centre for Drugs and Drug Addiction) (2008) *Annual Report: The State of the Drugs Problem in Europe* (Lisbon: ECMDDA).

Energy and Climate Change Committee (2010) *5th Report session 2009-10: Fuel Poverty* HC 242 (London: TSO).

English Nature (2003) *Nature and Psychological Well-Being* (London: English Nature).

Enstrom, J. and Kabat, G. (2003) 'Environmental Tobacco Smoke and Tobacco Related Mortality in a Prospective Study of Californians, 1960–98', *British Medical Journal,* 326(7398): 1057 (doi: 10.1136/bmj.326.7398.1057 accessed 18.5.10)

Entwhistle, T. (2006) 'The Distinctiveness of the Welsh partnership Agenda', *International Journal of Public Sector Management,* 19(3): 228–37.

Environment Agency (2002) *Agriculture and Natural Resources: Benefits, Costs and Potential Solutions* (London: Environment Agency).

Environment, Transport and Regional Affairs Committee (2000) *6th Report 1999–2000: The Environment Agency,* HC 34 (London: TSO).

Environmental Health Commission (1997) *Agendas for Change* (London: Chadwick House).

Epstein, E. (1977) *Agency of Fear* (New York: G.P. Putnam).

Epstein, L. and Ogden, J. (2005) 'A Qualitative Study of General Practitioners' View of Treating Obesity', *British Journal of General Practice,* 55: 750–4.

Epstein, S.S. (1992) 'Mammography Radiates Doubts', *International Journal of Health Services,* 22(3): 463–4.

Erickson, K. and Kramer, A.F. (2008) 'Exercise Effects on Cognitive and Neural Plasticity in Older Adults', *British Journal of Sports Medicine,* 43: 22–4 (doi: 10.1136/bjsm.2008.052498 accessed 15.5.10).

Ereaut, G. and Segnit, N. (2006). *Warm Words: How are We Telling the Climate Story and Can We Tell it Better?* (London: Institute for Public Policy Research).

ESRC (Economic and Social Research Council) (2005) *Devolution is a Process Not a Policy: The New Governance of the English Regions ESRC Programme on Devolution and Constitutional Change Briefing no 18* (available at www.devolution.ac.uk).

ESRC (2008) *ESRC Society Today: Violence Fact Sheet* (www.esrc.ac.uk/ESRCInfoCentre accessed 15.09.08).

EU Health Policy Forum (2003) *Recommendations on Health and EU Social Policy* (Brussels: EHPF).

Eurohealth (2005) 'Mythbusters: An Ounce of Prevention Buys a Pound of Cure', 11(4): 25–6.

Europa (2007) 'Environment: Commission Takes Steps to Cut Industrial Emissions Further' (press release IP/07/1985) www.europa.eu/rapid/searchAction.do (accessed 24.6.08).

European Charter on Alcohol (1995) European Conference on Health, Society and Alcohol Paris, 12–12 December 1995.

European Commission (2005) *Green Paper: Improving the Mental Health of the Population: Towards a Strategy on Mental Health for the European Union* (Brussels: Health and Consumer Protection Directorate-General).

European Commission (2007) *Reach in Brief* (Brussels: European Commission).

European Commission, Health and Consumer Directorate General (2007) *Green Paper Towards a Europe Free From Tobacco Smoke*

– *Policy Options at EU Level* COM 2007 Final (Brussels: European Commission).

European Environment Agency (2009) EU Greenhouse Gas Emissions Fall for the Third Consecutive Year' Press Release (Copenhagen: EEA) (www eea.europa.eu accessed 19.3.10).

European Health Policy Forum (2003) *Recommendations on Health and EU Social Policy* (Brussels: EHPF).

European Pact for Mental Health and Wellbeing (2008) EU High Level Conference: Together for Mental Health and Wellbeing (Brussels) 12–13 June 2008.

European Parliament (1997) *Report on Alleged Contraventions or Maladministration in the Implementation of Community Law in Relation to BSE*, Committee of Inquiry into BSE, Europe Parliament, Session Documents DOC-EN/RR/3191/319544 and DOC-EN/RR/319/319579.

European Parliament (1999) Report 0082/99, (the Needle report), February (Luxembourg: Office for Official Publications of the European Communities).

European Parliament and Council of the European Union (2001) *Directive 2001/37/EC on the Approximation of Laws, Regulations and Administrative Provisions of the Member States Concerning the Manufacturing, Presentation and Sale of Tobacco Products*.

European Parliament and Council of the European Union (2003) *Directive 2003/22/EC on the Approximation of Laws, Regulations and Administrative Provisions of the Member States Relating to the Advertising and Sponsorship of Tobacco Products*.

European Union (1997) *The Treaty of Amsterdam* (Luxembourg: European Commission, Office for Official Publications of the European Community).

European Union (2002) Organic Farming in the EU: Facts and Figures (www.europa.eu.int/Comm.agriculture/qual/organic/factors_en.pdf).

Evans, A.J., Pinder, S., Ellis, I.O. and Wilson, A.R. (2001) 'Screen Detected Ductal Carcinoma In Situ (DCIS): Over-diagnosis or an Obligate Precursor of Invasive Disease?', *Journal of Medical Screening*, 8(3): 149–51.

Evans, D. (2003) 'Taking Public Health Out of the Ghetto: The Policy and Practice of Multi-disciplinary Public Health in the United Kingdom', *Social Science & Medicine*, 57(6): 959–67.

Evans, D. (2004) 'Shifting the Balance of Power? UK Public Health Policy and Capacity Building', *Critical Public Health*, 14(1): 63–75.

Evans, D. (2006) 'We Do Not Use The Word "Crisis" Lightly', *Policy Studies*, 27(3): 235–52.

Evans, G., Wells, N. and Moch, A. (2003) 'Housing and Mental Health: A Review of the Evidence and a Methodological and Conceptual Critique', *Journal of Social Issues*, 59(3): 475–500.

Evans, J. and Hesmondhalgh, D. (eds) (2005) *Understanding Media: Inside Celebrity* (Maidenhead: Open University Press).

Eve, R., Hodgkin, P., Quinney, D. and Waller, J. (2000) *What do Practice Nurses do?* (Sheffield: Centre for Innovation in Primary Care).

Ewles, L. (1993) 'Hope Against Hype', *Health Service Journal*, 26 August, 30–1.

Ewles, L. and Simnett, I. (2003) *Promoting Health* (5th edn) (London: Balliere Tindall).

Exworthy, M., Stuart, M., Blane, D. and Marmott, M. (2003) *Tackling Health Inequalities since the Acheson Inquiry* (Bristol: Policy Press).

Faculty of Public Health (2008) *Specialist Public Health Workforce in the UK* (Grey, S.) (London: FPH).

Faculty of Public Health and the Royal Society of Public Health (2010) *12 Steps to Better Public Health: A Manifesto* (London: FPH, RSPH).

Faculty of Public Health Medicine (FPHM) (undated) *Carrying Out a Health Impact Assessment of a Transport Policy* (London: FPHM).

Fahey, D., Carson, E., Cramp, D. and Muir Gray, J. (2003) 'User Requirements and Understanding of Public Health Networks in England', *Journal of Epidemiology and Community Health*, 57: 938–44.

Fairclough, N. (2000) *New Labour, New Language?* (London: Routledge).

Falck, P., Ricci, A., Wolff, M. et al. (1992) 'Elevated Levels of PCBS and Other Organochlorides, *Archives of Environmental Health*, 47(2): 143–6.

Family and Parenting Institute (FPI) (2009) *Health Visitors: A Progress Report* (London: FPI).

Family Planning Association (2009) *Statistics on Teenage Pregnancy* (www.fpa.org.uk accessed 5.11.09).

FAO (Food and Agriculture Organization) (2002) *Report of the World Food Summit: Five Years Later* (www.fao.org accessed 16.10.08).

FAO/WHO (2000) *Safety Aspects of Genetically Modified Foods of Plant Origin: Report of a Joint FAO/WHO Expert Consultation on Foods Derived from Biotechnology* (Geneva: FAO/WHO).

FAO/WHO (2002) *Report of the Evaluation of the Codex Alimentarius and Other FAO and WHO Food Standards Work* (Geneva: WHO) (http://www.who.int/foodsafety/codex/en/ accessed 13.05.10).

FAO/WHO (Food and Agriculture Organization and World Health Organization) (WHO) (2003)

Diet, Nutrition and the Prevention of Chronic Diseases (Geneva: WHO).

Farooqi, I.S. and Hopkin, J.M. (1998) 'Early Childhood Infection and Atopic Disorder', *Thorax*, 53(11): 927–32.

Farrell, C. (2004) *Patient and Public Involvement in Health: The Evidence for Policy Implementation* (London: DoH).

Farrell, M., Bebbington, P., Brugha, T., et al. (2002) 'Psychosis and Drug Dependence: Results From a National Survey of Prisoners', *British Journal of Psychiatry*, 181: 393–8.

Farrell, M., Ward, J. and Mattick, R. (1994) 'Methadone Maintenance Treatment in Opiate Dependence: A Review', *British Medical Journal*, 309: 997–1001.

Feder, G., Crook, A., Magee, P. et al. (2002) 'Ethnic Differences in Invasive Management of Coronary Disease: Prospective Cohort Study of Patients Undergoing Angiography', *British Medical Journal*, 324(7336): 115–16.

Fee, E. and Porter, D. (1992) 'Public Health, Preventive Medicine and Professionalisation: England and America in the Nineteenth Century' in Wear, A. (ed.) *Medicine and Society: Historical Essays*, (Cambridge: Cambridge University Press), pp. 249–75.

Fehily, J., Yarnell, J.W., Sweetnam, P.M. and Ellwood, P.C. (1993) 'Diet and Ishaemic Heart Disease: The Caerphilly Study', *British Journal of Nutrition*, 69(2): 303–14.

Feinstein, A. (1999) 'Biases Introduced by Confounding and Imperfect Retrospective and Prospective Exposure Assessments' in Bate, R. (ed.) *What Risk* (London: Butterworth), pp. 37–48.

Felce, D. and Perry, J. (1995) 'Quality of Life: Its Definition and Measurement', *Research and Developmental Disabilities*, 16(1): 51–74.

Fergusson, D., Horwood, L.J. and Ridder, E. (2005) 'Tests of Causal Linkages Between Cannabis Use and Psychotic Symptoms', *Addiction*, 100(3): 354–66.

Fernie, J. (2004) *The Whitehall II Study* (London: Council of Civil Service Unions/Cabinet Office).

Ferrie, J., Martikainen, P., Shipley, M. et al. (2001) 'Employment Status and Health after Privatisation in White Collar Civil Servants: Prospective Cohort Study', *British Medical Journal*, 322(7287): 647.

Ferrie, J., Shipley, M., Newman, K. et al. (2005) 'Self-Reported Job Insecurity and Health in the Whitehall II Study: Potential Explanations of the Relationship', *Social Science & Medicine*, 60: 1593–602.

File on 4 (2007) 'Occupational Health' 9 October, BBC Radio Four.

Finer, S. (1962) *The Life and Times of Sir Edwin Chadwick* (London: Methuen).

Finkel, M. (2005) *Understanding the Mammography Controversy: Science, Politics, and Breast Cancer Screening* (Westport, CT: Praeger Publishers).

Finlayson, A. (1999) 'Third Way Theory', *Political Quarterly*, 70: 42–51.

Fischer, F. (1990) *Technocracy and the Politics of Expertise* (Newbury Park: Sage).

Fischer, J., Koch, L., Emmerling, C. et al. (2009) 'Inactivation of the Fto Gene Protects from Obesity', *Nature*, 458(7240): 894–8.

Fish, J. (2006) *Hetrosexism in Health and Social Care* (Basingstoke: Palgrave Macmillan).

Fisher, R.B. (1991) *Edward Jenner* (London: Andre Deutsch).

Fitzpatrick, M. (2001) *The Tyranny of Health* (London: Routledge).

Flegal, K., Graubard, B., Williamson, D. and Mitchell, G. (2005) 'Excess Deaths Associated with Underweight, Overweight, and Obesity', *The Journal of the American Medical Association*, 293(15): 1861–7.

Flinn, M.W. (ed.) (1965) *Report on the Sanitary Condition of the Labouring Population of Great Britain by Edwin Chadwick, 1842* (Edinburgh: Edinburgh University Press).

Flinn, M.W. (1968) *Public Health Reform in Britain* (London: Macmillan – now Palgrave Macmillan).

Florin, D. and Dixon, J. (2004) 'Public Involvement in Health Care', *British Medical Journal*, 328: 159–61.

Flynn, R., Williams, G. and Pickard, S. (1996) *Markets and Networks: Contracting in Community Health Services* (Buckingham: Open University).

Food and Drink Federation (FDF) (2008) *Our Five Fold Environmental Ambition* (London: FDF).

Food Commission (2002) *Attitudes to Food Irradiation in Europe* (London: Food Commission).

Food Commission (2004a) *Going Hungry* (London: Food Commission).

Food Commission (2004b) *Food Commission Guide to Food Additives* (London: Food Commission).

Foresight (2007) *Tackling Obesities: Future Choices* (London: Government Office for Science).

Foresight (2009) *Tackling Obesities: Future Choices* (2nd edn) (London: Government Office for Science).

Fort, M., Mercer, M. and Gish, O. (eds) (2004) *Sickness and Wealth: The Corporate Assault on Global Health* (Cambridge MA: South End Press).

Fotaki, M. (2007) 'Can Directors of Public Health Implement the New Public Agenda in Primary Care? A Case Study of Primary Care Trusts in the North West of England', *Policy and Politics*, 35(2): 311–19.

Follett, G. (2000) 'Antibiotic Resistance in the EU: Science, Politics and Policy' *AGbioforum* 3(2-

3), article 13 (www.agbioforum.org accessed 13.8.10).

Fowler, N. (1991) *Ministers Decide* (London: Chapman).

Fox, J., Goldblatt, P. and Jones, D. (1990) 'Social Class Mortality Differentials: Artefact, Selection, or Life Circumstances?' in Goldblatt, P. (ed.) *Longitudinal Study: Mortality and Social Organisation 1971–81*, OPCS LS 6 (London: HMSO), pp. 100–8.

Frank, L., Saelens, B., Powell, K. and Chapman, J. (2007) 'Stepping Towards Causation: Do Built Environments or Neighbourhood and Travel Preferences Explain Physical Activity, Driving, and Obesity?', *Social Science & Medicine*, 65(9): 1898–914.

Frankl, P. (2008) *Deploying Renewables* (Paris: International Energy Agency/OECD).

Fraser, D. (1973) *The Evolution of the British Welfare State: A History of Social Policy Since the Industrial Revolution* (London: Macmillan – now Palgrave Macmillan).

Frazer, W.M. (1950) *A Study of English Public Health 1834–1939* (London: Balliere, Tindall, Cox).

Freedman, B. (1977) 'Asthma Induced by Sulphur Dioxide, Benzoate and Tartrazine Contained in Orange Drinks,' *Clinical and Experimental Allergy*, 7(5): 407–15.

Freeman, R. (1992) 'The Idea of Prevention: A Critical Overview' in Scott, S., Williams, G., Platt, S. and Thomas, H. (eds) *Private Risks and Public Dangers* (Aldershot: Avebury), pp. 34–56.

Freeman, R. (1995) 'Prevention and Government: Health Policy Making in the UK and Germany', *Journal of Health Politics, Policy and Law*, 20(3): 745–65.

Freeman, R. (2000) *Prevention and Government: Health Policy Making in the UK and Germany* (Manchester: Manchester University Press).

French, J. (2007) 'The Market-dominated Future of Public Health?' in Douglas, J., Earle, S., Handsley, S. et al. *A Reader in Promoting Public Health: Challenge and Controversy (Published in association with The Open University)* (London: Sage Publications), pp. 19–25.

Frenk, J. (1992) 'The New Public Health in Pan-American Health Organisation', in *The Crisis of Public Health: Reflections for Debate* (Washington: PAHO, WHO), pp. 68–85.

Friedli, L. (2007) 'Mental Health Promotion' in Douglas, J., Earle, S., Handsley, S. et al. *A Reader in Promoting Public Health: Challenge and Controversy (Published in association with The Open University)* (London: Sage Publications), pp. 273–80.

Friedli, L. (2009) *Mental Health, Resilience and Inequalities* (Copenhagen: WHO Regional Office for Europe).

Friel, S., Dangour, A., Garnett, T. et al. (2009) 'Public Health Benefits of Strategies to Reduce Greenhouse Gas Emissions: Food and Agriculture', *The Lancet*, 374: 2016–25.

Friends of the Earth (2001) Endocrine Disrupting Pesticides Briefing (http://www.foe.co.uk/resource/briefings/endocrine_disrupting.html accessed 1.5.10).

Friends of the Earth (2008) *Budget 2008 and Climate Change* (London: FOE).

FSA (Food Standards Agency) (2002) *Survey for Irradiated Foods: Herbs and Spices, Dietary Supplements, Prawns and Shrimps* (London: FSA).

FSA (2007) *Dioxins and Dioxin-like PCBs in Foods – EU Monitoring 2006* (London: FSA).

FSA (2008a) *FSA Attitudes Public Survey 2007* (London: FSA).

FSA (2008b) *UK Food Establishment Survey 2007* (London: FSA).

FSA (2008c) *Paper for Information: Local Authority Monitoring Data on Food Law Enforcement April 2006 – March 2007 info 08/03/02* (London: FSA).

FSA/Welsh Assembly Government (2003) *Food and Wellbeing: Reducing Inequalities Through a Nutrition Strategy for Wales* (Cardiff: FSA/Welsh Assembly Government).

Fuchs, C., Giovannucci, E., Colditz, G. et al. (1999) 'Dietary Fiber and the Risk of Colorectal Cancer and Adenoma in Women', *New England Journal of Medicine*, 340(3): 169–76.

Fuchs, V. (1974) *Who Shall Live?* (New York: Basic).

Fuel Poverty Advisory Group (2008) *Sixth Annual Report 2007* (London: Department for Business Enterprise and Regulatory Reform).

Fulop, N. and Hunter, D. (1999) 'Editorial: Saving Lives or Sustaining the Public's Health?', *British Medical Journal*, 323: 89–92.

Funatogawa, I., Funatogawa, T. and Yano, E. (2008) 'Overweight Children do not Necessarily Make Overweight Adults: Repeated Cross Sectional Annual Nationwide Survey of Japanese Females over Nearly Six Decades', *British Medical Journal*, 337: a802.

Fung, T., Stampfer, M., Manson, J. et al. (2004) 'Prospective Study of Major Dietary Patterns and Stroke Risk in Women', *Stroke*, 35(9): 2014–19.

Furedi, F. (1997) *Culture of Fear* (London: Cassell).

Future Foundation (2005) *The Assault on Pleasure* (London: Future Foundation).

Galbraith, J.K. (1992) *The Culture of Contentment* (London: Sinclair-Stevenson).

Gallerani, M., Manfredini, R., Caracuolo, S. et al. (1995) 'Serum Cholesterol Concentrations in Parasuicide', *British Medical Journal*, 310: 1632–6.

Gamble, A. (1994) *The Free Economy and the Strong State: The Politics of Thatcherism* (2nd edn) (London: Macmillan – now Palgrave Macmillan).

Gard, M. and Wright, J. (2005) *The Obesity Epidemic, Science, Morality and Ideology* (London and New York: Routledge).

Gardner, P. (2008) 'A Brief History of the Rise and Fall of the School Medical Service in England', *Public Health*, 122(3): 261–7.

Garfield, S. (1994a) *Britain in the Time of AIDS* (London: Faber and Faber).

Garfield, S. (1994b) *The End of Innocence: Britain in the time of AIDS* (London: Faber and Faber).

Garnett, T. (2008) *Cooking up a Storm: Food, Greenhouse Gas Emissions and our Changing Climate* (Food Climate Research Network Centre, Centre for Environmental Strategy, University of Surrey).

Garrett, L. (1994) *The Coming Plague* (Harmondsworth: Penguin).

Gauderman, W., Vora, H., McConnell, R. et al. (2007) 'Effect of Exposure to Traffic on Lung Development from 10 to 18 Years of Age: A Cohort Study', *The Lancet*, 369: 571–7.

Geddes, M., Davies, J. and Fuller, C. (2007) 'Evaluating Local Strategic Partnerships: Theory and Practice of Change' *Local Government Studies*, 33(1): 97–116.

Gelling, L. (2007) 'Legal Issues and Young People's Health', in D. DeBell (ed.) *Public Health Practice and the School-age Population* (London: Hodder Arnold), pp. 21–36.

Gerrard, M. (2006) *A Stifled Voice. Community Health Councils in England 1974–2003* (Brighton: Pen Press).

Gibson, S. (1997) 'Obesity: Is it Related to Sugar in Children's Diets?' *Nutrition and Food Science*, 97(5): 184–7.

Giddens, A. (1991) *Modernity and Self-Identity: Self and Society in the Late Modern Age* (Cambridge: Polity).

Giddens, A. (1998) *The Third Way: The Renewal of Social Democracy* (Cambridge: Polity).

Gidley, B. (2007) 'Sure Start: An Upstream Approach to Reducing Health Inequalities?' in Scriven, A. and Garman, S. *Public Health: Social Context and Action* (Maidenhead: Open University Press), pp. 144–53.

Gilbert, B. (1970) *British Social Policy 1914–1939* (London: Batsford).

Gilchrist, A. (2003) 'Community Development and Networking for Health' in Orme, J., Powell, J., Harrison, T. and Grey, M. *Public Health for the 21st Century: New Perspectives on Policy, Participation and Practice* (Maidenhead: Open University Press), pp. 145–59.

Gilchrist, A. (2006) 'Partnership and Participation: Power in Process', *Public Policy and Administration*, 21(3): 71–85.

Gillam, S., Abbott, S. and Banks-Smith, J. (2001) 'Can Primary Care Groups and Trusts Improve Health?', *British Medical Journal*, 323: 89–92.

Gillies, R., Schoen-Angerer, T. and t'Hoen, E. (2006) 'Historic Opportunity for WHO to Reassert Leadership', *The Lancet*, 368: 1405–6.

Gillman, M.W., Cupples, L.A., Millen, B.E. et al. (1997) 'Inverse Associates of Dietary Fat with the Development of Ischaemic Stroke in Men', *Journal of the American Medical Association*, 278(24): 2145–50.

Gilmore, A., Fooks, G. and MecKee, M. (2009) 'The IMF and Tobacco: a Product like any Other?', *International Journal of Health Services*, 39(4): 789–93.

Giovannucci, E. (2003) 'Diet, Body Weight, and Colorectal Cancer: A Summary of the Epidemiologic Evidence', *Journal of Women's Health*, 12(2): 173–82.

Givel, M. (2007) 'A Comparison of the Impact of US and Canadian Cigarette Pack Warning Label Requirements on Tobacco Industry Profitability and the Public Health', *Health Policy*, 83(2–3): 343–52.

Glaister, S., Burnham, J., Stevens, H. et al. (2006) *Transport Policy in Britain* (Basingstoke: Palgrave Macmillan).

Glantz, S.A., Slade, J., Bero, L. et al. (1996) *The Cigarette Papers* (Los Angeles: University of California Press).

Glasby, J. and Dickinson, H. (2008) *Partnership Working in Health and Social Care* (Bristol: Policy Press).

Glasby, J. and Littlechild, R. (2004) *The Health and Social Care Divide: The Experiences of Older People* (2nd edn) (Bristol: Policy Press).

Glasby, J., Smith, J. and Dickinson, H. (2006) *Creating NHS Local: A New Relationship Between PCTs and Local Government* (Birmingham: Health Services Management Centre).

Glass, N. (1999) 'Sure Start: the Development of an Early Intervention Programme for Young Children in the UK', *Children and Society*, 13(4): 257–64.

Glendinning, C. and Coleman, A (2003) 'Joint Working: The Health Service Agenda', *Local Government Studies*, 29(3): 51–72.

Glynn, M.K., Bopp, C., Dewitt, W. et al. (1998) 'Emergence of Multidrug Resistant Salmonella Enterica Serotype Typhimurium DT104 Infections in the United States', *New England Journal of Medicine*, 338(19): 1333–8.

GM Science Review Panel (2003) *First Report* (London: Department of Trade and Industry).

GM Science Review Panel (2004) *Second Report* (London: Department of Trade and Industry).

Godber, G. (1986) 'Medical Officers of Health and Health Services', *Community Medicine*, 8(1): 1–14.

Godeau, E., Gabhainn, S., Vignes, C. et al. (2008) 'Contraceptive Use by 15-Year-Old Students at Their Last Sexual Intercourse', *Archives of Paediatrics and Adolescent Medicine*, 162(1): 66–73.

Godfrey, C., Parrott, S. and Coleman, T. (2005) 'The Cost-Effectiveness of English Smoking Treatment Services – Evidence from Practice', *Addiction*, 100: 70–83.

Godlee, F. (1992) 'The Dangers of Ozone Depletion' in Godlee, F. and Walker, A. *Health and the Environment* (London: BMJ Publications), pp. 27–33.

Goldacre, B. (2008) *Bad Science* (London: Fourth Estate).

Goldblatt, P. (1989) 'Mortality by Social Class 1871–85'. In Population Trends (London: HMSO), pp. 6–15.

Goldblatt, P., Fox, J. and Leon, D. (1990) 'Mortality of Employed Men and Women', in Goldblatt, P. (ed.) *Longitudinal Study: Mortality and Social Organisation, 1971–81*, OPCS (London: HMSO), pp. 67–80.

Goldstein, A. and Kalant, H. (1993) 'Drug Policy: Striking the Right Balance' in Bayer, R. and Oppenheim, G. (eds) *Confronting Drugs Policy* (Cambridge: Cambridge University Press), pp. 78–114.

Goldthorpe, J. and Mills, C. (2008) 'Trends in Intergenerational Class Mobility in Modern Britain: Evidence from National Surveys, 1971–2005', *National Institute Economic Review*, 205(1): 83–100.

Golomb, B., Dimsdale, J., White, H.L. et al. (2008) 'Reduction in Blood Pressure with Statins', *Archives of Internal Medicine*, 168(7): 721–7.

Golub, A. and Johnson, B. (2001) 'Variation in Youthful Risks of Progression from Alcohol and Tobacco to Marijuana and to Hard Drugs Across Generations', *American Journal of Public Health*, 91(2): 225–32.

Gonzalez-Suarez, C., Worley, A., Grimers-Somers, K. and Dones, V. (2009) 'School-Based Interventions on Childhood Obesity – A Meta-Analysis', *American Journal of Preventive Medicine*, 37: 418–27.

Goodchild, B. (1998) 'Poor Housing – Poor Health: What is the Relationship?', *International Journal of Health Promotion and Education*, 36(3): 84–6.

Goodin, R. (1991) 'Permissable Paternalism: In Defence of the Nanny State', *The Responsive Community*, 1: 42–51.

Goodin, R. (1995) *Utilitarianism as a Public Philosophy* (Cambridge: Cambridge University Press).

Goodman, A., Johnson, P. and Webb, S. (1997) *Inequality in the UK* (Oxford University Press)

Goodwin, A. (2007) *Measuring the Harm from Illegal Drugs: The Drug Harm Index 2005* (London: Home Office).

Goraya, A. and Scambler, G. (1998) 'From Old to New Public Health: Role, Tensions and Contradictions', *Critical Public Health*, 8(2): 141–51.

Gordon, R., McDermott, L., Stead, M. and Angus, K. (2006) 'The Effectiveness of Social Marketing Interventions for Health Improvement: What's the Evidence?,' *Public Health*, 120(12): 1133–9.

Gorman, D., Douglas, M., Conway, L. et al. (2003) 'Transport Policy and Health Inequalities: A Health Impact Assessment of Edinburgh's Transport', *Public Health*, 117: 15–24.

Gossop, M. (1996) *Living with Drugs* (4th edn) (Aldershot: Arena/Ashgate).

Gostin, L. (2007) 'General Justifications for Public Health Regulation', *Public Health*, 121: 829–34.

Gothenburg European Council (2001) Prediemcy Conclusions: Gothenurg European Council 15–16 June 2001 (http://ec.europa.eu/governance/impact/background/docs/goteborg_concl_en.pdf accessed 5.5.10).

Gotzsche, P.C. and Nielsen, M. (2006) 'Screening for Breast Cancer with Mammography', *Cochrane Database of Systematic Reviews* 2006, Issue 3.

Graham, B., Normand, C. and Goodall, Y. (2002) *Proximity to Death and Acute Health Care Utilisation* (Information and Statistics Division, ISD, NHS Scotland).

Graham, H. (1993) *When Life's A Drag: Women, Smoking and Disadvantage*, Department of Health (London: HMSO).

Graham, H. (2004) 'Tackling Inequalities in Health in England: Remedying Health Disadvantages Narrowing Health Gaps or Reducing Health Gradients?', *Journal of Social Policy*, 33(1): 115–31.

Graham, H. (2007) *Unequal Lives, Health and Socio-economic Inequalities* (Maidenhead: McGraw Hill).

Graham, H. (2009) 'Health Inequalities, Social Determinants and Public Health Policy', *Policy and Politics*, 37(4): 463-79.

Graham, H. and Power, C. (2004) *Childhood Disadvantage and Adult Health: A Lifecourse Framework* (London: Health Development Agency).

Grandjean, P. and Landrigan, P. (2006) 'Developmental Neurotoxicity of Industrial Chemicals', *The Lancet*, 368: 2167–78.

Grant, C., Nicholas, R., Moore, L. and Salisbury, C. (2002) 'An Observational Study Comparing Quality of Care in Walk-in Centres with General Practice Using Standardised Patients', *British Medical Journal*, 324: 1556–62.

Grant, W. (2000) *Pressure Groups and British Politics* (Basingstoke: Macmillan – now Palgrave Macmillan).

Gravelle, H. (1998) 'How Much of the Relation between Population Mortality and Unequal Distribution of Income is a Statistical Artefact', *British Medical Journal*, 316: 382–5.

Gravelle, H., Wildman, J. and Sutton, M. (2002) 'Income, Income Inequality and Health: What can we Learn From Aggregate Data?', *Social Science & Medicine*, 54: 577–89.

Gray, D. and Hicks, N. (2007) 'The Contribution of the Acute Sector to Promoting Public Health' in Griffiths, S. and Hunter, D. (eds) *New Perspectives in Public Health* (London: Routledge), pp. 251–9.

Gray, S. (2007) 'Academic Public Health' in Griffiths, S. and Hunter, D. (eds) *New Perspectives in Public Health* (London: Routledge), pp. 285–93.

Gray, S. and Sandberg, E. (2006) *The Specialist Public Health Workforce in the UK 2005 Survey* (London: Faculty of Public Health).

Green, A., Ross, D. and Mirzoev, T. (2007) 'Primary Health Care and England: The Coming of Age of Alma Ata', *Health Policy*, 11–31.

Green, D. (1987) *The New Right: The Counter Revolution in Political, Economic and Social Thought* (Brighton: Wheatsheaf).

Green, G. (1992) 'Liverpool' in Ashton, J. (ed.) *Healthy Cities* (Milton Keynes: Open University Press), pp. 88–95.

Green, H., McGinnity, A., Meltzer, H. et al. (2005) *Mental Health of Children and Young People in Great Britain, 2004* (Office for National Statistics) (Basingstoke: Palgrave Macmillan).

Green, J. (2008) 'Health Education: The Case for Rehabilitation', *Critical Public Health*, 18(4): 446–56.

Green, T.H. (1911) 'Lecture on Liberal Legislation and Freedom of Contract' in *Works*, Volume 3, (London: Longmans Green).

Greenaway, J. (2003) *Drink and British Politics Since 1830: A Study in Policy-Making* (Basingstoke: Palgrave Macmillan).

Greer, S. (2005) 'The Territorial Bases of Health Policy Making in the UK After Devolution', *Regional and Federal Studies*, 15(4): 501–18.

Greer, S. (2007) 'Public Health Policy Making in a Disunited Kingdom' in Griffiths, S. and Hunter, D. (eds) *New Perspectives in Public Health* (London: Routledge), pp. 55–60.

Greer, S. (2009a) *Territorial Politics and Health Policy* (Manchester: Manchester University Press).

Greer, S. (2009b) *The Politics of European Union Health Policies* (Maidenhead: Open University Press).

Griffith, G. (2002) *Assessing the Needs of Rough Sleepers* (London: ODPM Homelessness Directorate).

Griffiths, J. and Dark, P. (2006) *The Future of Public Health Promoting Health in the NHS* (London: DoH).

Griffiths, S. and Hunter, D. (eds) (1999) 'Introduction', *Perspectives in Public Health* (Oxford: Radical Medical Press), pp. 3–10.

Griffiths, S., Jewell, T. and Donnelly, P. (2005) 'Public Health in Practice: The Three Domains of Public Health', *Public Health*, 119: 907–13.

Grubb, M., Koch, M., Munson, A. et al. (1993) *The Earth Summit Agreements: A Guide and Assessment* (London: Earthscan).

Grund, A., Krause, H., Siewers, M. et al. (2001) 'Is TV Viewing an Index of Physical Activity and Fitness in Overweight and Normal Weight Children?', *Public Health and Nutrition*, 4(6): 1245–51.

Grundy, C., Steinbach, R., Edwards, P. et al. (2009) 'Effect of 20 MPH Traffic Speed Zones on Road Injuries in London: 1986–2006: Controlled Time Series Analysis', *British Medical Journal*, 339 (doi: 10.1136/bmj.b4469) accessed 17.3.10).

Guardian (2009) 'Drug Busts Force Price of Cocaine to Record Levels', 12 May (www.guardian.co.uk accessed 17.05.10).

Guardian (2010) 'Anger over Weight Watchers Endorsement of McDonald's' (www.guardian.co.uk accessed 3.3.10).

Guillot, C. and Greenway, D. (2006) 'Recreational Ecstasy Use and Depression', *Journal of Psychopharmacology*, 20(3): 411–16.

Gustafson, U. (2002) 'School Meals Policy: The Problem with Governing Children', *Social Policy and Administration*, 26(6): 685–97.

Gustafson, U. and Driver, S. (2005) 'Parents, Power and Public Participation: Sure Start, An Experiment in New Labour Governance', *Social Policy and Administration*, 39(5): 528–43.

Guthrie, B., Inkster, M. and Fahey, T. (2007) 'Tackling Therapeutic Inertia Role of Treatment Data in Quality Indicators', *British Medical Journal*, 335: 542–4.

Gwyn, R. (1999) '"Killer Bugs", "Silly Buggers" and "Politically Correct Pals": Competing Discourses in Health Care Reporting', *Health*, 3 March, 335–45.

Gyngell, K. (2009) *The Phoney War on Drugs* (London: Centre for Policy Studies).

Habermas, J. (1976) *Legitimation Crisis* (London: Heinemann).

Haines, A., Kovats, R., Campbell-Lendrum, D. and Corvalan, C. (2006) 'Climate Change and Human Health: Impacts, Vulnerability and Mitigation', *The Lancet*, 367: 2109–9.

Hall, D. and Elliman, D. (2002) *Health for All Children: 4th Report* (Oxford: Oxford University Press).

Hall, D. and Elliman, D. (2006) *Health for All Children* (Revised 4th edn) (Oxford: Oxford University Press).

Hall, P. and Lamont, M. (eds) (2009) *Successful Societies: How Institutions and Culture Affect Health* (Cambridge: Cambridge University Press).

Hall, W.D. and Lynskey, M. (2005) 'Is Cannabis a Gateway Drug? Testing Hypotheses about the Relationship Between Cannabis Use and the Use of Other Illicit Drugs', *Drug and Alcohol Review*, 24(1): 39–48.

Ham, C. and Mitchell, J. (1990) 'A Force to Reckon With', *Health Service Journal*, 1 February, 164–5.

Hamer, L. (2000) *A National Review and Analysis of Health Improvement Programmes 1999–2000* (London: Health Development Agency).

Hamer, L. and Easton, N. (2002) *Community Strategies and Health Improvement: A Review of Policy and Practice* (London: Health Development Agency).

Hamer, M. and Chida, Y. (2008) 'Waling and Primary Prevention: A Meta-Analysis of Prospective Cohort Studies', *British Journal of Sports Medicine*, 42: 238–43.

Hammersley, R., Forsyth, A. and Morrison, V. (1989) 'The Relationship Between Crime and Opoid Use', *British Journal of Addiction*, 84: 1029–43.

Hammond, R.J. (1951) *Food: The Growth of Policy, Volume I* (London: HMSO).

Hampton, K. (2001) *Developing Success Criteria for Joint Appointments Between the NHS and Local Government* (London: Office for Public Management).

Hancock, T. (1985) 'The Mandala of Health: A Model of the Human Ecosystem', *Family and Community Health*, 8: 1–10.

Hancock, T. (1992) 'The Healthy City from Concept to Application: Implications for Research' in Davies, J. and Kelly, M. *Healthy Cities* (Buckingham: Open University Press), pp. 14–24.

Handsley, S. (2007a) 'Community Involvement and Civic Engagement in Multidisciplinary Public Health' in Lloyd, C., Handsley, S., Douglas, J., Earle, S., and Spurr, S. (eds) *Policy and Practice in Promoting Public Health* (London: Sage/Open University Press), pp.223–56.

Handsley, S. (2007b) 'Promoting Mental Health and Social Inclusion' in Lloyd, C.E., Handsley, S., Douglas, J. et al. (eds) *Policy and Practice in Promoting Public Health* (London: Sage).

Handy, S., Boarnet, M., Ewing, E. and Killingsworth, R. (2002) 'How the Built Environment Affects Physical Activity: Views from Urban Planning', *American Journal of Preventative Medicine*, 23(2S): 64–73.

Hann, A. (1996) *The Politics of Breast Cancer Screening* (Aldershot: Avebury).

Hann, A. and Peckham, S. (2010) 'Politics, Ethics and Evidence: Immunisation and Public Health Policy' in Hann, A. and Peckham, S. *Public Health Ethics and Practice* (Bristol; Policy Press), pp. 117–36.

Hansard (1957) Session 1956/7, 1 March, volume 565, column 1640.

Hansard (2006) Commons, 21 March, part 23, column 262 w.

Hansen, J. (2004) 'Defusing the Global Warming Time Bomb', *Scientific American,* 290(3): 68–77.

Hansen, S., Carlsen, L. and Tickner, J. (2007) 'Chemicals Regulation and Precaution: Does REACH Really Incorporate the Precautionary Principle?', *Environmental Science and Policy*, 10(5): 395–404.

Hantrais, L. (2007) *Social Policy in the European Union* (3rd edn) (Basingstoke: Palgrave Macmillan).

Hardy, L., Dobbins, T., Denney-Wilson, E. et al. (2009) 'Sedentariness, Small-Screen Recreation, Fitness in Youth', *American Journal of Preventive Medicine*, 36(2): 120–5.

Harling, K. (2007) 'Work and Health: What Direction for Occupational Health Practice?' in Griffiths, S. and Hunter, D.J. *New Perspectives in Public Health* (Oxford: Radcliffe Publishing), pp. 194–200.

Harrabin, R., Coote, A. and Allen, J. (2003) *Health in the News: Risk Reporting and Media Influence* (London: King's Fund).

Harrison, B. (1971) *Drink and the Victorians* (London: Faber and Faber).

Harrison, L. (1986) 'Tobacco Battered and the Pipes Shattered: A Note on the Fate of the First British Campaign Against Smoking', *British Journal of Addiction*, 81: 553–8.

Harrison, S., Hunter, D., Johnson, I., Nicholson, N. and Thunhurst, C. and Wistow, G. (1994) *Health Before Healthcare*, Social Policy Paper No. 4 (London: Institute for Public Policy Research).

Harrow, J. (1991) 'Local Authority Health Strategies' in McNaught, A. (ed.) *Managing Community Health Services* (London: Chapman and Hall), pp. 3–16.

Hart, C. (2004) *Nurses and Politics: The Impact of Power and Practice* (Basingstoke: Palgrave Macmillan).

Harvie, M., Hooper, L. and Howell, A.H. (2003) 'Central Obesity and Breast Cancer Risk: A Systematic Review', *The International Association for the Study of Obesity. Obesity Reviews*, 4: 157–73.

Hastings, G. (2007) *Social Marketing* (London: Butterworth-Heinmann).

Hastings, G. and Stead, M. (2006) 'Social Marketing', Chapter 10 in Macdowall, W., Bonell, C. and Davies, M. (eds) *Health Promotion*

Practice (Maidenhead: Open University Press), pp. 139–51.

Hastings, G., Stead, M., McDermott, L. et al. (2003) *Review of Research on the Effects of Food Promotion to Children: Final Report* (Glasgow: Centre for Social Marketing).

Havel, P. (2002) 'Control of Energy Homeostasis and Insulin Action by Adipocyte Hormones: Leptin, Acylation Stimulating Protein, and Adiponectin', *Current Opinion in Lipidology*, 13(1): 51–9.

Havelock Ellis, H. (1892) *The Nationalisation of Health* (London: Fisher Unwin).

Haw, S. and Gruer, L. (2007) 'Changes in Exposure of Adult Non-Smokers to Second-Hand Smoke after Implementation of Smoke-Free Legislation in Scotland: National Cross Sectional Survey', *British Medical Journal*, 335: 549–52.

Hayek, F. (1976) *The Constitution of Liberty* (London: Routledge).

Hayek, F. (1988) *The Fatal Conceit: The Errors of Socialism* (London: Routledge).

Hayes, B. and Prior, P. (2003) *Gender and Healthcare in the UK* (Basingstoke: Palgrave Macmillan).

Haynes, R., Bentham, G., Lovett, A. and Gale, S. (1999) 'Effects of Distances to Hospital and GP Surgery on Hospital Inpatient Episodes, Controlling for Needs and Provision', *Social Science & Medicine*, 49: 425–33.

HDA (Health Development Agency) (2000) *Participatory Approaches in Health Promotion and Planning: A Literature Review* (London: HDA).

HDA (2002) *National Healthy School Standard – Report* (Yorkshire: Health Development Agency).

HDA (2003) 'Healthy Communities Collaborative Launches Nationally: 60% Reduction in Falls Achieved in Pilot Sites', Press Release 24-9-03.

HDA (2004) *Lessons from Health Action Zones* (London: HDA).

He, F., Nowson, C. and MacGregor, G. (2006) 'Fruit and Vegetable Consumption and Stoke: Meta-Analysis of Cohort Studies', *The Lancet*, 367: 320–6.

He, J., Vupputuri, S., Allen, K. et al. (1999) 'Passive Smoking and the Risk of Coronary Heart Disease – A Meta-Analysis of Epidemiologic Studies', *New England Journal of Medicine*, 340(12): 920–6.

He, K., Merchant, A., Rimm, E. et al. (2003) 'Dietary Fat Intake and Risk of Stoke in Male US Healthcare Professionals: 14 Year Prospective Cohort Study', *British Medical Journal*, 327.

Health Committee (1990) *Food Poisoning: Listeria and Listeriosis*, 1st Report 1989/90, HC 93,

Health Committee (1999) *The Relationship Between Health and Social Services*, 1st Report 1998/99, HC 74-I (London: HMSO).

Health Committee (2000) 2nd Report 1999–2000 *The Tobacco Industry and the Health Risks of Smoking*, HC 27 (London: TSO).

Health Committee (2001) 2nd Report 2000–1 *Public Health*, HC 30 (London: TSO).

Health Committee (2002) 2nd Report 2001–2 *The National Institute for Clinical Excellence*, HC 515 (London: TSO).

Health Committee (2003a) 7th Report 2002–3 *Patient and Public Involvement*, HC 697 (London: TSO).

Health Committee (2003b) 3rd Report 2002–3, *Sexual Health*, HC 69 (London: TSO).

Health Committee (2003c) 4th Report 2002–3 *Provision of Maternity Services*, HC 464 (London: TSO).

Health Committee (2004) 3rd Report 2003–4 *Obesity*, HC 23 (London: TSO).

Health Committee (2005a) The Government's Public Health White Paper Minutes of Evidence, HC 358i, Session 2004–5 (London: TSO).

Health Committee (2005b) 1st Report 2005–6 *Smoking in Public Places*, HC 485 (London: TSO).

Health Committee (2006a) 2nd Report 2005–6 *Changes to Primary Care Trusts*, HC 646 (London: TSO).

Health Committee (2006b) 4th Report 2006–7 *Workforce Planning*, HC 171 (London: TSO).

Health Committee (2006c) 3rd Report 2006–7 *Patient and Public Involvement in the NHS* (London: TSO).

Health Committee (2009) 3rd Report 2008–9 *Health Inequalities* HC 286 (London: TSO).

Health Committee (2010) 1st Report 2009–10 *Alcohol*, HC 151 (London: TSO).

Health England (2009) *Public Health and Prevention Expenditure in England: Health England Report No 4* (London: DoH, Butterfield, R., Henderson, J. and Scott, R.).

Health Promotion Agency (HPA) (1999) *Mental Health Promotion: A Database of Initiatives in Northen Ireland* (Belfast: HPA).

Health Promotion Agency for Northern Ireland (1996a) *Eating and Health: A Food and Nutrition Strategy for Northern Ireland* (Belfast: HPA).

Health Promotion Agency for Northern Ireland (1996b) *Be Active Be Healthy* (Belfast: HPA).

Health Protection Agency (HPA) (2007a) *All New STI Episodes Made at Genitourinary Medicine (GUM) Clinics in the United Kingdom: 1997–2006* (London: HPA).

Health Protection Agency (2007b) *GUM Waiting Times Audits May 2006 – August 2007* (London: HPA).

Health Protection Agency (2009) *HIV in the United Kingdom 2009 Report* (London: HPA).

Health Visitors' Association (1996) *HVA Centenary Survey: Return of Diseases and Social Conditions of the Nineteenth Century* (London: HVA).

Healthcare Commission (2006) *State of Health Care 2006* (London: Healthcare Commission).

Healthcare Commission (2007a) *Performing Better: A Focus on Sexual Health Services in England* (London: Healthcare Commission).

Healthcare Commission (2007b) *No Ifs, No Buts – Improving Services for Tobacco Control* (London: Commission for Healthcare Audit and Inspection).

Healthcare Commission (2007c) *Audit of Equalities Publications* (London: Healthcare Commission).

Healthcare Commission (2007d) *Summary of Intervention at Bromley Primary Care Trust* (London: Healthcare Commission).

Healthcare Commission and Audit Commission (2008) *Are We Choosing Health? The Impact of Policy on the Delivery of Health Improvement Programmes and Services* (London: Commission for Healthcare Audit and Inspection).

Healthwork UK (2001) Project to Develop National Standards for Specialist Practice in Public Health

Hearnden, I. and Magill, C. (2004) *Decision-making by Burglars: Offenders' Perspectives* (London: Home Office).

Heenan, D. and Birrell, D. (2006) 'The Integration of Health and Social Care: The Lessons from Northern Ireland', *Social Policy and Administration*, 40(1): 47–66.

Heinz, J., Laumann, E., Nelson, R. and Salisbury, R. (1993) *The Hollow Core: Private Interests in National Policy Making* (Cambridge, MA: Harvard University Press).

Heller, R., Heller, T. and Pattison, S. (2003) 'Putting the Public Back into Public Health Part 1: A Redefinition of Public Health: *Public Health*, 117: 62–5.

Helm, D., Smale, R. and Phillips, R. (2007) Too Good to be True? The UK's Climate Change Record (http://www.dieterhelm.co.uk/sites/default/files/Carbon_record_2007.pdf accessed 5.5.10).

Help the Aged (2005) 'Memorandum' in Health Committee (2005) Health – Minutes of Evidence HC 358i, session 2004/5 (London: TSO).

Henderson, J., North, K., Griffiths, M. et al. (1999) 'Pertussis Vaccination and Wheezing Illnesses in Young Children: Prospective Cohort Study: The Longitudinal Study of Pregnancy and Childhood Team', *British Medical Journal*, 318: 1173–6.

Henderson, M., Wight, D., Raab, G. et al. (2006) 'Impact of a Theoretically Based Sex Education Programme (SHARE) Delivered by Teachers on NHS Registered Conceptions and Terminations: Final Results of Cluster Randomised Trial', *British Medical Journal*, (334): 133.

Henderson, P. (1975) The School Health Service 1908–74 (London: Department of Education and Science).

Hendrick, H. (2005) 'Children and Social Policies' in Hendrick, H. *Child Welfare and Social Policy: An Essential Reader* (Bristol: Policy Press), pp. 31–50.

Henquet, C., Krabbendam, L., Spauwen, J. et al. (2005) 'Prospective Cohort Study of Cannabis Use, Predisposition for Psychosis and Psychotic Symptoms in Young People', *British Medical Journal*, 330(7841): 11.

Henry, L. (2005) 'Fall Prevention Programmes in Older People', *Evidence Based Healthcare and Public Health*, 9(5): 349–50.

Hens, L. and Nath, B. (2003) *The World Summit on Sustainable Development: The Johannesburg Conference* (New York: Springer).

Hesketh, K., Wake, M., Graham, M. and Waters, E. (2007) 'Stability of Television Viewing and Electronic Game/Computer Use in a Prospective Cohort of Australian Children: Relationship with Body Mass Index', *International Journal of Behavioural Nutrition and Physical Activity*, 4: 60 (doi: 10.1186/1479-5868-4-60 accessed 15.5.10).

Hibbeln, J.R. (2002) 'Seafood Consumption, the DHA Content of Mothers' Milk and Prevalence Rates of Postpartum Depression: A Cross-national, Ecological Analysis', *Journal of Affective Disorders*, 69: 15–29.

Higgins, J. (1989) 'Defining Community Care: Realities and Myths', *Social Policy and Administration*, 23(1): 3–16.

Hildebrand, P. (2005) 'The European Community's Environmental Policy, 1957 to "1992": From Incidental Measures to an International Regime?' in Jordan, A. (ed.) *Environmental Policy in the EU* (2nd edn) (London: Earthscan), pp. 19–41.

Hill, M. and Hupe, P. (2002) *Implementing Public Policy* (London: Sage).

Hills, J. (1997) *The Future of Welfare* (York: Joseph Rowntree Foundation).

Hills, J., Le Grand, J. and Piachaud, D. (eds) (2002) *Understanding Social Exclusion* (Oxford: Oxford University Press).

Hills, J., Sefton, T. and Stewart, K. (2009) *Poverty, Inequality and Policy Since 1997* (York: Joseph Rowntree Foundation).

Hillsdon, M., Foster, C., Cavill, N. et al. (2005) *The Effectiveness of Public Health Interventions for Increasing Physical Activity Among Adults:*

A Review of Reviews, Evidence Briefing (2nd edn), February 2005 (London: Health Development Agency).

Hippisley-Cox, J., Hardy, C., Pringle, M. et al. (1997) 'The Effect of Deprivation on Variations in General Practitioners Referral Rates: A Cross Sectional Study of Computerised Data on New Medical and Surgical Out Patient Referrals in Nottinghamshire', *British Medical Journal*, 314: 458–61.

Hirsch, D. (2006) *What Will it Take to End Child Poverty? Firing on all Cylinders* (York: Joseph Rowntree Foundation).

Hirsch, D. (2009) *Ending Child Poverty in a Changing Economy* (York: Joseph Rowntree Foundation).

Hitchman, C., Christie, I., Harrison, M. and Lang, T. (2002) *Inconvenience Food – The Struggle to Eat Well on a Low Income* (London: Demos).

HM Government (2002) *Updated Drug Strategy 2002* (London: HM Government).

HM Government (2005a) *Extended Schools – Building on Experience* (Nottingham: Department of Children, Schools and Families).

HM Government (2005b) *Health, Work and Well-Being: Caring for our Future. A Strategy for the Heath and Well-Being of Working Age People* (London: TSO).

HM Government (2007a) *PSA Delivery Agreement 18: Promote Better Health and Wellbeing for All* (London: HM Treasury).

HM Government (2007b) *PSA Delivery Agreement 5, Deliver Reliable and Efficient Transport Networks that Support Economic Growth* (London: HM Government).

HM Government (2007c) *PSA Delivery Agreement 28, Secure a Healthy Natural Environment for Today and the Future* (London: Cabinet Office).

HM Government (2007d) *PSA Delivery Agreement 27, Lead the Global Effort to Avoid Dangerous Climate Change* (London: Cabinet Office).

HM Government (2007e) *Safe. Sensible. Social. Next Steps in the National Alcohol Strategy* (London: DoH).

HM Government (2007f) *PSA Delivery Agreement 25: Reduce the Harm Caused by Alcohol and Drugs* (London: HM Government).

HM Government (2007g) *PSA Delivery Agreement 12 Improve the Health and Wellbeing of Children and Young People* (London: HM Government).

HM Government (2008a) *Health is Global: A UK Government Strategy 2008–13* (London: TSO).

HM Government (2008b) *Healthy Weight, Healthy Lives: A Cross-Government Strategy for England* (London: Cross-Government Obesity Unit, Department of Health and Department of Children, Schools and Families)

HM Government (2008c) *Drugs: Protecting Families and Communities – The 2008 Drug Strategy* (London: HM Government).

HM Government (2009a) *The UK Low Carbon Transition Plan* (London: TSO).

HM Government (2009b) *Be Active Be Healthy: A Plan for Getting the Nation Moving* (London: Department of Health (DoH).

HM Government (2009c) *New Opportunities – Fair Chances for the Future* (London: TSO).

HM Government (2010a) *Food 2020* (London: TSO).

HM Government (2010b) *A Smoke-free Future* (London: TSO).

HM Government (2010c) *The Coalition: Our Programme for Government* (London: Cabinet Office).

HM Government/Department of Health (2006) *Health Challenge England: Next Steps for Choosing Health* (London: DoH).

HM Treasury (2001) *Tackling Child Poverty; Giving Every Child the Best Possible Start in Life: A Pre-budget Report* (London: HM Treasury).

HM Treasury (2004) *Public Service Agreements 2005–08* (London: TSO)

HM Treasury (2006a) *The Climate Change Levy Package* (London: HM Treasury).

HM Treasury (2006b) *New Responses to New Challenges: Reinforcing the Tackling Tobacco Smuggling Strategy* (London: HM Treasury).

HM Treasury and DfES (2007) *Policy Review of Children and Young People: A Discussion Paper* (London: HM Treasury).

HM Treasury, Department for Work and Pensions, Department for Children, Schools and Families (2008) *Ending Child Poverty: Everybody's Business* (London: HM Treasury).

HM Treasury/DoH (2002) *Tackling Health Inequalities: Summary of the 2002 Cross Cutting Review* (London: DoH).

Hobson-West, P. (2004) *The Construction of Lay Resistance to Vaccination* in Shaw, I. and Kauppinen, K. (eds) *Constructions of Health and Illness* (Aldershot: Ashgate).

Hockley, T. and Bosanquet, N. (1998) *New Dynamics in Public Health Policy* (London: Social Market Foundation).

Hodgett, G. (1998) 'Ethics, Science and the Social Management of Risk; the BSE Epidemic', *Biosciences and the Law*, 1: 359–86.

Hodgkinson, R. (1967) *The Origins of the NHS: The Medical Services of the New Poor Law* (London: Wellcome Foundation).

Hogg, C. (1999) *Patients, Power and Politics* (London: Sage).

Hogg, C. (2008) *Citizens, Consumers and the NHS: Capturing Voices* (London: Palgrave Macmillan).

Hogg, C. and Williamson, C. (2001) 'Whose Interests do Lay People Represent? Towards an Understanding of the Role of Lay People as Members of Committees', *Health Expectations*, 4(2): 2–9.

Hogwood, B. and Gunn, L. (1984) *Policy Analysis for the Real World* (Oxford: Oxford University Press).

Hole, D., Perkins, A., Wilson, J. et al. (2005) 'Does Organic Farming Benefit Biodiversity?', *Biological Conservation*, 122: 113–30.

Holland, W. and Stewart, S. (1990) *Screening in Health Care: Benefit or Bane?* (London: NPHT).

Holland, W. and Stewart, S. (1998) *Public Health: The Vision and the Challenge* (London: Nuffield Trust).

Holland, W. and Stewart, S. (2005) *Screening in Disease Prevention: What Works?* (Oxford: Radcliffe/Nuffield Trust).

Hollis, P. (1974) *Pressure from Without in Early Victorian England* (London: Edward Arnold).

Holm, S. (2007) 'Should Genetic Information be Disclosed to Insurers? Yes', *British Medical Journal*, 334(7605): 1196.

Holtzman, N.A. and Shapiro, D. (1998) 'Genetic Testing and Public Policy', *British Medical Journal*, 316: 852–6.

Home Affairs Committee (2002) *3rd Report 2001–2: the Government's Drug Policy: Is It Working?*, HC 318 (London: TSO).

Home Affairs Committee (2005) *5th Report 2004–5: Anti-Social Behaviour*, HC 80-1 (London: TSO).

Home Affairs Committee (2008) *Policing in the 21st Century: 7th Report 2007–8*, HC 364 (London: TSO).

Home Affairs Committee (2010) *7th Report 2009–10: The Cocaine Trade*, HC 74 (London: TSO).

Home Office (1985) *Tackling Drug Misuse* (London: Home Office).

Home Office (1999) *Cardiff Violence Prevention Group: Cutting Crime Building Communities* (London: Home Office).

Home Office (2007) *Press Release: Underage Sales Down* (London: Home Office).

Home Office (2009) *Blueprint Drugs Education: The Response of Pupils and Parents to the Programme* (London: Home Office).

Home Office, DoH, DFES (2006) *FRANK Review* (London: Home Office).

Honingsbaum, F. (1970) *The Struggle for the Ministry of Health* (London: Social Administration Research Trust).

Hood, C., Rothstein, H. and Baldwin, R. (2004) *The Government of Risk* (Oxford: Oxford University Press).

Hooper, L., Summerbell, C., Higgins, J. et al. (2001) 'Dietary Fat Intake and Prevention of Cardiovascular Disease: Systematic Review', *British Medical Journal*, 322: 757–63.

Hooper, L., Thompson, R., Harrison, R. et al. (2006) 'Risks and Benefits of Omega 3 Fats for Mortality, Cardiovascular Disease, and Cancer: Systematic Review', *British Medical Journal*, 332: 752–60.

Hope, S. and Neville, S. (2008) 'Councils Dumping Recycled Rubbish in Landfill', *Daily Telegraph* 20.12.08 p.1.

Hornsby, D., Summerlee, S. and Woodside, K. (2007) 'NAFTA's Shadow Hangs Over Kyoto's Implementation', *Canadian Public Policy*, 33(3): 285–98.

Horton, R. (2004) *Measles-Mumps-Rubella Science and Fiction* (London: Granta).

Horton, R. (2006) 'WHO: Strengthening the Road to Renewal' (www.thelancet.com) 367: 1793–5.

Hou, F. and Myles, J. (2005) 'Neighbourhood Inequality, Neighbourhood Affluence and Population Health', *Social Science & Medicine*, 60: 1557–69.

Hough, M., Clancy, A., McSweeney, T. and Turnbull, P. (2003) *The Impact of Drug Treatment and Testing Orders on Offending: Two-Year Reconviction Results* (London: Home Office).

Hough, M., Hunter, M., Jacobson, J. and Cossalter, S. (2008) *The Impact of the Licensing Act 2003 on Levels of Crime and Disorder: An Evaluation* (London: Home Office).

House of Commons (1977) *1st Report from the Select Committee on Expenditure Together with the Minutes of Evidence Taken Before the Social Services and Employment Sub-Committee in Sessions 1975–76 and 1976–77 Preventive Medicine* (London: Her Majesty's Stationery Office).

House of Lords (1998a) *7th Report of the Science and Technology Committee 1997–1998: Resistance to Antibiotics and Other Microbial Agents*, HL 81 (London: TSO).

House of Lords (1998b) *9th Report of the Science and Technology Select Committee 1997–1998: Cannabis: The Scientific and Medical Evidence*, HL 151 (London: TSO).

House of Lords (2000) *3rd Report of the Science and Technology Committee 1999–2000: Science and Society* (London: TSO).

House of Lords (2001a) *3rd Report of the Science and Technology Committee 2000–2001: Resistance to Antibiotics* (London: TSO).

House of Lords (2001b) *2nd Report of the Science and Technology Committee 2000–2001: Therapeutic Uses of Cannabis,* HL 50 (London: TSO).

House of Lords (2003) *4th Report of the Science and Technology Committee 2002–2003: Fighting Infection*, HL 138 (London: TSO).

House of Lords (2006) *5th Report from the Economic Affairs Select Committee 2005–06 on Government Policy on the Management of Risk,* HL 183-I (London: TSO).

House of Lords (2008a) *6th Report of the Science and Technology Committee 2007–2008: Waste Reduction,* HL 163 (London: TSO).

House of Lords (2008b) *7th Report from the European Union Committee 2007–2008: The Future of the Common Agricultural Policy* HL 54 (London: TSO).

House of Lords (2008c) *33rd report of the European Union Committee 2007–2008: The Revision of the EU's Emissions Trading System,* HL 197 (London: TSO).

House of Lords (2010) *1st Report from the Science and Technology Committee 2009–10 on Nanotechnologies and Food,* HL 22 (London: TSO).

Houston, A. (2008) 'Complex Community Based Initiatives' in Cowley, S. (ed.) *Community Public Health in Policy and Practice* (London: Balliere Tindall Elsevier), pp.129–60.

Howard, B., Van Horn, L., Hsia, J. et al. (2006) 'Low-Fat Dietary Pattern and Risk of Cardiovascular Disease', *Journal of American Medical Association,* 295: 655–6.

Howden-Chapman, P., Matheson, A., Crane, J. et al. (2007) 'Effect of Insulating Existing Houses on Health Inequality: Cluster Randomised Study in the Community', *British Medical Journal* (doi: 10.1136/bmj.39070.573021.80).

Hoyer, A.P., Grandjean, P., Jorgensen, T. et al. (1998) 'Organochloride Exposure and Risk of Breast Cancer', *The Lancet,* 352: 1816–20.

Hoyer, A.P., Jorgensen, T., Grandjean, P. and Hartvig, H.B. (2000) 'Repeated Measurements of Organochlorine Exposure and Breast Cancer Risk (Denmark)', *Cancer Causes and Control,* 11(2): 177–84.

HSE (Health and Safety Executive) (2007) *Workplace Stress Costs Great Britain in Excess of £530m* (London: HSE).

HSE (2008) *Statistics* (www.hse.gov.uk/statistics accessed 29.08.08).

Hu, F., Stampfer, M., Manson, J. et al. (1997) 'Dietary Fat Intake and the Risk of Coronary Heart Disease in Women', *New England Journal of Medicine,* 337(21): 1491–9.

Hu, F.B., Stampfer, F.B., Manson, J. et al. (1998) 'Frequent Nut Consumption and Risk of Coronary Heart Disease in Women: Prospective Cohort Study', *British Medical Journal,* 317: 1341–5.

Hu, G., Tuomilehto, J., Silventoinene, K. et al. (2007) 'Body Mass Index, Waist Circumference, and Waist-Hip Ratio on the Risk of Total and Type-Specific Stroke', *Archives of Internal Medicine,* 167(13): 1420–7.

Hudson, B. (2006) 'Children and Young People's Strategic Plans: We Have Been Here Before Haven't We?', *Policy Studies,* 27(2): 87–99.

Hudson, B. and Hardy, B. (2002) 'What is a Successful Partnership and How Can it be Measured?' in Glendinning, C., Powell, M. and Rummery, K. (eds) *Partnerships, New Labour and Governance* (Bristol: Policy Press), pp. 51–66.

Hudson, B. and Henwood, M. (2002) 'The NHS and Social Care: The Final Countdown', *Policy and Politics,* 30: 153–66.

Hudson, J. and Lowe, S. (2004) *Understanding the Policy Process* (Bristol: Policy Press).

Hughes, K., MacKintosh, A.M., Hastings, G. et al. (1997) 'Young People, Alcohol and Designer and Drinks: Quantitative and Qualitative Study', *British Medical Journal,* 314: 416–18.

Hughes, L. (2009) *Joint Strategic Needs Assessment: Progress So Far* (London: IDeA).

Huisman, M., Kunst, A. and Mackenbach, J. (2003) 'Socioeconomic Inequalities in Morbidity Among the Elderly: A European Review' *Social Science & Medicine,* 57(5): 861–73.

Human Genetics Advisory Commission (1997) *The Implications of Genetic Testing for Insurance* (London: Office of Science and Technology).

Human Genetics Commission (2001) *The Use of Genetic Information in Insurance: Interim Recommendations* (London: DoH).

Hume Hall, R. (1990) *Health and the Global Environment* (Oxford: Polity).

Hung, H.C., Joshipura, K., Jiang, R. et al. (2004) 'Fruit and Vegetable Intake and Risk of Major Chronic Disease', *Journal of the National Cancer Institute,* 96(21): 1577–84.

Hunt, K., Ford, G., Harkins, L., and Wyke, S. (1999) 'Are Women More Ready to Consult Than Men?', *Journal of Health Services Research,* 4(2): 96–100.

Hunt, S. (1997) 'Housing-Related Disorders' in Charlton, J. and Murphy, M. *The Health of Adult Britain 1841–1994 Volume 1* (London: TSO), pp. 156–70.

Hunter, D. (2003) *Public Health Policy* (Cambridge: Polity).

Hunter, D. (2009) 'Relationship between Evidence and Policy: A Case of Evidence-Based Policy or Policy-Based Evidence?', *Public Health,* 123: 582–6.

Hunter, D. and Marks, L. (2005) *Managing for Health: What Incentives Exist for NHS Managers to Focus on Wider Health Issues?* (London: King's Fund).

Hunter, D., Wilkinson, J. and Coyle, E. (2005) 'Would Regional Government Have Been Good for Your Health?', *British Medical Journal,* 330: 159–60.

Hunter, D., Marks, L. and Smith, K. (2007a) *The Public Health System in England: A Scoping Study*. Part 1 (Centre for Public Policy in Health: Durham University).

Hunter, D., Marks, L. and Smith, K. (2007b) *The Public Health System in England: A Scoping Study*. Part 2 (Centre for Public Policy in Health: Durham University).

Hunter, D., Marks, L. and Smith, K. (2010) *The Public Health System in England*, Bristol: Policy Press.

Huntington, R. (2004) *The Nanny State* (London: Artnik).

Huppert, F., Baylis, N. and Keverne, B. (2005) *The Science of Wellbeing* (Oxford: Oxford University Press).

Hutton, W. (1996) *The State We're In* (London: Vintage).

Hyde, H.M. (1976) *Neville Chamberlain* (London: Weidenfeld and Nicolson).

Ibarluzea, J.J., Fernandez, M.F., Santa-Marina, L. et al. (2004) 'Breast Cancer Risk and the Combined Effects of Environmental Oestrogens', *Cancer Causes Control*, 15: 591–600.

Iliffe, S. and Lenihan, P. (2003) 'Integrating Primary Care and Public Health: Learning from the Community Oriented Primary Care Model', *International Journal of Health Services*, 33(1): 85–98.

Illich, I. (1977) *Limits to Medicine* (Harmondsworth: Penguin).

Illsley, R. (1986) 'Occupation Class Selection and the Production of Inequalities in Health', *Quarterly Journal of Social Affairs*, 2(2): 151–65.

ILO (International Labour Organisation) (2007) *Working Time Around the World: Trends in Working Hours, Laws and Policies in a Global Comparative Perspective* (ILO).

Independent Advisory Group on Sexual Health and HIV (2006) *Annual Report 2005/6* (London: Department of Health).

Independent Advisory Group on Sexual Health and HIV (2007) *Sex, Drugs, Alcohol and Young People's Sexual Behaviour* (London: Department of Health).

Independent Advisory Group on Sexual Health and HIV and Medical Foundation for AIDS and Sexual Health (2008) *Progress and Priorities – Working Together for High Quality Sexual Health* (London: Medical Foundation for AIDS and Sexual Health).

Independent Commission on Social Mobility (2009) *Report* (London: Independent Commission on Social Mobility).

Independent Inquiry into Inequalities in Health (1998) *Report* (Acheson Report) (London: TSO).

Independent Inquiry on BSE (2000) *Report* (The Phillips Inquiry) (London: TSO).

Independent on Sunday (1994) 'Drink Companies Pay Dons to Rubbish Alcohol Report', 4th December.

Independent Working Group on Drug Consumption Rooms (2006) *Report* (York: Joseph Rowntree Foundation).

Inglis, B. (1965) *A History of Medicine* (London: Weidenfield & Nicolson).

Ingram, D., Sanders, K., Kolybaba, M. and Lopez, D. (1997) 'Case Control Study of Phyto-oestrogens and Breast Cancer', *The Lancet*, 305(9083): 990–4.

Institute for Alcohol Studies (2009) *Alcohol and Accidents*. IAS Factsheet (St Ives: IAS).

Institute of Medicine (1988) *The Future of Public Health* (Washington DC: The National Academies Press).

Institute of Medicine (2004) *Immunisations, Safety Review: Vaccines and Autism* (Immunization Safety Review Committee).

Institute of Medicine (2009) *Secondhand Smoke Exposure and Cardiovascular Effects* (Washington DC: National Academies Press).

Interdepartmental Committee on Drug Addiction (1961) *Report* (London: HMSO).

Interdepartmental Committee on Drug Addiction (1965) *Report* (London: HMSO).

Interdepartmental Expert Group on Mobile Phones (2000) *Report: The Stewart Report* (www.iegmp.org.uk accessed 17.06.08).

International Agency for Research into Cancer (2002) *Effectiveness of Screening: Breast Cancer Screening* (Lyon: International Agency for Research into Cancer).

International Agency for the Research on Cancer (2002) *Monograph on Tobacco Smoke and Involuntary Smoking* (International Agency for the Research on Cancer).

International Commission on the Future of Food and Agriculture (2003) *Manifesto on the Future of Food* (San Rossore: ICFFA).

International Obesity Taskforce (IOTF) Consumers International and International Association for the Study of Obesity (IASO) (2008) *Recommendations for an International Code on Marketing of Foods and Non-Alcoholic Beverages to Children* (London: IOTF, IASO).

Intersalt Cooperatives Research Group (1988) 'Intersalt: An International Study of Electrolyte Excretion and Blood Pressure. Results for 24 Hour Urinary Sodium and Potassium Excretion', *British Medical Journal*, 297: 319–28.

IPCC (Intergovernmental Panel on Climate Change) (2007) *Climate Change 2007: The Physical Science Basis* (Geneva: IPPC).

Irvine, F. and Kenkre, J. (2004) Review of Primary Care and Community Nursing in Wales: Summary and Recommendations (unpublished).

Irwin, A. and Wynne, B. (1996) 'Conclusion'. In Irwin, A. and Wynne, B. (eds) *Misunderstanding Science? The Public Reconstruction of Science and Technology* (Cambridge: Cambridge University Press), pp. 214–21.

Jacobs, D., Blackburn, H., Higgins, M. et al. (1992) 'Report of the Conference on Low Blood Cholesterol: Mortality Associations', *Circulation*, 86: 1046–60.

Jacobson, J. and Jacobson, S. (1997) Evidence for PCBs as Neurodevelopmental Toxicants in Humans', *Neurotoxicology*, 18(2): 415–24.

James, O. (2007) *Affluenza* (London: Vermillion).

Jamrozik, K. (2005) 'Estimate of Deaths Attributable to Passive Smoking Among UK Adults: Database Analysis', *British Medical Journal,* Online (doi: 10.1136/bmj.38370.496632.8F accessed 18.5.10).

Jansen, M.C., Bueno-de-Mesquista, H.B., Budna, R. et al. (1999) 'Dietary Fibre and Plant Foods in Relation to Colorectal Cancer Mortality: The 7 Countries Study', *International Journal of Cancer*, 81(2): 174–9.

Jarup, L., Wolfgang, B., Houthuijs, D. et al. on Behalf of the HYENA Study Team (2008) 'Hypertension and Exposure to Noise Near Airports: The HYENA Study', *Environmental Health Perspectives*, 116(3): 329–33.

Jefferson, T., Dietrantonj, C., Al-Ansory, L. et al. (2010) *Vaccines for Preventing Influenza in the Elderly (Review) Cochrane Collaboration* The Cochrane Library Issue 2 (Chichester: John Wiley and Sons).

Jeffreys, M., Davey-Smith, G., Martin, R. et al. (2004) 'Childhood Body Mass Index and Later Cancer Risk: A 50-Year Follow-Up of the Boyd Orr Study', *International Journal of Cancer*, 122: 348–51.

Jenkins, G., Perry, M. and Prior, M. (2008) *The Climate of the UK: Recent Trends* (Exeter: Met Office).

Jenkins-Smith, H. and Sabatier, P. (1994) 'Evaluating the Advocacy Coalition Framework', *Journal of Public Policy*, 14(2): 175–203.

Jerrett, M., Burnett, R., Pope, C. et al. (2009) 'Long-term Ozone Exposure and Mortality', *New England Journal of Medicine*, 360: 1085–95.

Jewkes, R. and Murcott, A. (1998) 'Community Representatives: Representing the Community?', *Social Science & Medicine*, 46(7): 843–58.

Jha, P. and Chaloupka, F. (1999) *Curbing the Epidemic: Governments and the Economics of Tobacco Control* (Washington: World Bank).

Jit, M., Vyse, A., Borrow, R. et al. (2007) 'Prevalence of Human Papillomavirus Antibodies in Young Female Subjects in England', *British Journal of Cancer*, 97: 989–91.

Jochelson, K. (2005) 'Nanny or Steward? The Role of Government in Public Health', *Public Health,* 120: 1149–55 (London: Kings Fund).

John, P. (1998) *Analysing Public Policy* (London: Pinter).

Johnson, M. (1993) 'Equal Opportunities in Service Delivery. Responses to a Changing Population?' in Ahmad, W. (ed.) *Race and Health in Contemporary Britain* (Buckingham: Open University Press).

Joint Working Group of the Human Genetics Commission and the UK National Screening Committee (2005) *Profiling the Newborn: A Prospective Gene Technology* (London: Human Genetics Commission).

Jones, F., Annan, D. and Shah, S. (2008) 'The Distribution of Household Income 1977 to 2006/07', *Economic & Labour Market Review*, 2(12): 18–31.

Jones, F., Annan, D. and Shah, S. (2009) 'The Redistribution of Household Income 1977 to 2006/07', *Economic and Labour Market Review*, 3(1): 31–43.

Jones, N. (2002) *The Control Freaks: How New Labour Gets Its Own Way* (London: Politicos).

Joossens, J. and Raw, M. (2000) 'How Can Cigarette Smuggling be Reduced?', *British Medical Journal*, 321: 947–50.

Joossens, J. and Raw, M. (2006) 'The Tobacco Control Scale: A New Scale to Measure Country Activity', *British Medical Journal*, 15: 247–53.

Joossens, J.V., Hill, M.J., Elliott, P. et al. (1996) 'Dietary Salt, Nitrate and Stomach Cancer Mortality in 24 Countries. European Cancer Prevention (ECP) and the INTERSALT Cooperative Research Group', *International Journal of Epidemiology*, 25: 494–504.

Jordan, A. (ed.) (2005) *Environmental Policy in the EU* (2nd edn) (London: Earthscan).

Jordan, G. and Maloney, W. (1997) *The Protest Business: Mobilising Campaign Groups* (Manchester: Manchester University Press).

Jordan, H., Roderick, P. and Martin, D. (2004) 'The Index of Multiple Deprivation 2000 and Accessibility Effects on Health', *Journal of Epidemiology and Community Health*, 58: 250–7.

Joseph Rowntree Foundation (1995) *Income and Wealth* (York: Joseph Rowntree Foundation).

Judd, D. (1977) *Radical Joe: A Life of Joseph Chamberlain* (London: Hamish Hamilton).

Judge, K. (1995) 'Income Distribution and Life Expectancy: A Critical Appraisal', *British Medical Journal*, 311: 1282–5.

Judge, K. and Bauld, L. (2007) 'Learning from Policy Failure? Health Action Zones in England', *European Journal of Public Health*, 16(4): 341–4.

Judge, K., Platt, S., Costongs, C. and Jurczak, K. (2005) *Health Inequalities: A Challenge for Europe* (London: COI).

Juniper, T. (1999) 'Unfair Trade Sparks New World War', *Guardian*, 17 August, 14.

Juster, H., Loomis, B., Hinman, T. et al. (2007) 'Declines in Hospital Admissions for Acute Myocardial Infarction in New York State After Implementation of a Comprehensive Smoking Ban', *American Journal of Public Health*, 97(11): 2035–9.

Kahn, E., Ramsey, L., Brownson, R. et al. and the Task Force on Community Preventative Services (2002) 'The Effectiveness of Interventions to Increase Physical Activity', *American Journal of Preventative Medicine*, 22(4S): 73–107.

Kahn, R., Wise, P., Kennedy, B. and Kawachi, I. (2000) 'State Income Inequality, Household Income, and Maternal Mental and Physical Health: Cross Sectional National Survey', *British Medical Journal,* 321: 1311–15.

Kahneman, D., Diener, E. and Schwartz, N. (eds) (2003) *Wellbeing: The Foundations of Hedonic Psychology* (New York: Russell Sage).

Kaiser, S. and Mackenbach, J. (2008) 'Public Health in Eight European Countries: An International Comparison of Terminology', *Public Health,* 122: 211–16.

Kammerling, R. and Kinnear, D. (1996) 'The Extent of the Two Tier Service for Fundholders', *British Medical Journal*, 312: 1399–401.

Kane, P. (2008) 'Sure Start Local Programmes in England', *The Lancet*, 372: 1610–11.

Kaplan, G.A., Pamuk, E.R., Lynch, J.W. et al. (1996) 'Inequality in Income and Mortality in the United States: Analysis of Mortality and Potential Pathways', *British Medical Journal*, 312: 999–1003.

Kasperson, J.X., Kasperson, R., Pidgeon, N.F. and Slovic, P. (2003) 'The Social Amplification of Risk: Assessing Fifteen Years of Research and Theory' (Cambridge: CUP), pp. 13–46.

Kawachi, I. and Berkman, L. (eds) (2003) *Neighbourhoods and Health* (Oxford: Oxford University Press).

Kawachi, I. and Kennedy, B. (1997) 'Health and Social Cohesion. Why Care About Income Inequality?', *British Medical Journal*, 314: 1037–40.

Kawachi, I., Kennedy, B., Lochener, K. and Prothrow-Stith, D. (1997) 'Social Capital, Income Inequality, and Mortality', *American Journal of Public Health*, 87(9): 1491–8.

Kay, J. (1832) The Moral and Physical Condition of the Working Classes of Manchester (London: Ridgeway).

Kaye, J., Del Mar Melero-Montes, M. and Jick, H. (2001) 'Mumps Measles and Rubella Vaccine and the Incidence of Autism Recorded by General Practitioners: A Time Trend Analysis', *British Medical Journal*, 322(7284): 460–3.

Keithley, J. and Robinson, F. (2000) 'Violence as a Public Health Issue', *Policy and Politics*, 28(1): 67–77.

Kelly, M.P., Davies, J.K. and Charlton, B.G. (1992) 'Healthy Cities?' in Davies, J. and Kelly, M. *Healthy Cities: Policy and Practice* (London: Routledge), pp. 1–14.

Kemm, J., Parry, J. and Palmer, S. (ed.) (2007) *Health Impact Assessment* (Oxford: Oxford University Press).

Kemp, T., Pearce, N., Fitzharris, P. et al. (1997) 'Is Infant Immunisation a Risk Factor for Childhood Asthma or Allergy?', *Epidemiology*, 8(6): 678–80.

Kendall, J. (2003) *The Voluntary Sector* (London: Routledge).

Kendall, L. (2001) *The Future Patient* (London: Institute for Public Policy Research).

Kennedy, B.P., Kawachi, I. and Prothrow-Stith, D. (1996) 'Income Distribution and Mortality: Cross-Sectional Ecological Study of the Robin Hood Index in the United States', *British Medical Journal*, 312: 1004–7.

Kerlikowske, K., Grady, D., Rubin, S.M. et al. (1995) 'Efficacy of Screening Mammography. A Meta-Analysis', *Journal of the American Medical Association,* 273(2): 149–54.

Key, T., Allen, N., Spencer, E. and Travis, R. (2002) 'The Effect of Diet on Risk of Cancer', *The Lancet*, 360(9336): 861–8.

Key, T., Thorogood, M., Appleby, P. and Burr, M. (1996) 'Dietary Habits and Mortality in 11,000 Vegetarians and Health Conscious People: Results of a 17 Year Follow Up', *British Medical Journal*, 313: 775–9.

Keys, A. (1980) *Seven Countries: A Multi Analysis of Death and CHD* (Cambridge, MA: Harvard University Press).

Khan, R., Wise, P., Kennedy, B. and Kawachi, I. (2000) 'State Income Inequality, Household Income, and Maternal Mental and Physical Health: Cross Sectional National Survey', *British Medical Journal*, 321: 1311–15.

Khaw, K.T., Wareham, N., Bingham, S. et al. (2008) 'Combined Impact of Health Behaviours and Mortality in Men and Women: The EPIC-Norfolk Perspective Population Study', *PLoS Medicine*, 5(1): e12.

Khoury, M., Burke, W. and Thomson, E. (2000) *Genetics and Public Health in the 21st Century: Using Genetic Information to Improve Health and Prevent Disease* (Oxford: Oxford University Press).

Kickbusch, I. (1986) 'Health Promotion Strategies for Action', *Canadian Journal of Public Health*, 77: 321–6.

Kickbusch, I. (2002) Influence and Opportunity: Reflections on the US Role in Public Global Public Health, *Health Affairs*, 21(6): 131–41.

Kickbusch, I. (2003) 'The Contribution of the World Health Organisation to the New Public Health and Health Promotion', *American Journal of Public Health*, 93(3): 383–7.

Kim, D., Kawachi, I., Vander Hoorn, S. and Ezzati, M. (2008) 'Is Inequality at the Heart of it? Cross-Country Associations of Income Inequality with Cardiovascular Diseases and Risk Factors', *Social Science & Medicine*, 66: 1719–32.

King James I (1616) 'A Counterblaste to Tobacco'. In James I (ed.) *The Works of the Most High and Mighty Prince, James* (London: Barker & Bill), pp. 214–22.

King, D. (1987) *The New Right: Politics, Markets and Citizenship* (London: Macmillan – now Palgrave Macmillan).

King, D. (2004) 'Policy Forum: Environment: Climate Change Science Adapt, Mitigate, or Ignore?', *Science*, 9: 176–7.

King, M., McKeown, E., Warner, J. et al. (2003) 'Mental Health and Quality of Life of Gay Men and Lesbians in England and Wales', *British Journal of Psychiatry*, 183(6): 552–8.

King's Fund (2004) *Public Attitudes to Health Policy* (London: King's Fund).

King's Fund (2005) 'Memorandum' in Health Committee (2005) Health – Minutes of Evidence, HC 358i, session 2004/5 (London: TSO).

Kingdon, J. (1984) *Agendas, Alternatives and Public Policy* (Boston: Little Brown).

Kinghorn G. (2001) 'A Sexual Health and HIV Strategy for England', *British Medical Journal*, 323(7307): 243–4.

Kinlen, L. (1988) 'Evidence for an Infective Cause of Childhood Leukaemia', *The Lancet*, 2: 1323–7.

Kinlen, L. (1995) 'Epidemiological Evidence for and Infective Basis in Childhood Leukaemia', *British Journal of Cancer*, 71: 1–5.

Kipping, R., Jago, R. and Lawlor, D. (2008) 'Obesity in Children Part 1: Epidemiology, Measurement, Risk Factors and Screening', *British Medical Journal*, 337: a1824 (doi: 10.1136/bmj.a1824).

Kisely, S. and Jones, J. (1997) 'Acheson Revisited: Public Health Medicine Ten Years After the Acheson Report', *Public Health*, 111(6): 361–4.

Kitto, H.D.F. (1957) *The Greeks* (London: Pelican).

Kitzinger, J. and Reilly, J. (1997) 'The Rise and Fall of Risk Reporting: Media Coverage of Human Genetics Research, False Memory Syndrome and Mad Cow Disease', *European Journal of Communication*, 12: 319–49.

Kivimaki, M., Leino-Arjas, P., Luukkonen, R. et al. (2002) 'Work Stress and Risk of Cardiovascular Mortality: Prospective Cohort Study of Industrial Employees', *British Medical Journal*, 325: 857–60.

Klein, R. (1980) 'Between Nihilism and Utopia in Health Care', Lecture at Yale University, New Haven (Unpublished).

Knoops, K., de Groot, L., Kromhout, D. et al. (2004) 'Mediterranean Diet, Lifestyle Factors, and 10-Year Mortality in Elderly European Men and Women', *Journal of the American Medical Association*, 292(12): 1433–9.

Knox, E. (2005) 'Childhood Cancers and Atmospheric Carcinogens', *Journal of Epidemiology and Community Health*, 59: 101–5.

Koivusalo, M. (2005) 'The Future of European Health Policies', *International Journal of Health Services*, 35(2): 325–42.

Koivusalo, M. (2006) 'The Impact of Economic Globalisation on Health', *Theoretical Medicine and Bioethics*, 27: 1–34.

Koivusalo, M. and Ollila, E. (1997) *Making a Healthy World* (London: Zed).

Kondo, N., Kawachi, I., Subramanian, S.V. et al. (2008) 'Do Social Comparisons Explain the Association Between Income Inequality and Health?: Relative Deprivation and Perceived Health Among Male and Female Japanese Individuals', *Social Science & Medicine*, 67: 982–7.

Kortenkamp, A. (2006) *Environmental Contaminants and Breast Cancer. The Growing Concerns About Endocrine Disrupting Chemicals. A Briefing Paper for WWF-UK*.

KPMG (2008) *Review of the Social Responsibility Standards for the Production and Sale of Alcoholic Drink* (London: Home Office).

Krause, R. (ed.) (1998) *Emerging Infections* (New York: Academy Press).

Krieger, N., Wolff, M.S., Hiatt, R. et al. (1994) 'Breast Cancer and Serum Organochlorines: A Prospective Study among White, Black and Asian Women', *Journal of the National Cancer Institute*, 86: 589–99.

Kriemler, S., Zahner, L., Schindler, C. et al. (2010) 'Effect of a School-Based Physical Activity Programme (KISS) on Fitness and Adiposity in Primary Schoolchildren: Cluster Randomised Controlled Trial', *British Medical Journal*, 340: c785 accessed 9.3.10.

Krug, E., Dahlberg, L., Mercy, J. et al. (eds) (2002) *World Report on Violence and Health* (Geneva: World Health Organization).

Kuh, D. and Ben-Schlomo, Y. (2004) *A Life Course Approach to Chronic Disease Epidemiology* (2nd edn) (Oxford: Oxford University Press).

Kuh, D., Ben-Shlomo, Y., Lynch, J. et al. (2003) 'Life Course Epidemiology', *Journal of Epidemiology and Community Health*, 57: 778–83.

Kunst, A.E., Groenhof, F. and Mackenbach, J. (1998) 'Occupational Class and Cause Specific

Mortality in Middle Aged Men in 11 European Countries: Comparison of Population Based Studies', *British Medical Journal*, 30 May, 1636–42.

Kunzli, N., Kaiser, R., Medina, S. et al. (2000) 'Public Health Impact of Outdoor and Traffic Related Air Pollution: A European Assessment', *The Lancet*, 356: 795–801.

Kuper, H., Singh-Manoux, J., Sigrist, J., and Marmot, M. (2002) 'When Reciprocity Fails; Effort-Reward Imbalance in Relation to CHD and Health Functioning Within the Whitehall II Study', *Occupational and Environmental Medicine*, 59: 777–84.

Labonte, R. (1998) 'Health Promotion and the Common Good', *Critical Public Health*, 8(2): 107–23.

Labonte, R. (2008) 'Global Health in Public Policy: Finding The Right Frame?', *Critical Public Health*, 18(4): 467–82.

Labonte, R. and Schrecker, T. (2004) 'Committed to Health for All?: How the G7/G8 Rate', *Social Science & Medicine*, 59: 1661–76.

LACORS (2008a) *Licensing Act 2003 and the Effects of Alcohol* (London: TNS/LGA).

LACORS (2008b) *Test Purchasing of Tobacco Products – Results From Local Authority Trading Standards 1st October – 31st March 2008* (London: LACORS and DoH).

Lakey, J. (2001) *Youth Employment, Labour Market Programmes and Health* (London: Policy Studies Institute).

Lalonde, M. (1974) *A New Perspective on the Health of Canadians* (Ottawa: Ministry of National Health and Welfare).

Lambert, J. (2002) *Refugees and the Environment* (Brussels: European Parliament).

Lambert, R. (1963) *Sir John Simon* (London: Magibbon and Kee).

Lancet, The (2007) 'Child Well-being in Rich Countries', *The Lancet*, 369(9562): 616.

Lancet, The /UHL Institute for Global Health Commission (2009) 'Managing the Health Effects of Climate Change', *The Lancet,* 373: 1693–73.

Landon, M. (2006) *Environment, Health and Sustainable Development* (Maidenhead: Open University Press).

Lang, T. and Heasman, M. (2004) *Food Wars: The Global Battle for Mouths, Minds, and Markets* (London: Earthscan).

Lang, T. and Rayner, G. (2002) *Why Health is the Key to the Future of Food and Farming: A Report on the Future of Farming and Food* (London: Health Development Agency).

Lang, T. and Rayner, G. (2007) 'Overcoming Policy Cacophony on Obesity: An Ecological Public Health Framework for Policymakers', *Obesity Reviews*, 8(Supp. 1): 165–81.

Lang, T., Barling, D. and Caraher, M. (2001) 'Food, Social Policy and the Environment: Towards a New Model', *Social Policy and Administration*, 35(5): 538–58.

Lang, T., Barling, D. and Caraher, M. (2009) *Food Policy: Integrating Health, Society and the Environment* (Oxford: Oxford University Press).

Lang, T., Rayner, G. and Kaelin, E. (2006a) *The Food Industry, Diet, Physical Activity and Health: A Review of Reported Commitments and Practice of 25 of the World's Largest Food Companies* (London: Centre for Food Policy).

Lang, T., Dowler, E. and Hunter, D. (2006b) *Review of the Scottish Diet Action Plan 1996–2005: Progress and Impacts* (Edinburgh: NHS Scotland).

Langford, A. and Johnson, B. (2009) *Social Inequalities in Adult Female Mortality by the National Statistics Socio-economic Classification, England and Wales, 2001–03* (London: Office for National Statistics).

Lanser, S. and Pless-Mulloli, T. (2003) 'Integrated Pollution Prevention and Control: A Review of Health Authorities' Experience', *Journal of Public Health Medicine*, 25(3): 234–6.

Lansley, A. (2010a) *A New Approach to Public Health*, UK Faculty of Public Health Conference 7 July 2010 (www.dh.gov.uk/en/mediaCentre/speeches/DH_117280 accessed 8.7.10)

Lansley, A. (2010b) 'Health Secretary Sets Out Future of Public Health' (Press release 7/7/10 (www.dh.gov.uk/en/MediaCentre/PressReleases/DH_117228 accessed 8.7.10).

Larsen, K. and Gilliland, J. (2008) 'Mapping the Evolution of Food Deserts in a Canadian City: Supermarket Accessibility in London, Ontario, 1961–2005', *International Journal of Health Geographies*, 7(16).

Lash, M., Szerszynski, S. and Wynne, B. (1996) *Risk, Environment and Modernity* (London: Sage).

Laukkanen, J., Rauramaa, R., Makikallio, T., Toriola, A. and Kurl, S.(2009) 'Intensity of Leisure Time Physical Activity and Cancer Mortality in Men', *British Journal of Sports Medicine* (doi: 10.1136/bjsm.2008.056713 accessed 15.5.10).

Laverack, C. (2005) *Public Health: Power, Empowerment and Professional Practice* (London: Palgrave Macmillan).

Law, J. and Faulkner, K. (2001) 'Cancers Detected and Induced, and Associated Risk and Benefit, in a Breast Screening Programme', *British Journal of Radiology*, 74(888): 1121–7.

Law, M.R., Morris, J.K. and Wald, N.J. (1997) 'Environmental Tobacco Smoke Exposure and Ischaemic Heart Disease: An Evaluation of the Evidence', *British Medical Journal*, 315: 973–80.

Law, M.R., Thompson, S.G. and Wald, N.J. (1994) 'Assessing Possible Hazards of Reducing Serum Cholesterol', *British Medical Journal*, 308: 373–9.

Lawrence, M. (ed.) (1987) *Fed Up and Hungry: Women, Oppression and Food* (London: Women's Press).

Lawrence, R. and Fudge, C. (2007) 'Health Cities: Key Principles for Professional Practice' in Scriven, A. and Garman, S. *Public Health: Social Context and Action* (Maidenhead: Open University Press), pp. 180–92.

Layard, R. (2006) *Happiness* (London: Penguin).

Le Fanu, J. (ed.) (1994a) 'Prevention: Wishful Thinking of Hard Science: The Exaggerated Claims of Health Promotion' in Le Fanu (ed.) *Preventionitis* (London: Social Affairs Unit), pp. 23–35.

Le Fanu, J. (ed.) (1994b) *Preventionitis* (London: Social Affairs Unit).

Le Grand, J. (1987) 'Equity, Health and Health-care', *Social Justice Research*, 1: 257–74.

Le Touze, S. and Calnan, M. (1996) 'The Banding Scheme for Health Promotion in General Practice', *Health Trends*, 28/3: 100–5.

Lee, C.D., Blair, S.N. and Jackson, A.J. (1999) 'Cardiorespiratory Fitness, Body Composition, and All Cause and Cardiovascular Disease Mortality in Men', *American Journal of Clinical Nutrition*, 69(3): 373–80.

Lee, K. and Collin, J. (eds) (2005) *Global Change and Health* (Maidenhead: Open University Press).

Lee, K. and Collin, J. (2006) '"Key to the Future": British American Tobacco and Cigarette Smuggling in China', *Public Library of Science (PLoS) Medicine*, 3(7): e228.

Lee, K. and Koivusalo, M. (2005) 'Trade and Health: Is the Community Ready for Action', *Public Library of Science (PLoS) Medicine*, 2(1): 8.

Lee, K., Sridhar, D. and Patel, M. (2009) 'Bridging the Divide: Global Governance of Trade and Health', *The Lancet*, 373: 416–22.

Lee, P. (1994) 'The Need for Caution in Interpreting Low Level Risks Reported by Epidemiologists' in Le Fanu, J. (ed.) *Preventionitis* (London: Social Affairs Unit), pp. 36–45.

LeFebvre, R. (2002) 'Social Marketing and Health Promotion' in Bunton, R. and Macdonald, G. (eds) *Health Promotion: Disciplines and Diversity* (2nd edn) (London: Routledge), pp. 218–45.

Leff, S. and Leff, V. (1959) *The School Health Service* (London: HK Lewis).

Lehtinen, M., Dillner, J., Knekt, P. et al. (1996) 'Serologically Diagnosed Infection with Human Papillomavirus Type 16 and Risk for Subsequent Development of Cervical Carcinoma: Nested Case Control Study', *British Medical Journal*, 312: 537–9.

Leichter, H. (1991) *Free to be Foolish* (New York: Princeton).

Leitzman, M., Moore, S., Peters, T. et al. (2008) 'Prospective Study if Physical Activity and Risk of Postmenopausal Breast Cancer', *Breast Cancer Research*, 10(R92).

Levenson, R., Joule, N. and Russell, J. (1997) *Developing Public Health in the NHS – The Multidisiplinary Contribution* (London: King's Fund).

Levitas, R. (1998) *The Inclusive Society? Social Exclusion and New Labour* (London: Macmillan – now Palgrave Macmillan).

Levitt, R., Nason, E. and Hallsworth, M. (2006) *The Evidence Base for the Classification of Drugs* (Europe: RAND).

Levy, M., Price, D., Zheng, X. et al. (2004) 'Inadequacies in UK Primary Care Allergy Services: National Survey of Current Provisions and Perceptions of Need', *Clinical and Experimental Allergy*, 34(4): 518–19.

Lewin, A., Lindstrom, L. and Nestle, M. (2006) 'Food Industry Promises to Address Childhood Obesity: Preliminary Evaluation', *Journal of Public Health Policy*, 27: 327–48.

Lewis, C. (2003) 'Chewing the Fat', *Health Service Journal*, 113(5881): 28–31.

Lewis, E. and National Children's Bureau (2006) *Children's Views on Non-Broadcast Food and Drink Advertising* (London: Office of the Children's Commissioner).

Lewis, J. (1986) *What Price Community Medicine?* (Brighton: Wheatsheaf).

Lewis, J. (1992) 'Providers, "Consumers": the State and the Delivery of Health-Care Services in Twentieth Century Britain' in Wear, A. (ed.) *Medicine in Society: Historical Essays* (Cambridge: Cambridge University Press), pp. 317–45.

Lewis, J. and Kijn, T. (2002) 'The Politics of Sex Education Policy in England and Wales and The Netherlands Since the 1980s', *Journal of Social Policy*, 31(4): 669–94.

Lewis, S.A. and Britton, J.R. (1998) 'Measles Infection, Measles Vaccination and the Effect of Birth in the Aetiology of Hay Fever', *Clinical and Experimental Allergy*, 28(12): 1493–500.

LGA (Local Government Association) (2000) *Partnerships with Health: A Survey of Local Authorities* (London: LGA).

LGA (2008) *Report of the LGA Commission on Health* (London: LGA).

LGA/UK Public Health Association (2000) *Joint Response to the Public Health White Paper 'Saving Lives'* (London: LGA).

LGA/UK Public Health Alliance/NHS Confederation (2004) *Releasing the Potential for the*

Public's Health (London: LGA, UKPHA, NHS Confederation).

LGA Climate Change Commission (2007) *A Climate of Change: Final Report of the Local Government Association Climate Change Commission* (London: Local Government Association).

Li, Y. (2007) 'Social Capital, Social Exclusion and Wellbeing' in Scriven, A. and Garman, S. *Public Health: Social Context and Action* (Maidenhead: Open University Press), pp. 60–75.

Liberal Democrats (2010) *Manifesto 2010* (London: Liberal Democrats).

Lieberman, S. and Gray, T. (2006) 'The So-called "Moratorium" on the Licensing of New Genetically Modified (GM) Products by the European Union 1998–2004: A Study in Ambiguity', *Environmental Politics*, 15(4): 592–609.

Lin, J., Zhang, S., Cook, N. et al. (2004) 'Body Mass Index and Risk of Colorectal Cancer in Women (United States)', *Cancer Causes and Control*, 15(6): 581–9.

Lincoln, P. (2007) 'Healthy Childhood and a Life Course Approach to Public Health' in Griffiths, S. and Hunter, D.J. *New Perspectives in Public Health* (2nd edn) (Oxford: Radcliffe), pp. 149–57.

Lindblom, C. (1959) 'The Science of Muddling Through', *Public Administration Review*, 19(2): 78–88.

Ling, T. (2000) 'Unpacking Partnership: The Case of Health Care' in Clarke, J., Gewirtz, S. and McLaughlin, E. (eds) *New Managerialism, New Welfare* (London: Sage), pp. 82–101.

Lipsky, M. (1979) *Street-Level Bureaucracy* (New York: Russell Sage).

Lisbon European Council (2000) An Agenda of Economic and Social Renewal for Europe: (The Commissions Contribution to the Lisbon Special European Council Contribution of the European Commission and the Special European Council in Lisbon 23–4 March 2000) (http://ec.europa.eu/growthandjobs/pdf/lison_en.pdf).

Lister-Sharp, D., Chapman, S., Stewart-Brown, S. and Sowden, A. (1999) 'Health Promoting Schools and Health Promotion in Schools: Two Systematic Reviews', *Health Technology Assessment*, 3 (22).

Lister, R. (2005) 'Investing in the Citizen-workers of the Future: Transformations in Citizenship and the State under New Labour' in Hendrick, H. *Child Welfare and Social Policy: An Essential Reader* (Bristol: Policy Press), pp. 449–2.

Littlewood, S. and While, A. (1997) 'A New Agenda for Governance? Local Agenda 21 and the Prospects for Holistic Local Decision Making', *Local Government Studies*, 23(4): 111–23.

Lloyd, N., O'Brien, M. and Lewis, C. (2003) *Fathers in Sure Start by The National Evaluation of Sure Start (NESS)* (London: Institute for Study of Children, Families and Social Issues).

Lobmayer, P. and Wilkinson, R. (2000) 'Income Inequality and Mortality in 14 Developed Countries', *Sociology of Health and Illness*, 22(4): 401–44.

Lock, K. and McKee, M. (2005) 'Health Impact Assessment: Assessing Opportunities and Barriers to Intersectoral Health Improvement in an Expanded European Union', *Journal of Epidemiological and Community Health*, 59: 356–60.

Lock, K., Stuckler, D., Charlesworth, K. and McKee, M. (2009) 'Potential Causes and Health Effects of Rising Global Food Prices' *British Medical Journal,* 339, doi:10.1136/bmj.b2403 accessed 13/8/2010.

Logan, W.P.D. (1950) 'Mortality in England and Wales from 1848–1947', *Population Studies*, 4: 132–78.

Longmate, N. (1966) *King Cholera: The Biography of a Disease* (London: Hamish Hamilton).

Longmate. N. (2003) *The Workhouse* (London: Pimlico).

Loos, R. and Bouchard, C. (2003) 'Obesity – Is It a Genetic Disorder?', *Journal of Internal Medicine*, 254(5): 401–25.

Lopez-Cervantes, M., Torres-Sanchez, L., Tobias, A. and Lopez-Carrillo, L. (2004) 'Dichlorodiphenyldicloroethane Burden and Breast Cancer Risk: A Meta-Analysis of the Epidemiological Evidence', *Environmental Health Perspectives*, 112(2).

Lord Laming (2009) *The Protection of Children in England: A Progress Report,* HC 330 (London: TSO).

Loughborough University (2008) *Well@Work Evaluation* (London: British Heart Foundation).

Low, A. (2004) 'Measure for Measure', *Health Service Journal*, 6th May 2004.

Low, N. (2007) 'Screening Programmes for Chlamydial Infection: When Will We Ever Learn?', *British Medical Journal*, 334: 725–8.

Lowe, R. (2007) *Facing the Future A Review of the Role of Health Visitors* (London: Department of Health).

Lowndes, V. and Skelcher, C. (1998) 'The Dynamics of Multi-organisational Partnerships: An Analysis of Changing Modes of Governance', *Public Administration*, 76: 313–33.

Lowndes, V., Pratchett, L. and Stoker, G. (2001a) 'Trends in Public Participation: Part 1: Citizen's Perspectives', *Public Administration*, 79(1): 205–22.

Lowndes, V., Pratchett, L. and Stoker, G. (2001b) 'Trends in Public Participation: Part 2: Citizen's Perspectives', *Public Administration*, 79(2): 445–55.

Lucas, K. and Lloyd, B. (2005) *Health Promotion: Evidence and Experience* (London: Sage).

Ludvigsen, A. and Sharma, N. (2004) *Burger Boy and Sporty Girl: Children and Young People's Attitudes Towards Food in School* (Essex: Barnardo's).

Lukes, S. (1974) *Power: A Radical View* (London: Macmillan – now Palgrave Macmillan).

Lund, B. (2006) *Understanding Housing Policy* (Bristol: Policy Press).

Lundberg, O. (1993) 'The Impact of Childhood Living Conditions on Illness and Mortality in Adulthood' *Social Science & Medicine*, 36(8): 1047–52.

Lynch, J. and Kaplan, G. (1997) 'Understanding How Inequality in the Distribution of Income Affects Health', *Journal of Health Psychology*, 2(3): 297–314.

Lynch, J., Smith, G., Harper, S. et al. (2004) 'Is Income Inequality a Determinant of Population Health? Part One: A Systematic Review', *Milbank Quarterly*, 82(2): 5–99.

McAllister, F. (2005) *Wellbeing Concepts and Challenges: Discussion Paper* (London: Sustainable Development Research Network).

McCallum, A. (1997) 'Public Health, Health Promotion and Broader Health Strategy' in Iliffe, S. and Munro, J. (eds) *Healthy Choices: Future Options for the NHS* (London: Lawrence and Wishart), pp. 94–119.

McCann, D., Barrett, A., Cooper, A. et al. (2007) 'Food Additives and Hyperactive Behaviour in 3 Year Old 8/9 Year Old Children in the Community: A Randomised, Double-Blinded, Placebo-controlled Trial', *The Lancet* (doi: 10.1016/SO140-6736(07)613063-3 accessed 11.5.10).

McCarthy, M. (2002) 'What's Going on at the World Health Organisation?', *The Lancet*, 360: 1108–12.

McClure, R., Turner, C., Peel, N. et al. (2008) 'Population-Based Interventions for the Prevention of Fall-Related Injuries in Older People', *The Cochrane Database of Systematic Reviews*, 2008, Issue 4.

McColl, K. (2008) 'The Fattening Truth About Restaurant Food', *British Medical Journal*, 337: a2229.

MacCoun, R. and Reuter, P. (2001) 'Evaluating Alternative Cannabis Regimes', *British Journal of Psychiatry*, 178: 123–8.

McCulloch, A. (2001) 'Social Environments and Health: Cross Sectional National Survey', *British Medical Journal*, 323: 208–9.

McCurry, J. (2008) 'G8 Meeting Disappoints on Global Health', *The Lancet*, 372: 191–4.

McDermott, L. (2005) Systematic Review of Social Marketing Nutrition and Food Safety Standards (University of Stirling, Institute of Social Marketing).

McDonagh, M., Whiting, P., Wilson, P. et al (2000) 'Systematic Review of Water Fluorida-tion', *British Medical Journal*, 321: 7 October, 855–9.

MacDonagh, O. (1977) *Early Victorian Government* (London: Weidenfield & Nicolson).

MacDonald, T. (1998) *Rethinking Health Promotion* (London: Routledge).

MacDonald, Z., Tinsley, L., Collingwood, J. et al. (2005) *Measuring the Harm from Illegal Drugs Using the Drug Harm Index* (London: Home Office).

MacDowall, W., Bonell, C. and Davies, M. (2006) *Health Promotion Practice* (Maidenhead: Open University).

McGrath, K. (2003) 'An Earlier Age of Breast Cancer Diagnosis Related to more Frequent use of Antiperspirants/Deodorants and Underarm Shaving', *European Journal of Cancer Prevention*, 12(6): 479–85.

MacGregor, A. (2006) *Evaluation of the Public Health Practitioner Initiative in Scotland* (Edinburgh: NHS Scotland).

McGregor, D., Partensky, C., Wilburn, J. and Rice, J. (1998) 'An IARC Evaluation of Polychlorinated Dibenzo-P-Dioxins and Polychlorinated Dibenzofurans as Risk Factors in Human Carcinogenesis', *Environmental Health Perspectives*, 106(Supp 2): 755–60.

McGregor, J.A. (2006) *Researching Well-being: From Concepts to Methodology*, WeD Working Paper 20 (Bath: ESRC Research Group on Well-being in Developing Countries).

McInnes, A. and Barrett, A. (2007) 'Drug Education' in Simpson, M., Shildrick, T. and Macdonald, R. *Drugs in Britain – Supply, Consumption and Control* (Basingstoke: Palgrave Macmillan), pp. 125–40.

Macintyre, S., Ellaway, A. and Cummins, S. (2002) 'Place Effects on Health: How Can We Conceptualise, Operationalise and Measure Them?', *Social Science & Medicine*, 55(1): 125–39.

Macintyre, S., Hiscock, R., Kearns, A. and Ellaway, A. (2001) 'Housing Tenure and Car Access: Further Exploration of the Nature of their Relationships with Health in a UK Setting', *Journal of Epidemiology and Community Health*, 55(5): 330–1.

Macintyre, S., Macdonald, L. and Ellaway, A. (2008) 'Do Poorer People Have Poorer Access to Local Resources and Facilities? The Distribution of Local Resources by Area Deprivation in Glasgow, Scotland', *Social Science & Medicine*, 67: 900–14.

Macintyre, S., McIver, S. and Soomans, A. (1993) 'Area, Class and Health: Should We Be Focusing on Places or People?', *Journal of Social Policy*, 22: 213–34.

McKee, M. (2005) 'European Health Policy: Where Now?', *European Journal of Public Health*, 15(6): 557–8.

McKee, M. (2006) 'A European Alcohol Strategy,' *British Medical Journal,* 333: 871–2.

McKee, M. (2007) 'International Public Health' in Hunter, D. and Griffiths, S. (eds) (2007) *New Perspectives in Public Health* (2nd edn) (Oxford: Radcliffe), pp. 71–6.

McKee, M. and Raine, R. (2005) 'Choosing Health? First Choose your Philosophy', *The Lancet,* 365: 29 January, 369–71.

McKeganey, N. (2005) *Random Testing of Schoolchildren: A Shot in the Arm or a Shot in the Foot for Drug Prevention?* (York: Joseph Rowntree Foundation).

McKeganey, N., Forsyth, A., Barnard, M. and Hay, G. (1996) 'Designer Drinks and Drunkenness amongst a Sample of Scottish Schoolchildren', *British Medical Journal,* 313: 401.

Mackenbach, J. and Stronks, K. (2002) 'A Strategy for Tackling Health Inequalities in the Netherlands', *British Medical Journal,* 325: 1029–32.

Mackenbach, J.P. (2005) *Health Inequalities: Europe in Profile* (Rotterdam: Eramus).

Mackenzie, M. (2008) 'Doing Public Health and Making Public Health Practitioners: Putting Policy into Practice in Starting Well', *Social Science & Medicine,* 67: 1028–37.

Mackenzie, M., Shute, J., Berzins, K. and Judge, K. (2004) *The Independent Evaluation of 'Starting Well: Final Report* (Edinburgh: Scottish Executive).

McKeown, T. (1976) *The Role of Medicine: Dream, Mirage or Nemesis* (London: Nuffield Provincial Hospital Trust).

Mackereth, C. (2006) *Community Development: New Challenges, New Opportunities* (London: Community Practitioners and Health Visitors' Association).

McKinlay, J.B. (1979) 'Epidemiological and Political Developments of Social Policies Regarding Public Health', *Social Science & Medicine,* 13A: 541–8.

McKinlay, J.B. (2005) 'A Case for Refocusing Upstream: The Political Economy of Illness' in Conrad, P. (ed.) *The Sociology of Health and Illness: Critical Perspectives* (7th edn) (New York: Worth Publishers), pp. 551–64.

McMillan, D., Sattar, N., Lean, M. and McArdle, C. (2006) 'Obesity and Cancer', *British Medical Journal,* 333: 1109–11.

McPherson, K., Taylor, S. and Coyle, E. (2001) For and Against: Public Health Does not Need to be Led by Doctors,' *British Medical Journal,* 323: 1593–6.

Macran, S., Clark, L. and Joshi, H. (1996) 'Women's Health: Dimensions and Differentials', *Social Science & Medicine,* 42: 1203–16.

McSweeney, T., Hough, M. and Turnbull, P.J. (2007) 'Drugs and Crime: Exploring the Links' in Simpson, M., Shildrick, T. and MacDonald, R. (eds) *Drugs in Britain: Supply, Consumption and Control* (Basingstoke: Palgrave MacMillan).

McTiernan, A., Kooperberg, C., White, E. et al. 2003) 'Recreational Physical Activity and the Risk of Breast Cancer in Postmenopausal Women', *The Journal of the American Medical Association,* 290(10): 1331–6.

Madsen, K., Hviid, A., Vestergaard, M. et al. (2002) A Population-based Study of Measles, Mumps and Rubella Vaccination and Autism', *The New England Journal of Medicine,* 347(19): 1477–82.

MAFF (Ministry of Agriculture Fisheries and Food) (1998) *A Review of Antimicrobial Resistance in the Food Chain. A Technical Report for MAFF* (London: MAFF).

MAFF and HSE (Health and Safety Executive) (1999) *Annual Report of the Working Party on Pesticide Residues* (London: MAFF).

Maheswaran, R., Pearson, T., Munro, J. et al. (2007) 'Impact of NHS Walk in Centres on Primary Care Access Times: Ecological Study', *British Medical Journal* Online (doi: 10.1136/bmj.39122.704051.55 (9 March) accessed 18.09.07).

Majone, G. (1989) *Evidence, Argument and Persuasion in the Policy Processes* (New Haven: Yale University Press).

Makela, A., Nuorti, J.P. and Peltola, H. (2002) 'Neurologic Disorders after Measles-Mumps-Rubella Vaccination', *Paediatrics,* 110(5): 957–63.

Malik, V., Schulze, M. and Hu, F. (2006) 'Intake of Sugar-Sweetened Beverages and Weight Gain: A Systematic Review', *The American Journal of Clinical Nutrition,* 84(2): 274–88.

Mallam, K., Metcalf, B., Kirkby, J. et al. (2003) 'Contribution of Timetabled Physical Education to Total Physical Activity in Primary School Children: Cross Sectional Study', *British Medical Journal,* 327: 529–93.

Mallinson, S., Popay, J., Kowarzik, U. and Mackian, S. (2006) 'Developing the Public Health Workforce: A Communities of Practice Perspective', *Policy and Politics,* 34(2): 265–85.

Maloney, W., Jordan, G. and McLaughlin, A. (1994) 'Interest Groups and the Policy Process: The Insider/Outsider Model revisited', *Journal of Public Policy,* 14(1): 17–38.

Mamudu, H., Hammond, R. and Glantz, S. (2008) 'Tobacco Industry Attempts to Counter the World Bank Report Curbing the Epidemic and Obstruct the WHO Framework Convention on Tobacco Control', *Social Science & Medicine,* 67: 1690–9.

Mangtani, P., Jolly, D., Watson, J. and Rodrigues, L. (1995) 'Socioeconomic Deprivation and Notification Rates for Tuberculosis in London During 1982–91', *British Medical Journal,* 310: 963–6.

Mann, M., Bradley, R. and Hughes, K. (1998) 'Global Scale Temperature Patterns and Climate Forcing Over the Past Six Centuries', *Nature*, 392: 779–92.

Marks, L. (2006) 'An Evidence Base for Tackling Inequalities in Health: Distraction or Necessity?', *Critical Public Health*, 16(1): 61–71.

Marmot, M. (2004) *Status Syndrome* (London: Bloomsbury).

Marmot, M.G. and Shipley, M.J. (1996) 'Do Socioeconomic Differences in Mortality Persist After Retirement? 25 Year Follow Up of Civil Servants from the First Whitehall Study', *British Medical Journal*, 313: 1177–80.

Marmot, M., Rose, G., Shipley, M. and Hamilton, P. (1978) 'Employment Grade and Coronary Heart Disease in British Civil Servants', *Journal of Epidemiology and Community Health*, 32: 244–9.

Marmot, M., Stansfield, S., Patel, C. et al. (1991) 'Health Inequalities Among British Civil Servants: The Whitehall II Study', *The Lancet*, 337: 1387–93.

Marquand, D. (1988) *The Unprincipled Society* (London: Fontana).

Marsh, A. (2007) 'Housing, Health and Wellbeing' in Scriven, A. and Garman, S. *Public Health Social Context and Action* (Maidenhead: Open University), pp. 207–18.

Marsh, A. and McKay, S. (1994) *Poor Smokers* (London: Policy Studies Institute).

Marsh, A., Gordon, D., Pantazis, C. and Heslop, P. (1999) *Home Sweet Home? The Impact of Poor Housing on Health* (Bristol: The Policy Press).

Marsh, D. and Rhodes, R. (eds) (1992) *Policy Networks in British Government* (Oxford: Clarendon).

Marsh, D. and Smith, M. (2005) 'Understanding Policy Networks: Towards a Dialectical Approach', *Political Studies*, 48(4): 4–21.

Martin, J. (2006) 'Overview and Scrutiny as a Dialogue of Accountability for Democratic Local Government', *Public Policy and Administration*, 21(3): 57–69.

Mathiason, N. (2008) 'HSE's "Shocking" Failure Costs Lives, Says Union', *Observer*, May 11.

Matka, E., Barnes, M. and Sullivan, H. (2002) 'Health Action Zones: Creating Alliances to Achieve Change', *Policy Studies*, 23: 97–106.

Maynard, M., Gunnell, D., Emmett, P. et al. (2003) 'Fruit, Vegetables, and Antioxidants in Childhood and Risk of Adult Cancer: The Boyd Orr Cohort', *Journal of Epidemiology and Community Health*, 57: 218–25.

Mayor of London (2004) *The London Plan* (London: Mayor of London).

Mayor of London (2006) *Healthy and Sustainable Food for London: The Mayor's Food Strategy Summary* (London: London Development Agency).

Mayor of London and London Sustainable Development Commission (2003) *A Sustainable Development Framework for London* (London: Mayor of London).

Mayor, S. (1999) 'Swedish Study Questions Mammography Screening Programmes', *British Medical Journal*, 6 March, 621.

Mayor, S. (2004) 'Researcher Objects to Drink Industry Representative Sitting on Alcohol Research Body', *British Medical Journal*, 329: 10 July, 71.

Meads, G., Killoran, A., Ashcroft, J. and Cornish, Y. (1999) *Mixing Oil and Water* (London: Health Education Authority).

Mechanic, D. (2003) Who Shall Lead? Is There a Future for Population Health? *Journal of Health Politics, Policy and Law*, 28(2–3): 214–42.

Medical Research Council (MRC) Human Nutrition Research (2007) *The 'Healthy Living' Social Marketing Initiative: A Review of the Evidence* (London: Department of Health).

Melhuish, E., Belsky, J., Leyland, A. and Barnes, J. (2008) 'Effects of Fully-Established Sure Start Local Programmes on 3 year old Children and Their Families Living in England: A Quasi-Experimental Observational Study', *The Lancet*, 372: 1641–7.

Melhuish, E., Belsky, J., Leyland, A. et al. (2005) *Early Impacts of Sure Start Local Programmes on Children and Families* (London: Institute for Study of Children, Families and Social Issues).

Mellor, J. and Milyo, J. (2001) 'Reexamining the Evidence of an Ecological Association Between Income Inequality and Health', *Journal of Health Politics*, 26(3): 487–522.

Meltzer, D., Fryers, T. and Jenkins, R. (2004) *Social Inequalities and the Distribution of Common Mental Disorders* (Hove: Psychology Press).

Melzer, D. (2008) 'Genetic Tests for Common Diseases: New Insights, Old Concerns', *British Medical Journal*, 336: 590–1.

Melzer, D. and Zimmern, R. (2002) 'Genetics and Medicalisation', *British Medical Journal*, 324(7342): 863–4.

Mencap (2007) *Death by Indifference* (London: Mencap).

Mental Health Foundation and Sustain (2006) *Feeding Minds: The Impact of Food on Mental Health* (London: Mental Health Foundation).

Metcalf, B., Voss, L., Jeffrey, A. et al. (2004) 'Physical Activity Cost of the School Run: Impact on Schoolchildren of Being Driven to School (EarlyBird 22)', *British Medical Journal*, 329: 832–3.

Metcalfe, O. and Higgins, C. (2009) 'Healthy Public Policy – Is Health Impact Assessment the Cornerstone?', *Public Health*, 123: 296–301.

Micha, R., Wallace, S. and Mozaffarian, D. (2010) 'Red and Processed Meat Consumption and Risk of Incident Coronary Heart Disease, Stroke And Diabetes Mellitus', *Circulation*, 121: 2271-83.

Midgley, J. (2009) *Just Desserts? Securing Global Food Futures* (Newcastle: Institute for Public Policy Research).

Milburn, A. (2000) 'A Healthier Nation and a Healthier Economy: The Contribution of a Modern NHS (LSE Health annual lecture) 8 March (London: London School of Economics).

Miles, A. (1991) *Women, Health and Medicine* (Buckingham: Open University Press).

Milewa, T., Valentine, J. and Calnan, M. (1998) 'Managerialism and Active Citizenships in Britian's Reformed Health Service: Power and Community in an Era of Decentralisation', *Social Science & Medicine*, 47: 507–17.

Milio, N. (1986) *Promoting Health Through Public Policy* (Ottawa: Canadian Public Health Association).

Mill, J.S. (1974) *On Liberty* (Harmondsworth: Pelican).

Miller, A. (1980) 'The Canadian National Breast Cancer Screening Study', *Clinical Investigative Medicine*, 4: 227–58.

Miller, K., Siscovick, D., Sheppard, L. et al. (2007) 'Long-term Exposure to Air Pollution and Incidence of Cardiovascular Events in Women', *New England Journal of Medicine*, 356(5): 447–58.

Mills, M. (1992) *The Politics of Dietary Change* (Aldershot: Dartmouth).

Mills, M. and Saward, M. (1993) 'Liberalism, Democracy and Prevention' in Mills, M. (ed.) (1993) *Prevention, Health and British Politics* (Aldershot: Avebury), pp. 161–73.

Millstone, E. and van Zwanenberg, P. (2002) 'The Evolution of Food Safety Policy-Making Institutions in the UK, EU and Codex Alimentarius', *Social Policy and Administration*, 36(6): 593–609.

Millward, L., Kelly, P. and Nutbeam, D. (2003) *Public Health Intervention Research – The Evidence* (London: Health Development Agency).

Milne, E. (2005) 'NHS Smoking Cessation Services and Smoking Prevalence: Observational Study', *British Medical Journal*, 330: 760.

MIND (2005) *Stress and Mental Health in the Workplace* (London: MIND).

Ministry of Social Affairs and Health (2001) *Government Resolution to the Health 2015 Public Health Programme* (Helsinki: Ministry of Social Affairs and Health).

Mirick, D., Davis, S. and Thomas, D. (2002) 'Antiperspirant Use and the Risk of Breast Cancer', *Journal of the National Cancer Institute*, 94: 1578–80.

Mishan, E.J. (1990) 'Narcotics: The Problem and the Solution', *Political Quarterly*, 61(4): 441–62.

Mitchell, R., Dorling D. and Shaw, M. (2000) *Inequalities in Life and Death: What if Britain Were More Equal?* (Bristol: The Policy Press).

Mitchell, R. and Popham, F. (2008) 'Effect of Exposure to Natural Environment on Health Inequalities: An Observational Population Study', *The Lancet*, 372(9650): 1655–60.

Monaghan, L. (2008a) *Men and the War on Obesity: A Sociological Study* (London: Routledge).

Monaghan, M. (2008b) 'The Evidence Base in UK Drug Policy: The New Rules of Engagement', *Policy and Politics*, 36(1): 145–50.

Montgomery, J. (2003) *Health Care Law* (2nd edn) (Oxford: Oxford University Press).

Moon, A., Mullee, M., Thompson, R. et al. (1999) 'Helping Schools to Become Health Promoting Environments: An Evaluation of the Wessex Healthy Schools Awards', *Health Promotion International*, 14(2): 111–22.

Moon, G. and Lupton, C. (1995) 'Within Acceptable Limits: Health Care Provider Perspectives on Community Health Councils in the Reformed British National Health Service, *Policy and Politics*, 23(4): 335–46.

Moon, G., Quarendon, G., Barnard, S. et al. (2007) 'Fat Nation: Deciphering the Distinctive Geographies of Obesity in England', *Social Science & Medicine*, 65: 20–31.

Mooney, G. and Healey, A. (1991) 'Strategy Full of Good Intentions', *British Medical Journal*, 303: 1119–20.

Mooney, H. (2006a) 'Sir Liam: Public Health was Rushed', *Health Service Journal*, 7 December, p. 7.

Mooney, H. (2006b) 'London PCTs Expect to Spend a Sixth of Choosing Health Cash', *Health Service Journal* 27 July, p. 5.

Moore, T., Zammit, S., Lingford-Hughes, A. et al. (2007) 'Cannabis Use and the Risk of Psychotic or Affective Mental Health Outcomes: A Systematic Review', *The Lancet*, 370: 319–28.

Moran, G. (1989) 'Public Health at Risk', *Health Service Journal*, 1 June, 668–9.

Morgan, A. and Popay, J. (2007) 'Community Participation for Health: Reducing Health Inequalities and Building Social Capital' in Scriven, A. and Garman, S. *Public Health: Social Context and Action* (Maidenhead: Open University Press), pp. 154–65.

Morgan, K. (2006) 'School Food and the Public Domain: The Politics of the Public Plate', *Political Quarterly*, 77(3): 379–87.

Morgan, M. (2000) 'Ecstasy (MDMA): A Review of its Possible Persistent Psychological Effects', *Psychopharmacology*, 152: 230–48.

Morison, J. (2000) 'The Government Voluntary Sector Compacts: Governance, Governmentality and Civil Society', *Journal of Law and Society*, 27: 98–132.

Morley, A. and Campbell, F. (2003) *People, Power and Health: A Green Paper on Democratising the NHS* (London: Democratic Health Network).

Morris, J.K. (1980) 'Are Health Services Important to People's Health?', *British Medical Journal*, 280: 167–8.

Morris, J.K., Cook, D.G. and Shaper, A.G. (1994) 'Loss of Employment and Mortality', *British Medical Journal*, 308: 1135–9Morris, R.J. (1976) *Cholera 1832: A Social Response to an Epidemic* (London: Croom Helm).

Morris, S., Sutton, M. and Gravelle, H. (2005) 'Inequity and Inequality in the Use of Health Care in England: An Empirical Investigation', *Social Science & Medicine*, 60: 1251–66.

Moynihan, D. (1998) *Too Much Medicine: The Business of Health and its Risks* (Sydney: ABC Books).

Moynihan, R. (2006) 'Obesity Task Force Linked to WHO Takes "Millions" From Drug Firms', *British Medical Journal*, 332: 1412 (doi: 10.1136/bmj.332.7555.1412a accessed 14.5.10).

MRC (Medical Research Council) Working Group (2002) *Water Fluoridation and Health* (London: MRC).

Mullins, D., Lee, P., Murie, A. et al. (2006*) Housing Policy in the UK* (Basingstoke: Palgrave Macmillan).

Mulvihill, C. and Quigley, R. (2003) *The Management of Obesity and Overweight* (London: Health Development Agency).

Muntaner, C., Lynch, J. and Davey Smith, G. (2001) 'Social Capital, Disorganised Communities and the Third Way', *International Journal of Health Services,* 31(2): 213–37.

Murali, V. and Oyebode, F. (2004) 'Poverty, Social Inequality and Mental Health', *Advances in Psychiatric Treatment*, 10: 216–24.

Murdock, G., Petts, J. and Horlick-Jones, T. (2003) 'After Amplification: Rethinking the Role of the Media in Risk Communication' in Pidgeon, N., Kasperson, R. and Slovic, P. (eds) *Social Amplification of Risk* (Cambridge: Cambridge University Press), pp. 156–78.

Muscat, J., Britton, J., Djordjevic, M.V. et al. (2003) 'Adipose Concentrations of Organochlorine Compounds and Breast Cancer Recurrence in Long Island, New York', *Cancer Epidemiology Biomarkers Prevention*, 12(12): 1474–8.

Myers, P., Barnes, J. and Brodie, I. (2004) *Partnership Working In Sure Start Local Programmes. Synthesis of Early Findings from Local Programme Evaluations* (London: Institute for the Study of Children, Families and Social Issues).

Mytton, O., Gray, A., Rayner, M. and Rutter, H. (2007) 'Could Targeted Food Taxes Improve Health?', *Journal of Epidemiology and Community Health*, 61: 689–94.

NACNE (National Advisory Committee on Nutrition Education) (1983) *A Discussion Paper on Proposals for Nutrition Guidelines for Health Education in Britain* (London: Health Education Council).

NAfW (National Assembly for Wales) (1998) Strategic Framework: Better Health, Better Wales (Cardiff, NAfW).

NAfW (1999a) *Realising the Potential: A Strategic Framework for Nursing, Midwifery and Health Visiting on Wales into the 21st Century* (Cardiff: NAfW).

NAfW (1999b) *Developing Health Impact Assessment in Wales* (Cardiff: NAfW).

NAfW (2000a) *A Strategic Framework for Promoting Sexual Health in Wales* (Cardiff: National Assembly for Wales).

NAfW (2000b) *Tackling Substance Misuse in Wales: A Partnership Approach* (Cardiff: NAfW).

NAfW (2001) *Improving Health in Wales* (Cardiff: National Assembly for Wales).

Nagle, D.L., McGrail, S.H., Vitale, J. et al. (1999) 'The Mahogany Protein is a Receptor Involved in Suppression of Obesity', *Nature*, 398: 148–52.

Naidoo, J. and Wills, J. (2000a) *Health Promotion: Foundations for Practice* (2nd edn) (London: Balliere Tindall).

Naidoo, J. and Wills, J. (2000b) 'Health Promotion in Schools' in Naidoo, J. and Wills, J. *Health Promotion Foundations for Practice* (2nd edn) (London: Bailliere Tindall), pp. 281–94.

Naidoo, J. and Wills, J. (2005) *Public Health and Health Promotion: Developing Practice* (2nd edn) (London: Balliere Tindall).

Naidoo, J., Orme, J. and Barrett, G. (2003) 'Capacity and Capability in Public Health' in Orme, J., Powell, J., Taylor, P. et al. *Public Health for the 21st Century* (Berkshire: Open University Press), pp. 79–92.

Naish, J. (2006) 'Our Health, Our Care, Our Say', *Journal of Medical Screening*, 13(2): 56–7.

Nakajima, K., Dharmage, S., Carlin, J. et al. (2007) 'Is Childhood Immunisation Associated with Atopic Disease from Age 7 to 32 Years?' *Thorax*, 62: 270–5.

NAO (National Audit Office) (1996a) *Health of the Nation: A Progress Report,* HC 656 Session 1995–6 (London: HMSO).

NAO (1996b) *Improving Health in Wales*, HC 633 Session 1995–6 (London: HMSO).

NAO (2000) *The Management and Control of Hospital Acquired Infections in Acute NHS Trusts in England,* HC 230 Session 1999–2000 (London: TSO).

NAO (2001) *Tackling Obesity in England,* HC 220 Session 2000–01 (London: TSO).

NAO (2002) *NHS Direct in England,* HC 505 2001–2 (London, TSO).

NAO (2004a) *Getting Citizens Involved: Community Participation in Neighbourhood Renewal,* HC 1070 Session 2002–03 (London: TSO).

NAO (2004b) *Improving Patient Care by Reducing the Risk of Hospital Acquired Infection: A Progress Report,* HC 876 Session 2003–4 (London: TSO).

NAO (2004c) *The Drug Treatment and Testing Order: Early Lessons,* HC 366 Session 2003–4 (London: The National Audit Office).

NAO (2006) *Sure Start Children's Centres,* HC 104 Session 2006–07 (London: TSO).

NAO (2008a) *The Home Office: Reducing the Risk of Violent Crime,* HC 241 Session 2007–08 (London: NAO).

NAO (2008b) *Reducing Alcohol Harm: Health Services in England for Alcohol Misuse,* HC 1049 (London: TSO).

NAO (2009a) *Reducing Healthcare Associated Infections in Hospitals in England,* Session 2008–09, HC 812 (London: TSO).

NAO (2009b) *Managing the Waste PFI Programme,* Session 2008–09, HC 66 (London: TSO).

NAO (2009c) *Air Quality* (London: NAO).

NAO (2010a) *Tackling Problem Drug Use,* Session 2009–10, HC 297 (London: TSO).

NAO (2010b) *Government Funding for Developing Renewable Energy Technologies,* HC 35 Session 2010-11 (London: NAO).

NAO, Healthcare Commission, Audit Commission (2006) *Tackling Child Obesity – First Steps,* HC 801 Session 2005–06 (London: TSO).

National Center for Health Statistics (2001) *Healthy People 2000 Final Review* (Hyattsville, MD: Public Health Service).

National Consumer Council (2006) *It's Our Health! Realising the Potential of Social Marketing* (London: NCC).

National Equality Panel (2010) *Report of the National Equality Panel* (London: Government Equalities Office).

National Statistics and Department for Transport (DfT) (2007) *Transport Trends* (London: TSO).

National Statistics and Department for Transport (DfT) (2010) *Transport Trends* (London: TSO).

National Statistics Online (2009) *Household Income – Top Fifth Four Times Better off Than Bottom Fifth* (London: TSO).

Navarro, V. (1976) *Medicine Under Capitalism* (London: Croom Helm).

Navarro, V. (1978) *Class, Struggle, the State and Medicine* (Oxford: Martin Robertson).

Nazroo, J.Y. (1998) 'Genetic, Cultural or Socio-economic Vulnerability? Explaining Ethnic Inequalities in Health', *Sociology of Health and Illness,* 20(5): 710–30.

Neal, M. and Davies, C. (1998) *The Corporation Under Siege?* (London: Social Affairs Unit).

Needham, C. (2003) *Citizens-Consumers: New Labour's Marketplace Democracy* (London: Catalyst).

Nelson, M., Nicholas, J., Suleiman, S. et al. (2006) *School Meals in Primary Schools in England* (London: Department for Education and Skills).

Neovius, M., Sundstrom, J. and Rasmussen, F. (2009) 'Combined Effects of Overweight and Smoking in Late Adolescence on Subsequent Mortality: Nationwide Cohort Study', *British Medical Journal,* 338: b496.

Neroth, P. (2004) 'Fat of the Land' (www.thelancet.com) 364: 651–2.

Nestle, M. (2003) *Food Politics* (Berkeley, CA: University of California Press).

Nettleton, S. and Burrows, R. (1997) 'Knit Your Own Without a Pattern: Health Promotion Specialists in an Internal Market', *Social Policy and Administration,* 31(2): 191–201.

Neuman, M., Bitton, A. and Glantz, S. (2002) 'Tobacco Industry Strategies for Influencing European Community Tobacco Advertising Legislation', *The Lancet,* 359(9314): 1323–30.

Neumann, I., Elian, R. and Nahum, H. (1978) 'The Danger of Yellow Dyes (Tartrazine) to Allergic Subjects', *Clinical Allergy,* 8: 65–8.

Neustaedter, R. (2002) *The Vaccine Guide: Risks and Benefits for Children and Adults* (Berkeley, CA: North Atlantic Books).

New Economics Foundation (NEF) (2003) *The Politics of Happiness: A NEF Discussion Paper* (London: NEF).

New Economics Foundation (2004) *A Well-being Manifesto for a Flourishing Society* (London: NEF).

New Economics Foundation (2009) The *Unhappy Planet Index 2.0: Why Good Lives Don't Cost the Earth* (www.neweconomics.org/projects/happy-planet-index accessed 21.5.10).

New Economics Foundation (2010) *Growth Isn't Possible: Why We Need a New Economic Direction* (London: NEF).

Newburn, T. and Elliott, J. (1998) *Police Anti-Drugs Strategies: Tackling Drugs Three Years On,* Crime Detection and Prevention Series 89 (London: Home Office).

Newby, J. and Howard, C. (2005) 'Environmental Influences in Cancer Aetiology', *Journal of Nutritional and Environmental Medicine,* 15: 56–114.

Newcombe, R. (1996) 'Live and Let Die: Is Methadone More Likely to Kill You Than Heroin?', *ISDD Druglink*, 11(1): 9–12.

Newcombe, R. (2006) *A Review of the UK Drug Strategy PSA Targets and Drug Harm Index* (Manchester: Lifeline).

Newcombe, R. (2007) 'Trends in the Prevalence of Illicit Drug Use in Britain' in Simpson, M., Shildrick, T. and Macdonald, R. *Drugs in Britain – Supply, Consumption and Control* (Basingstoke: Palgrave Macmillan).

Newman, J. (2001) *Modernising Governance: New Labour Policy and Society* (London: Sage).

Newman, T.B. and Hulley, S.B. (1996) 'Carcinogenicity of Lipid Lowering Drugs', *Journal of American Medical Association*, 275(1): 55–60.

NFER (National Foundation for Education Research) (1998) *The Health Promoting School: A Summary of the ENHPS Evaluation Project in England* (London: Health Education Authority).

NHS Alliance (2002) *The Vision in Practice* (Retford: NHS Alliance).

NHS Centre for Reviews and Dissemination (1999) 'Preventing the Uptake of Smoking in Young People', *Effective Health Care*, 5(5): 12.

NHS Confederation (2004) *Making a Difference: How Primary Care Trusts are Transforming the NHS* (London: NHS Confederation).

NHS Health Scotland (2005) *Competencies for Health Promotion Practitioners: Report of Working Group* (Edinburgh: NHS Health Scotland).

NHS Information Centre (2007) *Drug Use, Smoking and Drinking among Young People in England in 2007* (Leeds: NHS Information Centre).

NHS Information Centre (2008a) *National Child Measurement Programme: 2007/08 School Year Headline Results* (London: Department for Health, Department for Children, Schools and Families).

NHS Information Centre (2008b) *Statistics on Drug Misuse, England* (Leeds: NHS Information Centre).

NHS Information Centre (2008c) *Statistics on Alcohol, England* (Leeds: NHS Information Centre).

NHS Information Centre (2009a) *Statistics on Obesity, Physical Activity and Diet; England* (Leeds: NHS Information Centre) (www.ic.nhs.uk).

NHS Information Centre (2009b) *Statistics on Smoking, England* 2009 (Leeds: NHS Information Centre).

NHS Information Centre (2009c) *Statistics on Alcohol, England* (Leeds: NHS Information Centre).

NHS Information Centre (2010) *Statistics on Obesity, Physical Activity and Diet; England* (Leeds: NHS Information Centre) (www.ic.nhs.uk).

NHS Workforce Review Team (2009) *Assessment of Workforce Priorities 2009/10* (Winchester: NHSWRT) (http://www.wrt.nhs.uk/ accessed 4.5.10)

NHSE (1996) *Promoting Clinical Effectiveness* (Leeds: NHSE).

NHSE/IHSM/NHS Confederation (1998) *In the Public Interest* (London: DoH).

NICE (National Institute for Health and Clinical Excellence) (2004) *The Assessment and Prevention of Falls in Older People* (London: NICE).

NICE (2005) *Housing and Public Health: A Review of Reviews of Interventions for Improving Health* (London: NICE).

NICE (2006a) *Cardiovascular Disease: Statins* (London: NICE).

NICE (2006b) *Obesity: The Prevention, Identification, Assessment and Management of Overweight and Obesity in Adults and Children* (London: NICE).

NICE (2006c) *Four Commonly Used Methods to Increase Physical Activity: Brief Interventions in Primary Care, Exercise Referral Schemes, Pedometers and Community-Based Exercise Programmes for Walking and Cycling* (London: NICE).

NICE (2006d) *Brief Interventions and Referral for Smoking Cessation in Primary Care and Other Settings* (London: NICE).

NICE (2007a) *Community-Based Interventions to Reduce Substance Misuse Among Vulnerable and Disadvantaged Children and Young People* (London: NICE).

NICE (2007b) *Drug Misuse: Psychosocial interventions* (London: NICE).

NICE (2007c) *Drug Misuse: Opioid Detoxification* (London: NICE).

NICE (2007d) *Workplace Health Promotion: How to Help Employees to Stop Smoking* (London: NICE).

NICE (2007e) *Behaviour Change at Population, Community and Individual Levels* (London: NICE).

NICE (2008a) *An Assessment of Community Engagement and Community Development Approaches Including the Collaborative Methodology and Community Champions* (London: NICE).

NICE (2008b) *Promoting Physical Activity in the Workplace* (London: NICE).

NICE (2008c) *Lipid Modification* (London: NICE).

NICE (2008d) *Promoting and Creating Built or Natural Environments That Encourage and Support Physical Activity* (London: NICE).

NICE (2008e) *Smoking Cessation Services in Primary Care, Pharmacies, Local Authorities and Workplaces, Particularly for Manual Working*

Groups, Pregnant Women and Hard to Reach Communities (London: NICE).

NICE (2009a) *Managing Long-term Sickness Absences and Incapacity for Work* (London: NICE).

NICE (2009b) *Promoting Mental Wellbeing Through Productive and Healthy Working Conditions: Guidance for Employers* (London: NICE).

NICE (2009c) *Promoting Physical Activity, Active Play and Sport for Pre-School and School-Age Children and Young People in Family, Pre-School, School and Community Settings* (London: NICE).

Nicoll, A., Jones, J., Aavitsland, P. and Giesecke, J. (2005) 'Proposed New International Health Regulations', *British Medical Journal*, 330: 321–2.

Nilsson, R. (1999) 'Is Environmental Tobacco Smoke a Risk Factor for Lung Cancer?' in Bate, R. (ed.) *What Risk: Science, Politics and Public Health* (London: Butterworth Heinemann), pp. 96–150.

Nilsson, L., Kjellman, N. and Bjorkstein, B. (1998) 'A Randomised Controlled Trial of the Effect of Pertussis Vaccines on Atopic Disease', *Archives of Paediatric and Adolescent Medicine*, 152(8): 734–8.

NIMHE (National Institute for Mental Health in England) (2003) *Inside Outside: Improving Mental Health Services for Black and Minority Ethnic Communities in England* (Leeds: NIMHE).

NIHME (2005) *Making it Possible: Improving Mental Health and Wellbeing in England* (London: NIMHE/Department of Health).

NIMHE (National Institute for Mental Health in England) (2006) *Reaching Out: Evaluation of Three Mental Health Promotion Pilots to Reduce Suicide Among Young Men* (London: NIMHE).

Nocon, A. (1993) 'Made in Heaven', *Health Service Journal*, 2 December, 24–6.

Nolte, E. and McKee, M. (2004) *Does Health Care Save Lives? Avoidable Mortality Revisited* (London: The Nuffield Trust).

Noppa, H., Gengtsson, C., Wedel, H. and Wilhemson, L. (1980) 'Obesity in Relation to Morbidity and Mortality from Cardio-Vascular Disease', *American Journal of Epidemiology*, 111: 682–92.

Northern Ireland Executive (2008) *Programme for Government* (Belfast: NIE).

Northern Ireland Office (2006) *Sustainable Development Strategy for Northern Ireland: First Steps Towards Sustainability* (Belfast: Northern Ireland Office).

Nottingham, C. (1999) *The Pursuit of Serenity: Havelock Ellis and the New Politics* (Amsterdam University Press).

Nozick, R. (1974) *Anarchy, State and Utopia* (London: Blackwell).

NPCRDC (National Primary Care Research and Development Centre) (2006) *The Implementation of Local Authority Scrutiny of Primary Health Care 2002–2005* (NPCRDC: Manchester).

NRPB (National Radiological Protection Board) (2001) 'ELF Electromagnetic Fields and the Risk of Cancer. Report of an Advisory Group on Non-Ionising Radiation', *Doc NRPB*, 12(1): 1–179.

NSC (National Screening Committee) (2000) *Second Report of the UK National Screening Committee* (London: DoH).

NSC (2010) *Advice on Private Screening Being Offered Through GP Practices* (London: NSC) (http://www.screening.nhs.uk/private-screening accessed 10.5.10).

Nuffield Council on Bioethics (1993) *Genetic Screening: Ethical Issues* (London: Nuffield Council on Bioethics).

Nuffield Council on Bioethics (2006) *Genetic Screening: A Supplement to the 1993 Report by the Nuffield Council on Bioethics* (London: Nuffield Council on Bioethics).

Nuffield Council on Bioethics (2007) Public Health Ethical Issues (London: Nuffield Council on Bioethics).

Nugent, N. (2003) *The Government and Politics of the European Union* (5th edn) (Basingstoke: Palgrave Macmillan).

Nugent, N. (2006) *The Government and Politics of the European Union* (6th edn) (Basingstoke: Palgrave Macmillan).

Nursing and Midwifery Council (2004) *Standards of Proficiency for Specialist Community Public Health Nurses* (London: NMC).

Nutt, D., King, L., Saulsbury, W. and Blakemore, C. (2007) 'Development of a Rational Scale to Assess the Harm of Drugs of Potential Misuse', *The Lancet*, 369: 1047–53.

O'Dowd, A. (2008) 'Deaths from Drug Poisoning in English and Welsh Men Reach Five Year Peak', *British Medical Journal*, 337 (doi: 10.1136/bmj.a1521 accessed 17.10.10).

O'Dwyer, L., Baum, F., Kavanagh, A. and Macdougall, C. (2007) 'Do Area-Based Interventions to Reduce Health Inequalities Work? A Systematic Review of Evidence', *Critical Public Health*, 17(4): 317–35.

O'Riordan, T. and Cameron, J. (1994) *Interpreting the Precautionary Principle* (London: Earthscan).

O'Riordan, T. and Weale, A. (1989) 'Administrative Reorganisation and Policy Change: The

Case of Her Majesty's Inspectorate of Pollution', *Public Administration*, 67: 277–94.

Odent, M., Culpin, E. and Kimmel, T. (1994) 'Pertussis Vaccination and Asthma: Is There a Link?', *Journal of the American Medical Association*, 272(8): a-593.

ODPM (Office of Deputy Prime Minister) (2003a) *Evaluation of Local Strategic Partnerships* (London: ODPM).

ODPM (2003b) *Sustainable Communities: Building for the Future* (London: ODPM).

ODPM (2003c) English House Conditions Survey 2001 (London: TSO).

ODPM (2004a) *Mental Health and Social Exclusion: Social Exclusion Unit* (London: ODPM).

ODPM (2004b) *The Impact of Overcrowding on Health & Education: A Review of Evidence and Literature* (London: ODPM).

ODPM (2005a) *Process Evaluation of Plan Rationalisation: Formative Evaluation of Community Strategies* (London: ODPM).

ODPM (2005b) *Planning Policy Statement 1: Delivering Sustainable Development* (London: ODPM).

ODPM (2006) *National Evaluation of Local Strategic Partnerships: Formative Evaluation and Action Research Programme 2002–2005* (London: ODPM).

ODPM and DoH (2004) *Achieving Positive Shared Outcomes in Health and Homelessness* (London: ODPM/DoH).

ODPM and DoH (2005) *Creating Healthier Communities: A Resource Pack for Local Patrnerships* (London: DoH).

OFCOM (Office of Communications) (2004) *Childhood Obesity – Food Advertising in Context: Children's Food Choices, Parents' Understanding and Influence, and the Role of Food Promotion* (London: OFCOM).

OFCOM (2008) *Changes in the Nature and Balance of Television Food Advertising to Children: A Review of HFSS Advertising Restrictions* (London: OFCOM).

Office of the First Minister and Deputy First Minister (OFMDFM) (2004) *Towards an Anti-poverty Strategy: New TSN - the way forward: a consultation document* (Belfast: OFMDFM)

Office of the First Minister and Deputy First Minister (OFMDFM) (2006) *Our Children and Young People – Our Pledge. A Ten Years Strategy for Children and Young People in Northern Ireland 2006–2016* (Belfast: OFMDFM).

Office of the First Minister and Deputy First Minister (OFMDFM) (2007a) *Our Children and Young People: Our Pledge. Action Plan 2007–8* (Belfast: OFMDFM).

Office of the First Minister and Deputy First Minister (OFMDFM) (2007b) *Government's anti poverty strategy and social inclusion strategy for Northern Ireland* (Belfast, OFMDFM).

Office of the First Minister and Deputy First Minister (OFMDFM) (2008) *Our Children and Young People: Our Pledge. Action Plan 2008–11* (Belfast: OFMDFM).Official Journal of the European Communities (1996) *Council Directive 96/61/EC Concerning Integrated Pollution Prevention and Control* (L257/27).

Official Journal of the European Communities (2000) *Proposal for a Decision of the European Parliament and of the Council Establishing a Programme of Community Action to Encourage Cooperation Between Members States to Combat Social Exclusion COM(2000) 368 final*.

Official Journal of the European Union (2008) *EU Drugs Action Plan for 2009–2012*.

Ofsted (2005a) *Every Child Matters: The Framework for the Inspection of Children's Services* (London: Ofsted).

Ofsted (2005b) *Drug Education in Schools* (London: Ofsted).

Ofsted (2006) *Healthy Schools, Healthy Children?* (Manchester: Ofsted).

Ofsted (2007a) *Time for Change? Personal, Social and Health Education* (Manchester: Ofsted).

Ofsted (2007b) *Joint Area Review of Children's Services from April 2007* (London: Ofsted).

Ofsted (2007c) *Food in Schools: Encouraging Healthier Eating* (London: Ofsted).

Ofsted (2008) *How Well Are They Doing? The Impact of Children's Centres and Extended Schools* (London: Ofsted)

Ofsted (2010) *Food in Schools: Progress in Implementing the New School Food Standards* (London: Ofsted).

Ogilvie, D., Egan, M., Hamilton, V. and Petticrew, M. (2004) 'Promoting Walking and Cycling as an Alternative to Using Cars: Systematic Review', *British Medical Journal*, 329: 763.

Ogilvie, D., Gruer, L. and Haw, S. (2005) 'Young People's Access to Tobacco, Alcohol and Other Drugs', *British Medical Journal*, 331: 393–6.

Ollila, E. (2005) 'Global Health Priorities: Priorities of the Wealthy?', *Globalisation and Health*, 1(6): 1–6.

Olsen, A., Sisse, N., Vejborg, I. et al. (2005) 'Breast Cancer Mortality in Copenhagen After Introduction of Mammography Screening: Cohort Study', *British Medical Journal*, 330(7485): 220.

Olsen, O. and Gotzsche, P. (2000) 'Is Screening for Breast Cancer with Mammography Justifiable?', *The Lancet*, 355: 129–34.

Olsen, O. and Gotzsche, P. (2001) 'Cochrane Review on Screening for Breast Cancer with Mammography', *The Lancet*, 358(9290): 1340–2.

Olsson, P., Armelius, K., Nordahl, G. et al. (1999) 'Women With False Positive Screening Mammograms: How do They Cope?', *Journal of Medical Screening*, 6(2): 89–93.

Oneplace (2010) National Overview Report (Oneplace.direct.gov.uk accessed 8.5.10).

ONS (1998) *Social Trends 1997* (London: TSO).

ONS (2002) *Mortality Statistics: Cause Review of Registrar General on Deaths by Cause, Sex and Age in England and Wales* (Newport: ONS).

ONS (2004) *Focus on Ethnicity and Identity* (London: ONS).

ONS (2007) *Health Statistics Quarterly, 36(4): 3. Trends in Life Expectancy by Social Class 1972–2005* (London: ONS).

ONS (2008a) *Analytic Classes and Operational Categories and Sub-Categories of NS-SEC* (London: ONS).

ONS (2008b) *Inequalities in Life Expectancy at 65 in UK* (London: ONS).

ONS (2009a) 'Life Expectancy at Birth Remains Highest in the South of England', *News Release* 21.10.09.

ONS (2009b) *Income Inequality – Little Change since 1980s,* National Statistics online www. statistics.gov.uk (London: ONS).

ONS (2009c) *Mortality Statistics Deaths Registered in 2008* (Newport: ONS).

ONS (2010) 'Women More Likely to Report Poorer Health than Men' *News Release* (London: ONS).

Orbach, S. (1978) *Fat is a Feminist Issue* (London: Hamlyn).

Orbach, S. (2009) *Bodies* (London: Profile Books).

Orey, M. (1999) *Assuming the Risk: The Mavericks, The Lawyers and the Whistleblowers Who Beat Big Tobacco* (Boston: Little Brown).

Orpana, H., Berthelot, J.-M., Kaplan, M. et al. (2009) 'BMI and Mortality: Results From a National Longitudinal Study of Canadian Adults', *Obesity*_(doi: 10.1038/oby.2009.191 accessed 14.5.10).

Osborne, S. and McLaughlin, K. (2002) 'Trends and Issues in the Implementation of Local Voluntary Sector Compacts in England', *Public Money and Management*, 22(1): 55–63.

Osler, M., Prescott, E., Gronbaek, M. et al. (2002) 'Income Inequality, Individual Income and Mortality in Danish Adults', *British Medical Journal*, 324(7328): 13–16.

Ostry, A. (2001) 'International Trade Regulation and Publicly Funded Health Care in Canada', *International Journal of Health Services*, 31(3): 475–80.

Oswald, A. (1997) 'Happiness and Economic Performance,' *Economic Journal*, 107: 1815–31.

Ottewill, R. and Wall, A. (1990) *The Growth and Development of the Community Health Services* (Sunderland. Business Education Publishers).

Ovretveit, J. (1993) 'Purchasing for Health Gain' *European Journal of Public Health*, 392: 77–84.

Owen, J. (2006) 'Street Prices of Cannabis, Ecstasy and Cocaine at an All-time Low', *The Independent* 10 September (www.independent.co.uk accessed 17.5.10).

PAC (Public Accounts Committee) (1989) 26th Report 1988–9, *Coronary Heart Disease*, HC 249 (London: HMSO).

PAC (1992) 2nd Report 1992–3, *Cervical and Breast Screening in England,* HC 58 (London: HMSO).

PAC (2001) 9th Report 2001–2, *Department of Health: Tackling Obesity in England,* HC 421 (London: TSO).

PAC (2007) 8th Report 2006–7: *Tackling Child Obesity – First Steps,* HC 1108 (London: TSO).

PAC (2009a) 5th Report 2008–9: *Programmes to reduce Household energy consumption*, HC 228 (London: TSO).

PAC (2009b) *49th report 2008–9: Improving Road Safety for Pedestrians and Cyclists in Great Britain,* HC 665 (London: TSO).

PAC (2010) 7th Report 2009–10 *Young People's Sexual Health: The National Chlamydia Screening Programme,* HC 283 (London: TSO).

Paci, E. and Duffy, S.W. (2005) 'Overdiagnosis and Overtreatment of Breast Cancer: Overdiagnosis and Overtreatment in Service Screening', *Breast Cancer Research*, 7: 266–70.

Palmer, G., MacInnes, T. and Kenway, P. (2007) *Monitoring Poverty and Social Exclusion 2007* (York: Joseph Rowntree Foundation).

Palmer, G., MacInnes, T. and Kenway, P. (2008) *Monitoring Poverty and Social Exclusion 2008* (York: Joseph Rowntree Foundation).

Palmer, S., Dunstan, F., Fielder, H. et al. (2005) 'Risk of Congenital Anomalies After Opening of Landfill Sites', *Environmental Health Perspectives,* 113(10): 1362–5.

Panter, J. and Jones, A. (2008) 'Associations Between Physical Activity, Perceptions of the Neighbourhood Environment and Access to Facilities in an English City', *Social Science & Medicine*, 67: 1917–23.

Pappas, G. and Moss, N. (2001) 'Health for All in the 21st Century, World Health Organisation Renewal and Equity in Health: A Commentary', *International Journal of Health Services,* 31(3): 647–58.

Parker, H., Aldridge, J. and Measham, F. (1998) *Illegal Leisure: The Normalisation of Adolescent Recreational Drug Use* (London: Routledge).

Parry, G., Van Cleemput, P., Peters, J. et al. (2004) *The Health Status of Gypsies and Travellers in England* (Sheffield: The University of Sheffield).

Parry, N. and Parry, J. (1976) *The Rise of the Medical Profession* (London: Croom Helm).

Parsonnet, J. (1999) *Microbes and Malignancy* (Oxford: Oxford University Press).

Parsonnet, J., Friedman, G.D., Vandersteen, D.P. et al. (1991) 'Helicobacter Pylori Infection and the Risk of Gastric Carcinoma', *New England Journal of Medicine*, 325(16): 1127–31.

Parsons, W. (1995) *Public Policy* (Aldershot: Edward Elgar).

Patterson, R.G. (1948) 'The Health of Towns Association in Great Britain 1844–9', *Bulletin of the History of Medicine (USA)*, 22(4): 373–402.

Patton, G., Coffey, C., Carlin, J. et al. (2002) 'Cannabis Use and Mental Health in Young People: Cohort Study', *British Medical Journal*, 325: 1195–8.

Paxton, W. and Dixon, M. (2004) *The State of the Nation: An Audit of Injustice in the UK* (London: Institute for Public Policy Research (IPPR)).

Pearce, G., Mawson, J. and Ayres, S. (2008) 'Regional Governance in England: A Changing Role for the Government's Regional Offices?', *Public Administration*, 86(2): 443–63.

Pearce, N., Foliaki, S., Sporle, A. and Cunningham, C. (2004) 'Genetics, Race, Ethnicity, and Health', *British Medical Journal*, 328: 1070–2.

Peckham, S. (2003) 'Who Are the Partners in Public Health' in Orme, J. et al. *Public Health for the 21st Century: New Perspectives on Policy, Participation and Practice* (Maidenhead: Open University Press), pp. 59–77.

Peckham, S., and Exworthy, M. (2003) *Primary Care in the UK: Policy Organisation and Management* (Basingstoke: Palgrave Macmillan).

Peckham, S. and Hann, A. (2008) 'General Practice and Public Health: Assessing the Impact of the New GMS Contract', *Critical Public Health*, 18(3): 347–56 (September 2008).

Peckham, S. and Taylor, P. (2003) 'Public Health and Primary Care' in Orme, J., Powell, J., Taylor, P. et al. *Public Health for the 21st Century* (Berkshire: Open University Press), pp. 93–106.

Pekka, P., Pirjo, P. and Ulla, U. (2002) 'Part III. Can we Turn Back the Clock or Modify the Adverse Dynamics? Programme and Policy Issues: Influencing Public Nutrition for Non-Communicable Disease Prevention: From Community Intervention to National Programme – Experiences From Finland', *Public Health Nutrition*, 5(1A): 245–51.

Pell, J., Haw, S., Cobbe, S. et al. (2008) 'Smoke-Free Legislation and Hospitalization for Acute Coronary Syndrome', *The New England Journal of Medicine*, 359: 482–91.

Pelling, M. (1978) *Cholera, Fever and English Medicine 1825–65* (Oxford: Oxford University Press).

Pendleton, A. (2008) 'The Global Politics of Climate Change: After the G8', *Open Democracy* 7 August (www.ippr.org/articles/?id=3226).

Pennington, H. (2003) *When Food Kills: BSE, E Coli, and Disaster Science* (Oxford: Oxford University Press).

Pennington, H. (2009) *The Public Inquiry Into the Outbreak of E Coli O157 in South Wales* (Cardiff: Welsh Assembly Government).

Pereira, J. (1993) 'What Does Equity in Health Mean?', *Journal of Social Policy*, 22(1): 19–48.

Pereira, M., O'Reilly, E., Augustsson, K. et al. (2004) 'Dietary Fibre and Risk of Coronary Heart Disease', *Archives of Internal Medicine*, 164(4): 370–6.

Pereira, M.A., Kartashov, A.I., Ebbeling, C.B. et al. (2005) 'Fast-food Habits, Weight Gain, and Insulin Resistance (the CARDIA study): 15-year Prospective Analysis', *The Lancet*, 365: 36–42.

Perkins, N., Smith, K., Hunter, D. et al. (2009) 'What Counts is What Works? New Labour and Partnerships in Public Health', *Policy and Politics online*.

Perri 6., Leat, D., Seltzer, K. and Stoker, G. (2002) *Towards Holistic Governance: The New Reform Agenda* (Basingstoke: Palgrave Macmillan).

Perterson, A. and Lupton, D. (1996) *The New Public Health; Health and Self in the Age of Risk* (London: Sage).

Pesticide Residue Committee (2007) *Annual Report of the Pesticide Residue Committee 2006* (London: DEFRA).

Peters, A., Von Klot, M., Heier, M. et al. (2004) 'Exposure to Traffic and the Onset of Myocardial Infarction', *New England Journal of Medicine*, 351(17): 1721–30.

Pevalin, D., Taylor, M. and Todd, J. (2008) 'The Dynamics of Unhealthy Housing in the UK: A Panel Data Analysis', *Housing Studies*, 23(5): 679–95.

Pianezza, M., Sellers, G.M. and Tyndale, R.F. (1998) 'Genetics and Cancer', *Nature*, 393: 750.

Pickard, S. (1997) 'The Future Organisation of Community Health Councils,' *Social Policy and Administration*, 31: 274–89.

Pidgeon, N., Kasperson, R. and Slovic, P. (eds) (2003) *The Social Amplification of Risk* (London: Cambridge University Press).

Pielke, R., Wigley, T. and Green, C. (2008) 'Dangerous Assumptions', *Nature*, 452 April, 531–2.

Pietroni, P. (1991) *The Greening of Medicine* (London: Victor Gollance).

Pilkington, P. and Kinra, S. (2005) 'Effectiveness of Speed Cameras in Preventing Road Traffic Collisions and Related Casualties: Systematic Review', *British Medical Journal*, 330: 331–4

Pischon, L., Boying, H., Hoffmann, K' et al. (2008) 'General and Abdominal Adiposity and

Risk of Death in Europe', *The New England Journal of Medicine*, 359: 2105–20.

Plant, M. and Plant, M. (2006) *Binge Britain: Alcohol and the National Response* (Oxford: Oxford University Press).

Platz, E.A., Giovannuci, E., Rumm, E.B. et al. (1997) 'Dietary Fibre and Distal Colorectal Adenoma in Men', *Cancer Epidemiology Biomakers Preview*, 6: 661–70.

PMS National Evaluation Team (2002) National Evaluation of First Wave NHS Personal Medical Pilots. Summaries of Findings from Four Research Projects (University of Birmingham, University of Manchester, Queen Mary College, University of London, University of Nottingham, University of Southampton).

Police Foundation, The (2000) *Drugs and the Law – Report of the Independent Inquiry into the Misuse of Drugs Act 1971* (London: The Police Foundation).

Policy Commission on the Future of Farming and Food (2002) *Farming and Food: A Sustainable Future* Chair: Sir Donald Curry CBE (London: Cabinet Office).

Policy Innovation Unit (2005) *Partnerships in Northern Ireland* (Belfast: Office of First Minister and Deputy First Minister for Northern Ireland) (http://www.ofmdfmni.gov.uk/partnership-ni-report.pdf accessed 8.5.10).

Pollock, A. and Price, D. (2003) 'New Deal from the World Trade Organisation', *British Medical Journal*, 327: 571–2.

Pollock, A., Price, D., Viebrock, E. et al. (2007) 'The Market in Primary Care', *British Medical Journal*, 335: 475–7 (8 September) (doi: 10.1136/bmj.39303.425359.AD).

Pollock, D. (1999) *Denial & Delay* (London: Action on Smoking).

Popay, J., Mallinson, S., Kowarzik, U. et al. (2004) 'Developing Public Health Work in Local Health Systems', *Primary Health Care Research and Development,* 5: 338–50.

Pope, C., Burnett, R., Thun, M. et al. (2002) 'Lung Cancer, Cardiopulmonary Mortality and Long-Term Exposure to Fine Particulate Air Pollution', *Journal of the American Medical Association*, 287(9): 1132–41.

Popham, G.T. (1981) 'Government and Smoking: Policymaking and Pressure Groups', *Policy and Politics*, 9(3): 331–47.

Porritt, J. and Winner, M. (1989) *The Coming of the Greens* (London: Fontana).

Porter, D. (1990) 'How Soon Is Now? Public Health and the BMJ', *British Medical Journal*, 301: 738–40.

Porter, R. (1995) *Disease, Medicine and Society in England 1550–1880* (Cambridge: Cambridge University Press).

POST (Parliamentary Office of Science and Technology) (2005) *Binge Drinking and Public Health* (London: POST).

POST (2007) *Ethnicity and Health* (London: Parliamentary Office of Science and Technology).

Potischman, N., Coates, R., Swanson, C. et al. (2002) 'Increased Risk of Early-Stage Breast Cancer Related to Consumption of Sweet Foods Among Women Less Than Age 45 in the United States', *Cancer Causes and Control*, 13(10): 937–46.

Potts, L. (1999) 'Breast Cancer on the Map', *Health Matters*, 35: 10–11.

Poulton, R., Caspi, A., Milne, B. et al. (2002) 'Association Between Children's Experience of Socioeconomic Disadvantage and Adult Health: A Life-Course Study', *The Lancet,* 360: 1640–5.

Powell, M. (1990) 'Need and Provision in the NHS: An Inverse Care Law', *Policy and Politics*, 18: 31–8.

Powell, M. and Glendinning, C. (2002) 'Introduction' in Glendinning, C., Powell, M. and Rummery, K. (eds) *Partnerships, New Labour and Governance* (Bristol: Policy Press), pp. 1–15.

Powell, M. and Moon, G. (2001) 'Health Action Zones: The Third Way of a New Area- based Policy', *Health and Social Care in the Community*, 9: 43–50.

Power, C., Matthews, S. and Manor, O. (1996) 'Inequalities in Self-Related Health in the 1958 Birth Cohort: Lifetime Social Circumstance or Social Mobility?', *British Medical Journal*, 313: 449–53.

Power, M. (2004) *The Risk Management of Everything: Rethinking the Politics of Uncertainty* (London: Demos).

Powles, J. (1973) 'On the Limitations of Modern Medicine', *Science, Medicine and Man*, 1: 1–30.

Prah Ruger, J. and Yach, D. (2005) 'Global Functions at the World Health Organization', *British Medical Journal*, 330: 1099–100.

Prentice, A. and Jebb, S. (1995) 'Obesity in Britain: Gluttony or Sloth?', *British Medical Journal*, 311: 437–9.

Prentice, A. and Jebb, S. (2007) 'Fast Foods, Energy Density and Obesity: A Possible Mechanistic Link', *Obesity Reviews*, 4: 187.

Pressman, J.L. and Wildavsky, A.B. (1973) *Implementation* (Berkerley: University of California Press).

Preston, R. (1994) *The Hot Zone* (New York: Doubleday).

Pretty, J., Ball, A., Lang, T. and Morison, J. (2005) 'Farm Costs and Food Miles: An Assessment of the Full Cost of the UK Weekly Food Basket', *Food Policy*, 30: 1–19.

Price, D. (2002) 'How the WTO Extends the Rights of Private Property', *Critical Public Health*, 12(1): 55–63.

PricewaterhouseCoopers (2008) *Building the Case for Wellness* (London: PwC).

Prime Minister's Strategy Unit (2002) *Game Plan: A Strategy for Delivering Government's Sport and Physical Activity Objectives* (London: Cabinet Office).

Prime Minister's Strategy Unit (2003a) *Strategy Unit Drugs Report: Phase One: Understanding the Issues* (London: Cabinet Office).

Prime Minister's Strategy Unit (2003b) *Strategy Unit Alcohol Harm Reduction Project, Interim Analytical Report* (London: Cabinet Office).

Prime Minister's Strategy Unit (2004) *Alcohol Harm Reduction Strategy for England: Final Report* (London: Cabinet Office).

Prime Minister's Strategy Unit (2008a) *Food Matters: Towards a Strategy for the 21st Century Executive Summary* (London: Cabinet Office).

Prime Minister's Strategy Unit (2008b) *Getting On, Getting Ahead – A Discussion Paper: Analysing the Trends and Drivers of Social Mobility* (London: Cabinet Office).

Prince's Trust (2007) *Fit for the Future: Exploring the Health and Well-being of Disadvantaged Young People* (London: Prince's Trust).

Princen, S. (2007) 'Advocacy Coalition and the Internationalisation of Public Health Policies', *Journal of Public Policy*, 27(1): 13–33.

Prochaska, J. and DiClemente, C. (1983) 'Stages and Processes of Self-change of Smoking: Toward an Integrative Model of Change', *Journal of Consulting and Clinical Psychology*, 51(3): 390–5.

Proctor, R. (1988) *Racial Hygiene: Medicine Under the Nazis* (Cambridge, MA: Harvard University Press).

Prüss-Üstün, A. and Corvalan, C. (2006) *Preventing Disease through Healthy Environments* (Geneva: WHO).

Public Health Alliance (1988) *Beyond Acheson* (Birmingham: PHA).

Public Health Commission (2009) *We're All in This Together: Improving the Long-term Health of the Nation* (www.publichealthcommission. co.uk).

Public Health Sciences Working Group (2004) *Public Health Sciences: Challenges and Opportunities* (London: The Wellcome Trust).

Putnam, R. (2000) *Bowling Alone: America's Declining Social Capital* (New York: Simon & Schuster).

Quigley, R. and Taylor, L. (2004) 'Evaluating Health Impact Assessment', *Public Health*, 118(8): 544–52.

Quigley, R., den Broeder, L., Fur, P. et al. (2006) Health Impact Assessment International Best Practice Principles Special Publication Series 5 (Fargo, USA: International Association for Impact Assessment).

Rachet, B., Woods, L.M., Mitry, E. et al. (2008) 'Cancer Survival in England and Wales at the End of the 20th Century', *British Journal of Cancer*, 99: S2–10.

Radical Statistics Health Group (1991) 'Missing – A Strategy for the Health of the Nation', *British Medical Journal*, 303: 299–302.

Raine, R. (2000) 'Does Gender Bias Exist in the Use of Specialist Health Care?', *Journal of Health Services Research and Policy*, 5: 237–9.

Raine, R., Hutchings, A. and Black, N. (2003) 'Is Publicly Funded Health Care Really Distributed According to Need? The Example of Cardiac Rehabilitation in the UK', *Health Policy*, 63: 63–72.

Raine, R., Walt, G. and Basnett, I. (2004) 'The White Paper on Public Health', *British Medical Journal,* 329: 1247–8.

Ram, R. (2005) Income Inequality, Poverty, and Population Health: Evidence from Recent Data for the United States', *Social Science & Medicine*, 61: 2568–76.

Ramsay, L.E., Yeo, W.W. and Jackson, P.R. (1994) 'High Blood Cholesterol: A Problem with No Ready Solution' in Le Fanu, J. *Preventionitis* (London: Social Affairs Unit), pp. 64–80.

Randall, E. (2001) *The European Union and Health Policy* (Basingstoke: Palgrave Macmillan).

Raphael, D. (2006) 'Social Determinants of Health: Present Status, Unanswered Questions, and Future Directions', *International Journal of Health Services*, 36(4): 651–77.

Raphael, D. (2008) 'Shaping Public Policy and Population Health in the United States: Why Is The Public Health Community Missing In Action?', *International Journal of Health Services*, 38(1): 63–94.

Raphael, D. and Bryant T. (2006) 'The State's Role in Promoting Population Health: Public Health Concerns in Canada, USA, UK and Sweden', *Health Policy*, 78: 39–55.

Rasmussen, S., Prescott, E., Sorensen, T. and Sogaard, J. (2005) 'The Total Lifetime Health Cost Savings of Smoking Cessation to Society', *European Journal of Public Health*, 15(6): 601–6.

Ratzan, S. (ed.) (1998) *Mad Cow Crisis: Health and the Public Good* (London: University College London Press).

Ravnskov, U., Rosch, P., Sutter, M. and Houston, M. (2006) 'Should we Lower Cholesterol as Much as Possible?' *British Medical Journal*, 332: 1330–2.

Rawls, J. (1999) *A Theory of Justice* (revised edn) (Cambridge, MA: Harvard University Press).

Redgrave, P. (2007) 'Making Joint Public Health Director Posts Work' in Griffiths, S. and Hunter, D. (eds) *New Perspectives in Public Health* (London: Routledge), pp. 224–9.

Reed, M. (2009) 'For Whom? The Governance of Organic Food and Farming in the UK', *Food Policy*, 34: 280–6.

Rees, G., Richards, C. and Gregory, J. (2008) 'Food and Nutrient Intakes of Primary School Children: A Comparison of School Meals and Packed Lunches', *Journal of Human Nutrition and Disease*, 21: 420–7.

Reeves, G., Pirie, K., Beral, V. et al. (2007) 'Cancer Incidence and Mortality in Relation to Body Mass Index in the Million Women Study: Cohort Study', *British Medical Journal*, 335(7630): 1134.

Regen, E., Smith, J., Goodwin, N. et al. (2001) *Passing on the Baton: Final Report of a National Evaluation of Primary Care Groups and Trusts* (Health Service Management Centre: University of Birmingham).

Regional Policy Commission (1996) *Reviewing the Regions Strategies for Regional Economic Development* (Sheffield Hallam University, PAVIC Publications).

Reid, F., Cook, D. and Whincup, P. (2002) 'Use of Statins in the Secondary Prevention of Coronary Heart Disease: Is Treatment Equitable?', *Heart*, 88: 15–19.

Reilly, J. and Wilson, D. (2006) 'ABC of Obesity: Childhood Obesity', *British Medical Journal*, 333: 1207–10.

Reinarman, C., Cohen, P. and Kaal, H. (2004) 'The Limited Relevance of Drug Policy: Cannabis in Amsterdam and in San Francisco', *American Journal of Public Health*, 94(5): 836–42.

Renehan, A., Tyson, M., Egger, M. et al. (2008) 'Body-mass Index and Incidence of Cancer: A Systematic Review and Meta-Analysis of Prospective Observational Studies', *The Lancet*, 371: 569–78.

Review of the Major Outbreak of E. coli *O157 in Surrey, 2009.* Report of the Independent Investigation Committee, June 2010 (Griffin report) (London: Health Protection Agency).

Rethink (2005) 'Memorandum' in *Health Committee (2005) Health – Minutes of Evidence*, HC 358i, Session 2004/5 (London: TSO).

Reuter, P. and Stevens, A. (2007) *An Analysis of UK Drug Policy – A Monograph Prepared for the UK Drug Policy Commission* (London: UK Drug Policy Commission).

Reynolds, P., Hurley. S., Goldberg, D.E. et al. (2004) 'Active Smoking, Household Passive Smoking, and Breast Cancer: Evidence From the California Teachers Study', *Journal of the National Cancer Institute*, 96: 29–37.

Rice, V. and Stead, L. (2004) *Nursing Interventions for Smoking Cessation* (Cochrane Database of Systematic Reviews, Issue 1).

Rich, D., Demissie, K., Lu, S. et al. (2008) 'Ambient Air Pollutant Concentrations During Pregnancy and the Risk of Fetal Growth Rrestriction', *Journal of Epidemiology and Community*, 63: 488–96.

Richardson, J. (2000) 'Governments, Interest Groups and Policy Change', *Political Studies*, 48: 1006–25.

Richardson, J. and Jordan, G. (1979) *Governing Under Pressure* (Oxford: Martin Robertson).

Richardson, J. and Moon, J. (1984) 'The Politics of Unemployment in Britain', *Political Quarterly*, 55: 29–37.

Ridley, F. and Jordan, G. (1998) *Protest Politics: Cause Groups and Campaigns* (Oxford: Oxford University Press).

Ritchie, D., Parry, D., Gnich, W. and Platt, S. (2004) 'Issues of Participation, Ownership and Empowerment in a Community Development Programme: Tackling Smoking in a Low Income Area of Scotland', *Health Promotion International*, 19(1): 51–9.

Ritz, B., Yu, F., Fruin, S. et al. (2002) 'Ambient Air Pollution and Risk of Birth Defects in Southern California', *American Journal of Epidemiology*, 155(1): 17–25.

Roberts, D., Mohan, D. and Abbasi, K. (2002) 'War on the Roads' *British Medical Journal*, 324: 1107–8.

Roberts, E., Robinson, J. and Seymour, L. (2002) *Old Habits Die Hard: Tackling Age Discrimination in Health and Social Care* (London: King's Fund Publishing).

Roberts, M. and Eldridge, A. (2007) *Expecting 'Great Things'? The Impact of the Licensing Act 2003 on Democratic Involvement, Dispersal and Drinking Cultures* (London:University of Westminster).

Roberts, S.B. and Greenberg, A.S. (1996) 'The New Obesity Genes', *Nutrition Review*, 54(2 part 1): 41–9.

Robinson, W.S. (1950) 'Ecological Correlations and the Behaviour of Individuals', *American Sociological Reviews*, 15: 351–7.

Roche, J. (2005) 'The 1989 Children Act and Children's Rights: A Critical Reassessment' in Hendrick, H. *Child Welfare and Social Policy: An Essential Reader* (Bristol: Policy Press), pp. 223–42.

Rodgers, A. (1990) 'The UK Breast Cancer Screening Programme: An Expensive Mistake', *Journal of Public Health Medicine*, 12(3, 4): 197–204.

Rodmell, S. and Watt, A. (1986) *The Politics of Health Education: Raising the Issues* (London: Routledge Kegan Paul).

Rogers, A. and Pilgrim, D. (2001) *Mental Health Policy in Britain* (2nd edn) (Basingstoke: Palgrave Macmillan).

Rogers, A. and Pilgrim, D. (2003) *Mental Health and Inequality* (Basingstoke: Palgrave Macmillan).

Rogers, G., Elston, J. and Garside, R. (2009) *The Harmful Effects of Recreational Ecstasy: A Systematic Review of Observational Evidence: Health Technology Assessment* Report 13(6) (10.3310/hta13060 www.hta.ac.uk accessed 17.5.10).

Rogers, P. (2007) *National Enforcement Priorities for Local Authority Regulatory Services* (London: Cabinet Office).

Rogers, R. (1999) *Towards an Urban Renaissance: The Report of the Urban Task Force* (London: E and FN Spon).

Romieu, I., Hernandez-Avila, M., Lazcano-Ponce, E. et al. (2000) 'Breast Cancer, Lactation History, and Serum Organochlorines', *American Journal of Epidemiology*, 152(4): 363–70.

Rose, G. (1985) 'Sick Individuals and Sick Populations', *International Journal of Epidemiology*, 14(1): 132–8.

Rose, G. (1992) *The Strategy of Preventive Medicine* (Oxford: Oxford University Press).

Rose, R. (1984) *Do Parties Make a Difference?* (2nd edn) (London: Macmillan – now Palgrave Macmillan).

Rosen, F. and Burns, J. (eds) (1983) *The Collected Works of Jeremy Bentham: Constitutional Code Vol I* (Oxford: Oxford University Press).

Rosen, G. (1993) *A History of Public Health* (New York: John Hopkins University Press) edited by E. Fee.

Ross, W. and Tomaney, J. (2001) 'Devolution and Health Policy in England', *Regional Studies*, 35(3): 265–70.

Rowntree, J. (1901) *Poverty: A Study of Town Life* (London: Macmillan – now Palgrave Macmillan).

Royal College of Physicians (1962) *Smoking and Health* (London: Pitman).

Royal College of Physicians (1971) *Smoking and Health Now* (London: Pitman).

Royal College of Physicians (1977) *Smoking or Health?* (London: Pitman).

Royal College of Physicians (1983) *Health or Smoking?* (London: Pitman).

Royal College of Physicians (1994) *Homelessness and Ill Health: Report of a Working Party* (London: Royal College of Physicians).

Royal College of Physicians (2002) *Nicotine Addiction in Britain* (London: RSA).

Royal College of Physicians (2003) *Allergy: The Unmet Need* (London: Royal College of Physicians),

Royal College of Physicians (2005a) 'Memorandum' in *Health Committee (2005) Health –*

Minutes of Evidence, HC 358i, Session 2004/5 (London: TSO).

Royal College of Physicians (2005b) *Going Smoke-Free. The Medical Case for Clean Air in the Home, At Work and in Public Places* (London: Royal College of Physicians).

Royal College of Physicians (2010) *Passive Smoking and Children.* (London: Royal College of Physicians).

Royal College of Physicians, Royal College of Paediatrics and Child Health, Faculty of Public Health (2004) *Storing up Problems: The Medical Case for a Slimmer Nation* (London: RCP).

Royal Commission on the State of Large Towns and Populous Districts (1844/1970) First Report, HC 572, House of Commons Sessional Papers, Vol. 17, p. 1. (Shannon: Irish University Press).

Royal Commission on the State of Large Towns and Populous Districts (1845/1970) Second Report, HC 602 and 610, House of Commons Sessional Papers, Vol. 18, pp. 1, 299. (Shannon: Irish University Press).

Royal Society, The (2002) *Genetically Modified Plants for Food Use and Human Health – An Update* (London: The Royal Society).

Royal Society, The (2009) Reaping the Benefits: Science and the Sustainable Intensification of Global Agriculture (London: The Royal Society).

RSA Commission (2007) *Drugs – Facing Facts. The Report of the RSA Commission on Illegal Drugs, Communities and Public Policy* (London: RSA).

Rugg-Gunn, A.J. and Edgar, W.M. (1984) 'Sugar and Dental Cavities. A Review of the Evidence, *Community Dental Health*, 1: 85–92.

Rush, M. (ed.) (1990) *Parliament and Pressure Politics* (Oxford: Clarendon).

Russell, M. (2010) 'The Independent Climate Change E Mails Review' (http://www.cce-review.org/ accessed 12.8.2010).

Rutter, H. (2007) 'Transport' in Griffiths, S. and Hunter, D.J. *New Perspectives in Public Health* (Oxford: Radcliffe Publishing), pp. 183–93.

Ryle, M. (1988) *Ecology and Socialism* (London: Rodins).

Sabatier, P. (1987) 'Knowledge, Policy Orientated Learning and Policy Change', *Knowledge: Creation, Diffusion, Utilisation*, 8: 649–92.

Sabo, D. and Gordon, G. (1993) *Men's Health and Illness: Gender Power and the Body* (London: Sage).

Saegert, S., Klitzman, S., Freudenberg, N. et al. (2003) 'Healthy Housing: A Structured Review of Published Evaluations of US Interventions to Improve Health by Modifying Housing in the United States, 1990–2001', *American Journal of Public Health*, 93(9); 1471–7.

Saffer, H. and Uhaloupka, F. (2000) The Effects of Tobacco Advertising Bans on Tobacco

Consumption', *Journal of Health Economics*, 19: 1117–37.

Sagan, L. (1987) *The Health of Nations* (New York: Basic Books).

Sample, I. (2007) 'Birth of Cloned Calf Poses Test for Europe's Food Safety Regulations,' *The Guardian*, 11th January 2007, p. 15.

Sampson, A. (2004) *Who Runs this Place?* (London: John Murray).

Sargent, R., Shepherd, R. and Glantz, S. (2004) 'Reduced Incidence of Admissions for Myocardial Infarction Associated With Public Smoking Ban: Before and After Study', *British Medical Journal*, 328: 988–9.

Scally, G. (1996) 'Public Health Medicine in a New Era', *Social Science & Medicine*, 42(5): 777–80.

Scambler, G. and Scambler, S. (2007) 'Social Patterning of Health Behaviours' in Scriven, A. and Garman, S. *Public Health: Social Context and Action* (Maidenhead: Open University Press), pp. 34–47.

Scarre, G. (1996) *Utilitarianism* (London: Routledge).

Schattschneider, E. (1960) *The Semi-Sovereign People* (New York: Holt, Rinehart and Winston).

Schiffman, M.H., Bauer, H.M., Hoover, R.N. et al. (1993) 'Epidemiologic Evidence Showing that Human Papillomavirus Infection Causes Most Cervical Intraepithelial Neoplasia?', *Journal of the National Institute*, 85: 958–64.

Schilt, T., de Win, M., Jager, G. et al. (2008) 'Specific Effects of Ecstasy and Other Illicit Drugs on Cognition in Poly-substance Users', *Psychological Medicine*, 38: 1309–17.

Schlosser, E. (2002) *Fast Food Nation* (London: Penguin).

School Food Trust (2009) *Primary School Food Survey 2009* (London: School Food Trust).

School Meals Review Panel (2005) *Turning the Tables: Transforming School Food* (School Meals Review Panel).

School Travel Advisory Group (2000) *Report 1998–9* (London: DETR).

Schroder, F., Hugosson, J., Roobol, M. et al. (2009) 'Screening and Prostate Cancer Mortality in a Randomised European Study', *New England Journal of Medicine*, 360(13): 1320–8.

Science and Technology Committee (2001) *Fifth Report 2000/1 Genetics and Insurance HC 174* (London, TSO).

Science and Technology Committee (2006) *Drug Classification: Making a Hash of It? 5th Report 2005-2006* (HC 1031) (London, TSO).

Scott-Samuel, A. (1998) 'Concepts of Health and Regeneration' in Health Education Authority *Putting Health on the Regeneration Agenda* (London: HEA), pp. 4–6.

Scott, P., Gillett, N., Hegerl, G. et al. (2010) 'Detection and Attribution of Climate Change: A Regional Perspective' *WIREs Climate Change* (wires.wiley.com/climatechange doi: 10.1002/wcc.34 accessed 15.3.10).

Scottish Executive (1999a) *Review of the Public Health Function in Scotland* (Edinburgh: Scottish Executive).

Scottish Executive (1999b) *Social Inclusion: Opening the Door to a Better Scotland* (Edinburgh: Scottish Executive).

Scottish Executive (1999c) *Social Justice: A Scotland Where Everyone Matters* (Edinburgh: Scottish Executive).

Scottish Executive (2000a) *Our National Health: A Plan for Action, a Plan for Change* (Edinburgh: Scottish Executive).

Scottish Executive (2000b) *Social Justice: A Scotland Where Everyone Matters: Annual Report 2002* (London: Scottish Executive).

Scottish Executive (2001a) *Nursing for Health: A Review of the Contribution of Nurses, Midwives and Health Visitors to Improving the Public's Health in Scotland* (Edinburgh: Scottish Executive).

Scottish Executive (2001b) *For Scotland's Children* (Edinburgh: Scottish Executive).

Scottish Executive (2002a) *Report of Joint Future Group* (Edinburgh: Scottish Executive).

Scottish Executive (2002b) *Choose Life: A National Strategy and Action Plan to Prevent Suicide in Scotland* (Edinburgh: Scottish Executive).

Scottish Executive (2002c) *Plan for Action on Alcohol Problems* (Edinburgh: Scottish Executive).

Scottish Executive (2002d) *Closing the Opportunity Gap; Scottish Budget for 2003–6* (Edinburgh: Scottish Executive).

Scottish Executive (2003a) *Improving Health in Scotland: The Challenge* (Edinburgh: Scottish Executive).

Scottish Executive (2003b) *Partnership for Care: Scotland's Health White Paper* (Edinburgh: Scottish Executive).

Scottish Executive (2003c) *National Programme for Improving Mental Health and Well-being: Action Plan 2003–06* (Edinburgh: Scottish Executive).

Scottish Executive (2003d) *Integrated Strategy for the Early Years* (Edinburgh: Scottish Executive).

Scottish Executive (2003e) *Hungry for Success: A Whole School Approach to School Meals in Scotland* (Edinburgh: Scottish Executive).

Scottish Executive (2003f) *Let's Make Scotland More Active: A Strategy for Physical Activity* (Edinburgh: Scottish Executive).

Scottish Executive (2004) *Closing the Opportunity Gap: Targets* (http://www.scotland.gov.uk/Topics/People/Social-Inclusion/17415/CtOG-targets/intro accessed 21.5.10).

Scottish Executive (2005a) Building a Health Service Fit for the Future (Edinburgh: Scottish Executive). The Kerr Report.

Scottish Executive (2005b) Getting it Right for Every Child: Proposals for Action (Edinburgh: Scottish Executive).

Scottish Executive (2005c) Respect and Responsibility: A Strategy and Action Plan for Improving Sexual Health (Edinburgh: Scottish Executive).

Scottish Executive (2006) Delivery of Mental Health (Edinburgh: Scottish Executive).

Scottish Executive (2007) Delivering a Healthy Future: An Action Framework for Children and Young People's Health in Scotland (Edinburgh: Scottish Executive).

Scottish Executive and Convention of Scottish Local Authorities (COSLA) (2008) Early Years and Early Interventions: A Joint Scottish Government and COSLA Policy Statement (Edinburgh: Scottish Executive).

Scottish Government (2005) Choosing Our Future: Scotland's Sustainable Development Strategy, Making the Links: Food (Edinburgh: Scottish Government).

Scottish Government (2006) Changing Our Ways: Scotland's Climate Change Programme (Edinburgh: Scottish Executive).

Scottish Government (2007a) Better Health, Better Care: A Discussion Document (Edinburgh: Scottish Government).

Scottish Government (2007b) Better Health, Better Care: Action Plan (Edinburgh: Scottish Government).

Scottish Government (2008a) The Road to Recovery: A New Approach to Tackling Scotland's Drug Problem (Edinburgh: Scottish Government).

Scottish Government (2008b) Equally Well: Report of the Ministerial Task Force on Health Inequalities (Edinburgh: Scottish Government).

Scottish Government (2008c) Equally Well: Implementation Plan (Edinburgh: Scottish Government).

Scottish Government (2008d) Achieving our Potential (Edinburgh: Scottish Government).

Scottish Government (2009a) Towards a Mentally Flourishing Scotland Policy and Action Plan 2009–11 (Edinburgh: Scottish Executive).

Scottish Government (2009b) Recipe for Success: Scotland's National Food and Drink Policy (Edinburgh: Scottish Government).

Scottish Government (2009c) Changing Scotland's Relationship with Alcohol: A Framework for Action (Edinburgh: Scottish Government).

Scottish Health Council (2007) Public Partnership Forums: What Direction and Support is Needed for the Future? (Glasgow: FMR Research).

Scottish Office (1991) Health Education in Scotland: A National Policy Statement (Edinburgh: HMSO).

Scottish Office (1992) Scotland's Health: A Challenge To Us All (Edinburgh: HMSO).

Scottish Office (1994) Scotland's Health. A Challenge to us all. The Scottish Diet, Report of a Working Party to the Chief Medical Officer for Scotland (Edinburgh Scottish Office).

Scottish Office (1996) Eating for Health: A National Diet Action Plan for Scotland (Edinburgh Scottish Office).

Scottish Office (1997) The Pennington Group Report (Edinburgh: TSO).

Scriven, A. (ed.) (1998) Alliances in Health Promotion Theory and Practice (London: Macmillan – now Palgrave Macmillan).

Searle, B. (2008) Wellbeing: In Search of a Good Life (Bristol: Policy Press).

Searle, G.R. (1971) The Quest for National Efficiency. A Study in British Politics and British Political Thought 1899–1914 (Oxford: Blackwell).

Searle, G.R. (1976) Eugenics and Politics in Britain 1900–14 (Leydon: Noordhoff International).

Sears, A. (1992) 'To Teach Them How to Live. The Politics of Public Health from TB to AIDS', Journal of Historical Sociology, 5(1): 61–83.

Secrett, C. and Bullock, S. (2002) 'Sustainable Development and Health' in Adams, L., Amos, M. and Munro, J. (eds) Promoting Health (London: Sage), pp. 34–45.

See, R., Abdullah, S., McGuire, D. et al. (2007) 'The Association of Differing Measures of Overweight and Obesity with Prevalent Atherosclerosis: The Dallas Heart Study', Journal of the American College of Cardiology, 50(8): 752–9.

Select Committee on Drunkenness (1834/1968) Report, HC 559/1834 (Shannon: Irish University Press).

Select Committee on Public Administration (2001) Innovations in Citizen Participation in Government 6th Report 2000–1, HC 373 (London: TSO).

Self, P. and Storing, H. (1962) The State and the Farmer (London: Allen and Unwin).

Selin, H. and Eckley, N. (2003) 'Science, Politics and Persistent Organic Pollutants: The Role of Scientific Assessments in International Environmental Co-operation', International Environmental Agreements: Politics, Law and Economics, 3(1): 17–42.

Sen, A. (1985) Commodities and Capabilities (Amsterdam and Oxford: North Holland).

Seth, A. and Randall, G. (2001) The Grocers (London: Kogan Page).

Shapiro, S., Venet, W., Strax, P. et al. (1982) 'Ten to Fourteen Year Effect of Breast Cancer Screening on Mortality', Journal of the National Cancer Institute, 69(2): 349–55.Sharma, N.

(2007) *It Doesn't Happen Here: The Reality of Child Poverty in the UK* (Essex: Barnardo's).

Sharpley, M., Hutchinson, G. and McKenzie, K. (2001) 'Bringing in the Social Environment: Understanding the Excess of Psychosis Among the African-Carribean Population in England', *The British Journal of Psychiatry*, 178: 60–8.

Shaw, M., Davey Smith, G. and Dorling, D. (2005) 'Health Inequalities and New Labour: How the Promises Compare with Real Progress', *British Medical Journal*, 330: 1016–21.

Shaw, M., Dorling, D., Gordon, D. and Davey Smith, G. (1999) *The Widening Gap: Health Inequalities and Policy in Britain* (Bristol: The Policy Press).

Shaw, M., Maxwell, R., Rees, K. et al. (2004) 'Gender and Age Inequity in the Provision of Coronary Revascularisation in England in the 1990s. Is it Getting Better?' *Social Science & Medicine*, 59(12): 2499–507.

Shaw, S., Ashcroft, J. and Petchey, R. (2006) 'Barriers and Opportunities for Developing Sustainable Relationships for Health Improvement: The Case of Public Health and Primary Care in the UK', *Critical Public Health*, 16(1): 73–88.

Sheaff, R. and Lloyd-Kendall, A. (2000) 'Principal-Agent Relationships in General Practice: The First Wave of English Personal Medical Services Pilot Contracts', *Journal of Health Services Research and Policy*, 5: 153–63.

Sheard, S. and Donaldson, L. (2006) *The Nation's Doctor: The Role of the Chief Medical Officer 1855–1998* (Oxford: Radcliffe).

Sheiham, A., Marmot, M., Rawson, D. and Ruck, N. (1987) 'Food Values: Health and Diet' in Jowell, R., Witherspoon, S. and Brook, L. *British Social Attitudes, The 1987 Report*, Social and Community Planning Research (Aldershot: Gower), pp. 97–112.

Shelter (2006) *Chance of a Lifetime: The Impact of Bad Housing on Children's Lives* (London: Shelter).

Shepherd, J. and Farrington, D. (1993) 'Assault as a Public Health Problem: Discussion Paper', *Journal of the Royal Society of Medicine*, 86: 89–92.

Shepherd, J., Sivarajasingham, V. and Rivara, F. (2000) 'Using Injury Data for Violence Prevention', *British Medical Journal*, 321: 1481–2.

Shibuya, K., Hashimoto, H. and Yano, E. (2002) 'Individual Income, Income Distribution, and Self-rated Health in Japan', *British Medical Journal*, 324(7324): 16–19.

Shiner, M. and Newburn, T. (1997) 'Definitely, Maybe Not: The Normalisation of Recreational Drug Use Amongst Young People', *Sociology*, 31(3): 511–29.

Shouls, S., Congden, P. and Curtis, S. (1996) 'Modelling Inequality in Reported Long-term Illness in the UK: Combining Individual and Area Characteristics', *Journal of Epidemiology and Community Health*, 50(3): 366–76.

Shryock, R. (1979) *The Development of Modern Medicine* (Madison, WI: University of Wisconsin Press).

Siegler, V., Langford, A. and Johnson, B. (2008) *Regional Differences in Male Mortality Inequalities Using the National Statistics Socio-economic Classification, England and Wales, 2001–03* (London: Office for National Statistics).

Siegrist, J. and Marmot, M. (2006) *Social Inequalities in Health: New Evidence and Policy Implications* (Oxford: Oxford University Press).

Signal, L. (1998) 'The Politics of Health Promotion: Insights from Political Theory', *Health Promotion International*, 13(3): 257–63.

Silagy, C., Lancaster, T., Stead, L. et al. (2004) 'Nicotine Replacement Therapy for Smoking Cessation', *Cochrane Database of Systematic Reviews* 3.

Simon, H. (1945) *Administrative Behaviour* (Glencoe: Free Press).

Simon, J. (1890) *English Sanitary Institutions* (London: Cassell and Co).

Sims, M., Maxwell, R., Bauld, L. and Gilmore, A. (2010) 'Short Term Impact of Smoke Free Legislation in England: Retrospective Analysis of Hospital Admissions for Myocardial Infarction' *British Medical Journal* 340, c2161, doi:10.1136/bmj.c2161 (accessed 24.11.10).

Sinclair, S. and Winkler, J.T. (2008) *The School Fringe: What Pupils Buy and Eat From Shops Surrounding Secondary Schools* (London Metropolitan University, Nutrition Policy Unit).

Singh-Manoux, A. and Marmot, M. (2005) 'Role of Socialization in Explaining Social Inequalities in Health', *Social Science & Medicine*, 60: 2129–33.

Singh, T. and Sweetman, T. (2008) *Green Dreams A Decade of Missed Targets* (London: Policy Exchange).

Singleton, N., Bumpstead, R., O'Brien, M. et al. (2001) *Psychiatric Morbidity among Adults Living in Private Households* (London: TSO).

Sinkler, P. and Toft, M. (2000) 'Raising the National Healthy School Standard (NHSS) Together', *Health Education*, 100(2): 68–73.

Sivarajasingam, V., Shepherd, J., Matthew, K. and Jones, S. (2002) 'Trends in Violence in England and Wales 1995-2000 An Accident and Emergency Perspective', *Journal of Public Health Medicine*, 24: 219–26.

Sjonell, G. and Ståhl, L. (1999) 'Mammographic Screening Does Not Reduce Breast Cancer Mortality', *Lakartidningen*, 96(8): 904–5, 908–13.

Skegg, D. (1991) 'Multiple Sclerosis: Nature or Nuture?', *British Medical Journal*, 302: 247–8.

Skidmore, P. and Harkin, J. (2003) *Grown-up Trust* (London: Demos).

Skidmore, P., Bound, K. and Lownsborough, H. (2006) *Community Participation: Who Benefits?* (York: Joseph Rowntree Foundation).

Skills for Health (2004) *Sector Skills Agreement for Health: Delivering a Flexible Workforce to Support Better Healthcare and Healthcare Services* (Bristol: Skills for Health).

Skills for Health (2007) Public Health (www. Ukstandards.org accessed 27.9.07).

Skills for Health/Public Health Resource Unit (2008) The Public Health Skills and Career Framework (http://www.phru.nhs.uk/ accessed 4.5.10).

Skrabanek, P. (1988) 'The Debate Over Mass Mammography in Britain', *British Medical Journal*, 297: 970–1.

Skrabanek, P. (1994) *The Death of Humane Medicine* (London: Social Affairs Unit).

Slattery, M., Benson, J., Berry, T. et al. (1997) 'Dietary Sugar and Colon Cancer', *Cancer Epidemiology Biomarkers and Prevention*, 6: 677.

Sloggett, A. and Joshi, H. (1994) 'High Mortality in Deprived Areas: Community or Personal Disadvantage?', *British Medical Journal*, 309: 1470–4.

Slovenian Presidency of the EU (2008) European Pact for Mental Health and Wellbeing, EU High Level Conference: Together for Mental Health and Wellbeing, Brussels 12–13 June 2008.

Smaje, C. (1995) *Health, 'Race' and Ethnicity: Making Sense of the Evidence* (London: King's Fund).

Smaje, C. and Le Grand, J. (1997) 'Ethnicity, Equity and the Use of Health Services in the British NHS', *Social Science & Medicine*, 45: 485–96.

Smed, S., Jensen, J. and Denver, S. (2007) 'Socio-economic Characteristics and the Effect if Taxation as a Health Policy Instrument', *Food Policy*, 624–39.

Smith, A. and Jacobson, B. (1988) The Nation's Health: A Strategy for the 1990s (London: King Edward's Hospital Fund).

Smith, F.B. (1979) *The People's Health 1830–1910* (London: Croom Helm).

Smith, M. (1993) *Pressure, Power and Policy* (Brighton: Harvester Wheatsheaf).

Smith, P. (1967) *Disraelian Conservatism and Social Reform* (London: Routledge, Kegan Paul).

Smith, R., Beaglehole, R., Woodward, D. and Drager, N. (2003) *Global Public Goods for Health; a Health Economic and Public Health Perspective* (Oxford: Oxford University Press).

Smith, R., Chanda, R. and Tangcharosathien, V. (2009) 'Trade in Health-Related Services', *The Lancet*, 373: 593–601.

Snape, S. (2004) 'Partnerships Between Health and Local Government: The Local Government Policy Context' in Snape, S. and Taylor, P. (eds) *Partnerships Between Health and Local Government* London: Frank Cass), pp. 73–98.

Social Exclusion Unit (1999) *Teenage Pregnancy* (London: TSO).

Social Exclusion Unit (2000) *National Strategy for Neighbourhood Renewal: A Framework for Consultation* (London: Cabinet Office).

Social Exclusion Unit (2001) *A New Commitment to Neighbourhood Renewal: National Strategy Action Plan* (London: Cabinet Office).

Social Issues Research Centre (2005) *Obesity and the Facts* (Oxford: SIRC).

Social Trends (2007) Environment Highlights (www.statistics.gov).

Socialist Health Association (2005) Government White Paper on Public Health (www.sochealth. co.uk/Policy/choosinghealth.htm accessed 11/7/2007).

Sofi, F., Cesari, F., Abbate, R. et al. (2008) 'Adherence to a Mediterranean Diet and Health Status: A Meta-Analysis', *British Medical Journal*, 337: a1344.

Soil Association (2000) *The Biodiversity Benefits of Organic Farming* (Bristol: Soil Association).

SOLACE (2001) *Healthy Living: The Role of Modern Local Authorities in Creating Healthy Communities* (London: SOLACE).

Sondik, E., Huang, D., Klein, R. and Satcher, D. (2010) 'Progress Toward the Healthy People 2010 Goals and Objectives', *Annual Review of Public Health*, 31: 271–81.

Sowden, A. and Arblaster, L. (1998) 'Mass Media Interventions for Preventing Smoking in Young People', *Cochrane Database of Systematic Reviews* 1.

Sowden, A., Arblaster, L. and Stead, L. (2003) 'Community Interventions for Preventing Smoking in Young People', *Cochrane Database System Reviews 1*.

Spence, J., Cutumisu, N., Edwards, J. et al. (2009) 'Relation Between Local Food Environments and Obesity Among Adults BMC', *Public Health*, 9: 192 (doi: 10.1186/1471-2458-9-192).

Spencer, N. and Law, C. (2007) 'Inequalities in Pregnancy and Early Years and the Impact Across the Life Course: Progress and Future Challenges' in Dowler, E. and Spencer, N. (2007) *Challenging Health Inequalities – From Acheson to 'Choosing Health'* (Bristol: Policy Press), pp. 69–94

Springett, J. (2001) 'Appropriate Approaches to the Evaluation of Health Promotion', *Critical Public Health*, 11(2): 139–51.

Sproston, K. and Mindell, J. (2006) *The Health of Minority Ethnic Groups* (London: The Information Centre).

Spruit, I. (1998) 'Deviant of Just Different?' Dutch Alcohol and Drug Policy' in Bloor, M. and Wood, F. *Addictions and Problem Drug Use: Issues in Behaviour, Policy and Practice* (London: Jessica Kingsley), pp. 107–21.

Sram, I. and Ashton, J. (1998) 'Millennium Report to Sir Edwin Chadwick', *British Medical Journal*, 317: 592–5.

Staley, K. (2003) *Genetic Testing in the Workplace* (Buxton: Genewatch).

Stallibrass, A. (1989) *Being Me and Also Us: Lessons from the Peckham Experiment* (Edinburgh: Scottish Academic Press).

Standerwick, K., Davies, C., Tucker, L. and Sheron, N. (2007) 'Binge Drinking, Sexual Behaviour and Sexually Transmitted Infection in the UK', *International Journal of STD and AIDS*, 18(12): 810–13.

Standing Conference for Community Development (2001) *Strategic Framework for Community Development* (Sheffield: SCCD).

Standing Nursing and Midwifery Advisory Committee (1995) *Making it Happen: Public Health The Contribution, Role and Development of Nurses, Midwives and Health Visitors* (London: DoH).

Stanistreet, D., Scott-Samuel, A. and Bellis, M.A. (1999) 'Income Inequality and Mortality in England', *Journal of Public Health Medicine*, 21(2): 205–7.

Stansfield, S., Fuhrer, R., Shipley, M. and Marmot, M. (1999) 'Work Characteristics Predict Psychiatric Disorder: Prospective Results from the Whitehall II Study', *Occupational and Environmental Medicine*, 56: 302–7.

Starr, P. (1982) *The Social Transformation of American Medicine* (New York: Basic Books).

Stead, L. and Lancaster, T. (2005) 'Intervention for Preventing Tobacco Sales to Minors', *Cochrane Database of Systematic Reviews*, Issue 1.

Steering Board of the Public Debate on GM and GM Crops (2003) *GM Nation? The Findings of the Public Debate* (London: Department of Trade and Industry).

Stefan, N., Kantartzis, K., Machaan, J. et al. (2008) 'Identification and Characterization of Metabolically Benign Obesity in Humans', *Archives of Internal Medicine*, 168(15): 1609–16.

Stern, J. (1983) 'Social Mobility and the Interpretation of Social Class Mortality Differentials', *Journal of Social Policy*, 12(1): 27–49.

Stern, N. (2006) *The Economics of Climate Change* (London: HM Treasury).

Stewart-Brown, S. (2006) *What is the Evidence on School Health Promotion in Improving Health or Preventing Disease and, Specifically, What is the Effectiveness of the Health Promoting Schools Approach?* (Copenhagen: WHO Regional Office for Europe).

Stewart-Brown, S. and Farmer, A. (1997) 'Screening Could Seriously Damage Your Health', *British Medical Journal*, 314: 533–4.

Stewart, J. (2004) *Taking Stock: Scottish Welfare After Devolution* (Bristol: Policy Press).

Stewart, J. (2005) 'A Review of UK Housing Policy: Ideology and Public Health', *Public Health*, 119: 525–34.

Stiller, C.A. and Boyle, P.J. (1996) 'Effect of Population Mixing and Socioeconomic Status in England and Wales 1979–85 on Lymphoblastic Leukaemia in Children', *British Medical Journal*, 313: 1297–300.

Stimson, G.V. and Oppenheimer, E (1982) *Heroin Addiction: Treatment and Control in Britain* (London: Tavistock).

Stockholm Network (2008) *Carbon Scenarios: Blue Sky Thinking for a Green Future* (Stockholm Network).

Stolze, M. and Lampkin, N. (2009) 'Policy for Organic Farming: Rationale and Concepts', *Food Policy*, 34: 237–44.

Stone, D. (2006) 'Sustainable Development: Convergence of Public Health and Natural Environment Agendas Nationally and Locally', *Public Health*, 120: 1110–13.

Strang, J. and Gossop, M. (eds) (1994) *Heroin Addiction and Drug Policy: The British System* (Oxford: Oxford University Press).

Strategic Review of Health Inequalities in England (2010) *Fair Society, Healthy Lives* (London: DoH).

Strazullo, P., Kerry, S., Barbato, A. et al. (2007) 'Do Statins Reduce Blood Pressure? A Meta-analysis of Randomised Controlled Trials', *Hypertension*, 49: 792.

Strong, P. and Robinson, J. (1990) *The NHS: Under New Management* (Buckingham: Open University Press).

Stuckler, D. and Basu, S. (2009) 'The International Monetary Fund's Effects on Global Health: Before and After the 2008 Financial Crisis', *International Journal of Health Studies*, 39(4): 771–81.

Sturm, R. and Gresenz, C. (2002) 'Relations of Income Inequality and Family Income to Chronic Medical Conditions and Mental Health Disorders', *British Medical Journal*, 324(7328): 20–3.

Subramanian, S.V. and Kawachi, I. (2004) 'Income Inequality and Health: What Have We Learned So Far?', *Epidemiologic Reviews*, 26: 78–91.

Subramanian, S.V. and Kawachi, I. (2004) 'Income Inequality and Health: What Have We Learned So Far?', *Epidemiologic Reviews*, 26: 78–91.

Subramanian, S.V. and Kawachi, I. (2007) 'Commentary: Chasing the Elusive Null – The Story of Income Inequality and Health', *International Journal of Epidemiology* (doi: 10.1093/ije/dym102).

Subramanian, S.V., Blakely, T. and Kawachi, I. (2003) 'Commentary: Income Inequality as a Public Health Concern: Where Do We Stand? Commentary on "Is Exposure to Income Inequality a Public Health Concern?"', *Health Services Research*, 38(1): 153–67.

Sui, X., LaMonte, M., Laditka, J. et al. (2007) 'Cardiorespiratory Fitness and Adiposity as Mortality Predictors in Older Adults', *Journal of the American Medical Association*, 298(21): 2507–16.

Sullivan, H. (2007) 'Interpreting Community Leadership in English Local', *Government Policy and Politics*, 35(1): 141–61.

Sullivan, H. and Gillanders, G. (2005) 'Stretched to the Limit: The Impact Local Public Service Agreements on Service Improvement and Central-Local Relations', *Local Government Studies*, 31(5): 555–74.

Sullivan, H. and Skelcher, C. (2002) *Working Across Boundaries: Collaboration in Public Services* (Basingstoke: Palgrave Macmillan).

Sullivan, H., Knops, A., Barnes, M. and Newam, J. (2004) 'Central Local Relations in an Era of Multilevel Governance: The Case of Public Participation Policy in England 1997–2001', *Local Government Studies*, 30(2): 245–65.

Sundh, M. and Hagquist, C. (2006) 'Does a Minimum-Age Law for Purchasing Tobacco Make Any Difference? Swedish Experiences Over Eight Years', *European Journal of Public Health*, 17(2): 171–7.

Sunstein, C. and Thaler, R. (2003) Libertarian Paternalism is not an Oxymoron, Working Paper 03-2, Joint Center, AEI-Brookings Joint Center for Regulatory Studies (www.aei.brookings.org).

Sunyer, J., Ballester, F., Tetre, A. et al. (2003) 'The Association of Daily Sulphur Dioxide Air Pollution Levels with Hospital Admissions for Cardiovascular Diseases in Europe (The Aphea II study)', *European Heart Journal*, 24(8): 752–60.

Sustainable Development Commission (2005) *Climate Change Programme Review: Sustainable Development Commission Submission* (London: Sustainable Development Commission)

Sustainable Development Commission (2009) *Breakthrough for the 21st Century* (London: Sustainable Development Commission).

Sutherland, H. and Piachaud, D. (2001) 'Reducing Child Poverty in Britain: An Assessment of Government Policy 1997–2001', *The Economic Journal*, 111: 85–101.

Sutherland, I. (1987) *Health Education – Half a Policy, 1968–86. Rise and Fall of the Health Education Council* (Cambridge: NEC).

Suzuki, S., Kojima, M., Tokudome, S. et al. (2008) 'Effect of Physical Activity on Breast Cancer Risk: Findings of the Japan Collaborative Cohort Study', *Cancer Epidemiology Biomarkers and Prevention*, 17(3396): 401.

Swithers, S. and Davidson, T. (2008) 'A Role of Sweet Taste: Calorie Predictive Relations in Energy Regulation by Rats', *Behavioural Neuroscience*, 122(1): 161–73.

Szreter, S. (1988) 'The Importance of Social Intervention in Britain's Mortality Decline c1850–1914', *Social History of Medicine*, 1(1): 1–38.

Tabar, L., Gad, A., Holmberg, L.H. et al. (1985) 'Reduction on Mortality From Breast Cancer After Mass Screening with Mammography. Randomised Trial from the Breast Cancer Screening Working Group of the Swedish National Board of Health and Welfare', *The Lancet*, I: 829–32.

Tabar, L., Vitak, B., Chen, H. et al. (2001) 'Beyond Randomized Controlled Trials: Organized Mammographic Screening Substantially Reduces Breast Carcinoma Mortality', *Cancer*, 91(9): 1724–31.

Tall, A.R. (1990) 'Plasma High Density Lipoprotein: Metabolism and the Relationship to Atherogenesis', *Journal of Clinical Investigation*, 86(1): 37–84.

Tanner, C., Ross, G.W., Jewell, S. et al. (2009) 'Occupationism and the Risk of Parkinsonism: A Multi-centre Case Control Study', *Archives of Neurology*, 66(9): 1106–13.

Tansey, G. and Worsley, T. (1995) *The Food System* (London: Earthscan).

Tanskanen, A., Hibbeln, J., Tuomilehto, J. et al. (2001) 'Fish Consumption and Depressive Symptoms in the General Population in Finland', *Psychiatric Services*, 52: 529–31.

Tarrow, S. (1998) *Power in Movement* (Cambridge: Cambridge University Press).

Taubert, K.A. and Shulman, S.T. (1999) 'Kawasaki Disease', *American Family Physician*, 59(11): 3093–102, 3107–8.

Taylor, B., Miller, E., Farrington, C.P. et al. (1999) 'Autism and Measles, Mumps and Rubella Vaccine?: No Epidemiological Evidence for a Causal Association, *The Lancet*, 353: 2626–9.

Taylor, E., Burley, V., Greenwood, D. and Cade, J. (2007) 'Meat Consumption and Risk of Breast Cancer in the UK Women's Cohort Study', *British Journal of Cancer*, 96: 1139–46.

Taylor, G. and Hawley, H. (2006) 'Health Promotion and the Freedom of the Individual', *Health Care Analysis*, 14: 15–24.

Taylor, G. and Millar, M. (2004) 'The Politics of Food Regulation and Reform in Ireland', *Public Administration*, 83(3): 585–603.

Taylor, M. (1999) 'Between Public and Private: Accountability in Voluntary Organisations', *Policy and Politics*, 2491: 57–72.

Taylor, M. (2006) 'Communities in Partnership: Developing a Strategic Voice', *Social Policy and Society*, 5(2): 269–79.

Taylor, P. (1984) *The Smoke Ring: Tobacco, Money and Multi-National Politics* (London: Bodley Head).

Taylor, P. (2003) 'The Lay Contribution to Public Health' in Orme, J., Powell, J., Harrison, T. and Grey, M. *Public Health for the 21st Century: New Perspectives on Policy, Participation and Practice* (Maidenhead: Open University Press), pp. 128–44.

Taylor, P., Peckham, S. and Turton, P. (1998) *A Public Health Model of Primary Care: From Concept to Reality* (Birmingham: Public Health Alliance).

Terrence Higgins Trust (THT), British HIV Association (BHIVA), Providers of AIDS Care and Treatment (PACT) and British Association for Sexual Health and HIV (2006) *Disturbing Symptoms 4: How Primary Care Trusts Managed Sexual Health Services in 2005 and How Specialist Clinicians Viewed Their Progress* (London: THT).

Terrence Higgins Trust (THT), British HIV Association (BHIVA), Providers of AIDS Care and Treatment (PACT) and British Association for Sexual Health and HIV (2007) Disturbing Symptoms 5: *How Primary Care Trusts Managed Sexual Health Services in 2006 and How Specialist Clinicians Viewed Their Progress* (London: THT).

Tervonen-Gonçalves, L. and Lehto, J. (2004) 'Transfer of Health for All Policy: What, How and Which Direction? A Two-Case Study', *Health Research Policy and Systems*, 2(1): 8.

Tesh, S. (1988) 'Political Ideology and Public Health in the Nineteenth Century', *International Journal of Health Services*, 12(2): 321–42.

Thiébaut, A., Kipnis, V., Chang, S.C. et al. (2007) 'Dietary Fat and Postmenopausal Invasive Breast Cancer in the National Institutes of Health–AARP Diet and Health Study Cohort', *Journal of the National Cancer Institute*, 99: 451–62.

Thomas, B., Dorling, D. and Davey Smith, G. (2010) 'Inequalities in Premature Mortality in Britain: Observational Study From 1921 to 2007' *British Medical Journal* 341: c3639 (doi: 10.1136/bmj.c3639 accessed 24.8.10).

Thomas, H. (1998) 'Reproductive Health Needs Across the Lifespan' in Doyal, L. (ed.) *Women and Health Services* (Maidenhead: Open University Press) pp. 39–53.

Thompson, J. and Anthony, H. (2005) 'The Health Effects of Waste Incinerators', *Journal of Nutritional and Environmental Medicine,* 15(2–3): 115–56.

Thomson, H. (2007) 'Housing and Health', *British Medical Journal* (doi: 10.1136/bmj.39133.558380.BE).

Thomson, H., Petticrew, M. and Morrison, D. (2001) 'Health Effects if Housing Improvement: Systematic Review of Intervention Studies', *British Medical Journal*, 323: 187–90.

Thorpe, G., Kirk, S. and Whitcombe, D. (2002) *The Impact of the National Healthy School Standard on School Effectiveness and Improvement* (London: Department for Education and Skills (DfES).

Tilson, H. and Berkowitz, B. (2006) 'The Public Health Enterprise: Examining our Twenty First Century Policy Challenges', *Health Affairs*, 24(4): 900 (doi: 10.1377/hlthaff 25.4.900).

Tinsley, R. and Luck, M. (1998) 'Fundholding and the Community Nurse', *Journal of Social Policy,* 27(4): 471–87.

Tocque, K., Edwards, R. and Fullard, B. (2005) 'The Impact of Partial Smoke-Free Legislation on Health Inequalities? Evidence From a Survey of 1150 Pubs in North West England', *BMC Public Health*, 5(91).

Toke, D. (2002) 'UK GM Crop Policy: Relative Calm Before the Storm?', *The Political Quarterly*, 73(1): 67–75.

Tones, K. (1987) 'Devising Strategies for Preventing Drug Abuse: The Role of Health Action Model' *Health Education Research Theory and Practice*, 2(4): 305–17.

Tones, K. and Green, J. (2004) *Health Promotion: Planning and Strategies* (London: Sage).

Townend, L. (2009) 'The Moralising of Obesity: A New Name for an Old Sin?', *Critical Social Policy*, 29(2): 171–90.

Towner, E. (2005) 'Injuries and Inequalities: Bridging the Gap', *Injury Control and Safety Promotion*, 12(3): 79–84.

Townsend, J., Roderick, P. and Cooper, J. (1994) 'Cigarette Smoking by Socioeconomic Group, Sex and Age: Effects of Price Income and Health Publicity', *British Medical Journal*, 309: 923.

Townsend, P. (2001) *Targeting Poor Health* (Cardiff: National Assembly for Wales).

Townsend, P., Davidson, N. and Whitehead, M. (eds) (1992) *Inequalities in Health* (Harmondsworth: Penguin).

Transform Drug Policy Foundation (2009) *A Comparison of the Cost-Effectiveness of the Prohibition and Regulation of Drugs* (Bristol: TDPF).

Transport Committee (2006) *10th 2005/2006: Road Policing and Technology: Getting the Right Balance*, HC 975 (London: TSO).

Transport Committee (2008a) *11th Report 2007/8: Ending the Scandal of Complacency: Road Safety Beyond 2010*, HC 460 (London: TSO).

Transport Committee (2008b) *School Travel plans 2007/8* (London: TSO).

Transport, Local Government and Regions Committee (2002) *9th Report 2001/2: Road Traffic Speed*, HC 557 (London: TSO).

Travis, R. and Key, T. (2003) 'Oestrogen Exposure and Breast Cancer Risk', *Breast Cancer Research*, 5: 239–47.

Treasury Committee (2006) *The Administration of Tax Credits, 6th Report of Session 2005–6, Volume 1*, HC 811 (London: TSO).

Treaty Establishing a Constitution for Europe (2004) (http://europa.eu/constituition/en/lstoc1_en.htm).

Treaty on European Union (1992) *Official Journal of the European Communities*, C244, 31 August (http://europa.eu.int/en/record/mt/top.html accessed 19.03.07).

Trevelyan, G.M. (1973) *English Social History: A Survey of Six Centuries* (London: Longman).

Trevett, N. (1997) 'Injecting New Life into the Wirral', Healthlines, 39(February): 20–1.

Trichopoulou, A., Bamia, C. and Trichopoulos, D. (2009) 'Anatomy of Health Effects of a Mediterranean Diet: Greek EPIC Prospective Cohort Study', *British Medical Journal*, 338: b2337.

Tritter, J. and McCallum, A. (2006) 'The Snakes and Ladders of User Involvement: Moving Beyond Arnstein', *Health Policy*, 76: 156–68.

Tsouros, A. (1990) *World Health Organisation Healthy Cities Project. A Project Becomes a Movement (Review of Progress 1987–1990)* (Copenhagen: WHO).

Tucker, J., Fitzmaurice, A., Imamura, M. et al. (2006) 'The Effect of the National Demonstration Project Healthy Respect on Teenage Sexual Behaviour', *European Journal of Public Health*, 17(1): 33–41.

Tudor Hart, J. (1971) 'The Inverse Care Law', *The Lancet*, 427: February, 405–12.

Tudor Hart, J. (2006) *The Political Economy of Health Care: A Clinical Perspective* (Bristol: The Policy Press).

Tudor, K. (1996) *Mental Health Promotion* (London: Routledge).

Turning Point (2004) *Turning 40* (London: Turning Point).

Tutt, D., Bauer, L. and Di Franza, J. (2009) 'Restricting the Supply of Tobacco to Minors', *Journal of Public Health Policy*, 30(1): 68–82.

UKCRC (2008) *Strengthening Public Health Research in the UK – Report of the UK Clinical Research Collaboration Public Health Strategic Planning Group* (UK CRC).

UK Drug Policy Commission (2009) *Refocusing Drug-related Law Enforcement to Address Harms* (London: UK Drug Policy Commission).

UK Scientific Committee on Tobacco and Health (1998) *Report* (London: HMSO).

UK Scientific Committee on Tobacco and Health (2004) *Update of Evidence on Health Effects of Secondhand Smoke* (London: DoH).

UKPHA (UK Public Health Association) (undated) *Health Visiting and the Public Health: A Paper by the UKPHA Special Interest Group on Health Visiting and Public Health* (London: UKPHA).

UKPHA (2004) Choosing Health or Losing Health (Birmingham: UKPHA).

UKPHA (2009) *Health Visiting Matters: Re-establishing Health Visiting* (London: UKPHA).

UKTED (UK Trial of Early Detection Cancer Group) (1988) 'First Results on Mortality Reduction in the UK Trial of Early Detection of Breast Cancer', *The Lancet*, 2: 411–16.

UKTED (UK Trial of Early Detection Cancer Group) (1999) '16 Year Mortality from Breast Cancer in the UK Trial of Early Detection of Breast Cancer', *The Lancet*, 353: 1909–14.

UN (2002) *World Summit on Sustainable Development* (http://www.un.org/jsummit/html/basic_info/basicinfo.html accessed 5.5.10)

UN (2009) *Declaration on the Guiding Principles of Drug Demand Reduction* (Geneva: UN).

UN (United Nations) Commission for Narcotic Drugs (1999) *Report of the Meeting of the High Level Expert Group to Review the UN International Drug Control Program and to Strengthen the UN Machinery for Drug Control* (Vienna: Commission for Narcotic Drugs).

UN General Assembly (2000) 'United Nations Millennium Declaration: Resolution Adopted by the General Assembly. 55th Session 18 September 2000 A/res/55/2.

UNDCP (UN Drug Control Programme) (1998) Economic and Social Consequences of Drug Abuse and Illicit Trafficking (UNDCP technical series) (www.unodc.org/pdf/technical_series_1998-01-01_1.pdf accessed 17.5.10).

UNEP (United Nations Environment Programme0 (1992) Environmental Effects of Ozone Regulation: 1991 Update (Nairobi: UNEP).

UNEP (2007) *Global Environment Outlook 4* (Nairobi: UNEP).

UNICEF (United Nations International Children's Emergency Fund) (1989) *Convention on the Rights of the Child* (Switzerland: Office of the United Nations High Commissioner for Human Rights).

UNICEF (2005) *Child Poverty in Rich Countries 2005* (New York: UNICEF).

UNICEF (2007) *Child Poverty in Perspective: An Overview of Child Well-being in Rich Countries: A Comprehensive Assessment of the Lives and Well-being of Children and Adolescents in the Economically Advanced Nations* (Florence: UNICEF Innocenti Research Centre).

University of East Anglia and National Children's Bureau (2007) *Children's Trust Pathfinders: Innovative Partnerships for Improving the Well-being of Children and Young People* (Norwich: University of East Anglia).

UNODC (2008) *World Drug Report* (Vienna: UNDOC).

UN World Commission on Environment and Development (1987) *Our Common Future* (Oxford: Oxford University Press).

Upshur, R. (2002) Principles for the Justification of Public Health Intervention', *Canadian Journal of Public Health*, 93(2): 101–3.

US Department of Health and Human Services (1980) *Promoting Health/Preventing Disease: Objectives for the Nation* (Washington: Public Health Service).

US Department of Health and Human Services (1986) *The Heath Consequences of Involuntary Smoking: A Report of the Surgeon General* (Washington DC: US Government Printing Office).

US Department of Health and Human Services (1991) *Healthy People 2000* (Washington: Public Health Service).

US Department of Health and Human Services (2000) *Healthy People 2010* (2nd edn) (Washington: Public Health Service).

US Environmental Protection Agency (1992) *Respiratory Effects of Passive Smoking, Lung Cancer and Other Disorders* (Washington DC: Office of Health and Environment Assessment, Office of Research & Development, USEPA).

Van Baal, P., Polder, J., Ardine de Wit, G. et al. (2008) 'Lifetime Medical Costs of Obesity: Prevention no Cure for Increasing Health Expenditure', *PLoS Medicine* (www.plosmedicine.org), 5(2): 0242–9.

Van Dam, R., Spiegelman, D., Franco, O. and Hu, F. (2008) 'Combined Impact of Lifestyle Factors on Mortality: Prospective Cohort Study in US Women', *British Medical Journal*, 337: a1440.

Van den Berg, G. (2009) 'Inequality in Individual Mortality and Economic Conditions Earlier in Life', *Social Science and Medicine*, 69: 1360-7.

van de Mheen, H.D., Stronks, K. and Mackenbach, J. (1998) 'A Lifecourse Perspective on Socio-economic Inequalities in Health: The Influence of Childhood Socio-economic Conditions and Selection Processes', *Sociology of Health and Illness*, 20(5): 754–77.

van Os, J., Bak, M., Hanssen, M. et al. (2002) 'Cannabis Use and Psychosis: A Longitudinal Population Based Study', *American Journal of Epidemiology*, 156: 319–27.

van Ours, J. (2003) Is Cannabis a Stepping Stone for Cocaine?' *Journal of Health Economics*, 22(4): 539–54.

Van Sluijs, E., McMinn, A. and Griffin, S. (2007) 'Effectiveness of Interventions to Promote Physical Activity in Children and Adolescents: Systematic Review of Controlled Trials', *British Medical Journal*, 335: 703 (doi: 10.1136/bmj.39320.843947.BE accessed 15.5.10).

Van Zwanenberg, P. and Millstone, E. (2003) 'BSE: A Paradigm of Policy Failure', *The Political Quarterly*, 74(1): 27–37.

Van't Veer, P., Lobbezoo, I., Martin-Moreno, J. et al. (1997) 'DDT (Dicophane) and Postmenopausal Breast Cancer in Europe: A Case Control Study', *British Medical Journal*, 315: 81–5.

Vartiainen, E., Puska, P., Jousilahti, P. et al. (1994) 'Twenty-Year Trends in Coronary Risk Factors in North Karelia and Other Areas of Finland', *International Journal of Epidemiology*, 23(3): 495–504.

Veenstra, G., Luginaah, I., Wakefield, S. et al. (2005) 'Who You Know, Where You Live: Social Capital, Neighbourhood and Health', *Social Science & Medicine*, 60: 2799–818.

Veerman, J., Van Beeck, E., Barendregt, J. and Mackenbach, J. (2009) 'By How Much Would Limiting TV Food Advertising Reduce Childhood Obesity?', *European Journal of Public Health*, (doi: 10.1093/eurpub/ckp039).

Venn, A., Lewis, S., Cooper, M. et al. (2001) 'Living near a Main Road and the Risk of Wheezing Illness in Children', *American Journal of Respiratory and Critical Care Medicine*, 164(12): 2177–80.

Verbeek, A., Holland, R., Sturmans, F. et al. (1984) 'Reduction of Breast Cancer Mortality Through Mass Screening with Modern Mammography', *The Lancet,* I: 1222–6.

Verschuren, W., Jacobs, D., Bloemberg, B. et al. (1995) 'Serum Total Cholesterol and Long-term Coronary Heat Disease Mortality in Different Cultures. Twenty-Five Year Follow Up of the 7 Countries Study', *Journal of the American Medical Association*, 274(2): 131–6.

Vetter, N. (1998) The Public Health and the NHS (Oxford: Radcliffe Medical Press).

Vineis, P., Schulte, P. and McMichael, A. (2001) 'Misconceptions about the Use of Genetic Tests in Populations', *The Lancet*, 357(9257): 709–12.

Violence Reduction Unit (2007) *Violence Reduction Unit Strategic Plan* (Glasgow: Violence Reduction Unit).

Visram, S. and Drinkwater, C. (2005) *Health Trainers: A Review of the Evidence* (Newcastle: Primary Care Development Centre University of Northumbria).

Vostanis, P. and Cumella, C. (1999) *Homeless Children: Problems and Needs* (London: Jessica Kinsgley).

Vrijheid, M., Dolk, H., Armstrong, B. et al. (2002) 'Chromosomal Congenital Anomalies and Residence near Hazardous Waste Landfill Sites', *The Lancet*, 359: January 320–2.

Waddell, G. and Burton, K. (2006) *Is Work Good for Your Health and Wellbeing?* (London: TSO).

Wade, E., Smith, J., Peck, E. and Freeman, T. (2006) *Commissioning in the Reformed NHS: Policy into Practice* (Birmingham: Health Service Management Centre, University of Birmingham).

Wainwright, D. and Calnan, M. (2002) *Work Stress: The Making of a Modern Epidemic* (Buckingham: Open University Press).

Wait, S. and Nolte, E. (2006) 'Public Involvement Policies in Health: Exploring Their Conceptual Basis', *Health Economics Policy and Law*, 1: 149–62.

Waitzkin, H., Jasso-Aguilar, R., Landwehr, A. and Mountain, C. (2005) 'Global Trade, Public Health, and Health Services: Stakeholder's Constructions of the Key Issues', *Social Science & Medicine*, 61: 893–906.

Wakefield, A.J., Murch, S.H., Anthony, A. et al. (1998) 'Ileal-lymphoid-nodular Hyperplasia, Non-specific Colitis, and Pervasive Development Disorder in Children', *The Lancet*, 351: 637–41.

Walker, A., Maher, J., Coulthard, M., et al. (2001) *Living in Britain: Results from the 2000/1 General Household Survey* (London: TSO).

Walkowiak, J., Wiener, J., Fastabend, A. et al. (2001) 'Environmental Exposure to Polychlorinated Biphenyls and Quality of the Home Environment: Effects on Psychodevelopment in Early Childhood', *The Lancet*, 358: 10th November, 1602–7.

Walt, G. (1994) *Health Policy: An Introduction to Process and Power* (London: Zed Books).

Walters, R. (2009) *Crime is in the Air: Air Pollution and Regulation in the UK* (Centre for Crime and Justice Studies, King's College, University of London).

Walvin, J. (1987) *Victorian Values* (London: Deutsch).

Wang, J., Liu, R., Liu, L. et al. (1999) 'The Effect of Leptin on Lep Expression is Tissue-Specific and Nutritionally Regulated', *Nature Medicine*, 5(8): 895–8.

Wanless, D. (2002) *Securing our Future Health: Taking a Long term View Final Report* (London: HM Treasury).

Wanless, D. (2003) *The Review of Health and Social Care in Wales* (Cardiff: Welsh Assembly).

Wanless, D. (2004) *Securing Good Health for the Whole Population* (London: HM Treasury).

Wanless, D. (2007) *Our Future Health Secured* (London: King's Fund).

Wannamethee, G., Shaper, A.G., Whincup, P.H. and Walker, M. (1995) 'Low Serum Total Cholesterol Concentrations and Mortality in Middle-Aged British Men', *British Medical Journal*, 311: 409–13.

Wardle, J., Llewellyn, C., Sanderson, S. and Plomin, R. (2009) 'The Fto Gene and Measured Food Intake in Children', *International Journal of Obesity*, 33: 42–5.

Warhurst, M. (2005) *An Introduction to Current System for Regulating Chemicals in the European Union* (University of Massachusetts: Lowell Centre for Sustainable Production).

Warner, M., Eskenazi, B., Mocarelli, P. et al. (2002) 'Serum Dioxin Concentrations and Breast Cancer Risk in the Seveso Women's Health Study,' *Environmental Health Perspectives*, 110(7): 625–8.

Watmough, D., Bhargava, A., Syed, S.R. and Sharma, P. (1997) 'For Debate: Does Breast Cancer Screening Depend on a Wobbly Hypothesis?', *Journal of Public Health Medicine*, 19(4): 375–9.

Watson, M. (2003) Environmental Impact Assessment and European Community Law XIV International Conference 'Danube - River of Cooperation', Beograd 13-15 November, 2003 (www.members.tripod.com/~danubedita/library/2003watson2.htm accessed 10.9.08).

Watson, M. and White, J. (2001) 'Accident Prevention Activities: A National Survey of Health Authorities', *Health Education Journal*, 60(3): 275–83.

Watterson, A. (1995) *Breast Cancer and the Links with Exposure to Environmental and Occupational Carcinogens* (Leicester: Centre for Occupational and Environmental Health Policy Research).

Watterson, A. and O'Neill, R. (2007) *Burying the Evidence: How the UK is Prolonging the Occupational Cancer Epidemic Hazards Magazine On Line Briefing* (www.hazards.org).

WCRF (World Cancer Research Fund) (2007) *Food, Nutrition, Physical Activity and the Prevention of Cancer* (Washington DC: American Cancer Research Institute).

WCRF (World Cancer Research Fund) and America Institute for Cancer Research (2009) *Policy and Action for Cancer Prevention* (Washington DC: American Cancer Research Institute).

Weale, A. (1983) 'Invisible Hand or Fatherly Hand? Problems of Paternalism in the New Perspective on Health', *Journal of Health Politics, Policy and Law*, 7(4): 784–807.

Weare, K. (2002) 'The Contribution of Education to Health Promotion' in Bunton, R. and Macdonald, G. (eds) *Health Promotion: Disciplines, Diversity and Developments* (London: UK, Routledge), pp. 102–25.

Webb, P. (2000) *The Modern British Party System* (London: Sage).

Webster, C. (1986) 'MoHs – For the Record', *Radical Community Medicine,* autumn (3): 10–14.

Webster, C. (1988) *Health Services Since the War, Volume 1: Problems of Health Care. The National Health Service Before 1957* (London: HMSO).

Webster, C. (1990) *The Victorian Public Health Legacy: A Challenge to the Future* (London: Public Health Alliance).

Webster, C. (1996) *Government and Health Care, Volume II: The National Health Service 1958–79* (London: HMSO).

Webster, C. (2007) 'Drug Treatment' in Simpson, M., Shildrick, T. and Macdonald, R. *Drugs in Britain – Supply, Consumption and Control* (Basingstoke: Palgrave Macmillan), pp. 141–61.

Webster, D. and Mackie, M. (1996) *Review of Traffic Calming Schemes in 20 mph Zones* Transport Research Laboratory Study Group 215 (London: DoE).

Webster. C. and French, J. (2002) 'The Cycle of Conflict: The History of the Public Health and Health Promotion Movements' in Adams, L., Amos, M. and Munro, J. (eds) *Promoting Health* (London: Sage), pp. 5–12.

Weinser, R.L., Hunter, G.R., Hevic, A.F. et al. (1998) 'The Etiology of Obesity: Relative Contribution of Metabolic Factors, Diet and Physical Activity', *American Journal of Medicine*, 105(2): 145–50.

Wellcome Trust (2004) *Public Health Sciences: Challenges and Opportunities* (London: The Wellcome Trust).

Welsh Assembly Government (1999) *Developing Health Impact Assessment in Wales* (Cardiff: Welsh Assembly Government).

Welsh Assembly Government (2000) *Children and Young People: A Framework for Partnership* (Cardiff: Welsh Assembly Government).

Welsh Assembly Government (2002a) *Wellbeing in Wales* (Cardiff: Welsh Assembly Government).

Welsh Assembly Government (2002b) *Children and Young People: Framework Planning Guidance* (Cardiff: Welsh Assembly Government).

Welsh Assembly Government (2003a) *Wales: A Better Country* (Cardiff: Welsh Assembly Government).

Welsh Assembly Government (2003b) *Healthy and Active Lifestyles in Wales* (Cardiff: Welsh Assembly Government).

Welsh Assembly Government (2003c) *Child Wellbeing* (Cardiff: WAG).

Welsh Assembly Government (2004) *Children and Young People: Rights to Action* (Cardiff: Welsh Assembly Government).

Welsh Assembly Government (2005a) *Designed for Life: Creating World Class Health and Social Care for Wales in the 21st Century* (Cardiff: Welsh Assembly Government).

Welsh Assembly Government (2005b) *A Fair Future for our Children: The Strategy of the Welsh Assembly Government for Tackling Child Poverty* (Cardiff: Welsh Assembly Government).

Welsh Assembly Government (2005c) *Flying Start* (Cardiff: Welsh Assembly Government).

Welsh Assembly Government (2006a) *Making the Connections – Delivering Beyond Boundaries. Transforming Public Services in Wales* (Cardiff: Welsh Assembly Government).

Welsh Assembly Government (2006b) *Climbing Higher* (Cardiff: Welsh Assembly Government).

Welsh Assembly Government (2007) *Developing a Whole School Food and Fitness Policy* (Cardiff: Welsh Assembly Government).

Welsh Assembly Government (2008a) *Appetite for Life* (Cardiff: Welsh Assembly Government).

Welsh Assembly Government (2008b) *Working Together to Reduce Harm – The Substance Misuse Strategy for Wales 2008–2018* (Cardiff: Welsh Assembly Government).

Welsh Assembly Government (2009a) *Climate Change Strategy; Programme of Action Consultation* (Cardiff: Welsh Assembly Government).

Welsh Assembly Government (2009b) *A Community Nursing Strategy for Wales* (Cardiff: Welsh Assembly Government).

Welsh Office (1996) *Forward Together: A Strategy to Combat Drug and Alcohol Misuse in Wales* (Cardiff: Welsh Office).

Welsh Office (1998) *Strategic Framework Better Health, Better Wales* (Cardiff: Welsh Office).

Welsh Office, NHS Directorate (1989) *Welsh Health Planning Forum: Strategic Intent and Direction for the NHS in Wales* (Cardiff: Welsh Office).

Welsh Office, NHS Directorate (1992) *Caring for the Future* (Cardiff: Welsh Office).

Welshman, J. (1997) 'The Medical Officers of Health in England and Wales 1900–74: Watchdog or Lapdog?', *Journal of Public Health and Medicine*, 19(4): 443–50.

West, P., Sweeting, H. and Leyland, A. (2004) 'School Effects on Pupils' Health Behaviours: Evidence in Support of the Health Promoting School', *Research Papers in Education*, 19(3): 261–91.

West, R., Townsend, J., Joossens, L. et al. (2008) 'Why Combating Tobacco Smuggling is a Priority', *British Medical Journal*, 337: 1933.

Westin, J.B. (1993) 'Carcinogens in Israeli Milk: A Study in Regulating Regulatory Failure', *International Journal of Health Services*, 23(3): 497–517.

Weyman, A. and Davey, C. (2007) 'Sexual Health: The Challenges' in Griffiths, S. and Hunter, D.J. *New Perspectives in Public Health* (2nd edn) (Oxford: Radcliffe), pp. 158–65.

Whincup, P., Gilg, J., Emberson, J. et al. (2004) 'Passive Smoking and Risk of Coronary Heart Disease and Stroke: Prospective Study with Cotinine Measurement', *British Medical Journal Online*. 329: 200–5 (24 July) (doi: 10.1136/bmj.38146.427188.55 accessed 18.5.10).

White, C. (2002) 'Unacceptable Errors Found in Breast Screening Service', *British Medical Journal*, 324(7343): 933.

White, C., Edgar, G. and Siegler, V. (2008) *Social Inequalities in Male Mortality for Selected Causes of Death by the National Statistics Socio-economic Classification, England and Wales, 2001–03* (London: Office for National Statistics).

White, C., Glickman, M., Johnson, B. and Corbin, T. (2007) *Social Inequalities in Adult Male Mortality by the National Statistics Socio-Economic Classification, England and Wales, 2001–03* (London: ONS).

Whitehead, M. (1987) *The Health Divide* (London: Health Education Council).

Whitehead, M. (1992) 'The Concepts and Principles of Equity and Health', *International Journal of Health Services*, 22(3): 429–46.

Whitehead, M. and Drever, M. (1997) 'Health Inequalities: Main Findings and Implications for the Future' in Drever, M. and Whitehead, M. *Health Inequalities* (London: TSO), pp. 224–36.

Whitmer, R.E., Barrett-Connor, E., Queensberry, C. and Yaffe, C. (2005) 'Obesity in Middle Age and Future Risk of Dementia: A 27-year Longitudinal Population-based Study', *British Medical Journal*, 330 (doi: 10.1136/bmj.38446.466238.E0 accessed 11.9.10).

Whitty, P. and Jones, I. (1992) 'Public Health Heresy: A Challenge to the Purchasing Orthodoxy', British Medical Journal, 304: 1039–41.

WHO (World Health Organization) (1946) *Constitution: Basic Documents* (Geneva: WHO).

WHO (1981) *Global Health Strategy for Health for All by the Year 2000* (Geneva: WHO).

WHO (1986) First International Conference on Health Promotion. The Move Towards a New Public Health: Ottawa Charter for Health Promotion Ottawa Nov 17–21 (Ottawa: WHO/Health and Welfare Canada/Canadian Association for Public Health).

WHO (1988) *Second International Conference on Health Promotion: Adelaide Recommendations* (Adelaide: WHO/Australian Department of Community Services and Health).

WHO (1990) *Diet, Nutrition and the Prevention of Chronic Diseases. Report of a WHO Study Group* (Geneva: WHO).

WHO (1991) *Third International Conference on Health Promotion: Sundsvall Statement on Supportive Environments for Health* (Sundsvall: WHO, UNEP and Nordic Council of Ministers).

WHO (1996) *International Strategy for Tobacco Control* (Geneva: WHO).

WHO (1997a) *Fourth International Conference on Health Promotion: The Jakarta Declaration* (Jakarta: WHO).

WHO (1997b) *Tobacco or Health: A Global Status Report 1997* (Geneva: WHO).

WHO (1997c) *Cannabis: A Health Perspective and Research Agenda* (Geneva: WHO).

WHO (1998a) *Health for All for the 21st Century* (Geneva: WHO).

WHO (1998b) *Health Promotion Glossary* (Geneva: WHO).

WHO (1998c) *Obesity: Preventing and Managing The Global Epidemic: Report of a WHO Consultation* Interim Report (Geneva: WHO).

WHO (1999) *Removing Obstacles to Healthy Development* (Geneva: WHO).

WHO (2000a) *The Fifth Global Conference on Health Promotion. Health Promotion: Bridging the Equity Gap* 5–9th June Mexico City (http://www.who.int/healthpromotion/conferences/previous/mexico/en/hpr_mexico_report_en.pdf accessed 21.5.10).

WHO (2000b) *Obesity: Preventing and Managing the Global Epidemic Report of a WHO Consultation* (Geneva: WHO).

WHO (2002) *Global Strategy for Food Safety* (Geneva: WHO).

WHO (2003) *WHO Framework Convention on Tobacco Control* (Geneva: WHO).

WHO (2004a) *Fifty-Seventh World Health Assembly, Provisional Agenda Item 12.6: Global Strategy on Diet, Physical Activity ad Health* (Geneva: WHO).

WHO (2004b) *Global Status Report on Alcohol 2004* (Geneva: WHO).

WHO (2005a) *The Bangkok Charter for Health Promotion in a Globalised World* 6th Global Conference on Health Promotion, Bangkok, Thailand 7–11 August (http://www.who.int/healthpromotion/conferences/6gchp/hpr_050829_%20BCHP.pdf accessed 21.5.10).

WHO (2005b) *World Health Report: Making Every Mother and Child Count* (Geneva: WHO).

WHO (2006a) *Guidelines for Drinking-Water Quality* (Geneva: WHO).

WHO (2006b) *Air Quality Guidelines for Particulate Matter, Ozone, Nitrogen Dioxide and Sulphur Dioxide: Global Update* (Geneva: WHO).

WHO (2007) *WHO Expert Committee on Problems Related to Alcohol Consumption* (Geneva: WHO).

WHO (2008a) *2008–13 Action Plan for the Global Strategy for the Prevention and Control of Noncommunicable Diseases* (Geneva: WHO).

WHO (2008b) *Primary Health Care – Now More Than Ever* (Geneva: WHO).

WHO (2008c) *Strategies to Reduce the Harmful Use of Alcohol* (Sixty-first World Health Assembly).

WHO (2008d) *Report on the Global Tobacco Epidemic, 2008 – The MPOWER Package* (Geneva: WHO).

WHO (2009a) *Prevention and Control of Noncommunicable Diseases; Implementation of the Global Strategy* (Geneva: WHO).

WHO (2009b) *Interventions on Diet and Physical Activity: What Works* (Geneva: WHO).

WHO (2009c) *The Global Burden* (http://www.who.int/substance_abuse/facts/global_burden/en/index.html accessed 17.5.10).

WHO (2009d) *Promoting Health and Development: Closing the Implementation Gap 7th Global Conference on Health Promotion 26–30 October, Nairobi, Kenya.*

WHO (2010) *Draft Global Strategy to Reduce the Harmful Use of Alcohol* (revised version, February, 2010) (Geneva: WHO).

WHO and UNICEF (United Nations Children's Fund) (1978) *Declaration of Alma Ata*. Report of the International Conference on Primary Health Care (Geneva: WHO/UNICEF).

WHO and UNICEF (2008) *World Report on Child Injury Prevention* (Geneva: WHO).

WHO Regional Office for Europe (1985) *Targets for Health for All: Targets in Support of the European Regional Strategy for Health for All* (Copenhagen: WHO Europe).

WHO Regional Office for Europe (1987) *WHO Air Quality Guidelines for Europe* (Copenhagen: WHO Europe).

WHO Regional Office for Europe (1988) *Healthy Nutrition: Preventing Nutrition-Related Disease in Europe* (Copenhagen: WHO Europe).

WHO Regional Office for Europe (1990) *Health and Environment: Charter and Commentary* (Copenhagen: WHO Europe).

WHO Regional Office for Europe (1993a) *Health for All Targets: The Health Policy for Europe* (Copenhagen: WHO Europe).

WHO Regional Office for Europe (1993b) *Healthy Schools: The European Network of Health Promoting Schools* (Copenhagen: WHO, European Commission and Council of Europe).

WHO Regional Office for Europe (1993c) *European Alcohol Action Plan* (Copenhagen: WHO Europe).

WHO Regional Office for Europe (1993d) *Action Plan for a Tobacco Free Europe* (Copenhagen: WHO Europe).

WHO Regional Office for Europe (1994) *Environmental Health Action Plan for Europe* (Copenhagen: WHO Europe).

WHO Regional Office for Europe (1998) *Comparative Analysis of Nutrition Policies in WHO Member States* (Copenhagen: WHO Europe).

WHO Regional Office for Europe (1999a) *Health Impact Assessment: Main Concepts and Suggested Approach: The Gothenburg Consensus* (Copenhagen: WHO Europe).

WHO Regional Office for Europe (1999b) *Charter on Transport, Environment and Health* (Copenhagen: WHO Europe).

WHO Regional Office for Europe (1999c) *Health 21: The Health for All Policy Framework for the Twenty First Century* (Copenhagen: WHO Europe).

WHO Regional Office for Europe (2000a) *WHO Air Quality Guidelines for Europe* (2nd edn) (Copenhagen: WHO Europe).

WHO Regional Office for Europe (2000b) *First Action Plan for Food and Nutrition Policy* (Copenhagen: WHO Europe).

WHO Regional Office for Europe (2000c) *European Alcohol Action Plan 2000–2005* (Copenhagen– WHO Europe).

WHO Regional Office for Europe (2001) *Declaration on Young People and Alcohol* (Adopted in Stockholm on 21 February 2001).

WHO Regional Office for Europe (2002) *Review of National Finnish Health Promotion Policies and Recommendations for the Future* (Copenhagen: WHO Europe).

WHO Regional Office for Europe (2004) *Children's Environment and Health Action Plan for Europe. Fourth Ministerial Conference on Environment and Health* (Copenhagen: WHO Europe).

WHO Regional Office for Europe (2005) *Mental Health Action Plan for Europe: Facing the Challenges, Building Solutions* (Copenhagen: WHO Europe).

WHO Regional Office for Europe (2006a) *Health Risks of Particulate Matter From Long Range Transboundary Air Pollution* (Copenhagen: WHO Europe).

WHO Regional Office for Europe (2006b) *European Charter on Counteracting Obesity* (Istanbul, Turkey: WHO European Ministerial Conference on Counteracting Obesity, Diet and Physical Activity for Health 15–17 November).

WHO Regional Office for Europe (2008a) *The Talinn Charter: Health Systems for Health and Wealth*. Ministerial Conference on Health Systems, 25–27 June, Talinn, Estonia (Copena-hagen: WHO Europe).

WHO Regional Office for Europe (2008b) *WHO European Action Plan for Food and Nutrition Policy 2007–12* (Copenhagen: WHO Europe).

WHO Regional Office for Europe (2010) *Parma Declaration on Environment and Health*, Fifth Ministerial Conference on Environment and Health, Parma, Italy, 10-12 March 2010 (Co-penghagen: WHO Europe).

Wicklander, M. (2006) 'Implementing and Evaluat-ing the National Healthy School Program in England', *The Journal of School Nursing*, 22(5): 250–8.

Widgery, D. (1988) *The National Health: A Radical Perspective* (London: Hogarth).

Wiggins, M., Rosato, M., Austerberry, H. et al. (2005) *Sure Start Plus National Evaluation: Final Report* (London: Social Science Research Unit, Institute for Education, University of London).

Wikler, D. (1978) 'Coercive Methods in Health Promotion: Can They be Justified?', *Health Education Monographs*, 6(2): 223–41.

Wildavsky, A. (1988) *Searching for Safety* (New Brunswick: Transaction).

Wildavsky, A. (1991) 'If Claims of Harm from Technology are False, Mostly False or Unprov-en, What Does That Tell Us About Science?' in Berger, P. (ed.) *Health, Lifestyle and Environ-ment* (London: Social Affairs Unit).

Wilde, J. (2007) 'Public Health in a Changing Ireland: An All-Island Perspective' in Griffiths, S. and Hunter, D. (eds) *New Perspectives in Public Health* (London: Routledge), pp. 45–54.

Wildman, R., Muntner, P., Reynolds, K. et al. (2008) 'The Obese Without Cardiometabolic Risk Factor Clustering and the Normal Weight with Cardiometabolic Risk Factor Clustering and the Normal Wight with Cardiometabolic Risk Factor Clustering', *Archives of Internal Medicine*, 168: 1617–24.

Wilkin, D., Coleman, A., Dowling, B. and Smith, K. (eds) (2002) *The National Tracker Survey of Primary Care Groups and Trusts 2001/2002: Taking Responsibility?* (Manchester: University of Manchester).

Wilkin, T., Metcalf, B., Murphy, M. and Voss, L. (2005) 'Physical Activity and BMI in Adoles-cence', *thelancetcom*, 366.

Wilkinson, D. (1999) *Poor Housing and Ill Health: A Summary of Research Evidence* (Scottish Office).

Wilkinson, J. (2007) Public Health Intelligence and Public Health Observatories in Griffiths and Hunter *New Perspectives in Public Health* (2nd edn) (Oxford: Radcliffe), pp. 303–13.

Wilkinson, P., French, R., Kane, R. et al. (2006) 'Teenage Conceptions, Abortions, and Births in England, 1994–2003, and the National Teenage Pregnancy Strategy', *The Lancet*, 368(9550): 1879–86.

Wilkinson, R. (1996) *Unhealthy Societies: The Af-flictions of Inequality* (London: Routledge).

Wilkinson, R. (1997) 'Health Inequalities: Relative or Absolute Material Standards?', *British Medi-cal Journal*, 314: 591–5.

Wilkinson, R. and Pickett, K. (2006) 'Income Inequality and Population Health: A Review an Explanation of the Evidence', *Social Science & Medicine*, 62: 1768–84.

Wilkinson, R. and Pickett, K. (2007) 'The Prob-lems of Relative Deprivation: Why Some Socie-ties do Better Than Others', *Social Science & Medicine*, 65: 1965–78.

Wilkinson, R. and Pickett, K. (2009) '*The Spirit Level: Why More Equal Societies Almost Al-ways do Better* (London: Allen Lane).

Wilkinson, S. and Kitzinger, C. (eds) (1994) *Wom-en and Health* (London: Taylor and Francis).

Willemson, M. (2005) 'The New EU Cigarette Health Warnings Benefit Smokers Who Want to Quit The Habit: Results From the Dutch Continuous Survey of Smoking Habits', *Euro-pean Journal of Public Health*, 15(4): 389–92.

Williams, J. (2007) 'Inspecting, informing, improv-ing: public health within the Healthcare Com-mission', in Griffiths, S. and Hunter, D. (2007) *New Perspectives in Public Health*, (2nd edn) (London: Routledge) pp. 87–93.

Williams, S. and Calnan, M. (eds) (1996) *Modern Medicine: Lay Perspectives and Experiences* (London: UCL Press).

Williamson, C. (1992) *Whose Standards? Con-sumer and Professional Standards in Health Care* (Buckingham: Open University Press).

Willis, E. (1998) 'Public Health, Private Genes: The Social Contract and Genetic Biotechnolo-gies', *Public Health*, 8(2): 131–9.

Willis, R. (2008) What Price Carbon? *Green Futures* (http://www.forumforthefuture.org/greenfutures/articles/whatpricecarbon accessed 5.5.10).

Wills, J. and Earle, S. (2007) 'Theoretical Per-spectives on Promoting Public Health' in Earle, S., Lloyd, C., Sidell, M. and Spurr, S. *Theory and Research in Promoting Public Health* (London: Sage), pp. 129–61.

Wills, J., Evans, D. and Scott Samuel, A. (2008) 'Policies and Prospects for Health Promotion in England', *Critical Public Health*, 18(4): 521–31.

Wilson, J.M.G. and Jungner, G. (1968) *Principles and Practice of Screening for Disease* (Geneva: WHO).

Wilson, M.E. (1995) 'Infectious Diseases: An Eco-logical Perspective', *British Medical Journal*, 311. 1681–4.

Winslow, C.E.A. (1920) 'The Untilled Fields of Public Health', *Science*, 51: 23.

Winters, L., Gordon, U., Atherton, J. and Scott-Samuel, S. (2007) 'Developing Public Health Nursing: Barriers Perceived by Community Nurses', *Public Health*, 121: 623–33.

Wirrmann, E. and Carlson, C. (2005) 'Public Health Leadership in Primary Care Practice in England: Everybody's Business?', *Critical Public Health*, 15(3): 205–21.

Wisotsky, S. (1986) *Breaking the Impasse on the War on Drugs* (London & New York: Greenwood Press).

Wohl, A.S. (1984) *Endangered Lives, Public Health in Victorian Britain* (London: Unwin Methuen).

Wolfe, R. and Sharpe, K. (2002) 'Anti-vaccinations Past and Present', *British Medical Journal*, 325: 430–2.

Wolff, M.A., Toniolo, P.G., Lee, E. et al. (1993) 'Blood Levels of Organochlorine Residues and Risk of Breast Cancer', *Journal of the National Cancer Institute*, 85: 648–52.

Wolfson, M., Kaplan, G., Lynch, J. et al. (1999) 'Relation Between Income Inequality and Mortality: Empirical Demonstration', *British Medical Journal*, 319: 953–7.

Wolin, K.Y., Yan, Y., Colditz, G.A. and Lee. I.M. (2009) 'Physical Activity and Colon Cancer Prevention: A Meta-Anlaysis', *British Journal of Cancer*, 100: 611–16.

Wolk, A., Manson, J.E., Stampfer, M.J. et al. (1999) 'Long-term Intake of Dietary Fibre and Decreased Risk of Coronary Heart Disease Among Women', *Journal of the American Medical Association*, 281(21): 1990–2004.

Woodall, A., Sandbach, E., Woorward, C. et al. (2005) 'The Partial Smoking Ban in Licensed Establishments and Health Inequalities in England: Modelling Study', *British Medical Journal*, 331(7515): 488–9.

Woodhead, D., Jochelson, K. and Tennant, R. (2002) *Public Health in the Balance* (London: King's Fund).

Woodman, C.B.J., Threlfall, A.G., Boggis, C.R.M. and Prior, P. (1995) 'Is the Three-Year Breast Screening Interval Too Long? Occurrence of Interval Cancers in NHS Breast Screening Programme's NorthWest Region', *British Medical Journal*, 310: 224–6.

Woodward, L. (1962) *The Age of Reform 1815–1870* (2nd edn) (Oxford: Oxford University Press).

Woolf, S. (2000) 'Taking Critical Appraisals to Extremes: The Need for Balance in the Evaluation of Evidence', *Journal of Family Practice*, 49(12). 1081–5.

Work and Pensions Committee (2004) *Child Poverty in the UK, 2nd Report of Session 2003–4*, HC 85i (London: TSO).

Work and Pensions Committee (2008) *3rd Report of 2007/2008: The Role of the Health and Safety Commission and the Health and Safety Executive in Regulating Workplace Health and Safety*, HC 246 (London: TSO).

World Bank and World Health Organisation (WHO) (2004) *World Report on Road Traffic Injury Prevention* (Geneva: WHO).

Wright, C.J. (1986) 'Breast Cancer Screening. A Different Look at the Evidence', Surgery, 100(4): 594–8.

Wright, J. (2007) 'Developing the Public Workforce' in Griffiths, S. and Hunter, D.J. *New Perspectives in Public Health* (2nd edn) (Oxford: Radcliffe), pp. 217–23.

Wright, J., Somervaille, L. and Dunkley, R. (2006) *Review of the Public Health Function of National Health Organisations and Units in Wales* (Cardiff: Public Health Resource Unit).

WTO (1994) *The WTO Agreement on the Application of Sanitary and Phytosanitary Measures* (SPS Agreement), (Geneva: WTO).

www.bmj.com (2007) 'Medical Milestones' (accessed 23.01.07).

www.energysavingtrust.org.uk/nottingham/nottingham-declaration accessed 28.10.09 'Nottingham Declaration on Climate Change'

www.healthyschools.gov.uk, accessed 16.7.10.

www.poverty.org.uk (2009) Homelessness, accessed 14.9.10.

Wyatt, M. (2002) 'Partnership in Health and Social Care: The Implications of Government Guidance in the 1990s in England with Particular Relevance to Voluntary Organisations', *Policy and Politics*, 30(2): 167–82.

Yale Center for Environmental Law and Policy/Centre for International Earth Science Information Network, Columbia University (2005) *Sustainability Index: Benchmarking National Environmental Stewardship* (New Haven: Yale University).

Yamey, G. (2002a) 'Why Does the World Still Need WHO?', *British Medical Journal*, 325, 1294-8.

Yamey, G. (2002b) 'WHO's Management: Struggling to Reform a "Fossilised Bureaucracy"', *British Medical Journal*, 325, 1170-3.

Yarrow, A. (1986) *Politics, Society and Preventative Medicine*, Occasional Paper 6, (London: Nuffield Provincial Hospitals Trust).

Yates, J. (1996) 'Medical Genetics', *British Medical Journal*, 312: 1021–5.

Yates, L. (2008) *Cut-Price, What Cost? How Supermarkets Can Affect Your Chances of a Healthy Diet* (London: National Consumer Council).

Yen, C-L., Cheong, M., Grueter, C. et al. (2009) 'Deficiency of the Intestinal Enzyme acyl CoA: Monpacylglycerol Acyltransferase-2 protects Mice from Metabolic Disorders Induced by High Fat Feeding', *Nature Medicine*, 15: 442–6.

Young, K. (1985) 'Local Government and the Environment' in Jowell, R. and Witherspoon, S. *British Social Attitudes: The 1985 Report* (Aldershot: Gower), pp. 158–63.

Young, K. (1991) 'Shades of Green' in Jowell, R., Brook, L., Taylor, B. and Prior, G. (eds) *British Social Attitudes the 8th Report* (Aldershot: Dartmouth), pp. 107-30.

Young, S. (1996) 'Stepping Stones to Empowerment?: Participation in the Context of Local Agenda 21', *Local Government Policy Making*, 22(4): 25–31.

Yudkin, J. (1972) 'Sugar and Disease', *Nature*, 239: 197–9.

Yusuf, S., Hawken, S. and Ounpuu, S. (2005) 'Obesity and the Risk of Myocardial Infarction in 27,000 Participants from 52 Countries: a Case-Control Study', *The Lancet*, 366: 1640–9.

Zachariah, M. and Acharya, U. (2008) 'Obesity and Infertility, Behind the Medical Headlines', (http://behindthemedicalheadlines.com/articles/obesity-and-infertility).

Zackrisson, S., Andersson, I., Janzon, L. et al. (2006) 'Rates of Over-diagnosis of Breast Cancer 15 years After the end of Malmo Mammographic Screening Trial: Follow up Study', *British Medical Journal*, 332(7543): 689–92.

Zaninotto, P., Head, J., Stamatakis, E. et al. (2009) 'Trends in Obesity Among Adults in England from 1993 to 2004 by Age and Social Class and Projections of Prevalence to 2012', *Journal of Epidemiology and Community Health*, 63: 140–6.

Zhang, Y., Lin, L., Cao, Y. et al. (2009) 'Phthalate Levels and Low Birth Weight: a Nested Case Control Study of Chinese Newborns', *Journal of Paediatrics*, 155(4): 500–4.

Zhou, M., Offer, A., Yang, G. et al. (2008) 'Body Mass Index, Blood Pressure, and Mortality From Stroke', *Stroke*, 39: 753.

Zou, E. and Matsumura, F. (2003) 'Long-term Exposure to B-hexachlorocyclohexane (B-HCH) Promotes Transformation and Invasiveness of MCF-7 Human Breast Cancer Cells', *Biochemical Pharmacology*, 66(5): 831–40.

Index